DATE DUE

2-28-08 IL : 3825565I			

Contemporary Considerations in the Treatment and Rehabilitation of Head and Neck Cancer

Contemporary Considerations
in the Treatment
and Rehabilitation
of Head and Neck Cancer

Voice, Speech, and Swallowing

Edited by

Philip C. Doyle and Robert L. Keith

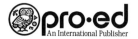

pro·ed
An International Publisher

8700 Shoal Creek Boulevard
Austin, Texas 78757-6897
800/897-3202 Fax 800/397-7633
www.proedinc.com

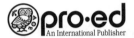

© 2005 by PRO-ED, Inc.
8700 Shoal Creek Boulevard
Austin, Texas 78757-6897
800/897-3202   Fax 800/397-7633
www.proedinc.com

Library of Congress Cataloging-in-Publication Data

Contemporary considerations in the treatment and rehabilitation of head and neck cancer :
  voice, speech, and swallowing / edited by Philip C. Doyle and Robert L. Keith.
      p. ; cm.
  Includes bibliographical references and indexes.
  ISBN 0-89079-988-1 (hardcover : alk. paper)
    1. Larynx—Cancer—Patients—Rehabilitation.   2.
  Larynx—Surgery—Patients—Rehabilitation.   3. Neck—Cancer—Patients—Rehabilitation.   4.
  Head—Cancer—Patients—Rehabilitation.   5. Voice disorders—Patients—Rehabilitation.   I.
  Doyle, Philip C.   II. Keith, Robert L.
    [DNLM: 1. Head and Neck Neoplasms—rehabilitation.   2. Laryngectomy—rehabilitation.
  3. Deglutition Disorders—therapy.   4. Head and Neck Neoplasms—therapy.   5. Speech,
  Alaryngeal.   6. Voice Disorders—therapy.   WE 707 C761 2004]
  RC280.T5C665   2004
  616.99'42203—dc22
                                                                              2004040146

Art Director: Jason Crosier
Designer: Nancy McKinney-Point
This book is designed in Bembo and Futura.

Printed in the United States of America

1   2   3   4   5   6   7   8   9   10   09   08   07   06   05

In honor of Frederic L. Darley, PhD

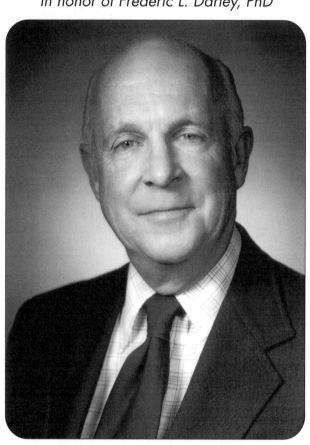

To the memory of Herbert A. (Andy) Leeper, PhD

Contents

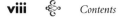

Chapter 14

PART III

Chapter 15

Chapter 16

Chapter 17

Chapter 18

Chapter 19

Chapter 20

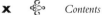

Foreword

Laryngeal or oral cancer is a diagnosis that often causes fear and trepidation in the patient, as well as for family members. Anyone facing the loss of his or her larynx or a major portion of the oral cavity is initially overwhelmed by the concerns of survival and the anticipation of changes in body image and function. *Contemporary Considerations in the Treatment and Rehabilitation of Head and Neck Cancer: Voice, Speech, and Swallowing* is a text designed to reduce these fears while providing information about the reality of cancer diagnosis and treatment. Dr. Philip C. Doyle from the University of Western Ontario in London, Ontario, Canada, and Mr. Robert L. Keith, a former speech–language pathologist at the Mayo Clinic in Rochester, Minnesota, have years of experience dealing with the most challenging of patients diagnosed and treated for head and neck cancer; together, Doyle and Keith have developed a unique understanding of the problems their patients face.

At the request of the late Dr. Frederic Darley, also from the Mayo Clinic, Doyle and Keith sought to provide a contemporary textbook that addressed many aspects of head and neck cancer, including its treatment and subsequent rehabilitation efforts. This new text certainly meets and likely surpasses Dr. Darley's desires and objectives. Doyle and Keith have organized a comprehensive collaborative effort by many experts who address the needs, both treatment and rehabilitative, of those individuals with malignant disease of the larynx or oral cavity. Those who are contributors to the text are recognized internationally and represent experts from the United States, Canada, and Europe. This new text provides the answers to many questions and concerns raised by patients and their families, as well as by clinicians who serve this clinical population. This book will be extremely important and informative to any member of the health care team who is involved in providing optimal treatment and rehabilitation.

Cancers of the larynx and oral cavity present unique challenges and mandate a special level of understanding by those who provide care for patients who face alterations in or loss of voice, speech, and swallowing. Fortunately, tumors in these regions are not all alike, and all are not treated the same. New operations, alternative therapies, and methods of rehabilitation continue to be developed almost daily. In my experience, patients are most satisfied when they are treated as individuals by knowledgeable and compassionate members of the health care team. This text will be an essential tool for members of that team to provide the best care. It will be shared with and used by my patients and peers to better understand the management of the disease and posttreatment rehabilitation. This book will also help patients and family members to become more confident in those who care for their future needs.

The text will help individuals treated by partial or total laryngectomy, those with minor and major oral cancer resections, and those treated with other forms of therapy to realize that they are not alone. Life can go on after the management of these malignancies and life can be lived richly and fully.

Kerry D. Olsen, MD
Rochester, Minnesota

Preface

It has been a privilege to be involved with this project from its inception in the summer of 1998 to its culmination as the subsequent 29 chapters. This book, although in fact a new text, has its origin in three earlier editions of *Laryngectomy Rehabilitation,* edited by Robert L. Keith and the late Frederic L. Darley from the Mayo Clinic in Rochester, Minnesota. In 1998, Keith and Darley asked whether I would consider assuming the primary responsibility for generating a new version of their book. Prior to his death in February 1999, Dr. Darley asked me whether a more contemporary book could be written to address a variety of issues that were emerging in what he termed the "new era" of rehabilitation following treatment for head and neck cancer. He also encouraged me to include, among the invited authors, a majority of new contributors who had not written for earlier editions or similar collections from other publishers and, therefore, offered fresh insights, ideas, and approaches. After considerable discussion with valued colleagues and members of my family, I decided the project was an important one and I consented to undertake editing the book with initial input from Bob Keith. In my opinion, the chapters that follow represent Darley's vision and ideals, and I am honored that I was asked to assume the primary responsibility for coordinating, organizing, and editing this text. I believe the chapters in this book will serve students at various levels in their education, as well as clinicians and scientists from multiple disciplines and professions. Ultimately, the objectives of this book will be successfully achieved if it positively influences the care and rehabilitation of those diagnosed and treated for head and neck cancer.

The contributors to this book have made a difficult task much easier. The interest, commitment, and passion of each contributor have provided an ideal representation of the "new era" in the care of individuals who experience voice, speech, and swallowing problems secondary to head and neck cancer and its treatment. These outstanding professionals have significant and extensive expertise in myriad domains of head and neck cancer treatment and rehabilitation. Additionally, many of these individuals maintain significant research profiles in this important clinical area. Each chapter not only presents valuable, contemporary, and relevant information to the reader, but perhaps more important, provides a unique perspective about a topic of clinical importance. I would like to offer my sincere and heartfelt thanks to all who contributed to this project. Collectively, these authors have made the experience of editing this text a rewarding one; I have benefited from working with each and every one of them.

In this book, numerous and complex issues related to voice, speech, swallowing, and the resultant quality of life for those diagnosed with and treated for head and neck cancer are addressed. The chapters contained in this book provide comprehensive coverage of the changes that individuals experience following treatment for malignancies of the head and neck. It is clear that the challenges faced by such individuals are significant. Treatment for head and neck cancer challenges an individual physically, physiologically, psychologically, emotionally, communicatively, and socially. These challenges also affect family members, friends, and coworkers, and seldom do such challenges exist in isolation. More often that not, the problems experienced are multidimensional and inherently complex, and simple answers do not suffice. Although the disease may be eliminated, the consequences of cancer as a disease and its treatment will always persist, sometimes with serious and devastating effects. Although distinct topic areas and perspectives are covered in each chapter, the intricate relationships across multiple domains of functioning are acknowledged throughout the book. Where appropriate, chapter authors cite other chapters to aid the reader in integrating information about related topics.

The book is divided into four sections, Parts I through IV. Although contributions included in each subdivision share some commonalities, each chapter and section should not be viewed as mutually exclusive because they are not independent entities. Part I includes six chapters that provide an overarching context for multiple and diverse issues that impact the individual treated for head and neck cancer, as well as the manner and comprehensiveness with which care and rehabilitation are provided. Chapter 1, authored by Philip Doyle, presents an overview of multiple factors that must be considered relative to postlaryngectomy rehabilitation. Although a number of these factors have been identified previously in the literature, the full impact of such considerations has been inadequately considered relative to the care of those with head and neck cancer in general, and laryngeal cancer specifically. Chapter 2, coauthored by Bob Keith, James Shanks, and Philip Doyle, presents an updated version of the historical progression of postlaryngectomy rehabilitation that previously appeared in Keith and Darley's third edition (1994). In Chapter 3, Shirley Salmon provides an interesting and insightful review of the commonalities among the methods of alaryngeal speech. Her review provides an ideal opportunity for clinicians to consider modes of alaryngeal speech within a broader based framework of communication and the postlaryngectomy challenges that the individual encounters. Chapter 4, coauthored by Robert Hillman, Michael Walsh, and James Heaton, provides a comprehensive and contemporary review of outcomes following treatment for laryngeal cancer and allows clinicians to reconsider the past literature with care. This chapter allows the clinician to better evaluate speech rehabilitation outcomes and more fully understand posttreatment changes that may exist over the long term. In Chapter 5, William Ryan provides an excellent and timely review of the long-term success experienced by alaryngeal speakers. He offers a considerable opportunity for the reader to reevaluate misconceptions and biases that may exist in previous literature. Chapter 6, coauthored by Philip Doyle and Tanya Eadie, concludes Part I with a comprehensive review of information related to the perceptual nature of laryngeal voice and speech, with the goal of identifying the value of assessing the multidimensional character of postlaryngectomy voice and speech in an effort to better address rehabilitation outcomes.

Part II includes eight chapters that address a variety of topics that focus on medical treatment interventions and related topics, as well as the influence of treatment on voice, speech, and swallowing. In Chapter 7, Howard Lampe and Wayne Matthews outline the details of evaluating individuals with head and neck cancer, with considerations of related issues secondary to medical treatment and long-term health considerations and outcomes of those with upper aerodigestive tract malignancies. Chapter 8, coauthored by Matthews and Lampe and a companion to the previous chapter, addresses a range of topics, including principles of treatment and a discussion of radiotherapy and surgery, along with information on basic surgical procedures and subsequent reconstructive options that are currently available. Chapter 9, written by Steven Zeitels, provides a thorough presentation of information on the treatment of malignant conditions of the larynx and contemporary methods of surgical intervention. In Chapter 10, Robert Orlikoff provides a lucid and comprehensive review of the literature related to nonsurgical treatment for cancer of the larynx and the influence of such treatment on vocal function. Chapter 11 by Gail Kempster offers information pertaining to recent advances in conservation laryngectomy procedures, the application of such conservative approaches to treatment, and a summary of outcomes secondary to the application of this treatment option. Chapter 12, authored by Daniel Deschler, provides a summary of the history and application of reconstructive surgical methods used in association in total laryngectomy with extended or total pharyngectomy. Chapter 13, coauthored by my late friend and colleague Andy Leeper and his dental colleagues, David Gratton, Henry Lapointe, and Joseph Armstrong, presents a comprehensive review of information on maxillofacial rehabilitation for individuals treated for oral cancer, including discussions of surgical resection and associated prosthodontic management and the effects on speech. Finally, in Chapter 14, Cathy Lazarus provides essential information related to the identification and management of swallowing disorders that are commonly observed in individuals treated for head and neck cancer.

Part III includes nine chapters that focus primarily on numerous issues and concerns secondary to medical management of head and neck cancer and the posttreatment process of voice and speech management and rehabilitation. This section also includes multiple perspectives on tracheoesophageal (TE) voice restoration (Chapters 17, 18, and 19). Chapter 15, authored by Leslie Glaze, provides information related to counseling the individual treated for laryngeal cancer and his or her family members; this includes a discussion of concerns that exist prior to and during treatment, as well as long-term considerations. In Chapter 16, Minnie Graham outlines a comprehensive approach to teaching esophageal speech and working toward proficient verbal communication using this alaryngeal method. Chapter 17, coauthored by Carla DeLassus Gress and Mark Singer, provides details of the tracheoesophageal puncture (TEP) voice restoration method; included is a discussion of assessment and candidacy issues, anatomical and physiological considerations, aspects of prosthesis fitting and patient instruction, and the variations in TEP prosthesis design. In Chapter 18, Frans Hilgers and Corina van As provide additional information on TEP voice restoration, with a unique perspective centered on use of the indwelling voice prosthesis. Chapter 19 is by Gail Monahan, who carefully outlines the procedures for clinical troubleshooting associated with TE voice restoration methods. In Chapter 20, Frans Hilgers and Annemieke Ackerstaff address the emerging and important issue of respiratory consequences secondary to total laryngectomy and the methods of postsurgical pulmonary rehabilitation. Chapter 21, written by Philip Doyle and Tanya Eadie, offers a provocative review of the literature in relation to pharyngoesophageal spasm; based on the literature, they suggest that a reconsideration of this physiological phenomenon is required in the context of contemporary rehabilitation programs. In Chapter 22, Philip Doyle presents a systematic program of instruction for use of the electronic artificial larynx. Chapter 23, the final chapter in this section, is coauthored by Geoff Meltzner, Robert Hillman, James Heaton, Kenneth Houston, James Kobler, and Yingyong Qi, who provide an excellent review and a compelling discussion of the state of the art concerning the electronic artificial larynx. This chapter includes a timely presentation of device development and future directions for modification of the electrolarynx using signal processing technology.

The final section, Part IV, comprises six chapters that address essential and critical issues that will influence postlaryngectomy outcomes and suggest the value of reconsidering what constitutes comprehensive programs of clinical care. Chapter 24, authored by Jan Lewin, provides information concerning impediments and obstacles to the success of alaryngeal speech acquisition, with a discussion of problems and solutions within the clinical environment. Lewin's chapter has been updated from a similar one that appeared in Keith and Darley's third edition (1994). In Chapter 25, Leslie Glaze carefully and elegantly outlines the value and importance of peer group support as a valuable component of comprehensive programs of postlaryngectomy rehabilitation. Chapter 26, authored by Candace Myers, outlines the structure and value of group treatment models for the rehabilitation of those treated for head and neck cancer and highlights the importance of such models in comprehensive programs of patient care. In Chapter 27, Minnie Graham addresses the important issue of accountability in clinical practice, with a particular focus on alaryngeal speech rehabilitation. The issue of accountability has not been addressed previously despite its obvious importance in clinical practice. Chapter 28, authored by Candace Myers, presents a detailed and compassionate review of the literature related to quality of life, the implications and impact of the disease and its treatment on those who are diagnosed with head and neck cancer, and the critical importance of understanding the multidimensional nature of the attributes that comprise quality of life. Finally, in Chapter 29, Philip Doyle seeks to provide the reader with an understanding of the relationship of some of the many facets that will impact the individual diagnosed and treated for head and neck cancer. Despite a wide range of clinical settings, the availability of multiple types and levels of service, the ever-changing health care environment at large, and the diverse needs of individuals and their family members, broadening clinical care in the hope of optimizing rehabilitation efforts can only be achieved through careful and critical evaluation of existing programs. Doyle's goal, in the last chapter, is to help the reader question and modify existing programs appropriately.

In summary, *Contemporary Considerations in the Treatment and Rehabilitation of Head and Neck Cancer: Voice, Speech, and Swallowing* provides a collection of comprehensive chapters that address many issues that influence the diagnosis, treatment, and rehabilitation, both short and long term, in persons with head and neck cancer. The perspectives provided are those of authors who are well versed in their topic area, as well as highly knowledgeable in the larger areas of head and neck cancer and its impact on the individual. I hope that the information included will guide a new generation of clinicians to offer the most comprehensive and compassionate care to those with whom they have the privilege to work. By doing so, the journey faced by those individuals who experience head and neck cancer may be made less arduous, and the opportunity of successful long-term rehabilitation may be enhanced considerably.

REFERENCE

Keith, R. L., & Darley, F. L. (1994). *Laryngectomee rehabilitation* (3rd ed.). Austin, TX: PRO-ED.

Acknowledgments

I would like to acknowledge the contributions of several individuals who have helped to shape my thinking on a variety of issues specific to this text, as well as those in complementary areas. First and foremost, a number of current and former students have greatly assisted me in rethinking a number of problem sets, discrepancies, and biases in the literature, in addition to weeding through and contextualizing the limitations found in the speech–language pathology literature. First, I wish to thank my mentor, Charles Reed, for his expert guidance and advice in the area of head and neck cancer that he provided more than 20 years ago; his teachings continue to inspire me today. My sincere thanks are extended to Candace Myers and Tanya Eadie, who have continually provided clear thinking and a fresh, enlightened perspective to the diverse and often overlooked problems that are faced by those with head and neck cancer—both of you are valued friends and colleagues. Several other current or former students have assisted me in reexamining "old" or persistent questions or in evaluating unique bodies of literature in an attempt to understand the "big picture" associated with head and neck cancer; thanks are extended to Sue Brown, Connie Ferri, Carla Anderson, Becky Hare, Fay Nascimento, Rhonda MacKinnon, Paul Beaudin, Mary Marven, Janice Wong, and Heather White. The always clear, expansive, well-reasoned, and visionary thinking of Elizabeth Skarakis-Doyle has significantly influenced the approach, organization, and breadth that emerges in the work I pursue specific to those with head and neck cancer. Needless to say, limitations in my thinking and any errors that emerge are my fault, not theirs! Prior to his untimely death, Andy Leeper provided valuable feedback on several of the chapters that I authored or coauthored, and his collegiality was and always will be appreciated—I think he would have liked the book!

It also is essential to acknowledge the patience, care, and professionalism of those involved in the publication process associated with this book. Specifically, I wish to express my gratitude to Peggy Kipping, Robin Spencer, and Dolly Jackson from PRO-ED. Your input and full support along the way, as well as constant patience and encouragement, have made a difficult task much easier—thank you.

Finally, and once again, I wish to thank my wife Betsy, our daughter Kate, and our son Peter for their tolerance, patience, and support, not to mention their care in moving among the piles and piles of paper at home. Bring in the hand-truck 'cause the boxes are getting stowed!

Philip C. Doyle

PART I

Chapter 1

Rehabilitation in Head and Neck Cancer

Overview

Philip C. Doyle

The diagnosis of cancer, the consequences of its treatment, and its long-term effects have tremendous impact on the individual's physical, physiological, psychological, social, and psychosocial levels of functioning. Because multiple levels of functioning may be affected with many cancer sites and types, the potential for secondary psychiatric influences is always present. In fact, Feinnmann and Happwood (1990) reported that up to 35% of all individuals diagnosed with cancer exhibit some type of psychiatric morbidity. In such circumstances, early professional intervention and counseling may reduce the potential for more significant, longer term problems. The ability to establish a dialogue between the individual with cancer and an appropriate professional resource is seen as one step toward the individual's acceptance of the problem and adjustment to this unfortunate situation.

In the case of cancer of the head and neck, however, treatment has a real and significant potential to impact the individual's ability to verbally communicate. This loss in and of itself may lead to withdrawal and isolation, with resulting negative impact on recovery and rehabilitation. When such withdrawal occurs, the effects may be pervasive throughout the posttreatment period. Bjordal and Kaasa (1995) reported that the negative effects of diagnosis and treatment for head and neck cancer and subsequent psychological changes may continue for some individuals for many years following treatment. Due to the reduction or elimination of verbal communication and the resulting limitations on accessing professional resources, the individual's ultimate health and well-being are clearly jeopardized in ways that may not commonly emerge in those with other cancers (e.g., lung, breast, colon, prostate).

The World Health Organization (WHO, 1999) defined *health* as "a state of complete physical, mental, and social well-being and not merely the absence of disease or infirmity" (WHO, 1999). The collective states of being are believed to coalesce at least in some form into the construct referred to as *quality of life* (QOL). Gritz et al. (1999) suggested that the multidimensional construct of QOL may also include dimensions such as spirituality, sexuality and intimacy, occupational functioning, and treatment satisfaction.[1] To say that the potential effect of a diagnosis of head and neck cancer and the subsequent treatment of such disease is anything but devastating to one's QOL is not unreasonable.

A rich and continuing literature documents that the treatment of head and neck cancer will create changes that cross one's physical, mental, and social well-being, broadly defined. This suggestion persists even if treatment is deemed to be "successful."[2] Because of this, rehabilitation efforts that consider multiple components of a person's health—components comprised of both independent and

---

[1]The dimension of treatment satisfaction must consider the patient's perspective as a formal outcome. Traditional measures of outcome are typically based on objective, instrumental measures or the clinician's perceptions. Consequently, the development of measures of dimensions such as treatment satisfaction indicate a belief that the individual who experiences the disease is in the best position to judge his or her own perception of satisfaction, success, rehabilitation, and so on, following treatment.

[2]Relative to cancer treatment, the term *success* may have multiple definitions. Thus, when this term is encountered in the literature, the reader is encouraged to identify the parameters or constructs underlying each author's definition.

interdependent constructs—are necessary to facilitate the best and most comprehensive approaches to pre- and posttreatment care. Effective cancer care must be multidimensional; hence, programs of care must always address physical, physiological, psychological, social, and psychosocial levels of functioning if treatment success is to be measured appropriately. Doing so increases the likelihood that those treatments offered or provided will have a positive impact on the person's ultimate health and posttreatment well-being (Hammerlid, Persson, Sullivan, & Westin, 1999).

Even though medical treatment is pursued in an effort to eliminate disease or decrease pain and suffering, the treatment itself may create significant levels of distress in many individuals. Although some differential levels of personal distress are to be expected across individuals, distress will nevertheless exist for all of those diagnosed with cancer in general and with head and neck cancers specifically. Any efforts to reduce such distress, therefore, are believed to be of value in facilitating the best possible posttreatment outcome. In actuality, reducing distress is probably the most critical prerequisite component of care in that it may facilitate active participation by the individual in the recovery and rehabilitation process.

The purpose of this introductory chapter is to briefly outline four key issues which, if recognized for their face validity, may help clinicians to modify or enhance existing programs of patient care.[3] First among these is the fact that a health-oriented model of care is replacing a disease-oriented model. Second, with the emergence of this new model, the acknowledgment that a wider array of professional expertise may be required if the best level of care is to be provided has also occurred. This recognition may be of particular relevance for those with head and neck cancer. Although collaborative care practices are long-standing and well recognized in the clinical area of head and neck cancer, this collaboration can be expanded further to address the psychological and psychosocial problems that may emerge in many individuals as a result of the disease and its treatment (Doyle, 1999; Gritz & Hoffman, 1996; Hammerlid et al., 1999). Third, concerns about how the individual responds to a cancer diagnosis also must be raised. In this regard, the importance of efforts to reduce the individual's "vulnerability" to psychological and psychiatric problems is discussed. Attempts to reduce vulnerability are viewed as essential if a comprehensive program of care is to be provided. At a minimum, and at least at some level, facilitating the individual's ability to express concerns about his or her situation may allow the individual to be actively involved in his or her own care. Reducing psychological burden is believed to be of substantial value in the care of those with cancer. Finally, when taken together, these three areas ultimately merge into the larger scale consideration of the impact of disease, in this case malignant disease, on the person. Hopefully, through raising and collectively discussing these key issues, professionals can work toward establishing an expanded, albeit cursory framework that seeks to address

---

[3]The issues raised in this discussion are not to be interpreted as comprehensive or exhaustive. The four areas discussed provide a cursory amalgamation of emerging issues that have the potential to directly influence health care models in head and neck cancer as well as other conditions or diseases.

more global dimensions influencing rehabilitation outcome following treatment for head and neck cancer.

DISEASE, ILLNESS, AND HEALTH: A CHANGING PARADIGM

In 1980, the World Health Organization (WHO) proposed the *International Classification of Impairments, Disabilities, and Handicaps* (ICIDH) as a means of classifying the consequences of a medically defined disease and its effects on the person who experiences it. Multiple revisions to this document since its inception have led to a more contemporary document titled the *International Classification of Functioning, Disability and Health* (ICIDH–2, 2001), now termed the *International Classification of Functioning,* or ICF. The premise of the more contemporary documents (ICIDH–2/ICF) was steeped in a desire to move from a biomedical model of illness to a model that focused on the biopsychosocial influences of disease, thus reflecting the effects of the condition on the individual.[4] As a result of this long-term process of reconsidering the original document and its inherent definitional strengths and limitations, health care may now move away from a *patient* care model, which has essentially been based on disease category and the elimination of disease, to one that places the *person* at the center of the model (Eadie, 2001). In essence, the new model has endeavored to address the body, mind, and social dimensions of a disease. This change has facilitated a new view of the impact of disease and treatment beyond that of the earlier view that focused solely on the entity of disease and its elimination.

Within the current framework of the ICF, the elimination of disease (e.g., excision of a malignant tumor) is now assessed in a context in which the impact of the disease has corollary potential on the individual; that is, even when the individual has been treated, the influence of the disease (diagnosis, consequences of treatment, prognosis, etc.) may remain a persistent problem that will influence the individual's health. The new WHO definition extends beyond the simple physical attributes of a problem (e.g., site of lesion, type of disease, histological character) to include how the person with a disease is perceived, how his or her inherent problems are addressed, and how the health care system provides service. The physical nature of a disease is no longer the sole attribute guiding the definition of health. As stated by Bill Moyers (1993) in his book *Healing and the Mind,* in relation to the structure and provision of health care practices,

> Talking with different doctors during this journey, I realized that we do need a new medical paradigm that goes beyond "body parts" medicine, and not only for the patient's sake…. Thinking about our medical system as a "health

---

[4]Relative to recent applications in the area of assessment and intervention in communication sciences and disorders, the reader is encouraged to consult Boswell (2000) and Threats (2001).

care" system rather than a "disease treatment" system would mean looking closely at medical education and our public funding priorities. (p. 5)

The need for such a paradigm shift at both practical and prepractical educational levels, as suggested by Moyers, evolves from many factors that influence how disease states have been viewed medically. The emerging taxonomy for health and well-being considers multiple factors and domains. In an excellent interpretation of the evolution of the WHO model since 1980 and its relationship to communication disorders with a specific focus on speech–language pathology, Eadie (2001) stated, "The original ICIDH, based on a biomedical model, could not explain how an individual could be treated medically and 'cured' of his or her impairment, and yet could be limited in activities of daily living" (p. 184).

The former biomedical model was insufficient in that it did not consider changes in function that were experienced by the individual; the disability associated with disease and its treatment was unrecognized (Bickenbach, 1993; Bickenbach, Chetterji, Badley, & Ustun, 1999). It is now clear that the biomedical model exhibited substantial limitations that subsequently resulted in an inadequate acknowledgment of the individual who experiences the disease. Again, health and well-being had previously been discarded from consideration; the disease and the person were disjoined. When constructs of health, well-being, quality of life, and other dimensions are considered, one can more fully appreciate the limitations of prior conceptual models of how "medical" care has been offered. Evaluating these concerns relative to the comprehensive care of those with head and neck cancer permits the opportunity for continued improvements and refinements in addressing the needs of this population. The biopsychosocial model will allow clinicians to rethink how rehabilitation of those with head and neck cancer is defined, to reconsider what constitutes best practice, to reassess the quality of services provided today, and, therefore, to better define the success or failure of rehabilitation efforts.

As an example, the success of treatment for cancer as a disease class has often been based on the temporal period of "survival" from the time of diagnosis to the time of death. Doyle (1994) suggested that this method of quantifying the success of treatment is a frail concept at best.[5] The period of survival postdiagnosis in no way correlates with qualitative components of one's health, well-being, or QOL (see Chapter 28 in this text). There is obviously no stepwise relationship between duration of survival and QOL. Statistical quantification of cancer treatment and its success or failure is indeed one dimensional when duration is used as an isolated measure. The following simple question refutes this numerical, biomedical index: Is 1 year of survival postdiagnosis less full or satisfying, or qualitatively worse than 3 years of survival postdiagnosis? This question is unanswerable without consideration of the individual's perception as captured

---

[5]Doyle did not suggest that survival data were unimportant, but rather that survival data are quantitative in the time domain without consideration of qualitative intrinsic perceptions of the individual.

through the biopsychosocial model. Treatment success can be defined in many ways, but it may best be represented if viewed as multidimensional in nature. As stated by Gritz and colleagues (1999), "Treatment of many malignancies of the head and neck may result in an adverse effect on patients' physical, functional, psychological, and social functioning, dimensions that cannot be equated with statistics on treatment response, disease progression, and survival" (p. 352).

Expanding this concept further, one can appreciate that efforts to assess the patient in a more global fashion will likely offer the potential to improve his or her life in the face of disease and treatment, and perhaps a poor prognosis (Terrell et al., 2004). Thus, revisions in the model proposed by the WHO (2001) now permit individual health care providers to redefine the roles and responsibilities of those on the rehabilitation team. Regarding the model's impact on those with head and neck cancer, Eadie (2001) explained that an adult who has lived for 5 years following removal of a malignant tumor would be considered disease-free, and therefore medically cured and healthy, according to the medical model. That person, however, may be living with scarring, stigma associated with altered physical appearance, and psychosocial factors related to treatment for cancer. Although the person may be limited in social activity involvement, which in turn affects his or her psychological and social well-being, the medical model does not consider this variation in functioning to be a "disability."

Optimal patient care will require that health and well-being move to the forefront of how the care process is initiated and progresses over time. The emerging model offered by WHO (2001) is applicable regardless of the class, subgroup, or type of "disease" because the individual remains at the core of the problem and its potential resolution or rehabilitation. The model does not negate the need for technical or essential procedural endeavors so often undertaken in health care. In many instances clinicians working with those with head and neck cancer must perform technical acts and procedures; such acts are a necessary and important component of the health care process in that they are believed to benefit the person receiving treatment.

Medical treatment is necessary in many cases to improve the patient's life. As with all medical treatments for cancer, however, side effects, complications, and morbidities do exist. The new WHO model suggests that those acts (i.e., treatments and their effects) must be viewed beyond the historic constraints of the "biomedical" model. Acts of this type are solely a component of a larger program of care; hence, professionals are required to view such acts in the larger context (i.e., how they affect the individual). Technical acts cannot be performed dispassionately because the influence of such acts ultimately emerges at the human level. Given that all professionals have specific areas of expertise, the model inferentially suggests that multiple professionals and services may be required to optimize the success of treatment or rehabilitation. Each professional discipline brings a unique knowledge base and skill to the cancer care process, but it is the collective attribute of the collaborative team that offers the most comprehensive level of care. Consequently, if care of the highest possible quality is desired, broad-based collaborative efforts are mandatory.

PATIENT CARE AS A COLLABORATIVE PROCESS

It is well documented in the clinical literature that the best level of care for those individuals who have undergone treatment for head and neck cancer involves the collaboration and cooperation of multiple professionals (see Doyle, 1994). Those professionals must have knowledge of what others bring to the "health care" process. These professionals must be readily available for communication and consultation about differences of opinion and areas of expertise.

Respect for others' areas of expertise is an essential component of good care throughout the process—at the time of diagnosis, immediately prior to the onset of primary treatment, during early medical treatments, and in the short- and long-term periods following treatment. In the ever-changing health care environment of the early part of the 21st century, this obligation is of even greater value because the demands on the system are often substantial. As with any complex and dynamic process, however, the "whole" of patient care is worth more that the "sum of its parts"; providing the most appropriate and thorough care for those with head and neck cancer demands that all of those involved participate actively and communicate directly with one another. What happens early in the collaborative process may indeed set the stage for the individual's longer term outcome. Professionals often communicate best with one another during the early care period; therefore, comprehensive, collaborative programs should be initiated at the time of diagnosis.

Because the stages of cancer treatment are often somewhat varied and because individual factors must always be considered, clinicians who serve those with head and neck cancer must bear the burden of understanding the "big picture" of what cancer as a disease class does to the individual and members of his or her family. Historically, the speech–language pathology literature has found itself mired in concerns related to the reacquisition of verbal communication. With that said, it must be clearly acknowledged that voice and speech rehabilitation is an essential and critical component of rehabilitation following head and neck cancer. The experience of many clinicians, however, will attest to the fact that retention of posttreatment oral speech functioning in those who have undergone the resection of an oral tumor, the ability to communicate without substantial reduction in speech intelligibility for those with mandibular or velopharyngeal defects, or the successful and functional acquisition of some method of alaryngeal speech (esophageal, tracheoesophageal, or artificial laryngeal voice) in those receiving total laryngectomy does not correlate well with what one might term rehabilitation "success" (Laverick, Lowe, Brown, Vaughan, & Rogers, 2004; Ramirez et al., 2003). Likewise, when disease and its treatment influence one's ability to manipulate food and drink and one's ability to swallow, positive improvements in such function, although important, do not always guarantee a successful posttreatment outcome. Some individuals may be fraught with fear about recurrent disease or the effects of treatment, have significant concerns about cosmesis, have problems with self-esteem, suffer the consequences of financial loss due to an inability to resume work, or ultimately isolate themselves from social activity. In almost every instance, self-induced isolation will negatively influence rehabilitation outcome with resultant decrements in one's QOL. These concerns, as well as many others, require thoughtful and careful consideration by multiple professionals if the care of individuals with head and neck cancer is to be enhanced (Doyle, 1999).

REDUCING VULNERABILITY IN HEAD AND NECK CANCER

Individuals treated for head and neck cancer are vulnerable to isolation when they cannot communicate easily or they fear the perception of others to their plight. Stigmatizing conditions, whether real or perceived, cannot be overlooked because they threaten the individual's judgment of self, which might then pose a risk to relationships within the individual's own social milieu (Goffman, 1963). Head and neck cancer and its treatment can be disfiguring, which further threatens the person's identity. Although other cancer treatment sites may be hidden, the sequelae of treatment for head and neck cancer may be easily observed both visually and auditorily. Furthermore, no other forms of cancer alter the structural integrity to effectively communicate, or in some instances render the individual unable to verbally communicate at all.

If verbal communication is viewed as a means of reducing fear, anxiety, and emotional burden, one can easily appreciate why those with head and neck cancer may be distinguished from other subgroups of malignant disease (based on site of lesion). In recent years, one of the major issues to emerge in regard to the reduction of anxiety pertains to what level of knowledge the person exhibits (Williams, 1993). The provision of information is reported to be a key factor in alleviating a person's unnecessary fear and anxiety. Simply stated, the more information one has about a health condition, the more capable he or she may be in coping with that problem.

Those diagnosed with head and neck cancer will almost certainly experience changes in verbal communication and cosmesis. These changes will also influence other areas, including self-concept, body image, and self-esteem. Therefore, some form of counseling relative to physical and communicative changes has been recommended as a vital element of direct patient care at both pre- and postoperative stages (see Chapter 15 in this text). Although the importance of providing essential and accurate information to those individuals who are diagnosed with head and neck cancer and who experience posttreatment communication disorders is well recognized, some concerns about the breadth and accuracy of information provided has been questioned.

For example, a recent study by Anderson and Doyle (2000) of 100 individuals who had undergone total laryngectomy across the United States and Canada indicated that the provision of information via counseling was characterized by numerous problems. Specifically, Anderson and Doyle found that many respondents to a survey on service provision reported receiving conflicting, incorrect, or unnecessary information as part of the pre- and postoperative counseling process. This finding suggests that, despite a professional recognition that such "counseling" is important, the ability of professionals to adequately and, perhaps more important, accurately present this information to those they serve may be problematic. When presented with inaccurate or inadequate information, a person is more likely to experience an increased level of anxiety or other related problems (e.g., maladaptive changes in the psychological or psychosocial domains). Similarly, increased levels of vulnerability may emerge, further limiting the individual's active participation in treatment. Therefore, all professionals involved in the care of those with head and neck cancer need to explore what and how information is provided in an attempt to reduce negative effects on the individual. All team members must have specific roles if the value of collaborative efforts is to be fully exploited (Doyle, 1999).

Reduced self-esteem also may increase the individual's vulnerability. Numerous authors have commented on how intrinsic responses to a cancer diagnosis and its treatment can influence the individual (e.g., Breitbart & Holland, 1988; Dhillon, Palmer, Pittam, & Shaw, 1982; Koster & Bergsma, 1990; West, 1977). The findings of such studies indicate that best practice requires that professionals formally address concerns of this type as part of a formal treatment program. Additionally, factors such as pain, physical symptoms and condition, fatigue, activity level, and psychological symptoms, to name a few, must be addressed (Jones, Lund, Howard, Greenberg, & McCarthy, 1992). Ongoing monitoring of all areas of concern—the physical, physiological, psychological, social, and psychosocial levels of functioning—increases the likelihood that when problems are identified, intervention can be initiated in a prompt and appropriate fashion. Factors of this type are collectively believed to influence the more global measure of QOL (see, e.g., Brinkley, 1985; DeHaes & Van Knippenberg, 1985; Drettner & Ahlbom, 1983; Maguire & Selby, 1989; Selby & Robertson, 1987; and Chapter 28 of this text).

THE IMPACT OF DISEASE

By disregarding the larger impact of the disease and its diagnosis, the clinician is unable to comprehensively care for the person with head and neck cancer and members of his or her family. Cancer knows no boundaries, and its impact is dramatic and far reaching. Thus, the continued expansion of the knowledge base regarding this clinical population is valuable and essential. Gross deficits at a physical level are often easily identified in individuals with head and neck cancer; however, the greatest impact is likely at the personal and social levels of performance and participation. The impact of disease may be reflected in the results of a variety of assessments and measures that fall in the category of QOL tools (e.g., Cella & Tulsky, 1990; Doyle, 1994; Hassan & Weymuller, 1993; Moore, Parsons, & Mendenhall, 1996; Schuster et al., 2004). Measures of QOL cut to the core of an individual's perception regarding his or her health status. Overall, these measures have been shown to have substantial value in treating those with head and neck cancer (deBoer, McCormick, Pruyn, Ryckman, & van den Borne, 1999); however, the successful application of such measures requires careful adherence to multiple methodological considerations (see Dijkers, 1999). Rehabilitation outcomes are contingent upon the ability of professionals to gather new data in this important area while considering past findings (Brockstein, 2003; see also Chapter 28 in this text). The chapters that follow in this text seek to encourage interested readers, including speech–language pathologists, head and neck surgeons, dentists, nurses, students from a variety of other professional disciplines, as well as many others, to continue efforts to provide better patient care.

SUMMARY

This chapter has briefly addressed four general areas that may influence the design of future programs of comprehensive rehabilitation for individuals with head and neck cancer. The topics included the changing paradigms and models of how professionals view illness and disease, the nature and importance of professional collaboration and cooperation in comprehensive programs of head and neck cancer care, personal vulnerability that follows a head and neck cancer diagnosis and an acknowledgment of factors that influence this behavior, and the impact of the disease at the human level. The issues raised in this chapter, as well as those discussed in the other chapters of this text, provide the reader with an expanded view of contemporary considerations of treatment and rehabilitation of this clinical population. The composite issues raised, however, are not exhaustive because professionals are continually learning more about the human condition when disease (regardless of etiology) occurs in the otherwise healthy human.

In the early 21st century, historic models of disease and treatment are already being revisited and changes have begun to emerge. A new model—one that considers a more comprehensive view of health via the biopsychosocial model—is now replacing the long-standing biomedical model of care. This change has direct implications for providing care and service to individuals who will experience alterations in voice, speech, and swallowing due to head and neck cancer and its treatment (Boswell, 2000). Through consideration of the larger biopsychosocial model of care, professionals will almost certainly develop proactive approaches to intervention and ultimately enhance them over time.

Future efforts that center on treating the individual who experiences the disease, rather than treating the disease as an isolated entity, will likely lead to the development of more extensive and effective rehabilitation programs. Although much work remains to be done in this important area of clinical care, those professionals who have been actively and prominently involved in the care of those with head and neck cancer have made substantial strides in recent years. Continued work in the future will help to provide greater insights into and understanding of the complexities associated with head and neck cancer, its medical management, and the rehabilitation and return to functioning of the individual.

REFERENCES

Anderson, C., & Doyle, P. C. (2000, July). *A retrospective examination of information provision following total laryngectomy.* Paper presented at the 5th International Conference on Head and Neck Cancer, San Francisco.

Bickenbach, J. E. (1993). The analysis of disablement. In J. E. Bickenbach (Ed.), *Physical disability and social policy* (pp. 20–58). Toronto, ON: University of Toronto Press.

Bickenbach, J. E., Chetterji, S., Badley, E. M., & Ustun, T. B. (1999). Models of disablement, universalism and the international classification of impairments, disabilities and handicaps. *Social Science and Medicine, 48,* 1173–1187.

Bjordal, K., & Kaasa, S. (1995). Psychological distress in head and neck cancer patients 7–11 years after curative treatment. *British Journal of Cancer, 71,* 592–597.

Boswell, S. (2000, May). WHO launches field trials, takes functional approach to disability. *The ASHA Leader,* pp. 3, 14.

Breitbart, W., & Holland, J. (1988). Psychosocial aspects of head and neck cancer. *Seminars in Oncology, 15,* 61–69.

Brinkley, D. (1985). Quality of life in cancer trials. *British Medical Journal, 291,* 685–686.

Brockstein, B. (2003). Organ preservation for advanced head and neck cancer concomitant chemoradiation. *Cancer Treatment Research, 114,* 235–248.

Cella, D. F., & Tulsky, D. S. (1990). Measuring quality of life today: Methodological aspects. *Oncology, 4,* 29–38.

deBoer, M. F., McCormick, L. K., Pruyn, J. F. A., Ryckman, R. N., & van den Borne, H. W. (1999). Physical and psychosocial correlates of head and neck cancer: A review of the literature. *Otolaryngology—Head and Neck Surgery, 120,* 427–436.

DeHaes, J. C. J. M., & Van Knippenberg, F. C. E. (1985). The quality of life of cancer patients. A review of the literature. *Social Science and Medicine, 20,* 809–817.

Dhillon, R. S., Palmer, B. V., Pittam, M. R., & Shaw, H. J. (1982). Rehabilitation after major head and neck surgery—The patient's view. *Clinical Otolaryngology, 7,* 319–324.

Dijkers, M. (1999). Measuring quality of life: Methodological issues. *American Journal of Physical Medicine and Rehabilitation, 78,* 286–300.

Doyle, P. C. (1994). *Foundations of voice and speech rehabilitation following laryngeal cancer.* San Diego, CA: Singular.

Doyle, P. C. (1999). Postlaryngectomy speech rehabilitation: Contemporary considerations in clinical care. *Journal of Speech–Language Pathology and Audiology, 23,* 109–116.

Drettner, B., & Ahlbom, A. (1983). Quality of life and state of health for patients with cancer in the head and neck. *Acta Otolaryngologica, 96,* 307–314.

Eadie, T. L. (2001). The ICIDH–2: Theoretical and clinical implications for speech–language pathology. *Journal of Speech–Language Pathology and Audiology, 25,* 181–200.

Feinnmann, C., & Happwood, P. (1990). Emotional disturbance of patients with functional symptoms. *Journal of the Royal Society of Medicine, 83,* 596–597.

Goffman, E. (1963). *Stigma: Notes on the management of spoiled identity.* Englewood Cliffs, NJ: Prentice Hall.

Gritz, E. R., Carmack, C. L., De Moor, C., Coscarelli, A., Schacherer, C. W., Meyers, E. G., & Abemayor, E. (1999). First year after head and neck cancer: Quality of life. *Journal of Clinical Oncology, 17,* 352–360.

Gritz, E. R., & Hoffman, A. (1996). Behavioral and psychosocial issues in head and neck cancer (pp. 1-14). In J. Beumer, T. Curtis, & M. Marunick (Eds.), *Maxillofacial rehabilitation: Prosthodontic and surgical considerations.* St. Louis, MO: Ishiyaku Euromica.

Hammerlid, E., Persson, L. O., Sullivan, M., & Westin, T. (1999). Quality-of-life effects of psychosocial intervention in patients with head and neck cancer. *Otolaryngology—Head and Neck Surgery, 120,* 507–516.

Hassan, S. J., & Weymuller, E. A. (1993). Assessment of quality of life in head and neck cancer patients. *Head and Neck, 15,* 485–496.

Jones, E., Lund, V. J., Howard, D. J., Greenberg, M. P., & McCarthy, M. (1992). Quality of life of patients treated surgically for head and neck cancer. *Journal of Laryngology and Otology, 106,* 238–242.

Koster, M., & Bergsma, J. (1990). Problems and coping behavior of facial cancer patients. *Social Science in Medicine, 5,* 569–578.

Laverick, S., Lowe, D., Brown, J. S., Vaughan, E. D., & Rogers, S. N. (2004). The impact of neck dissection on health-related quality of life. *Archives of Otolaryngology—Head and Neck Surgery, 130,* 149–154.

Maguire, P., & Selby, P. (1989). Assessing quality of life in cancer patients. *British Journal of Cancer, 60,* 437–440.

Moore, G. J., Parsons, J. T., & Mendenhall, W. M. (1996). Quality of life outcomes after primary radiotherapy for squamous cell carcinoma of the base of the tongue. *International Journal of Radiation Oncology and Biological Physics, 36,* 351–354.

Moyers, B. (1993). *Healing and the mind.* New York: Doubleday.

Ramirez, M. J., Ferriol, E. E., Domenech, F. G., Llatas, M. C., Suarez-Varela, M. M., & Martinez, R. L. (2003). Psychosocial adjustment in patients surgically treated for laryngeal cancer. *Otolaryngology—Head and Neck Surgery, 129,* 92–97.

Schuster, M., Lohscheller, J., Hoppe, U., Kummer, P., Eysholdt, U., Rosanowski, F. (2004). Voice handicap of laryngectomees with tracheoesophageal speech. *Folia Phoniatrica and Logopaedia, 56,* 62–67.

Selby, P., & Robertson, B. (1987). Measurement of quality of life in patients with cancer. *Cancer Surveys, 6,* 521–543.

Terrell, J. E., Ronis, D. L., Fowler, K. E., Bradford, C. R., Chepeha, D. B., Prince, M. E., Teknos, T. N., Wolf, G. T., & Duffy, S. A. (2004). Clinical predictors of quality of life in patients with head and neck cancer. *Archives of Otolaryngology—Head and Neck Surgery, 130,* 401–408.

Threats, T. T. (2001). New classifications will aid assessment and intervention. *The ASHA Leader, 6*(18), 12–13.

West, D. (1977). Social adaptation patterns among cancer patients with facial disfigurement resulting from surgery. *Archives of Physical Medicine and Rehabilitation, 58,* 473–479.

Williams, O. A. (1993). Patient knowledge of operative care. *Journal of the Royal Society of Medicine, 86,* 328–331.

World Health Organization. (1980). *International classification of impairments, disabilities and handicaps.* Geneva: Author.

World Health Organization. (1999). *Constitution of the World Health Organization.* Geneva: Author.

World Health Organization. (2001). *International classification of functioning, disability and health.* Geneva: Author.

Chapter 2

Historical Highlights
Laryngectomy Rehabilitation

Robert L. Keith, James C. Shanks, and Philip C. Doyle

History does not always do justice or provide ample credit to those individuals who have made important contributions to medical science and its evolution within specific areas. This is certainly true in relation to the history of the treatment for laryngeal cancer and the development and evolution of the laryngectomy procedure. Perhaps this sketchiness is due to the time and complexity involved in reviewing, analyzing, and differentiating individual contributions and the relative influences of those who have contributed in some way to a specific topic. In past retrospectives (Keith & Shanks, 1994) and in this chapter, our intent has not been to provide a detailed account of each historical event that has contributed to current laryngectomy procedures, but rather to provide a brief historical sketch of the most significant events that have led to present-day techniques. It is our opinion that new challenges always emerge and that such challenges are often met with novel approaches to address the problems. With that said, however, it is also important to note that careful exploration of the early historical literature on the surgical treatment of laryngeal cancer would show that current advances are almost always steeped in past endeavors. Sometimes early attempts proved unsuccessful and may in hindsight seem medieval at best. As information from inquiry at basic and applied levels has advanced, however, old methods have been "rediscovered" and outcomes have often differed appreciably.

One of the more contemporary examples of this evolution pertains to tracheoesophageal puncture (TEP) voice restoration following total laryngectomy. Although the general approach to this contemporary method of surgical voice restoration was not necessarily a new concept when introduced by Singer and Blom (1980), advances in materials science and related aspects of prosthesis design and fabrication permitted a prosthetic means to successfully merge with this surgical method of postlaryngectomy voice rehabilitation. One needs only to assess the variety of TEP voice prostheses that are currently available worldwide to confirm the timeliness of this advance. This example provides a framework for the review of the historical information to follow. We hope that future endeavors, through exposure to the past, will emerge with greater promise for the improved clinical care of those diagnosed with and treated for laryngeal cancer.

As is common with most of history, the past often provides an opportunity to assess new developments in a more all-encompassing context. This is particularly true as medical approaches to the treatment of myriad disorders and diseases continue to expand. By carefully evaluating the history of laryngeal cancer and laryngectomy, professionals in the future will almost certainly devise more knowledgeable approaches to treatment and patient care. Therefore, the purpose of this chapter is twofold. Initially, a summary of important events in the history of laryngectomy is presented. This summary provides an opportunity for the reader to understand the major changes that occurred relative to surgical treatment of laryngeal cancer, with a particular focus on the early evolution of total laryngectomy. Second, this chapter provides a similar review of information related to the development and evolution of the artificial larynx up to the modern era. In this review, the term *artificial larynx* will encompass a broad array of appliances that have existed over the years.

HISTORY OF LARYNGECTOMY
A Review of the Literature

There is some confusion in the historical literature relative to the surgical treatment of laryngeal cancer. Although timelines are in many respects quite closely aligned, some discrepancies in reports, or interpretations of reports, do exist. The idea of laryngeal extirpation seems to have its origins in animal work conducted in the late 1820s. In 1829, Albers (cited in Jackson & Jackson, 1939), while conducting experiments on the physiology of the larynx, removed the entire larynx from a dog. The dog lived for 9 days. Additional work with the canine model was performed in the 1870s by Czerny. Subsequent schemes for human laryngectomy were allegedly proposed by Eugene Keberle in 1856 and Baron Bernard R. K. von Langenbeck in 1875 (Rosenberg, 1971). In 1866, the actual operation was pioneered by Patrick H. Watson of Edinburgh. Watson's work apparently preceded that of Theodore Billroth, who has frequently been credited with performing the first laryngectomy in 1873 (see Güssenbauer, 1874). Furthermore, Billroth's work may have occurred in close proximity to that of Isambert (1876). Significantly, it does appear that Billroth was the first surgeon to pursue this method of surgical treatment for laryngeal cancer. Also of interest, it seems that the first conservation (partial) laryngectomy may have been undertaken by Sands in 1865, well before any understanding of laryngeal lymphatics and associated anatomical compartmentalization existed. Based on Sands's clinical report, he appears to have been the first to pursue thyrotomy with cordectomy for an apparent glottic carcinoma.

The removal of the entire laryngeal framework (i.e., total laryngectomy) set the stage for dramatic surgical advances relative to managing malignancies of the larynx in years to come. Regardless of who officially garners credit for the first laryngectomy, it is clear that the procedure raised many questions regarding the removal of such a critical structure of the upper airway, with multiple changes, complications, and related morbidities observed.

The following is an account of the earliest clinical case of a laryngectomy reported by Watson (1881, as cited in Jackson & Jackson, 1939):

> The first case was a gentleman, age 36, suffering from tertiary syphilis, with the destruction of the laryngeal cavity. I had previously, about a year before, opened his trachea to relieve him from the ulcerative condition. The larynx then healed, but the puckering gave rise to a condition of matters by which some portion of all fluid nutriment and saliva made its way into the trachea, and occasioned fits of spasmodic cough. Feeding by the tube did not prevent the saliva from passing down, and in almost every instance on its withdrawal some fluid regurgitated, and some of it passed into the trachea, etc. I operated by a linear incision, clearing the trachea, first above the tracheotomy opening, I cut it right across, introduced a gum elastic tube (a full-sized lithotomy tube) and tied the trachea upon it by a piece of silk ligature. I then cleared the soft parts from the larynx by means of the points of probe pointed scissors,

using them to pull away the structures when one could, and clipping with them when it was necessary. The patient rallied from the operation, but died some weeks afterward from pneumonia. (p. 255)

Because Watson's patient died, the surgical procedure was generally condemned; nevertheless, the idea of total laryngectomy had been instilled in the literature. The fundamentals of the procedure were grasped by Vincenz Czerny (1870) of Heidelberg, who then executed effective laryngectomies on dogs. Czerny was a young surgical assistant of Theodore Billroth (Donagan, 1965).

Early efforts at laryngectomy, therefore, were discouraging, and until 1900 progress was very slow. Glück and Soerensen (1920, 1922) in Berlin probably did the most to improve and develop the technical details of laryngectomy. Starting with and abandoning a two-stage operation, they developed a wide-field approach with open exposure of the neck. They also developed the plan of removing the larynx from above and downward and of closing the pharyngeal defect before amputation of the larynx (Jesberg, 1960).

The illustrious Theodore Billroth was born on an island in the Baltic Sea in 1829. Encouraged to study medicine by his family, Billroth enrolled at the University of Göttingen, where he became interested in surgical pathology and physiology. Billroth graduated in 1852; his thesis was titled, "The Nature and Cause of Pulmonary Affections Produced by Bilateral Vagal Section" (Weir, 1973).

At 25 years of age, Billroth was appointed to an assistantship at the Langenbeck Clinic. He remained there for 6 years, during which time he became engrossed in surgical pathology and published many papers. After many unsuccessful bids for surgical posts, he was eventually appointed chair of surgery in Zurich in 1859. In 1867, Billroth accepted the position of chair of surgery in Vienna. In the beginning, the Viennese were not favorably disposed to Billroth's ambitious nature. Students complained that he did not teach surgery as a complete science, but rather as having indefinite and unknown factors. Because Billroth tried to chart the unknown, his clinic became a surgical Mecca during the 26 years that he worked in Vienna. He performed the first excision of the esophagus in 1872, the first successful laryngectomy for cancer in 1873, the first subtotal colectomy in 1879, and the first gastrectomy in 1881.

For historical interest, the following is a review of the first successful laryngectomy as reported by Carl Güssenbauer, Billroth's assistant (Schechter & Morfit, 1965):

The entire procedure of total laryngectomy took Billroth one hour and 45 minutes. The patient, a 36-year-old teacher with a tumor below the true vocal cords, was first treated with multiple cauterizations and biopsies (microscopic report: epithelial carcinoma of the larynx). On November 21, 1873 (after a preliminary tracheotomy), Dr. Billroth performed a laryngofissure and removed the tumor with scissors and sharp curette. The main tumor was situated on the left side, so the surgeon was able to preserve the right vocal cord; the wound edges were approximated with tape. On the second postoperative day the patient began to have septic temperatures, and infection developed in the wound, which was treated with a preparation containing silver nitrate; on the seventh postoperative day the patient was up and about, and two days later a high degree of dyspnea developed. The wound was reopened and examination revealed that the growth had recurred.

In an attempt to curette the larynx, Dr. Billroth reopened the wound, but discovered that the malignant growth had invaded the cartilage. The patient was awakened, informed of the necessity to remove the larynx and again anesthetized. The technique consisted mainly in dull dissection of the larynx on both sides while the assistant exerted a pull on the larynx. The trachea was divided just below the cricoid, the larynx was pulled forward and up, and dissected from the anterior wall of the esophagus; the thyrohyoid membrane was divided last. The anesthesia was not sufficient, and the operative procedure was frequently interrupted by strong coughing spells during which blood in rather large amounts was expelled from the trachea. The bleeding was controlled by pressure with large sponges.

The growth must have been quite large since, after examining the specimen, Dr. Billroth decided to remove most of the epiglottis and the first two tracheal rings. The tracheal stoma was fixed to the skin with one suture on each side and the opening into the pharynx was made smaller by applying three sutures. Four hours later, during a bout of coughing, a profuse hemorrhage developed from the left superior laryngeal artery which required a ligature. Dr. Güssenbauer remarked about the large amounts of coagulated blood which the patient had coughed up without having had great signs of dyspnea. Three days after the operation the sutures and the ligatures were removed. The wound represented a groove with the tracheal stoma in the lower end and the opening into the pharynx on the upper end.

Fortunately, the patient escaped all secondary complications, such as shock, aspiration, pneumonia, mediastinitis, sepsis, meningitis, tetanus and large abscess. The pharyngeal fistula began to close early, and the patient was started on a soft diet on the eighth postoperative day; the gastric feeding tube was removed on the eighteenth day. The patient was dismissed on March 3, 1874, after he had learned how to use the artificial larynx designed by Dr. Güssenbauer.... Unfortunately, a recurrence of the lesion with metastatic nodes developed, and the patient died approximately one year after the operation. (p. 465)

The second recorded total laryngectomy for carcinoma of the larynx was performed in April 1874 by Heine of Prague (Schüller, 1880); the patient survived for 6 months. In June of the same year, Maas (1876b) of Breslau performed the third laryngectomy, but the patient died 2 weeks following the operation after developing pneumonia. Schmidt (1875) of Frankfurt performed the fourth laryngectomy in August of that year, but the 56-year-old patient survived only 4 days and died of collapse. Billroth performed his second total laryngectomy, combined with removal of a small goiter, on a 54-year-old man in November 1874.

The patient suffered preoperatively from bronchitis and died of bronchopneumonia 4 days after the operation.

The first successful laryngectomy reported with many years of survival was performed in 1875 by Bottini of Italy on a 24-year-old man (Schüller, 1880). The lesion was a mixed round and spindle cell sarcoma. The patient lost a large amount of blood and erysipelas developed, but he survived. For years postoperatively he was able to continue his work as a mail carrier in a mountainous region.

A notable advance in the technique of total laryngectomy was reported by von Langenbeck (1875). In July 1875, he presented an unusual specimen during the meeting of the Medical Society in Berlin. It included the entire larynx with epiglottis, hyoid, a third of the tongue, the anterior and lateral portion of the pharynx, a portion of the esophagus, both submaxillary glands, and lymphatic tissue from the submaxillary triangle. A 57-year-old man with carcinoma of the larynx had undergone tracheotomy but initially refused to have a laryngectomy. He returned 7 months after the operation, and in July was again operated on by von Langenbeck. The incision was T-shaped. The dissection was performed from above so that the trachea was severed last. The time involved for the surgery was a little more than 2 hours. It is recorded that the operation was done as exactly as an anatomic dissection, and in spite of the extensive region involved, blood loss was unusually small because each vessel was ligated prior to being cut. Forty-one ligatures were made, including both external carotid arteries; lingual, facial, and superior thyroids; and so on. The patient survived for 4 months but died of collapse during an attempt to remove the metastatically involved glands of the left side of the neck. The operation performed by von Langenbeck could be considered the forerunner of the combined wide-field laryngectomy with neck dissection.

In December 1887, the *Journal of Laryngology and Rhinology* published a review of the first 103 total laryngectomies for cancer. At least 40 (39%) of these patients died of the immediate effects of the operation within a period varying from a few hours to 8 weeks, over half of them as a result of pneumonia. Recurrence was noted in 21 (20%) of the patients, the shortest time being 2 months and the average being 6 months. One patient died suddenly of suffocation 8 months after laryngectomy; there was no evidence of recurrence at postmortem, but a feather used to clean the tracheostomy cannula reportedly was found in the trachea (Newman, 1886a).

Although Billroth was credited with the first total laryngectomy for cancer, he personally operated on only 4 patients out of the reported 103. He said, "At my years I can be regarded only as a useful direction pointer and who can point in the direction of the right way?" (Newman, 1886b). Nevertheless, Billroth drew some conclusions from his first experience with total laryngectomy. First, he believed it should have been performed at an earlier stage of the disease, and second, to prevent recurrence, the epiglottis should have been removed with the tumor. He believed strongly in the value of meticulous documentation of cases and pioneered the importance of accurate statistics. Billroth laid the foundations on which present-day surgery is built, and his teachings were furthered by his pupils, some of whom were Czerny, Gussenbauer, Mikulicz, and Woeffler; these men were later to hold chairs of surgery throughout Europe (Weir, 1973).

Following a severe attack of pneumonia in 1887, Billroth became increasingly troubled with congestive heart failure. He went to Italy in December 1893 in the hopes of regaining his health, but he never returned to his adopted Vienna. He died at Abbazia on the Adriatic in February 1894. Prior to his death, Billroth published 140 papers, and his major work, "Allgemeine Chirurgische Pathologie und Therapie," was translated into nine languages.

Based on the results of the first 103 cases, total laryngectomy was not regarded as successful unless the patient's life was extended at least 12 months. It was believed that this length of survival could be achieved by tracheotomy alone. Only 9 (8.5%) of the 103 cases fulfilled these criteria, the longest length of survival being 5 years. The surgeon in one third of the successful cases was Carl Güssenbauer.

The unusually high mortality rate and the minimal curative value of such procedures provoked a number of physicians to question seriously whether surgery for cancer of the larynx was justified. Such skepticism spread throughout Europe, painting a gloomy future for laryngectomy surgery. As Paul Kock, a noted authority, put it, "The surgeon's skill is sometimes shown by the patient not dying under his knife" (cited in Schechter & Morfit, 1965, p. 467). Some of the surgeons' comments portrayed an inauspicious beginning. In one survey, Solis-Cohen stated, "Laryngectomy has not tended to the prolongation of life; and the prolonged existence of a very few cases seemed purchasable only at the sacrifice of the remnant of existence of many others" (cited in Schechter & Morfit, 1965, p. 467).

At a meeting of the International Medical Congress, opinions on the merits of laryngectomy were sharply divided. Solis-Cohen reiterated,

> I am afraid that there is a tendency to the operation being overrated, if we do not appreciate the usually miserable conditions of the patients who have undergone it successfully, for there is an important difference between "recovery" and mere "survival after operation." (Schechter & Morfit, 1965, p. 467)

The renowned Sir Felix Semon of London remarked,

> I cannot help feeling that in the whole question one important fault is committed by a good many members of the profession, namely, that of confounding the two very different ideas of the "possibility" and of the "justifiability" of an operation. I am astonished to hear ... taken for granted that as the diagnosis of carcinoma of the larynx is established, under all circumstances extirpation should forthwith be proceeded with.... I desire to say that I have no theoretical objections against the operation as such ... but that I consider it a duty to protest against its indiscriminate recommendation in all cases of carcinoma, a recommendation which, I think, is with difficulty theoretically justifiable, and which is certainly practically not justified. I wish to protest still stronger against the operation in cases of recurrent papillomata, a

subject on which I shall have to say more on a future occasion. (Schechter & Morfit, 1965, p. 467)

Remarks made by Professor Burow refer not only to the choice of treatment, but also to information given the patient:

In my opinion it is better not to perform total extirpation on patients with carcinoma of the larynx, but if the case be a suitable one, to make endo-laryngeal, even if only partial, excision, and to tracheotomize if dyspnea makes its appearance. Such patients live on the average of two and a half years from the beginning of the affection, and one and a half after tracheotomy, and are frequently able to follow their vocation for a considerable time. If the operation of extirpation is to be performed at all in such cases, it certainly ought to be done at a very early period; but will we in such an early period, when the symptoms are still slight, get the patient's permission, unless we tell them the malignant nature of their affection? By doing so, we make the rest of their existence miserable, and deprive them of the desirable self-deception in which we can keep them for a long time if we only temporize—i.e., tra-cheotomize. These are my present views, but it is, of course possible that new observations in coming years may lead me to modify them. (Schechter & Morfit, 1965, p. 467)

Czerny's statements probably were as complete and encompassing as any made:

The question of extirpation of the larynx presents such difficulties that I have come here not to teach but to learn. Fully as I recognize the right of exis-tence of the skeptical party which has to separate the chaff from the grain, yet I must pertinently claim for my less skeptical party the recognition that we ask, quite as conscientiously as the other side, in every individual case:"What would you wish to be done unto yourself under the circumstances of the case?" If we look at Dr. Foulis' tables, it is true that we should come to the conclusion the extirpation of the larynx was but of little value, only five of all who had been operated on being alive now. But let us be true to ourselves, and confess that of all patients operated on for carcinoma but few have been permanently cured. As long as we do not possess a treatment as efficient against malignant tumors as the knife, we really must be consistent, and not refuse the patient, who is irreparably lost through his laryngeal carcinoma, the possible advantage of the operation. As to the permissibility of the extirpa-tion of the larynx, the state of the patient after the operation is, it is true, of decisive importance, and we have just heard that an American patient was very, very miserable after its performance. I have performed the operation three times on men, and do not consider it so very dangerous, but the after-treatment is one of the most difficult tasks that could be given to the surgeon, and the functional results vary very much according to the stage of the dis-ease. But even in my first two cases, in which I was only able to operate late, as the diagnosis was for a long time uncertain, yet there is the advantage that the pains, which before the operation rendered taking of food almost impossible, ceased afterwards. It is necessary to remove much skin, the cicatricial contraction is not sufficient to cover completely the space around the artificial larynx; under these circumstances, taking food, especially fluid, is often impeded. In my last case, which unfortunately is only of three months date, the state of affairs is so favorable, and the artificial vocal apparatus answers so admirably, that the patient is about to resume his duties as to superior judge. Let us hope that he may fulfill them for a long time! The question, in functional respects, as to the preservation of the epiglottis, is not yet decided. The results vary much according to the patient's individuality, which has the greatest influence upon the functional success. For all this it follows that the whole question is a most difficult one, and which will not be ripe for decision for a long time to come. I believe that extirpation of the larynx, apart from other indications, is demanded as soon as the diagnosis of a malignant new formation, be it by means of the laryngoscope or by microscopic examination of removed particles, is attained, and as soon as it becomes visible that after failure of other remedies the malady irresistibly progresses, and unquestionably endangers the life of the patient. (Schechter & Morfit, 1965, p. 468)

The postoperative treatment in those early days was to leave the wound wide open and pack it with sponges soaked in carbol solution to soak up wound secretions. The outer dressing produced counterpressure to eliminate dead space. The trachea was secured to the skin with silk sutures, and the tracheal cannula was inserted. The dressings were changed daily, and the wound was irrigated with carbol solution. The oral cavity was washed out several times daily with disinfectant solutions, and the patient was fed by a gastric tube. A steam kettle evaporating turpentine oil with carbolic acid and glycerin was placed in the room.

In January 1887, when he was 58 years old, the Emperor Frederick III of Germany developed the first symptoms of gradually increasing hoarseness following a common cold. Examination of the larynx was carried out in March by Professor Gerhardt of Berlin. His findings indicated a polypoidal swelling on the edge of the left vocal cord, slightly anterior to the vocal process, and redness of both vocal folds, but unimpaired mobility. Galvanocautery was used several times without improvement. After numerous biopsies and many problems with increasing obstruction and continued hoarseness, a tracheotomy became necessary in February 1888. In June of that year, Professor Gerhardt's patient died from complications secondary to tracheotomy, metastases, aspiration pneumonia, and pulmonary gangrene. In this case, the necessity for biopsy was argued. For the next 50 years, arguments against biopsy continued with a contention that biopsy contributed to the spread of cancer. This controversy influenced the course of laryngology through the first quarter of the 20th century (Holinger, 1975).

As is evident in the preceding historical review, the first laryngectomy was not an isolated event in the history of laryngology. Therapy was hampered by lack of adequate understanding of the pathology of laryngeal lesions. It should also be remembered that direct laryngoscopy and biopsy postdated the first laryngectomy by approximately 20 years. The first laryngectomy was actually the culmination of nearly half a century of groping toward an understanding of the pathology, its natural history, and a more effective management regimen for laryngeal cancer. This search continues today as knowledge of the larynx and its diseases continues to be gathered.

Predicting the future of laryngectomy in terms of surgical procedures and the nature of cancer at a fundamental and etiological level is impossible at this time. For the predictable future, fundamental advances will likely continue. At least one laryngeal transplantation in a human has taken place, although this was in the case of a total laryngectomy due to traumatic injury as opposed to malignant disease (Strome et al., 2001). Interestingly, it is noteworthy that the earliest operations were not applied to malignant neoplastic disease but were performed for nonmalignant conditions. It may be that the need for partial and total laryngectomy will outlast the application to carcinoma (Jesberg, 1960).

Historical Highlights of Laryngectomy to 1925

Although an exhaustive review is not possible, an outline of the major advances in laryngectomy is provided in this section. With the aid of a brief historical timeline and an extensive bibliography (see the References and Additional Historical Readings Sections at the end of this chapter), the reader who desires more information may delve into the topic in greater depth.

400 B.C.   Hippocrates said, in effect, "A tumor is a tumor, a superabundance of tissue, and therefore should be removed" (Jackson & Jackson, 1939, p. 214). Although many great clinicians of the time recognized differences in tumors when opened and during their clinical course, they did not have microscopes; thus, histological evaluation was impossible (Jackson & Jackson, 1939).

1743 A.D.   The first authenticated attempt at examining the larynx was by Leveret, a French *accoucheur* (obstetrician), who devised a bent mirror for examination of the throat (Albers, 1829; cited in Jackson & Jackson, 1939).

1829   Albers did experimental laryngectomies, partial and total, on dogs, but there is no record of his attempting the operation on human beings.

1829   Babington (1829; cited in Mackenzie, 1880) presented the first effective invention that could be called a laryngoscope to the Hunterian Society of London.

1833   The first laryngofissure was performed for tumor treated with cautery (Rosenberg, 1971).

1837   Trousseau, the great clinician and observer of diseases, reported a case of "carcinomatous laryngeal phthisis," making a distinction between tuberculosis and carcinoma (Jackson & Jackson, 1939).

1851   The first laryngofissure was performed for excision of a laryngeal tumor (Rosenberg, 1971).

1854   The method of indirect laryngoscopy was discovered by a Spanish singing teacher, Garcia (Rosenberg, 1971).

1858   Virchow's (1858) *Cellular Pathology* established the modern era of distinguishing tumors by their cellular structure.

1858   Krackowizer, an Austrian immigrant, introduced the art of laryngoscopy to North America when he moved to New York (Delavan, 1912).

1866   A laryngectomy was performed by Watson (1881; cited in Jackson & Jackson, 1939) of Edinburgh because of syphilis.

1867   Lister (1867) founded antiseptic surgery and laid the foundation for aseptic surgery. Although not generally accepted until about 1884, aseptic procedures soon thereafter had a marked effect on the results of laryngectomy, as on every other operation. Surgeons of today, for whom aseptic procedures and the use of sterile gloves are routine, shudder to read of an operation done in 1886 and described in a standard textbook of the time: "Laryngectomy was affected by (a) further careful and thorough separation of the attachments to the pharynx by raspatory, knife-handle, and fingernail; (b) division" and so on. That "fingernail" is haunting (Jackson & Jackson, 1939).

1870   Czerny (1870), who was interested in the total extirpation done by Patrick Watson, experimented with total laryngectomy on dogs and assisted Billroth in the first recorded laryngectomy for cancer.

1871   Mackenzie (1880) performed the first indirect laryngeal biopsy.

1873   Billroth (Billroth & Güssenbauer, 1874) performed total laryngectomy for cancer on a 36-year-old male. Cancer recurred and the patient died 7 months later.

1874   Heine (1876) performed a laryngectomy on a 50-year-old male patient due to carcinoma. Recurrence was fatal 6 months later.

1874   Schmidt (1875) performed a laryngectomy on a 56-year-old male patient with cancer. The patient died of surgery-related causes 5 days after the operation.

1875   Bottini (1875) performed a laryngectomy on a 24-year-old male with sarcoma. Two years later, the patient was well and at work as a mail carrier on a long rural route.

1875   Billroth (Billroth & Gussenbauer, 1874) performed a laryngectomy on a 54-year-old male due to carcinoma. The patient died from pneumonia 2 days later.

1875   Schönborn (1875) performed a laryngectomy on a 72-year-old male with carcinoma. The patient died a few days later.

1875   Von Langenbeck (1875) performed a laryngectomy on a
        57-year-old male due to carcinoma. Recurrence with cervical
        lymphatics was fatal 4 months later.

1876   Reyher (1877) performed a laryngectomy on a 60-year-old
        male with carcinoma of vocal cords. The patient died 11 days
        later due to hypostatic pneumonia.

1876   Gerdes (1877) performed a laryngectomy for carcinoma in a
        male patient, age 76. The patient died following collapse 4 days
        later.

1876   Maas (1876a) performed a laryngectomy on a 50-year-old male
        with epithelioma. The disease recurred at the base of the tongue
        3 months later, and the patient died 6 months postoperatively.
        In another case, the patient died 14 days after surgery (Maas,
        1876b).

1877   Bottini (1878) performed a laryngectomy on a 48-year-old male
        with epithelioma. The man died on the third postoperative day
        due to double pneumonia.

1877   Foulis (1877a) performed a laryngectomy on a 28-year-old male
        with mixed papilloma and spindle-cell sarcoma. The patient died
        due to phthisis pulmonalis $1\frac{1}{2}$ years later.

1877   Kosinski (1877) performed a laryngectomy on a 36-year-old
        female with epithelioma involving skin. The patient died due
        to recurrence 9 months after the operation.

1878   Billroth performed the first conservative hemilaryngectomy
        (Rosenberg, 1971).

1878   Von Bruns (1878) performed a laryngectomy on a 54-year-old
        male with epithelioma. Recurrence was fatal 9 months later.

1878   Bottini reported a bloodless laryngectomy by means of gal-
        vanocautery. The patient died 3 days later from double
        pneumonia (Jackson & Jackson, 1939).

1879   Lange (1880) became the first to perform laryngectomy in
        North America.

1879   The American Laryngological Association was founded, inau-
        gurating the study of the larynx as a specialty. In 1939, Jackson
        and Jackson reported that at almost every annual meeting since
        1879 something related to the study of laryngeal cancer was
        contributed.

1880   Schüller (1880) described his technique of laryngectomy from
        above downward, which included placing his finger in the pa-
        tient's mouth to guide the point of the knife so as to include
        the epiglottis with the resected larynx.

1880   Mackenzie (1880) summarized the results of laryngectomy by
        various surgeons. Of 19 patients, 1 died from the passage of a

bougie into the mediastinum, 8 died of collapse or pneumonia within a fortnight, 7 had recurrence within a few months, and 1 lived for 18 months postoperatively. Two cases out of 19 were lasting cures. Mackenzie thought this was good work and quoted Koch, "The skill of the surgeon is, in some cases, shown by the patient not dying under his knife."

1880s Glück recommended that the bottom of the pharynx be completely sewn up in laryngectomized patients to obviate aspiration pneumonia, the greatest hazard of laryngectomy (Glück & Zeller, 1881).

1881 Foulis (1881) undertook collective research. Of the first 25 laryngectomized patients, none survived a year.

1887 Mackenzie and Crown Prince Frederick of Germany. Biopsy by indirect laryngoscopy is benign, but the patient soon died of this malignancy (Rosenberg, 1971).

1892 Crile performed the first laryngectomy in the United States; he performed 34 surgeries in the next 20 years (Crile, 1913, 1947).

1892 Solis-Cohen (1892a, 1892b, 1892c) of Philadelphia performed the first successful laryngectomy in America.

1880– The operative mortality of total laryngectomy was nearly 50%
1900 (Rosenberg, 1971).

1925 Laryngectomy became accepted as a treatment procedure for laryngeal cancer (Rosenberg, 1971).

HISTORY OF THE ARTIFICIAL LARYNX

Not surprisingly, the development of the artificial larynx paralleled that of the laryngectomy as a procedure to preserve life. The total laryngectomy reported by Billroth in 1873 was followed in the early postoperative period by the fitting of an artificial larynx. Thus, concerns about restoring some form of verbal communication were raised early in the history of laryngectomy. What may be surprising is that the early versions of the artificial larynx also sought to preserve life. For example, laryngeal extirpation opened paths upward into the hypopharynx and downward into the respiratory tree. To restore voice, early laryngologists tried to dam the airstream up from the lungs. Blocking the route down from the throat also prevented aspiration of food and liquid. The hazard of aspiration still threatens efforts to establish connections between the respiratory and the alimentary systems. Nevertheless, restoration of verbal communication via alternative sources of voice was a clear priority.

Artificial larynxes have varied in form over the years. In comparing the types of artificial laryngeal appliances, multiple questions can be raised: What is the sound source? How is sound generated by the appliance delivered into the vocal tract? What, if any, health problems are created by using the device? How does the verbal signal sound? How does this signal influence the social dyad? and How can one make the artificial larynx sound more normal and natural? Although these are long-standing issues in the historical literature on postlaryngectomy speech rehabilitation, the potential for improving artificial laryngeal communication in these areas has reemerged as refinements in design and materials have occurred. Therefore, modifications that might have been improbable in the past, may now be pursued (see Chapter 23 in this text).

In the past century and a half, the engineer, surgeon, speech scientist, and others have collaborated in the pursuit of postlaryngectomy voice rehabilitation and improved quality of life for individuals following laryngectomy. The quest continues today, although professionals with engineering backgrounds, including electrical and computer engineers, as well as those with expertise in materials science, are now becoming valuable colleagues for the speech scientist and physician. The following account highlights some of the more memorable historical efforts involving the artificial larynx.

A Review of the Literature

The artificial larynx is a prosthesis meant to replace the diseased or damaged larynx when it has been surgically removed or when, as a result of a disease process, it can no longer produce phonation. The Czech physiologist Johann Nepomuk Czermak (1859) gave the first known description of a laryngeal prosthesis.

Various devices were developed and employed in the early period, characterized by considerable differences in design and materials. Despite the variations, the underlying premise of all the early devices was to restore speech through pneumatic means, that is, using an internal, pulmonary air source as a power supply. Although access to a pulmonary power supply was a commonality of all early devices, some unique aspects of each device are important to note. Some devices appear to have been designed so that tracheal (pulmonary) air could be diverted into the pharynx via a bivalved cannula type of system. This type of device appears to have been the precursor of more modern versions of hypopharyngeal prostheses, such as the Northwestern prosthesis (Sisson, McConnel, Logemann, & Yeh, 1975). For other devices, a cannula affixed with a reed type of device served to provide an externally generated voicing source (via the reed) into the pharyngeal region, where it could then be articulated in the vocal tract. In contrast, other devices were designed to transfer air from the trachea using an internal (pulmonary) source or via use of an external (bellows-type) power source. With these devices, the air source was directed through a tube into the pharyngeal region, where it appears that a "pharyngeal" sound source was generated. The latter two devices used transnasal methods of supplying air to the vocal tract. Many of these devices served as the early impetus for other pneumatic devices of the modern era, such as the air bypass voice prosthesis (Taub & Bergner, 1973), other reed–fistula methods of voice rehabilitation (Weinberg, Shedd, & Horii, 1978), and the Tokyo artificial larynx (see Weinberg & Riekena, 1973).

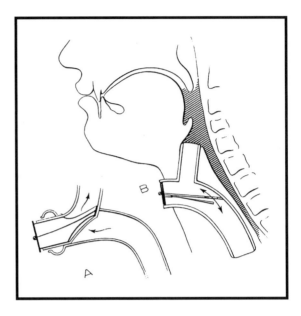

In 1859 at the Imperial Academy of Sciences in Vienna, Czermak reported on an 18-year-old woman who had been tracheotomized because of a complete laryngeal stenosis. Czermak provided her with an artificial larynx. In the tube was a reed, a small flexible tongue of metal that could be set into vibration by blowing air through the tube. Thus began the history of the artificial larynx. Also in 1859, while studying a case of complete laryngeal stenosis, Czermak conceived the idea that the expiratory current of air issuing from the tracheal cannula that the patient had in place could be used to produce voice and speech if it could be directed into the mouth through a tube containing a vibrating reed. Brucke (as cited by Czermak, 1859) constructed an apparatus based on Czermak's idea. Using it, the patient could, with sufficient effort, produce single syllables. A few years later, while experimenting with animals, Czerny (1870) contrived several different machines. Following Czerny's lead, Billroth, who in 1873 performed the first successful total extirpation of the larynx for cancer, worked with Eiselberg to design a laryngeal prosthesis in which the tone was conducted through the tracheal opening into the pharyngeal cavity. This artificial larynx consisted of three parts: tracheal, pharyngeal, and phonation cannulas. The phonation cannula was set inside the pharyngeal cannula. The tone-producing reed, which was thrown into vibration by the expiratory breath, was set in the phonation cannula. The tone, when projected into the resonating space above, could be transformed into the sounds of articulate value (Billroth & Gussenbauer, 1874).

Foulis (1877a) also developed a reed-based device for a patient (Figure 2.1). He used a vulcanite laryngeal tube that was fitted into the trachea. Within this tracheostoma tube and by means of a simple arrangement, a vibrating reed was introduced that took the place of the vocal cords. The patient reportedly spoke in a resonant, loud, and clear, but monotonous voice.

Within the year, this device was further improved. Trying to make the artificial tone sound like natural voice, von Bruns (1881) discarded the rigid laryngeal tube and replaced it with a flexible semi-rubber membrane. Stoerk (1880, 1887, 1896) used an ordinary reed pipe placed between the teeth and connected to the tracheal cannula by means of a rubber tube, through which the expiratory breath stream could be directed across the reed. The patient articulated at the same time that he produced the tone. If he wished, he could sound the reed by means of a double balloon bulb adapted for it. The purpose of some improvements, such as that of Wolff (1893a, 1893b), was to prevent the accumulation of secretions and particles of food on the device. Other improvements reduced irritation of adjacent tissues by the appliance. Cases of recurrence had been reported in which the irritation of tissue in contact with the apparatus was suspected as a contributing etiological factor.

With this in mind, Gottstein (1900) returned to the earlier ideas of Czermak and Stoerk. Gottstein's apparatus had an accessory piece adapted for the trachea that was connected to a flexible rubber tube. The wall of the tube was held rigid by means of a spiral wire housed within it. To the free end of this rubber tube was attached a metal piece that was placed so as to lie behind the last molar. Air from the trachea reached the pharyngeal cavity by this route. The voice-producing mechanism was placed in the rubber tube.

Without any knowledge of Stoerk's prior apparatus, which had already been described, and after some experiments, Hochenegg (1892) prepared an apparatus similar to Stoerk's but differing primarily in the manner of application. The artificial power source for activation of the reed was placed through the nose into the oropharynx; instead of a small balloon, the power source consisted of a bellows fastened to the side of the patient's thorax. Hochenegg had to abandon his first idea of activating the reed by the use of pulmonary air itself because the user was found to lack sufficient breath support to initiate a tone. Additionally, the instrument reportedly made the patient cough violently.

When Glück and his coworkers appeared on the scene, they established for themselves a place in the history of laryngeal surgery. They made fundamental modifications in the technique used for total extirpation of the larynx and invented and constructed laryngeal prostheses ingenious enough to radically influence the patient's postoperative social status. Glück (1899, 1904, 1908, 1913, 1921) constructed a whole series of cannulas and artificial larynxes activated by bellows. His later models, however, depended on the lungs for air, with the vibrating mechanism placed within an endonasal or endo-oral metal olive. He also prepared tiny artificial voice boxes connected to bellows and compression chambers that could be activated mechanically or electrically. These voice boxes permitted the production of speech by means of a similar sensitive vocal olive. Later, he prepared gramophone records on which was registered a sustained tone beautifully sung by a good singer; these gramophones were capable of amplification by means of a diaphragm. This tone was conducted through a tube in the patient's mouth that could then be articulated as speech. Interruption of the tone was controlled by special adjustments. Tests with this method showed much promise, but further development seemed to have met some obstacle. Perhaps the increasing evidence of the possibility of developing a vicarious physiological voice mechanism influenced its demise.

The problem of producing an artificial voice varied with the technique of laryngectomy. As it is now performed, laryngectomy excludes any communication between the trachea and the pharynx. Some of the early laryngeal prostheses were remarkably and skillfully contrived. Onodi (1918) constructed a model in which a tone was carried by means of a microphone into the nasopharynx. The devices of Tapia (1914), Casadesus (1923; cited in Snidecor, 1968), Hinojar (1923), Leyro Diaz (1924), and Mackenty (cited in Fletcher, 1929/1953), are based on the same fundamental idea, but naturally each developer considered his own device to be the best.

The disadvantages of the older laryngeal prostheses were many. Some of the devices were believed to irritate adjacent tissue and account for occasional cases of cancer recurrence (Kallen, 1931). Many devices produced shrill and squeaky sounds. Others caused respiratory complications, and all increased salivation. Speaking situations were rather painful and trying. Although later devices made things easier for the patient, the cost was prohibitive and likely limited their widespread use.

The prime reason for not using even the best of these devices is that most patients could be taught to use a vicarious voice source with some degree of modulation. This voice was often more natural and human sounding and may have been more clearly enunciated. Kallen (1931) noted that for psychological reasons the mastery of a vicarious voice is of great importance in maintaining the health of a patient's psyche following laryngectomy. He suggested that a mechanical device can never have the same psychological significance as a living organ with a newly developed function that becomes entirely identified with the individual personality.

In 1920, the first notable improvement in the United States was made by J. E. Mackenty of New York (Fletcher, 1929/1953). He used the rubber band as a reed, but discovered that a soft rubber mouthpiece greatly improved the speaker's vocal quality. The case of his instrument was made of hard rubber.

Pollock and Lederer (1922) described another artificial larynx:

> An artificial larynx was presented, which consisted in the main of a trachea cannula and a pharyngeal cannula, the latter being made of flexible rubber in order to prevent irritation of the epiglottis that results when a metallic tube, which does not give, is used. A diaphragm arrangement between the two allows for phonation. (p. 480)

In 1924, Mackenty enlisted the cooperation of the Western Electric Company in the development of an artificial larynx that overcame to a great extent the defects of the other devices. This device delivered a low-pitched, somewhat guttural, but strikingly human voice. Mackenty's idea on the best way to accomplish this was by using a transverse rubber band, but the Western Electric Company felt that a better voice could be developed with the use of reeds. Mackenty had tried reeds but they had failed; he told the company that the reed required too strong an air current to vibrate it, consequently tiring the patient. Furthermore, the voice it produced was reported to be a musical and singing tone, which was thought to be disagreeable to the ear. His plans were adopted, and the result was a very useful instrument, not embarrassing, burdensome, impractical, delicate, or difficult to repair (Fletcher, 1929/1953). In the hands of anyone of ordinary mechanical ability, it reportedly worked well.

In 1923, Brown (1925) attempted to fashion an artificial larynx by means of a "tube flap," from which very good voice resulted. The difficulty caused by the escape of saliva, however, made Brown discard the method. This device also required that the patient have both the pharyngeal opening and the tracheal opening. With considerable experimentation, Brown was able to control the leakage of saliva, and the device could be worn for up to 3 hours at a time.

In the late 1920s, the first Bell Telephone Laboratories instrument was made by George W. Burchett of New York, and it was patented in December 1931 (Hanson, 1940). The Laboratories' initial efforts resulted in an instrument, designated Type 1A, that employed rubber bands stretched in a manner to simulate the vocal cords. The rubber bands deteriorated rapidly, however, and were a source of considerable dissatisfaction. The second instrument invented was reported by Robert R. Riesz (1930) in the *Journal of the Acoustical Society of America*. Subsequently in 1929 a new larynx, designated Type 2A, was developed. This new device incorporated several refinements, including the substitution of a vibrating metallic reed for the elastic bands. This model, with minor changes, was manufactured by Western Electric Company for many years (Barney, Haworth, & Dunn, 1959). In 1932 and 1933, Bell Labs modified the instrument with reed-adjusting devices.

McKesson (1927) described a mechanical larynx in the *Journal of the American Medical Association*. This artificial larynx employed the reed element, which was a thin rubber band inserted transversely in the container. Details of how the source moved to the vocal tract are not available.

In 1931, Charles Sheard of the Mayo Clinic in Rochester, Minnesota, presented a new reed-type artificial larynx. He claimed that it could operate at all times and under all circumstances, would permit ordinary or loud speaking, would possess a given fundamental frequency that could be made as high or as low as desired, and could be replaced in case the reed was broken or damaged during cleaning (Sheard, 1931).

M. A. Goldstein (1932) described the modification of an artificial larynx to the American Laryngological Association. He also presented metal disks for the permanent recording or reproduction of a patient's speech. He additionally presented a new terminal on the rubber connecting tube to be applied to the device after removal of the tracheal cannula; it consisted of half a rubber sponge ball with the center punched out and adapted to a tracheal fistula. Goldstein removed the rubber flange underneath the metallic reed and substituted a small fiber-like flange with small holes in it to reduce adherence of the reed to the base by moisture.

In 1936, Iglauer presented a new artificial larynx with a patient demonstrating its use. It was similar to that made by the Bell Telephone Company except that a thumb screw regulated the movements of the reed.

The general principles of voice generation using the electronic larynx can be demonstrated by mouthing words while placing any vibrator source (e.g., an electric razor) on the neck. The vibrator serves as a sound source that is activated electrically. In 1942, Wright, using this principle with the Aurex Corporation and later the Kett Engineering Corporation, developed and manufactured electronic artificial larynx instruments (Rigrodsky, Lerman, & Morrison, 1971). The Aurex Model M 410 used a cord connecting the battery and the vibrator unit, whereas the Aurex Model M 520 eliminated the cord by encasing the battery in the instrument. Kett Mark III required a cord and C-2 batteries, whereas the Mark II and Mark III were cordless. The Mark III used a nickel cadmium battery capable of being recharged. In 1960, the Bell Telephone Company developed a cordless, transistorized electronic larynx that had an octave pitch range when the on switch was depressed completely (Haworth, 1960).

Cooper, a dentist, developed two variations of the electronic larynx (Cooper & Millard, 1959). The Cooper–Rand Speech Aid used the principle of electrically generated sound, with the sound conducted via a plastic tube inserted in the mouth. The other Cooper instrument used the principle of battery power carried by wire to a transducer located on a denture. V. Tait and Tait (1959) came out with a similar instrument known as the Oral Vibrator. Similarly, Ticchioni used an electromagnet fitted into the bowl of a pipe and powered with a battery source so that sound could be delivered through the pipe to the mouth (Lebrun, 1973).

Historical Highlights of Artificial Laryngeal Devices

Highlights of the development of the artificial larynx are provided in the following timeline. It is important to know about the evolution of this device. Today, many devices with many modifications are available to effectively serve the person following laryngectomy (see Chapters 22 and 23 in this text). The reader also is referred to Lebrun (1973) or Salmon and Goldstein (1978) for detailed histories of the development of the artificial larynx.

1859	Czermak described a laryngeal prosthesis used for an 18-year-old woman who had been tracheotomized because of laryngeal stenosis. A reed device used air from the lungs directed into the corner of the mouth via a thin tube.
1873	Leiter, an instrument maker, devised an artificial larynx for Billroth's patient that could be inserted between the trachea and the pharynx. Actually, it was an internal pneumatic laryngeal prosthesis.
1874	Gussenbauer (Billroth & Güssenbauer, 1874) improved on Leiter's prosthesis (Figure 2.1A) by replacing Leiter's fixed phonatory cannula with a reed case placed nearer to the tracheostoma and which could be easily withdrawn.

1877   Foulis (1877b) had a new voice tube designed with the help of Irvine, a doctor, and the assistance of a dentist named Fould. It was based on Gussenbauer's plan, but had essential modifications (Figure 2.1B).

1877   Stoerk in Vienna contrived an external prosthesis that was driven by air from a bulb that the patient, a tracheotomized girl with a laryngeal stenosis, had to squeeze with her hand. As the bulb did not produce enough air, Stoerk suppressed the bulb and connected the artificial larynx to the patient's tracheal cannula (Hochenegg, 1892).

1878 and 1881   Von Bruns (1878, 1881) substituted a flexible cannula for the rigid laryngeal cannula and discarded the artificial epiglottis, which had proved to be of little help. To prevent food from falling into the lungs, a plug fitted on a curved rod similar to the Irvine–Fould prosthesis could be introduced before each meal into the laryngeal cannula through the tracheostoma.

1885   Two French physicians, Labbe (1886) and Cadier, made a prosthesis seemingly modeled on Güssenbauer's artificial larynx.

1892   Hochenegg (1892) reduplicated Stoerk's appliance. The patient was unable to exhale with sufficient strength to cause the reed to vibrate. Moreover, the buccal tube interfered with articulation. Consequently, Hochenegg designed an artificial larynx powered by air from a pair of bellows that the patient held under his armpit. The resulting puffs of air were delivered into the pharynx through a nasal tube.

1893   Wolff (1893a, 1893b) felt that the von Bruns device had several drawbacks. Saliva dripped into the device during speech, the voice was monotonous, and the valve did not admit enough air. Wolff tried to remedy these flaws by shortening the laryngeal cannula and lengthening the phonatory cannula so that they were of equal length. According to Wolff, these changes improved the quality of the voice.

1897   Anderson-Stuart (1897), a professor of physiology at the University of Sydney, reported on an artificial larynx with a tracheal butt that could be inserted into the rubber cannula and which the patient wore permanently. This short tube was attached to a voice box provided at its base with a large opening for breathing. When the patient occluded this opening with a thumb and exhaled, air was forced into the superior part of the voice box, which contained a metallic reed taken from a mouth organ. The puffs of air delivered by the reed left the voice box through a wired rubber tube that entered the pharynx through a fistula cut below the hyoid bone. To prevent saliva and food from falling into the prosthesis, the top of the pharyngeal tube was provided with a valve made of kid leather. This valve, Anderson-Stuart (1897) wrote, "is absolutely efficient, for while wet it readily permits the sound-bearing air to pass into the pharynx, and it prevents anything from passing down into the artificial larynx, so that the patient wore the apparatus the livelong day" (p. 1081).

1900   Taptas (1900) wrote a paper in which he described an artificial larynx. The device comprised a tracheal cannula, a pharyngeal cannula, and a flexible tube. The pharyngeal cannula was inserted into a pharyngostoma and was connected with the tracheal cannula by the flexible tube. The upper end of the pharyngeal cannula had a valve that prevented food and saliva from entering the prosthesis. By this device, pulmonic air could be led to the vocal tract and the patient could produce an audible, whispered voice. Tissue-oscillated voice, however, could not be generated.

1902   The French phonetician Rousselot (1902) reported on an artificial larynx made by Martin. The appliance consisted of a tracheal cannula, a phonatory cannula, and a hood. The front part of the tracheal cannula was closed by an emergency valve, which could be opened in case the artificial larynx should become obstructed. The bottom of the phonatory cannula communicated with the tracheal cannula. It resulted in a truncated pyramid capped by a flat rubber tube.

1910   At the turn of the century, Glück was experimenting with various types of external artificial larynxes. In some of them, the reed was a bead placed in the patient's nose, and a small tube delivered air puffs to the pharynx. In others, the reed was attached to an upper denture (Glück, 1910). In still others, the rubber reed and the inhalatory valve sat in a cylindrical box just outside the patient's tracheostoma (Tapia, 1914).

1914   Pereda, a Spanish laryngectomee, attempted to remedy the flaws noted by Glück. He discarded the cylinder containing the reed and the inhalatory valve. The tracheal tube was left open and provided with a side butt. A rubber tube linked this butt with a voice box carried in the patient's pocket or held in a hand. Another rubber tube conducted puffs of air from the voice box to the mouth. When the patient wanted to speak, he had to close the opening in the front of his tracheal cannula with his finger (Tapia, 1914).

1918   Onodi and Stockman (Onodi, 1918) constructed a device similar to the one used by Glück in which the bellows were driven by an electromotor powered by batteries.

1920s   Mackenty, senior surgeon of the Manhattan Eye, Ear, and Throat
         Hospital in New York, together with Fletcher and Lane, two sci-
         entists of the Western Electric Company, developed an artificial
         larynx. The device consisted of a soft-rubber tracheal pad and
         a flexible tracheal connection that could be strapped over the
         tracheostoma; a silver cylinder containing a hard-rubber tube
         across which a rubber band was stretched; a thumb nut to adjust
         the tension of the membrane and, consequently, the pitch of
         the voice; and a mouthpiece that fitted in the metal stem in the
         top of the reed box. The cylinder had an inhalatory hole that
         the user occluded with a finger during speech (Barney, 1958;
         Barney et al., 1959).

1924   Leyro Diaz (1924) used a tube connecting the trachea with the
         nasopharynx. Near the lower end, the tube had a lateral opening
         through which the patient could breathe. When the patient com-
         municated, he had to exhale, close the breathing hole with a
         finger, and turn the pulmonic airstream into an audible whisper.

1925   The Australian surgeon Brown (1925) reported on an artificial
         larynx that resembled Anderson-Stuart's appliance of 1896.
         Brown had cut a pharyngostoma in a patient's neck just below
         the hyoid bone. An aural speculum made of gold and containing
         a violin pitch pipe was fitted into the pharyngostoma and held
         in a position by two tapes tied round the head. The patient
         was further provided with a thin shield of vulcanite that closely
         fitted the front of her neck except at its superior border, where a
         small gap was left between it and the neck. The shield was held
         in position by tapes that passed around the back of the neck.
         The loosely applied portion at the superior border allowed
         breathing to take place through the tracheostoma. When speech
         was required, the patient brought her head forward, producing
         an airtight space between the neck and the shield. The expired
         air entered the reed, which then delivered air puffs to the
         pharynx.

1925   Jewett, then–president of Bell Telephone Laboratories, cham-
         pioned the company's involvement in the design of the artifi-
         cial larynx. The company's first efforts employed rubber bands
         stretched in a manner to simulate the vocal cords and was desig-
         nated Type 1A (Riesz, 1930). Modifications in design and mate-
         rial advances continued over the next 30 years until the modern
         era of the contemporary electrolarynx with the work of Barney
         et al. (1959). At the same time, the Western Electric Company
         pursued similar work related to external pneumatic devices
         (L. P. Goldstein, 1982).

1927   McKesson (1927) described his device, christened the Vocophone, in the *Journal of the American Medical Association:*

> This instrument enables a patient whose larynx has been
> removed because of carcinoma to speak with a voice ap-
> proaching the normal in volume and quality. A neckpiece is
> held in place by means of the collar, to which it is attached
> by an ordinary collar button. A rubber tube connects the
> neckpiece with the trumpet, and a tube from the trumpet
> conducts the sound into the mouth. To speak, the neck-
> piece is pressed gently against the neck, and air is blown
> through the trumpet, setting up a sound resembling the
> normal voice. (p. 645)

1929   Bell Telephone Laboratories developed a new artificial larynx,
designated the Western Electric Type 2A, to incorporate several
refinements, including the substitution of a vibrating metallic
reed for the elastic bands (Riesz, 1930). The metallic reed was
connected by tubing to the tracheostoma so that the user's
breath could actuate the reed. The sound of the vibrating reed
was conducted through another tube into the mouth to be articulated into speech. In ensuing years, Riesz, a Bell Laboratories
engineer, patented other variations in Western Electric devices
(see Figures 2.2 through 2.5). Another variation is shown in
Figure 2.6 with a bellows for initiating voice, and in Figure 2.7
beside a Western Electric #2 for comparison (see L. P. Goldstein,
1982).

1929   Narro-Casadesus, an instrument maker from Barcelona, designed
a pneumatic artificial larynx. It consisted of an adjustable metallic reed whose housing was carried in the patient's pocket. A
flexible rubber tube connected the reed with the tracheal cannula and another tube connected it with the patient's mouth.
The reed box was provided with an inhalatory valve. The bottom of the box could be unscrewed to remove mucous deposits.

1931   Sheard (1931) designed a device (Figure 2.8) based on the Western Electric pneumatic device. The four essential parts of this artificial larynx included a rubber tube for insertion in the mouth
and one with a connection to the neck. The partially cupped
plate carried a valve for purposes of breathing in case the user
failed to remove a thumb from the voice box when he or she
needed to breathe. A few years after Riesz, a workable homemade device was made using strips of radiographic film as a
vibrator source (Figure 2.9).

1932   Lane (1932) applied for a patent for an improved larynx that
overcame the disadvantages of previous devices. A trachea connection was applied to the trachea opening in the user's neck.

(text continues on p. 44)

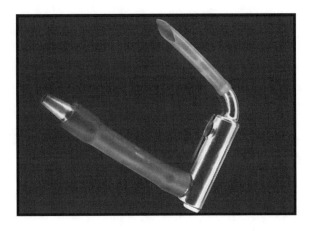

FIGURE 2.2. Western Electric 2A pneumatic mechanical larynx. (Courtesy of Roberta Rauch.)

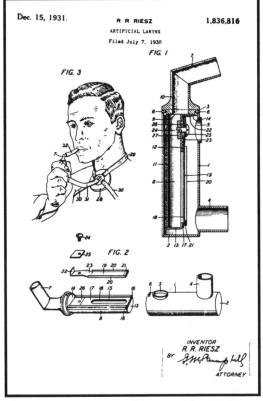

FIGURE 2.3. Variation of Western Electric 2A pneumatic mechanical larynx. (Courtesy of Roberta Rauch.)

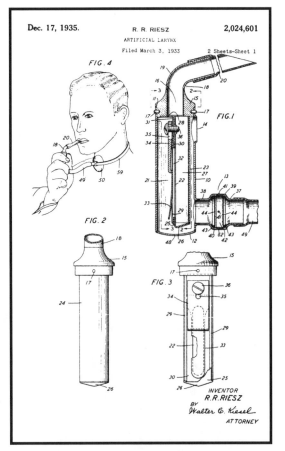

FIGURE 2.4. Later variation of Western Electric #2. (Courtesy of Roberta Rauch.)

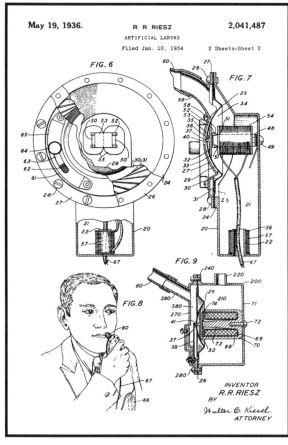

FIGURE 2.5. Western Electric #2 variation of pneumatic larynx by R. R. Riesz. (Courtesy of Roberta Rauch.)

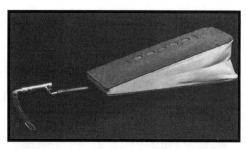

FIGURE 2.6. Early mechanical larynx with activating bellows. (Courtesy of Roberta Rauch.)

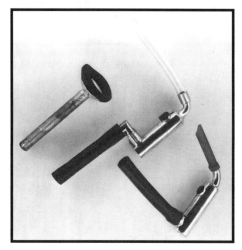

FIGURE 2.7. Original Western Electric #2 and subsequent variations of pneumatic artificial larynxes. (Courtesy of Roberta Rauch.)

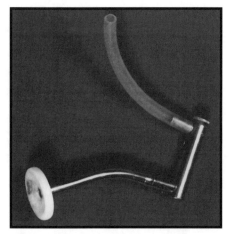

FIGURE 2.8. The Neher Pneumatic Larynx developed by Sheard. (Courtesy of James Shanks.)

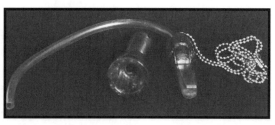

FIGURE 2.9. Vibrator using strip of radiographic film as sound source. (Courtesy of James Shanks.)

This connection was joined to a sound chamber through an air passageway so as to introduce air from the lungs into the sound chamber. This chamber contained a vibratory element in the form of a tubular elastic member rigidly supported at one end of the chamber and having its free end slightly open. After the air passed through the element, it was led to the user's mouth, where the sounds of speech were articulated.

1933   McKesson (1933) applied for a patent, which was assigned to the Vocophone Company of Toledo, Ohio. This invention relates to air handling, especially for oral resonance control. It had utility for mouth communication from the lungs, bypassing the larynx and throat as in Lane's (1932) device.

1936   Snidecor (1962) discussed a retired St. Louis policeman who was using a self-designed instrument:

> The source of power was the hand-squeezed bulb of an old automobile horn of the type that once graced the side of Stutz Bearcat. A tube led into the mouth where a reformed clarinet reed vibrated with ample power and complexity. (p. 149)

1936   Loring demonstrated the prosthesis he had made for himself (Iglauer, 1936). The device resembled the artificial larynx described by Riesz (1930). The reed worked in an open slot, however, whereas the Western Electric #2 had a reed cushion.

1937   Kellotat (1937) applied for a patent for a device consisting of a denture and a mechanism for producing voice. It included a sound chamber having outlets; a reed chamber having an inlet, the reed chamber being operatively associated with the sound chamber; a vibrating reed within the reed chamber; side extensions carried by the denture and conforming to the contour of the side of the mouth; and a flexible apron disposed between the side extensions and functioning therewith to seal the back of the throat and direct exhaled air into the inlet of the reed chamber. The entire assembly was adapted to be wholly contained within the oral cavity.

1939   Hanson (1940) and a patient named Roberts made an artificial larynx out of hard rubber. By means of this prosthesis, a voice could be produced that Hanson claimed was close to the natural laryngeal voice. In addition, the device was light, unbreakable, and moisture resistant.

1940   Firestone (1940) designed an instrument whereby voice could be generated via a diaphragm that was external to the oral cavity and connected with the mouth. This device comprised a relaxation oscillator and a receiver. The pulses delivered by the diaphragm of the receiver were introduced into the oral cavity

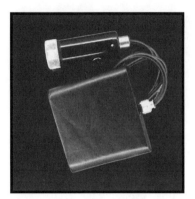

FIGURE 2.10. Wright Electrolarynx produced by Aurex. (Courtesy of James Shanks.)

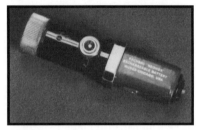

FIGURE 2.11. Aurex Neovox electrolarynx with rechargeable battery. (Courtesy of James Shanks.)

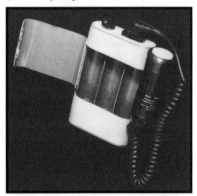

FIGURE 2.12. Wright Electrolarynx produced by Kett. (Courtesy of James Shanks.)

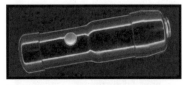

FIGURE 2.13. Cordless Electrolarynx, Kett Mark III, with rechargeable battery. (Courtesy of James Shanks.)

through an air-filled glass tube. Firestone recommended that the oscillator be provided with a continuous, rapidly operable control of frequency so as to permit inflection. He also suggested the use of a push-button volume control for distinguishing between voiced and unvoiced consonants.

1942   Wright (1942) probably should receive credit for the first electrolarynx. With separate power pack connected by cord, sound was introduced into the throat by transmission through the neck wall. The device was known as the Sonovox (which also let the train "talk" in the Walt Disney movie, *Dumbo*).

1945   Wright's (Luchsinger, 1949) artificial larynx was eventually produced by the Aurex Corporation of Chicago, Illinois, first as the Wright Electrolarynx (Figure 2.10) and then as the Aurex Neovox (Figure 2.11). Wright's design also inspired a similar electronic larynx (Figure 2.12), later known as the Kett Mark III (Figure 2.13), which was manufactured by the Kett Engineering Company.

1950   Dunn (1950) was the first to calculate the resonant function in an electronic vocal tract. This work served as impetus for the preliminary design of contemporary-era versions of the transcervical electronic artificial larynx. This work was expanded over the next several years in an attempt to develop a transistorized electronic artificial larynx. Dunn's work was later extended by Stevens, Kasowski, and Fant (1953), who developed electrical analogs of the vocal tract.

1955   Hyman (1955) comparatively studied speech of the Western Electric #2 and intrinsic alaryngeal (esophageal) speech.

1957   Pichler (1961a, 1961b) of Vienna invented an electrolarynx consisting of four parts: a battery-powered signal generator carried in the patient's pocket, an antenna worn around the patient's neck, a tiny receiver affixed to a denture, and a switch located in the tracheal cannula. When the patient exhaled with sufficient energy, the switch let the generator emit radio signals, which caused the diaphragm of the receiver to vibrate.

1957   Cooper (1958), head of the Cleft Palate Clinic in Lancaster, Pennsylvania, and electronic engineers of the Rand Development Corporation manufactured the Cooper–Rand electrolarynx (Figure 2.14) from 1957 until 1972. Subsequently, neck-type devices utilized the Cooper–Rand feature of independent controls for levels of loudness and pitch. These European models included the Servox (Figure 2.15), the Romet (Figure 2.16), and the Rehaton (Figure 2.17). The original development was initiated to meet a twofold need for a new artificial larynx: (a) to provide individuals following laryngectomy with a temporary means of speech, both in the interim period immediately following surgery and prior to esophageal speech lessons and also during the times when, due to a cold, digestive upset, or any other reason, esophageal speech was difficult or impossible, and (b) to provide individuals following laryngectomy with a compact instrument that would introduce sound into the mouth and be easy to use, especially for those who are weak or lying down.

1957   Cooper and Millard (1959) filed a patent for a mouth-type electronic artificial larynx. The device consisted of a battery pack carried in the pocket, an on–off switch located under the armpit, and a wire leading from the battery pack to a diaphragm that was plugged into the lateral aspect of an upper dental plate. A slight squeeze of the arm produced a sound in the mouth that could be articulated into speech. A modification of this device remains in use today.

1958   Barney and colleagues presented information on use of transistors and miniaturized components in a prototype transistorized artificial larynx (Barney, 1958; Barney et al., 1959). Barney and colleagues also introduced the concept of a potential pitch-changing mechanism for a mechanical device.

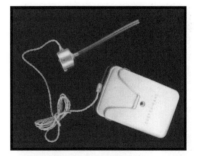

FIGURE 2.14. Cooper–Rand, a mouth-type electrolarynx. (Courtesy of James Shanks.)

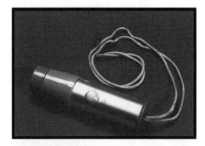

FIGURE 2.15. Servox electrolarynx. (Courtesy of James Shanks.)

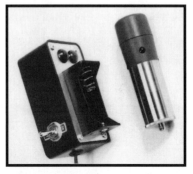

FIGURE 2.16. Romet electrolarynx, with battery charger. (Courtesy of James Shanks.)

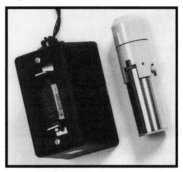

FIGURE 2.17. Rehaton electrolarynx. (Courtesy of James Shanks.)

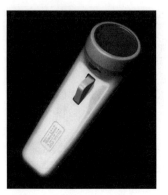

FIGURE 2.18. Early Western Electric #5 electrolarynx. (Courtesy of James Shanks.)

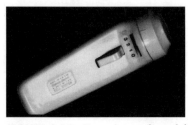

FIGURE 2.19. Experimental model of Western Electric #5 with variable intensity levels. (Courtesy of James Shanks.)

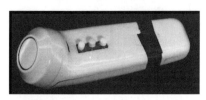

FIGURE 2.20. Experimental model of Western Electric #5 with continuous variable frequency. (Courtesy of James Shanks.)

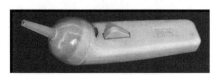

FIGURE 2.21. Experimental model of Western Electric #5 that directs sound into the mouth. (Courtesy of James Shanks.)

1958   Cooper (1958) was granted a U.S. patent for a prosthesis that differed from Tait's oral vibrator (R. Tait, 1959, 1960, 1962) in that the diaphragm was not attached to the center of the dental plate but at the side of it. When the diaphragm was energized, its vibrations were transmitted to the back of the mouth by the air column between the hard palate and the slightly concave dental plate. The general rationale behind this design was that speech is more intelligible when buccal air is set into vibration from behind, as in normal speakers.

1959   Bell Laboratories developed a transistorized electrolarynx. An early Western Electric #5 model (Figure 2.18), allowing frequency variation for inflected speech, used a modified telephone receiver. By 1964, the neck connector was reduced in size. Subsequent efforts were made by the company to alter intensity levels (Figure 2.19). Additional alterations were attempted by users for continuous frequency variation (Figure 2.20) and to deliver sound directly into the mouth (Figure 2.21). In the 1980s, Bell introduced Model 5C (Figure 2.22) using a 9-volt transistor battery but sacrificing frequency variation.

1959   The Cooper–Rand transoral artificial larynx was formally introduced (see Figure 2.14).

1963   The Laryngophone was made in Belgium, partly out of metal and partly out of flexible material. It had no inhalatory valves. The DSP #8 artificial larynx (Figure 2.23) was made in Holland. Made of nylon and weighing about 30 g, it consisted of a flexible plastic cup with an inflated collar, a sieve with staggered joints that prevented secretions from entering the prosthesis, an inhalatory valve, and a thin adjustable membrane disc that vibrated to create sound.

1964   Japanese inventors created pneumatic larynxes based on a different vibrator. An inch-long strip of rubber, 1/2 inch wide, is held taut by a rubber band. Brought to the United States by St. Germain, these devices (Figure 2.24) were popularized by "Red" Woodworth of Texas.

1965   Zerneri (1965) contrived a simple and cheap device. It consisted of a small rubber cup that was to be held over the tracheostoma and that contained a transverse rubber band stretched over the opening of a plastic tube. This tube passed through the top of the bell-like voice box and conducted puffs of air into the speaker's mouth.

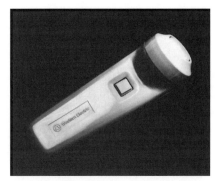

FIGURE 2.22. Western Electric artificial larynx Model 5C. (Courtesy of James Shanks.)

1972   Taub and Spiro (1972) made a device similar to the one created by the Australian surgeon, Brown. Taub used a U-shaped pneumatic prosthesis, one end of which was inserted into the trachea while the other end was introduced into the hypopharynx through a fistula surgically cut into the lateroanterior part of the neck. The tracheal butt of the artificial larynx was provided with a one-way valve for inspiration. Expiration took place through the prosthesis. The metal reed, like that in the Western Electric #2, vibrated in the U-shaped tube only when pressure was exerted on exhalation. This was consistent with the normal physiological process, in which quiet expiration is passive and the pressure drop through the respiratory tract is small. To produce audible speech, the pressure of exhalation had to be actively increased.

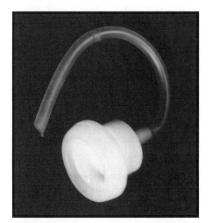

FIGURE 2.23. Dutch DSP 8 artificial larynx using a disc to create tone. (Courtesy of James Shanks.)

1972   Mueller and Kupperman (1972) reported on the first "contemporary" type of pneumatic artificial larynx that relied on diversion of pulmonary air through a tracheostoma housing with a self-contained reed system. A tube directed into the oral cavity permitted the externally generated voice source to be articulated into speech. This device, developed in Japan, later became known as the Tokyo pneumatic artificial larynx.

1974   The Danapipe was a Danish mouth-type electronic larynx consisting of miniaturized circuitry, a transducer, and a battery concealed in a bowl portion of a tobacco pipe. A switch on the side of the bowl activated the sound, which was transmitted through the stem of the pipe to the user's mouth. The same principle was employed earlier in the

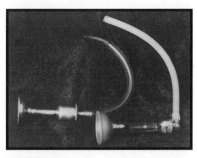

FIGURE 2.24. Japanese pneumatic larynxes, using strips of rubber to vibrate for tone. (Courtesy of James Shanks.)

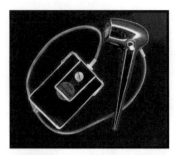

FIGURE 2.25. Pipa di Ticchioni electrolarynx. (Courtesy of James Shanks.)

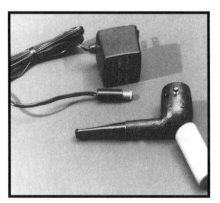

FIGURE 2.26. Artificial Larynx of North America. (Courtesy of James Shanks.)

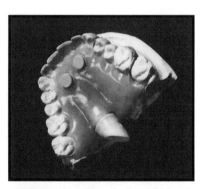

FIGURE 2.27. Speech-master electrolarynx providing tone at top of oral cavity. (Courtesy of James Shanks.)

Pipa di Ticchioni (Figure 2.25), made in Milan, and later in the Artificial Larynx of North America (Figure 2.26).

1975   The concept of merging an electronic artificial voice generator within a dental appliance emerged as a working model for postlaryngectomy voice restoration.

1976   The Speechmaster intraoral artificial larynx was developed to fit against the upper palate like a dental bridge. It operates on a 6-volt replaceable power supply. The on–off switch is controlled by the tongue (Figure 2.27).

1976   Griffiths, Fredrickson, and Bryce (1976) introduce use of electromagnetic sound sources that can be implanted. Materials limitations for bioimplantations clearly exist. Concerns related to biocompatibility are assessed using dogs.

1980   An implantable electronic artificial laryngeal transducer and prototype device continue to be conceptualized. Bioimplantation appears to be a viable alternative for voice rehabilitation (Young, Bailey, Everett, & Griffiths, 1980); therefore, assessment of biomaterials remains a prominent component of developing implantable devices.

1980   Charles, Fredrickson, and Bryce (1980) report on the first two humans who are implanted with a biocarbon electromagnetic device.

1982   Painter and colleagues present initial findings on a new implantable artificial larynx (Painter, Kaiser, Fredrickson, & Karzon, 1987).

1991   Qi and Weinberg (1991) report that reductions in low-frequency energy (<500 Hz) associated with electrolaryngeal speech have a potential influence on the overall speech sound quality.

1993   Vocal tract transfer function relative to artificial laryngeal speech is explored, and its influence on source characteristics and associated changes on formant characteristics are evaluated. Results indicate that specific characteristics of source and filter must be considered as researchers pursue further electroacoustic enhancement of electrolaryngeal speech (Myrick & Yantoro, 1993).

1994   Uemi and Ifukube (1994) of Japan explore the design of a potential electronic artificial larynx with pitch-changing mechanism.

1998   Espy-Wilson, Chari, MacAuslan, Huang, and Walsh (1998) explore the enhancement of electrolaryngeal speech through use of adaptive filtering.

1999   A prototype electronic artificial larynx is explored through combined efforts of professionals in Boston (see Chapter 23 in this text). This device has three modifications: improved acoustic characteristics of the electronic voice source, a signal-processing model to enhance the speech signal produced, and a physiologic control mechanism for pitch change.

1999   Pitch-control mechanism continues to be explored by Japanese group (Ifukube & Uemi, 1999).

2001   Dutch investigators assess the aeroacoustic characteristics of a silicone rubber lip reed that was used in a pneumatic type of artificial larynx (van der Torn, Mahieu, & Festen, 2001).

2004   Researchers at the Massachusetts Eye and Ear Infirmary, the Massachusetts Institute of Technology, and Harvard Medical School report on the design and implementation of a hands-free electrolarynx (E. A. Goldstein et al., 2004).

SUMMARY

This chapter has provided historical reviews of (a) surgical treatment for laryngeal cancer, with a detailed view of how total laryngectomy began and how it has evolved, and (b) the development and continuing evolution of the electronic artificial larynx. Whereas the review provided herein is not exhaustive, it serves to identify key points and developments in the history of total laryngectomy and the artificial larynx. Knowledge of these historical developments is essential if one is to understand the current state of the art.

The literature cited in this chapter provides information on the evolution of surgical techniques and methods that have led to current approaches to surgical treatment. The fact that methods of medical treatment for laryngeal cancer have remained relatively unchanged in the modern era suggests that knowledge of what has transpired previously may permit further refinements that lead to more positive posttreatment outcomes. Despite a number of advancements in the treatment of laryngeal cancer, surgery remains a primary method of medical management worldwide.

Similarly, the evolution of the artificial larynx provides a rich framework for understanding the long-standing problems inherent to many artificial laryngeal devices. As other areas of knowledge have emerged in recent years (e.g., more sophisticated computerized technology), the historical view allows professionals to reconsider how problems may be solved (e.g., miniaturization, computer chip technology). New opportunities for restoring functional communication for those individuals who undergo total laryngectomy are likely as significant technological and materials advances are introduced in the contemporary computerized era. Similarly, the ability to modify the acoustic properties of the sound source and source–filter relationships will likely have an impact on new advances (see Chapter 23 in this text). As noted early in this chapter, past experiences and ideas will likely continue to lead investigators from a variety of professions and disciplines to new concepts and prototype instruments. We believe that the historical information offered in this chapter will serve as a useful tool for future advances in the treatment and rehabilitation of those diagnosed with laryngeal malignancies.

REFERENCES

Anderson-Stuart, T. (1897, April 17). An artificial larynx. *The Lancet*, pp. 1081–1084.

Barney, H. L. (1958). A discussion of some technical aspects of speech aids for postlaryngectomized patients. *Annals of Otology, Rhinology and Laryngology, 67,* 558–570.

Barney, H. L., Haworth, F. E., & Dunn, H. K. (1959). An experimental transistorized artificial larynx (Monograph No. 3395). *The Bell System Technical Journal, 38,* 1337–1356.

Billroth, C. A. T., & Gussenbauer, C. (1874). Über die erste durch Th. Billroth am menschen ausgefuhrte kehlkopf extirpation und die anwendung eines kunstlichen kehlkopfes. *Archiv für die klinische Chirurgie, 17,* 343–356.

Bottini, E. (1875). Communicazione Letta Innanzi la R. *Giornale della academia di medicina di Torino,* pp. 418–434.

Bottini, E. (1878). Extirpation totale du larynx à l'aide du galvano-cautère. *Annales des Maladies de l'Oreille et du Larynx et des Organes, 4,* 182–186.

Brown, R. G. (1925). A simple but effective artificial larynx. *Journal of Laryngology, 40,* 793–797.

Charles, D. P., Fredrickson, J. M., & Bryce, D. P. (1980). An implantable electromagnetic sound source: Preliminary results of human implantation. In D. P. Shedd & B. Weinberg (Eds.), *Surgical and prosthetic approaches to speech rehabilitation* (pp. 247–257). Boston: G.K. Hall.

Cooper, H. K. (1958). *U.S. Patent No. 2,862,209.* Washington, DC: U.S. Patent and Trademark Office.

Cooper, H. K., & Millard, R. T. (1959). A dental approach to speech restoration in the laryngectomee: A preliminary report. *Dental Digest, 65,* 106–112.

Crile, G. W. (1913). Laryngectomy for cancer. *Transactions of the American Surgical Association, 31,* 259–276.

Crile, G. W. (1947). *George Crile: An autobiography* (Vols. 1 and 2). Philadelphia: Lippincott.

Czermak, J. N. (1859). Über die sprache bei luftdichter verschliessung des kehlkopfs, sitzungsberichte der kaiserlichen academie der wissenschaften mathematischnaturwissenschaftliche classe. *Wien, 35,* 65–72.

Czerny, V. (1870). Versuche über kehlkopf extirpation. *Wiener medizinische Wochenschrift, 24,* 557, 561.

Delavan, D. B. (1912). Laryngology: An historical sketch. In H. A. Kelly (Ed.), *Cyclopedia of American medical biography* (pp. lxiii–lxxi). Philadelphia: Saunders.

Donagan, W. L. (1965). An early history of total laryngectomy. *Surgery, 57,* 902–905.

Dunn, H. K. (1950). The calculation of vowel resonances and an electrical vocal tract. *Journal of the Acoustical Society of America, 22,* 740–750.

Espy-Wilson, C. Y., Chari, V. R., MacAuslan, J. M., Huang, C. B., & Walsh, M. J. (1998). Enhancement of electrolaryngeal speech by adaptive filtering. *Journal of Speech, Language, and Hearing Research, 41,* 1253–1264.

Firestone, F. (1940). An artificial larynx for speaking and choral singing by one person. *Journal of the Acoustical Society of America, 11,* 357–361.

Fletcher, H. (1953). Artificial larynx. In H. Fletcher (Ed.), *Speech and hearing communication* (pp. 12–13) New York: Van Nostrand. (Original work published 1929)

Foulis, D. F. (1877a). Excision of larynx, and use of artificial vocal apparatus. *British Medical Journal.* pp. 811–812.

Foulis, D. F. (1877b). Extirpation of the larynx. *Lancet, 2,* 530–532.

Foulis, D. F. (1881). Indications for the complete or partial extirpation of the larynx. *Proceedings of Sub-Section for Diseases of the Throat, Transactions of 7th Session, International Medical Congress, 3,* 251–258.

Gerdes, H. (1877). Total extirpation des kehlkopfes: Tod am vierten tage. *Archiv für die klinische Chirurgie, 21,* 473–477.

Glück, T. (1899). Flustersprache und phonationsapparate. *Berliner klinische Wochenschrift, 36,* 215–216.

Glück, T. (1904). Der gegenwartige stand der chirurgie des kehlkopfs, pharynx, oesophagus, und der trachea. *Monatsschrift für Orenheilkunde, 39,* 89, 141.

Glück, T. (1908). Verbandlungen des internationalen laryngo-rhinologen congresses. *Wien, 1,* 66–108.

Glück, T. (1910). Patienten mit totalexstirpation des pharynx, larynx und oesophagus, denen eine kunstliche stimme dutch einen automatisch arbeitenden apparat geliefert wird. *Berliner klinische Wochenschrift, 47,* 33–35.

Glück, T. (1913). Das techische und funktionelle problem bei den operationen und den obesen luft- und speisewegen. *Internationales Centrablatt für Laryngologie, Rhinologie, und verwandte Wissenschaften, 29,* 610.

Glück, T. (1921). Probleme und zeile der chirurgie der oberen luftwege und speiswege. *Monatschrift für Obrenheilkunde, 55,* 1150–1174.

Glück, T., & Soerensen, J. (1920). Ergebnisse einer neuen reihe von 100 total extirpationen des kehlkopfs. *Archives für Laryngologie und Rhinologie, 33,* 84–102.

Glück, T., & Soerensen, J. (1922). Die extirpation und resektion des kehlkopfes. *Handbuch der speziellen chirurgie des obres und der oberen luftwege* (3rd ed., Vol. 4, pp. 1–70). Würzburg, Germany: C. Kabisch.

Glück, T., & Zeller, A. (1881). Die prophylactische resektion der trachea. *Archiv für die klinische Chirurgie, 26,* 427–436.

Goldstein, E. A., Heaton, J. T., Kobler, J. B., Stanley, G. B., & Hillman, R. E. (2004). Design and implementation of a hands-free electrolarynx device controlled by neck strap muscle electromyographic activity. *IEEE Transactions on Biomedical Engineering, 51,* 325–332.

Goldstein, L. P. (1982). History and development of laryngeal prosthetic devices. In A. Sekey (Ed.), *Electroacoustic analysis and enhancement of alaryngeal speech* (pp. 137–165). Springfield, IL: Thomas.

Goldstein, M. A. (1932). Metal discs for permanent recording and reproduction of speech: Modification of the artificial larynx. *Transactions of the American Laryngological Association, 54,* 105–111.

Gottstein, G. (1900). Pseudo-stimme nach total extirpation des larynx. *Archiv für die klinische Chirurgie, 62,* 126–146.

Griffiths, C. M., Fredrickson, J. M., & Bryce, D. P. (1976). An implantable electromagnetic sound source for speech production. *Archives of Otolaryngology, 102,* 676–682.

Güssenbauer, T. (1874). Ueber die erste durch T. Billroth an menschen ge führte kehldopfextstripation, und die anwendung eines kunstlichen kehlkopfes. *Verhulh Deutsch Chirgurie.*

Hanson, W. L. (1940). A new artificial larynx with a historical review. *Illinois Medical Journal, 78,* 483–486.

Haworth, F. E. (1960). An electronic artificial larynx. *Bell Laboratories Recordings, 38,* 362–368.

Heine, C. (1876). Resection des kehlkopfes bei laryngostenose. *Archiv für die klinische Chirurgie, 19,* 514–526.

Hinojar, A. (1923). Simple phonetic apparatus. *Anales de la Academia Medico Quirúrgica Española, 10,* 93.

Hochenegg, J. (1892). Totale kehlkopf-exstirpation und resektion des oesophagus wegen carcinoma laryngis. Oesophagoplastick. Ein neuer spfechapparat. *Weiner klinische Wochenschrift, 5,* 123–127.

Holinger, P. H. (1975). The historical development of laryngectomy. *Laryngoscope, 85,* 287, 322–333.

Hyman, M. (1955). An experimental study of artificial-larynx and esophageal speech. *Journal of Speech and Hearing Disorders, 20,* 291–299.

Ifukube, T., & Uemi, N. (1999). A new electrical larynx with pitch control function. *Proceedings of the* 2nd *East Asian Conference on Phonosurgery,* pp. 1–5.

Iglauer, S. (1936). Artificial larynx, with patient demonstrating its use. *Annals of Otology, Rhinology and Laryngology, 45,* 1176–1177.

Isambert, E. (1876). Contribution a l'étude du cancer du larynge. *Annales des Maladies de l'Oreille et du Larynge, 2,* 1.

Jackson, C., & Jackson, C. L. (1939). *Cancer of the larynx.* Philadelphia: Saunders.

Jesberg, N. (1960). Laryngectomy: Past, present, and future. *Annals of Otology, Rhinology and Laryngology, 69,* 184–198.

Kallen, L. (1931). Vicarious vocal mechanisms. *Archives of Otolaryngology, 20,* 460–503.

Keith, R. L, & Shanks, J. C. (1994), Historical highlights: Laryngectomy rehabilitation (pp. 1–48). In R. L. Keith & F. L. Darley, (Eds.), *Laryngectomee rehabilitation* (3rd ed.), Austin, TX: PRO-ED.

Kellotat, W. F. (1937). *U.S. Patent No. 2,093,453.* Washington, DC: U.S. Patent and Trademark Office.

Kosinski, J. K. (1877). Vollstandige extirpation des kehlkopfs. *Centralblatt für Chirurgie, 4,* 401–406.

Labbe, L. (1886). Sur un cas d'extirpation totale du larynx. *Bulletin de l'Académe de Médicine, 50*(2), *15,* 159–162.

Lane, C. E. (1932). *U.S. Patent No. 1,840,112.* Washington, DC: U.S. Patent and Trademark Office.

Lange, F. (1880). Extirpation of the larynx and anterior wall of the oesophagus—Recovery. *Archives of Laryngology, 1,* 36–49.

Lebrun, Y. (1973). *The artificial larynx.* Amsterdam: Swets & Zeitlinger.

Leyro Diaz, J. (1924). Consideraciónes sobre laringectomia y aparato de fonacion en los laringectornizados. *La Semana Medica, 31,* 27–30.

Lister, J. (1867). Antiseptic principle in the practice of surgery. *Lancet, 1,* 353–356.

Luchsinger, R. (1949). Voice without a larynx: Alaryngeal dysphonia. In R. Luchsinger & G. E. Arnold (Eds.), *Voice–speech–language* (p. 288). Belmont, CA: Wadsworth.

Maas, H. (1876a). Extirpation des kehlkopfes; heilung. *Archiv für die klinische Chirurgie, 20,* 535–539.

Maas, H. (1876b). Vellständige extirpation des kehlkopfes; Tod nach 14 tagen. *Archiv für die klinische Chirurgie, 19,* 507–513.

Mackenzie, M. (1880). *Diseases of the pharynx, larynx and trachea.* New York: William Wood.

McKesson, E. I. (1927). A mechanical larynx. *Journal of the American Medical Association, 88,* 645–646.

McKesson, E. (1933). *U.S. Patent No. 1,922,385.* Washington, DC: U.S. Patent and Trademark Office.

Mueller, P. B., & Kupperman, G. L. (1972). Post-laryngectomy speech: An evaluation of a Japanese pneumatic speech aid. *Eye, Ear, Nose, and Throat Monthly, 51,* 478–481.

Myrick, R., & Yantoro, R. (1993). Vocal tract modeling as related to the use of an artificial larynx. *Proceedings of the IEEE Biomedical Conference,* pp. 75–77.

Newman, D. (1886a). Notes of a case of excision of the larynx for malignant disease. *Lancet, 2,* 159–161.

Newman, D. (1886b). Two lectures on tumors of the larynx, their pathology, symptoms and treatment; with illustrative cases. *British Medical Journal, 1,* 579–583, 769, 813, 865.

Onodi, A. (1918). Ergebnisse der Abteilung für Hör-Sprache-Stimmstorungen und Tracheotomierte. *Monatsschift für Ohrenheilkunde und Laryngo-Rhinologie, 52,* 85–102.

Painter, C., Kaiser, T., Fredrickson, J. M., & Karzon, R. (1987). Human speech development for an implantable artificial larynx. *Annals of Otology, Rhinology, and Laryngology, 96,* 573–577.

Pichler, H. (1961a). Klinische Erfahrungen mit einem neuen kunstlichen Larynx. *Monatsschift für Ohrenheilkunde, 95,* 299–301.

Pichler, H. (1961b). Ueber ein neuartiges automatisch gesteuertes elektronisches sprechgerat für laryngektomierte. *Acta Otolaryngologica, 53,* 374–380.

Pollock, H. L., & Lederer, F. L. (1922). Artificial larynx. *Transactions American Academy of Ophthalmology, 27,* 480.

Qi, Y. Y., & Weinberg, B. (1991). Low-frequency energy deficit in electrolaryngeal speech. *Journal of Speech and Hearing Research, 34,* 1250–1256.

Reyher, C. (1877). Die laryngotomie als diagnostischer und therapeutischer eingriff bei ulcerationen im kehlkopf; eine extirpation laryngis wegen karcinom der stimmbänder. *St. Petersburger medicinische Wochenschrift, 2,* 137, 149.

Riesz, R. R. (1930). Description and demonstration of an artificial larynx. *Journal of the Acoustical Society of America, 1,* 273–279.

Rigrodsky, S., Lerman, J., & Morrison, E. (1971). *Therapy for the laryngectomized patient.* New York: Teachers College Press.

Rosenberg, P. J. (1971). Total laryngectomy and cancer of the larynx. *Archives of Otolaryngology, 94,* 313–316.

Rousselot, J. (1902). La parole avec un larynx artificiel. *La Parole, 12,* 65–79.

Salmon, S. J., & Goldstein, L. P. (1978). *The artificial larynx handbook.* New York: Grune & Stratton.

Schechter, D. C., & Morfit, H. H. (1965). The evolution of surgical treatment of tumors of the larynx. *Surgery, 57,* 457–479.

Schmidt, M. (1875). Total extirpation des Kehlkopfes mit ungümstigem Ausgange. *Archiv für die klinische Chirurgie, 18,* 189–194.

Schönborn, K. W. E. J. (1875). Extirpatio laryngis. *Berliner klinische Wochenschrift, 12,* 525.

Schüller, H. (1880). *Die tracheotomie, laryngotomie, und extirpation des kehlkopfes* [Monograph]. Stuttgart, Germany: F. Enke.

Sheard, C. (1931). A new, simple artificial voice box and its use. *Proceedings of Staff Meetings at the Mayo Clinic, 6,* 253–256.

Singer, M. I., & Blom, E. D. (1980). An endoscopic technique for restoration of voice after laryngectomy. *Annals of Otology, Rhinology and Laryngology, 89,* 529–533.

Sisson, G. A., McConnel, F. M. S., Logemann, J. A., & Yeh, S. (1975). Voice rehabilitation after laryngectomy: Results with the use of a hypopharyngeal prosthesis. *Archives of Otolaryngology, 101,* 178–181.

Snidecor, J. C. (1962). *Speech rehabilitation of the laryngectomized.* Springfield, IL: Thomas.

Snidecor, J. C. (1968). *Speech rehabilitation of the laryngectomized* (2nd ed.). Springfield, IL: Thomas.

Solis-Cohen, J. (1892a). A case of laryngectomy. *Journal of Laryngology, 7,* 285–289.

Solis-Cohen, J. (1892b). Two cases of laryngectomy for adenocarcinoma of the larynx. *New York Medical Journal, 56,* 533–535.

Solis-Cohen, J. (1892c). Two cases of laryngectomy for adenocarcinoma of the larynx. *Transactions of the American Laryngological Association, 14,* 60–66.

Stevens, K. N., Kasowski, S., & Fant, G. M. (1953). An electrical analog of the vocal tract. *Journal of the Acoustical Society of America, 25,* 734–742.

Stoerk, K. (1880). *Klinik der krankheitendes kehlkopfs der nase, und des rachens* (pp. 546–555). Stuttgart, Germany: F. Enke.

Stoerk, K. (1887). Über larynxextirpation. *Weiner medizinische Wochenschrift, 37,* 1586–1590.

Stoerk, K. (1896). Über extirpation des larynx bei karzinom. *Archives of Laryngology and Rhinology, 5,* 22–31.

Strome, M., Stein, J., Esclamado, R., Hicks, D., Lorenz, R. R., Braun, W., et al. (2001). Laryngeal transplantation and 40-month follow-up. *New England Journal of Medicine, 344*(22), 1676–1679.

Tait, R. (1959). The oral vibrator. *British Dental Journal, 106,* 336–340.

Tait, R. (1960). The oral vibrator. *British Dental Journal, 109,* 506–507.

Tait, R. (1962). The oral vibrator. *British Dental Journal, 112,* 249–250.

Tait, V., & Tait, R. (1959). Speech rehabilitation with the oral vibrator. *Speech Pathology and Therapy, 2,* 64–69.

Tapia, A. G. (1914). Presentación de un laringuectomizado hablando con un sencillismo aparato artificial. *Revista Española de Laringologia, Otologia y Rhinologia, 5,* 48–55.

Taptas, N. (1900). Un cas de laryngectorme totale pour sarcome; larynx artificiel externe. *Annales des Maladies de l'Oreille et du Larynx, 26,* 37–45.

Taub, S., & Bergner, L. H. (1973). Air bypass voice prosthesis for vocal rehabilitation of laryngectomees. *American Journal of Surgery, 125,* 748–756.

Taub, S., & Spiro, R. H. (1972). Vocal rehabilitation of laryngectomees: Preliminary report of a new technique. *American Journal of Surgery, 124,* 87–90.

Uemi, N., & Ifukube, T. (1994). Design of new electrolarynx having pitch control function. *EEE International Workshop on Robots and Human Communication,* pp. 198–203.

van der Torn, M., Mahieu, H. F., & Festen, J. M. (2001). Aero-acoustics of silicone rubber lip reeds for alternative voice production in laryngectomees. *Journal of the Acoustical Society of America, 110,* 2548–2559.

Virchow, R. L. K. (1858). *Die cellular pathologie in thren begrundung auf physiologische und pathologische gewebelehre.* Berlin: A. Hirschwald.

von Bruns, P. (1878). *Die Laryngotomie zur Entfernung intralaryngealer Neubildungen.* Berlin: A. Hirschwald.

von Bruns, P. (1881). Ueber enige Verbesserungen des kunstlichen Kehlkopfes. *Archiv für die klinische Chirurgie, 26,* 780–782.

von Langenbeck, B. R. K. (1875). Total extirpation des kehlkopfs mit dem zungenbein, einem theil der zunge, des pharynx und esophagus. *Berliner klinishe Wochenschrift, 12,* 453–455.

Weinberg, B., & Riekena, A. (1973). Speech produced with the Tokyo artificial larynx. *Journal of Speech and Hearing Disorders, 38,* 383–389.

Weinberg, B., Shedd, D. P., & Horii, Y. (1978). Reed–fistula speech following pharyngolaryngectomy. *Journal of Speech and Hearing Disorders, 43,* 401–403.

Weir, N. F. (1973). Theodore Billroth: The first laryngectomy for cancer. *Journal of Laryngology and Otology, 87,* 1161–1169.

Wolff, J. (1893a). Über den künstlichen kehlkopf und die pseudo-stimme. *Berliner klinische Wochenschrift, 30,* 1009–1013.

Wolff, J. (1893b). Über den künstlichen und die pseudo-stimme. *Archiv für die klinische Chirurgie, 45,* 237–241.

Wright, G. M. (1942). *U.S. Patent No. 2,273,077.* Washington, DC: U.S. Patent and Trademark Office.

Young, K. E., Bailey, B. J., Everett, R., & Griffiths, C. M. (1980). Electronic laryngeal prosthesis for implantation: A progress report. In D. P. Shedd & B. Weinberg (Eds.), *Surgical and prosthetic approaches to speech rehabilitation* (pp. 231–245). Boston: G. K. Hall.

Zerneri, L. (1965). Su un nuovo apparecchio protesico per laringectomizzati. *Archivio Italiano di Otologia, Rinologia e Laringologia, 76,* 748–754.

ADDITIONAL HISTORICAL READINGS

Amatsu, M., Matsui, T., Maki, T., & Kanagawa, K. (1977). Voice rehabilitation after total laryngectomy: A new one-stage surgical technique. *Nippon Jibiinkoka Gakkai Kaiho, 80,* 779–785.

Arslan, M. (1975). Techniques of laryngeal reconstruction. *Laryngoscope, 85,* 862–865.

Arslan, M., & Serafini, I. (1972). Restoration of laryngeal function after total laryngectomy: Report of the first 25 cases. *Laryngoscope, 82,* 1349–1360.

Asai, R. (1972). Laryngoplasty after total laryngectomy. *Archives of Otolaryngology, 95,* 114–119.

Berlin, C. (1965). Clinical measurement of esophageal speech: III. Performance of non-biased groups. *Journal of Speech and Hearing Disorders, 30,* 174–183.

Braini, A. (1958). Il ricupero sociale dei laringectomizzati attraverso un metodo personale operatorio. *Medicina Sociale, 8,* 265–269.

Calcaterra, T. C., & Jafek, B. W. (1971). Tracheo-esophageal shunt for speech rehabilitation after total laryngectomy. *Archives of Otolaryngology, 94,* 124–128.

Conley, J. J. (1959). Vocal rehabilitation by autogenous vein graft. *Annals of Otology, Rhinology and Laryngology, 68,* 990–995.

Conley, J. J., DeAmesti, F., & Pierce, J. K. (1958). A new surgical technique for the vocal rehabilitation of the laryngectomized patient. *Annals of Otology, Rhinology, and Laryngology, 67,* 655–664.

Creech, H. B. (1966). Evaluating esophageal speech. *Journal of the Speech and Hearing Association of Virginia, 72,* 13–19.

Damsté, P. H. (1958). *Oesophageal speech after laryngectomy.* Groningen, The Netherlands: Hoitsema.

Damsté, P. H. (1975). Methods of restoring the voice after laryngectomy. *Laryngoscope, 85,* 649–655.

DiBartolo, R. (1971). Psychological considerations in the attainment of esophageal speech. *Journal of Surgical Oncology, 3,* 451–466.

Diedrich, W. M. (1968). The mechanism of esophageal speech. *Annals of the New York Academy of Science, 155,* 303–317.

Diedrich, W. M., & Youngstrom, K. (1966). *Alaryngeal speech.* Springfield, IL: Thomas.

Duguay, M. J. (1966). Preoperative ideas of speech after laryngectomy. *Archives of Otolaryngology, 83,* 69–72.

Edwards, N. (1974). Post-laryngectomy vocal rehabilitation. *Journal of Laryngology and Otology, 88,* 905–918.

Edwards, N. (1975). Post-laryngectomy rehabilitation by the external fistula method: Further experiences. *Laryngoscope, 85,* 690–699.

Edwards, N. (1976). New voices for old: Restoration of effective speech after laryngectomy by the pulmonary air-shunt vocal fistula principle. *Bristol Medico Chirurgical Journal, 90,* 11–17.

Foulis, D. F. (1878). Extirpation of the larynx. *Lancet, 1,* 118–120.

Foulis, D. F. (1879). Extirpation of the larynx. *Lancet, 1,* 436–437.

Gardner, W. H. (1966). Adjustment problems of laryngectomized women. *Archives of Otolaryngology, 83,* 31–42.

Gardner, W. H. (1971). *Laryngectomee speech and rehabilitation.* Springfield, IL: Thomas.

Goldberg, R. T. (1975). Vocational and social adjustment after laryngectomy. *Scandinavian Journal of Rehabilitative Medicine, 7,* 1–8.

Goode, R. (1973). The development of an improved artificial larynx. *Transactions of the American Academy of Ophthalmology and Otolaryngology, 73,* 279–287.

Güssenbauer, C. (1874). Ueber die erste durch Billroth am menschen ausgefiihrte kehlkopf-exstirpation und die anwendung eines kunstlichen kehlkopfes. *Archiv für die klinische Chirurgie, 17,* 343–356.

Guttman, M. R. (1932). Rehabilitation of the voice in laryngectomized patients. *Archives of Otolaryngology, 15,* 479.

Guttman, M. R. (1935). Tracheohypopharyngeal fistulization. *Transactions of the American Laryngology, Rhinology and Otology Society, 41,* 219–226.

Herzog, W., & Neumann, D. (1965). Ein kunstlicher elektronischer kehlkopf. *Phonetica, 13,* 117–133.

Johnson, J. T., Casper, J., & Lesswing, N. J. (1979). Toward the total rehabilitation of the alaryngeal patient. *Laryngoscope, 89,* 1813–1819.

Keith, R. L., & Darley, F. L. (1994). *Laryngectomee rehabilitation* (3rd ed.) Austin, TX: PRO-ED.

Kluyskens, P., & Ringoir, S. (1970). Follow-up of a human larynx transplantation. *Laryngoscope, 80,* 1244–1250.

Komorn, R. M. (1974). Vocal rehabilitation in the laryngectomized patient with a tracheoesophageal shunt. *Annals of Otology, Rhinology and Laryngology, 83,* 445–451.

Komorn, R. M., Weycer, J. S., Sessions, R. B., & Malone, P. E. (1973). Vocal rehabilitation with a tracheoesophageal shunt. *Archives of Otolaryngology, 97,* 303–335.

McConnel, F. M., Sisson, G. A., & Logemann, J. A. (1977). Three years experience with a hypopharyngeal pseudoglottis after total laryngectomy. *Transactions of the American Academy of Ophthalmology and Otolaryngology, 84,* 63–67.

McGrail, J. S., & Oldfield, D. L. (1971). One-stage operation for vocal rehabilitation at laryngectomy. *Transactions of the American Academy of Ophthalmology and Otolaryngology, 75,* 510–512.

Miller, A. H. (1967). First experiences with the Asai technique of vocal rehabilitation after total laryngectomy. *Annals of Otology, Rhinology and Laryngology, 76,* 829–833.

Miller, A. H. (1968). Further experiences with the Asai technique for vocal rehabilitation after laryngectomy. *Transactions of the American Academy of Ophthalmology and Otolaryngology, 72,* 779–781.

Miller, A. H. (1971). Four years experience with the Asai technique of vocal rehabilitation for the laryngectomized patient. *Journal of Laryngology and Otolaryngology, 85,* 567–576.

Montgomery, W. W., & Toohill, R. J. (1968). Voice rehabilitation after laryngectomy. *Archives of Otolaryngology, 88,* 499–506.

Moolenaar-Bijl, A. (1953). Connection between consonant articulation and the intake of air in oesophageal speech. *Folia Phoniatrica, 5,* 212–216.

Morrison, W. W. (1931). The production of voice and speech following total laryngectomy. *Archives of Otolaryngology, 14,* 413–431.

Panje, W. R. (1981). Prosthetic vocal rehabilitation following laryngectomy—The voice button. *Annals of Otology, Rhinology and Laryngology, 90,* 116–120.

Pearson, B. W. (1981). Subtotal laryngectomy. *Laryngoscope, 91,* 1904–1912.

Pearson, B. W., Woods, R. D., & Hartman, D. E. (1980). Extended hemilaryngectomy for T3 glottic carcinoma with preservation of speech and swallowing. *Laryngoscope, 90,* 1950–1961.

Shedd, D., Bakamjian, V., Sako, K., Mann, M., Barba, S., & Schaaf, N. (1972). Reed fistula method of speech rehabilitation after laryngectomy. *American Journal of Surgery, 124,* 510–514.

Shedd, D., Schaaf, N., & Weinberg, B. (1976). Technical aspects of reed fistula speech following pharyngolaryngectomy. *Journal of Surgical Oncology, 8,* 305–310.

Shipp, T. (1967). Frequency, duration, and perceptual measures in relation to judgments of laryngeal speech acceptability. *Journal of Speech and Hearing Research, 10,* 417–427.

Siegel, E., Konig, K., & Heidrich, R. (1969). Sociopsychiatric problems of laryngectomized patients. *Psychiatrie, Neurologie, und medizinische Psychologie, 21,* 330–336.

Singer, M. I, & Blom, E. D. (1981). A selective myotomy for voice rehabilitation after total laryngectomy. *Archives of Otolaryngology, 107,* 670–673.

Snidecor, J. C. (1969). *Speech rehabilitation of the laryngectomized* (2nd ed.). Springfield, IL: Thomas.

Snidecor, J. C. (1975). Some scientific foundations for voice restoration. *Laryngoscope, 85,* 640–647.

Vega, M. F. (1975). Larynx reconstructive surgery—A study of three-year findings: A modified surgical technique. *Laryngoscope, 85,* 866–881.

Wallen, V., & Webb, V. P. (1975). A survey of the background characteristics of 2000 laryngectomees: A preliminary report. *Military Medicine, 140,* 532–534.

Weinberg, B., & Westerhouse, J. (1973). A study of pharyngeal speech. *Journal of Speech and Hearing Disorders, 38,* 111–118.

Wolff, J. (1893). Über verbesserungen am kunstlichen kehlkopf. *Archiv für die klinische Chirurgie, 45,* 242–257.

Zwitman, D., & Calcaterra, T. (1973). Phonation using the tracheoesophageal shunt. *Journal of Speech and Hearing Disorders, 38,* 369–373.

Chapter 3

Commonalities Among Alaryngeal Speech Methods

Shirley J. Salmon

Many investigators have studied characteristics of the various types of alaryngeal speech. In general, their findings have stressed the differences among artificial larynx (AL), esophageal (ES), or tracheoesophageal (TE) speech. In compiling survey responses from 203 laryngectomized individuals about their preferred method(s) of alaryngeal speech (Salmon, 1999b), I found that most respondents used more than one mode of communication. Given this fact, in addition to what I have learned through clinical experience, it seems realistic to consider treatment techniques that may be applied to more than one type of alaryngeal communication.

In this chapter, I first report the survey data, which indicate that those having undergone laryngectomy frequently use more than one type of alaryngeal communication. I present information on commonalities among the three alaryngeal speech methods. Topics discussed are selection of communication method, placement of speech aids, distractors and frustrations, on–off timing, and speech parameters (i.e., articulation, loudness, pitch, and rate). Also, I suggest how to apply this information in individual treatment for each alaryngeal speech type, as well as in group settings where all three methods are represented. Finally, I compare the feelings and behaviors of those who have experienced loss of a larynx with those of terminally ill cancer patients, as described by Kubler-Ross (1974). Such information should prove helpful when counseling laryngectomized individuals and their families.

SURVEY DATA

Far too often, professionals in local, state, national, and international organizations tend to imply that use of *one* method of alaryngeal communication (AL, ES, or TE) is more desirable than either of the others. To find out which method or methods are most used in the United States, I conducted a survey (Salmon, 1999b) of 203 individuals who use alaryngeal speech and who either attended state laryngectomy meetings in California, Florida, or Texas, or attended the International Association of Laryngectomees (IAL) meeting in 1997 or 1998. I asked respondents to indicate their "primary" mode of communication and their backup mode of communication.

Table 3.1 shows the percentages of alaryngeal speech modes used based on respondents' states of residence. In California, TE is used more frequently as a primary method of alaryngeal communication, followed by AL and then ES. In Florida, Minnesota, and Texas, AL speech was used more frequently. In Florida and Texas, AL was followed by TE and then ES, whereas in Minnesota, AL was followed by ES and then TE. Data from the 19th IAL meeting in Indiana showed that a significantly higher number of those surveyed used TE followed by AL, and then ES.

When these data are combined with data from two other recent studies (Gelman, 1995; Hillman, Walsh, Wolf, Fisher, & Hong, 1998), one can determine that, of the 392 individuals surveyed between 1993 and 1998, approximately 44% used AL speech, 22% used ES, and 29% used TE speech as their *primary* method of communication. As a backup mode of alaryngeal communication,

TABLE 3.1

Primary Mode of Alaryngeal Speech (in Percentages) for Artificial Larynx (AL), Esophageal (ES), and Tracheoesophageal (TE) Speech

Survey Sites	Types of Alaryngeal Speech		
	AL	**ES**	**TE**
California	31	19	50
Florida	44	15	41
Indiana	28	26	46
Minnesota	67	26	7
Texas	48	17	35
Mean	43	20	36
Gelman (1995)[a]	38	46	13
Hillman et al. (1998)[a]	55	6	31
Combined mean	44	22	29

[a] These figures do not include respondents who used nonvocal communication.

approximately 40% of TE and 40% of ES speakers reported using AL speech, whereas about 10% of TE and 10% of AL speakers reported using ES.

Based on the survey data gathered, commonalities are evident in the use of various alaryngeal speech types. Thus, it might be reasonable and efficient to consider treatment techniques that can be used to achieve proficiency with any of the three common methods of alaryngeal communication.

SELECTION OF ALARYNGEAL SPEECH MODE

Following laryngectomy, individuals are faced with choices for both primary and secondary methods of alaryngeal communication. If, for example, a TE puncture (TEP) was performed as a primary surgical procedure, the person may not feel that the surgeon gave him or her much choice (Fagan, Lentin, Oyarzabel, Issacs, & Sellars, 2003). On the other hand, if the individual researched all possible methods of communication, he or she might have requested vocal restoration surgery as either a primary or secondary procedure. Persons who use standard ES (a) may have had surgery prior to the introduction of the TEP in the early 1980s (Singer & Blom, 1980) when choices were limited to two alaryngeal speech methods or (b) may have chosen to learn ES and acquired it successfully. These individuals may continue to be satisfied with ES for their everyday communication; they need not bother with any type of TE voice prosthesis and have both hands available while speaking. Those individuals using an artificial larynx may also have been involved in selecting an instrument from the wide variety available (Eksteen, Rieger, Nesbitt, & Seikaly, 2003; Salmon, 1999a).

In the ideal clinical environment, all individuals undergoing laryngectomy have been exposed to the communication alternatives and involved in making decisions about both their primary and backup methods of postsurgical communication. For many, making choices is a continuing process, because the selections made soon after surgery may, for a variety of reasons, seem inappropriate in the future.

PLACEMENT OF SPEECH AIDS

To a large extent, placement of the artificial larynx will determine the vocal tone. Because no current artificial laryngeal voice source can sound like voice produced with a larynx, the goal is to make the tone sound as good as possible (see Chapter 23 in this text). All artificial larynx users have dealt with issues concerning the best placement of the device (see Chapter 22 in this text). Location of the vibratory site and the air reservoir determine whether the new voice, and the resultant speech, will be referred to as buccal, pharyngeal, or esophageal. The site that typically produces the best sound is the esophagus. Those individuals using esophageal speech have learned how and where to inject or inhale air so that it is available to activate the vibratory source in the upper esophagus, as opposed to either the pharynx or the cheeks (see Weinberg & Westerhouse, 1971, 1973).

Artificial larynx speakers must learn proper placement of the intraoral tube or the vibrating head of a transcervical or neck-type device to achieve the best resonance and, consequently, the best tone (see Chapter 22 in this text). Inaccurate placement will cause poor resonance, resulting in a less than adequate voice quality and less proficient speech (Beaudin, Doyle, & Eadie, 2004; Beaudin, Meltzner, Doyle, & Hillman, 2004; see Chapter 6 in this text).

Those using TE speech without a tracheostoma breathing valve must accurately place the thumb or other fingers over the tracheostoma to achieve total occlusion. The same rule applies to TE speakers who may wear breathing valves that fail to maintain a tight seal for sufficient periods of time. Frequently, at the end of the day when a leak in the seal of the breathing valve may appear, these individuals may need a temporary "fix" through application of digital pressure against the valve housing and adhesive disc.

DISTRACTORS AND FRUSTRATION

Distractors are alaryngeal speaker behaviors that divert listeners' attention from what the speaker is trying to communicate. Common distractors of esophageal speakers include double or triple pumping maneuvers needed to insufflate the esophagus, chin tucking, klunking, invasion of the listener's personal space to compensate for the speaker's lack of vocal loudness, stoma noise, and facial grimaces. For the TE speaker, distractors include the elbow in the listener's face that results when the speaker places a thumb over the tracheostoma, the searching around in order to achieve adequate digital occlusion of the tracheostoma, or stoma noise. Additionally, the volume of speech may be too soft or too loud, and the listener may find it offensive when the speaker uses the dominant hand first to occlude the stoma and then to shake hands. For the AL speaker, a common distractor is the delay caused by a search for proper device placement in the mouth (intraoral artificial larynx) or along the neck (transcervical device), or for the instrument inside a purse or pocket. (Such a search often reminds me of myself or a friend frantically digging through a purse to locate a set of car keys, which can be very distracting!) Another distractor frequently observed in AL users is the extraneous noise from the device that occurs immediately before or after an utterance, or as a result of accidental pressure against the activation (on–off) button. Also, for listeners engaging with either TE speakers who use digital occlusion or AL users, the appearance of the hand up and tucked under the chin or the appearance of an artificial larynx device is considered a real visual distractor.

It is relevant to note here an investigation conducted by Williams and Watson (1987), who asked judges with no previous exposure to laryngectomized individuals to rate the speaking proficiency of all three types of alaryngeal speakers. On the factor of visual presentation, the judges rated the TE speakers similarly to those using laryngeal speech, which is not surprising because all TE speakers in this study were using a tracheostoma breathing valve. The judges also rated two groups—the esophageal and the artificial larynx speaker groups—similarly for visual presentation; this finding is interesting because many of those who are laryngectomized have expressed concerns about speaking with an artificial larynx because they assumed the appearance of such a device would be more distracting to listeners than would the use of esophageal speech. The findings by Williams and Watson, however, fail to support such an assumption. According to these investigators,

> naive judges, who likely resemble the general population, may not prefer the appearance of esophageal speech over electrolarynx speech. Apparently, the injection of air into the esophagus by esophageal speakers affects visual appearance just as much as does use of an electrolarynx. (p. 739)

That interesting finding presents a real challenge to both esophageal speakers and speech–language pathologists who are seeing them for therapy to eliminate those visible injection and inhalation behaviors that negatively influence judgments of the speakers' communicative proficiency (see Chapter 6 in this text).

There are other frustrations common to all alaryngeal speakers. Probably the most irritating is the inability to produce voice on demand. Most TE speakers have experienced prostheses that have become clogged or dislodged at exactly the wrong time; esophageal speakers have reported tremendous frustration when either intense emotion or pharyngoesophageal (PE) spasm prevents them from producing adequate esophageal voice; and artificial larynx devices are subject to mechanical breakdown or battery failure, either of which can cause the users to become voiceless without warning. With careful planning and management, many of these happenings can be avoided, but professional counseling must play an integral part. Clinicians must inform their clients that these types of occurrences are inevitable and discuss appropriate precautions or solutions. These discussions present an excellent opportunity to encourage consideration of a backup alaryngeal speech method. Because no one method is foolproof, persons who have been laryngectomized should realize that developing a backup method is *not* a sign of weakness. Rather, it indicates common sense and consideration for others.

In his discussion of listener preference and acceptability, Doyle (1994) summarized some of the audible distractors frequently associated with the various modes of alaryngeal speech. Reportedly, "listeners indicated that 'nonspeech noises,' 'slurring of words,' and poor control of 'loudness and rate' were judged as unacceptable features of speech" (p. 245). The distractors and frustrations noted herein suggest other areas of focus for treatment and self-help programs that should be directly considered as components of a comprehensive postlaryngectomy rehabilitation program (Doyle, 1999).

ON–OFF TIMING

At first thought, the parameter of on–off timing may seem to pertain only to those using an artificial larynx. When and how fast artificial larynx (electrolarynx) users start and stop the sound of their instrument are important factors. Timing is also a concern, however, for those using esophageal speech who might continue to pump air before they begin voicing, as well as for those using TE speech without a tracheostoma breathing valve who search for adequate digital placement before they can initiate voice. Such behaviors can cause noticeable silences before the initiation of voice from those using either esophageal or TE speech. Silence is not the problem with those using AL speech; the listener hears buzzing or extraneous noise from the instrument before or after the person speaks, which can be disruptive and confusing to the listener and negatively affect the speaker's communicative effectiveness.

SPEECH PARAMETERS

Articulation

Undoubtedly, articulation is the most important dimension to consider when teaching proficient use of any method of alaryngeal speech because it is the parameter most responsible for determining how well people understand the speech of a postlaryngectomy speaker. All individuals who use alaryngeal speech must pay close attention to delivering their message with clear, precise enunciation. Regardless of the alaryngeal speech type used, distinctions between voiced and voiceless consonants are not easily perceived by listeners (see, e.g., Doyle, Danhauer, & Reed, 1988; Sacco, Mann, & Schultz, 1967; Shames, Font, & Matthews, 1963; Tikofsky, 1965). For example, voiceless stop-plosives and affricates are particularly difficult to differentiate from their voiced cognates. Speakers using ES or AL speech are unable to access their own lung air for production of voiceless consonants. Consequently, ES and AL speakers whose intelligibility is perceived as either good or excellent have learned to compensate. Many have learned to build up enough intraoral and pharyngeal air pressure to produce voiceless consonants more clearly (Doyle & Haaf, 1989). The intelligibility of some speakers is often judged as poor because they have never learned how to differentiate between these voiced and voiceless productions.

TE speakers have the benefit of being able to use pulmonary air for voicing and, presumably, to better differentiate production of voiced and voiceless consonants (Merwin, Goldstein, & Rothman, 1985). Theoretically, a more powerful (i.e., larger volume) driving source should have a positive influence on phoneme productions (Doyle et al., 1988); however, numerous studies of alaryngeal speech intelligibility have failed to show significant intelligibility differences among the three modes at the whole word level (Doyle, 1994). It may be that the pulmonary air pressure used by TE speakers for voicing has no real impact on their ability to produce more intelligible speech at the more global level (e.g., words, sentences). Some work, however, has shown that TE speakers may exhibit unique attributes of phoneme intelligibility based on context. For example, Doyle et al. (1988) found that TE speakers exhibited a higher percentage of voiced for voiceless phoneme misperceptions when voiceless consonants were produced in an intervocalic context. In contrast, Doyle and Haaf (1989) found that TE speakers exhibited some advantage in producing voiceless phonemes in the initial position of targets. Regardless of these differences, it appears that TE speakers must achieve precise articulation in the same manner as do those using the other two types of alaryngeal speech. Although TE speakers may tend to produce voiced for voiceless errors in some contexts because they are unable to terminate PE segment vibration due to increased airflows through the sphincter, in other situations, they may perform differently. For example, they must learn to build up enough intraoral and pharyngeal air pressure to distinguish voiced and voiceless consonants. Their failure to do so may be caused by lack of effort or awareness. Many times individuals who have undergone TEP are only provided therapy that stresses care of the prosthesis for adequate voicing, and clinicians fail to address all of the various speech parameters, including articulation. Without training and awareness, these speakers are likely to have difficulty producing speech that is readily intelligible.

All alaryngeal speakers, therefore, should learn how to produce voiced and voiceless consonants and seek to use these strategies in everyday speech productions. During treatment, clinicians should stress techniques and tasks that aid the alaryngeal speaker in learning how to sustain voiced consonants and achieve buildup of intraoral and pharyngeal pressures for productions of voiceless consonants. The clinician should explain the importance of producing such distinctions so that the postlaryngectomy speakers can incorporate exercises that emphasize such contrasts as part of their home practice sessions.

Hearing is another factor that must be considered when discussing articulation and the precise production of the most difficult consonants. It is difficult for any speaker to tell whether he or she is producing sounds correctly if the individual has a hearing loss, and the type of hearing loss associated with aging is very likely to be prevalent both in the population of laryngectomized individuals and their spouses. An investigation by Clark (1985), in which he used both young and older judges, emphasizes the fact that older listeners have more difficulty understanding all modes of alaryngeal speech. Therefore, most individuals who are laryngectomized and their spouses should consider scheduling appointments with an otolaryngologist and a qualified audiologist to determine whether a hearing aid would improve their ability to hear their own speech and the speech of others.

Loudness

Access to the air supply from their lungs may not only, under specified circumstances, serve to help TE speakers distinguish between voiced and voiceless consonants, but also provide other benefits to these speakers. In general, compared with esophageal speakers, TE speakers can achieve a higher fundamental pitch level and greater pitch range, and can talk longer, louder, and faster and with improved speech prosody. The advantages of a pulmonary air source on pitch, loudness, rate, and stress enhance intelligibility and influence speech acceptability (Eadie & Doyle, 2004; van As, Koopmans-van Beinum, Pols, & Hilgers, 2003). Robbins, Fisher, Blom, and Singer (1984) found that TE speech was more intense (i.e., loud) than either esophageal or laryngeal speech. Such loudness, in some instances, can be perceived as inappropriate and not necessarily a desirable feature. Many AL speakers resemble TE speakers in that they sometimes speak more loudly than necessary. Spouses of some AL users have reported that their mates use excessive vocal loudness, and the resultant speech is frequently misinterpreted as representing extreme anger. Such a notion should be explained in treatment, and patients who speak too loudly should be discouraged from doing so if modifications can be achieved.

A lack of loudness can also be deleterious. Esophageal speech has been characterized as being low in intensity level (Smith, Weinberg, & Horii, 1980). This characteristic always is mentioned as a major disadvantage for esophageal speakers. At times, loudness level can be briefly enhanced with digital pressure against the PE segment, but for increased loudness over prolonged periods of time, esophageal speakers are encouraged to use other compensatory strategies. A select group of TE speakers may benefit from using similar strategies. Bosone (1999) speculated that some TE speakers who undergo a pharyngeal constrictor muscle relaxation procedure may exhibit a soft, breathy voice. In either instance, amplification or use of an artificial larynx might be advisable if loudness significantly affects communicative effectiveness. In this context, one investigation seems particularly relevant.

Clark and Stemple (1982) measured the intelligibility of three modes of alaryngeal speech (ES, TE, and AL) in the presence of three levels of background noise (i.e., signal-to-noise ratios). Both young and older listeners judged that, under all three noise levels, the AL speech mode was easier to understand than the other two. This finding is not surprising to many professionals. Nevertheless, many ES and TE speakers refuse to use an amplifier or an electrolarynx in situations where listeners may have trouble understanding low volume levels. It is difficult and frustrating for people who want to converse with these individuals but cannot hear what is said. I am reminded of my attempts, at a large laryngectomy rehabilitation convention, to converse with several attendees at a large hotel patio beside the pool. The acoustics were terrible in the open air, and the noise from the water fountains did not help. The only speakers who were easily heard that evening were those using an artificial larynx. I will always remember one TE speaker who came up to greet me while using an artificial larynx. He had purchased the device a couple of years earlier to demonstrate during hospital visitations and had brought it to use that evening because he knew his voice would be overridden with background noise. That man's speech clinician undoubtedly helped him realize that his purpose was to communicate rather than to favor any specific alaryngeal speech method. His is the type of motivation clinicians should try to instill during treatment sessions. Clinicians do have the opportunity and responsibility to anticipate problems their clients might encounter and to help them achieve logical solutions.

Pitch

Alaryngeal voices typically are produced at fundamental frequency levels lower than those of adult male laryngeal voices. Comparative mean frequency values for laryngeal, esophageal, and TE speakers were reported by Robbins et al. (1984). During sustained vowel phonation and oral reading, the frequency values for both alaryngeal types were lower than for the laryngeal speakers. Although more variable, TE values were closer than esophageal values to those measured for the laryngeal speakers. Pulmonary air supply offers a distinct advantage for the TE speakers—they should be encouraged to use it effectively and avoid monotonous, repetitive intonation patterns. This is true for ES speakers as well. The limited capacity of the esophagus restricts their potential for substantial pitch change, but there are some possibilities.

Many laryngectomized speakers, using any of the three alaryngeal speech modes, excel in speaking, singing, acting, and reading aloud. They practice by imitating radio announcers, singing scales, reading poetry or bedtime stories to their grandchildren, or recording and rerecording themselves on audio- or videotape in an effort to achieve more "normal" sounding pitch and intonation patterns. These individuals would surely support Shipp's (1967) contention that higher overall vocal frequencies for esophageal speech result in higher ratings of proficiency (Doyle, 1994; Chapter 6 in this text).

Additional research findings point out other commonalities among alaryngeal speakers relative to the parameter of pitch. For instance, female esophageal speakers seem capable of achieving a higher fundamental pitch than do male esophageal speakers, and the same holds true for female versus male TE speakers. To explain this phenomenon, Pauloski (1998) suggested possible differences in the phonatory physiology; for example, she speculated that, "For females there may be a smaller and thinner PE segment interacting with reduced air flow"

(p. 134). Regardless of the reasons, the potential apparently exists for females to have higher pitch, although practice and determination are required to achieve such pitch differences. Because many alaryngeal females are interested in obtaining a more feminine-sounding voice, clinicians should address this issue in speech therapy and suggest self-help exercises as part of a home program.

To date, there has been no getting around the fact that AL speech is mechanical sounding and usually produced in a monotone. According to Merwin et al. (1985), electrolarynx devices often have "high intensity upper harmonics present which give them a harsh and metallic quality" (p. 733). Professionals need to inform AL users that the fundamental frequency on AL devices is preset at the factory. For example, the frequency of the Tru-Tone II is set at 75 Hz, which approximates the frequency of esophageal tone, whereas the frequency for the Servox Inton is set at 110 Hz, considerably higher, because the manufacturers believe that the higher pitch is perceived as a better sounding tone. Speakers using instruments similar to the two described can change the fundamental frequency so that it more closely resembles the pitch of their prelaryngectomy voice and the frequency range so that they need not speak in a monotone. The frequency range of the Tru-Tone II is 40 to 200 Hz, but the usable range is about 60 to 180 Hz, whereas the frequency range for the Servox Inton is 50 to 170 Hz. There are other ways to achieve pitch changes if the AL speaker is willing to practice so that the intonation patterns sound more "normal" and not contrived (Salmon, 1999a). Instrumental manipulations may also be achieved (see Chapter 23 in this text).

With the increased acceptance of artificial larynx devices, speakers are becoming more interested in comparing the features of various instruments, and some purchase backup devices. As a subgroup of alaryngeal speakers, AL users are becoming larger in number and are demanding more from manufacturers. All have the same interest in common: to have an instrument that sounds less mechanical and more like a laryngeal voice (Beaudin, Doyle, & Eadie, 2004; see also Chapter 23 in this text). To date only one commercially available instrument, the Servox, has been redesigned to alter variable frequency control during speech. It will be interesting to note whether such a feature becomes valued by laryngectomized consumers and considered worthwhile by other manufacturers in the near future.

Rate

Artificial larynx speakers can talk faster than those using other types of alaryngeal speech. When they do so, they sometimes sacrifice various parameters of speech, and perceptual features may be introduced that can interfere with speech intelligibility and acceptability. They might fail to use pauses, to sustain some vowels to add meaning, to use interrupters, to add intonation, or to take turns in conversation. At times, they might activate and deactivate the control button so frequently that they sound as if they are sending a message in Morse code. None of these behaviors are desirable, and AL users should be counseled accordingly. Specific therapy tasks can be designed to encourage appropriate use of the device. Clinicians may wish to record a client's speech for playback and discuss the need to practice various improvement techniques.

The pulmonary air supply in TE speech allows for a rapid speaking rate more similar to that of laryngeal speech than esophageal speech (Pauloski, 1998; Robbins et al., 1984). TE speakers do not have to replenish their air supply as often as do ES speakers, so less time is lost to lengthy pauses or silence. The problems that TE speakers might encounter with rate are similar to those of AL users. Because speed is not always the most desirable feature of speech, TE speakers should learn attributes (e.g., normal speech rate, natural pauses during speech) that cause them to be perceived as proficient speakers. Periods of inappropriate silences by the TE speaker are usually due to problems related to the prosthesis, such as insufficient digital occlusion or failure of the tracheostoma breathing valve housing to remain sealed. With proper instruction, TE speakers can limit such inconveniences to a minimum.

Improving speech rate is a different issue for esophageal speakers; instead of reducing rate, as the other two groups of alaryngeal speakers might want to do, esophageal speakers should increase it. The best technique is to use consonant injection in conjunction with one of the other methods of air intake and to reduce the length of time between air intake and expulsion of air for speech purposes.

In summary, all alaryngeal speakers, whether they use ES, TE, or AL speech, need to attend to behaviors associated with the various speech parameters noted. To improve performance, one type of speaker may need to react in one way and another type of speaker may need to react in the opposite way. Some individuals will care enough to pursue change and improvement by gathering information about new alternatives, seeking different ways to improve their speech, and recording and rerecording their communication styles in order to produce speech that the public will perceive as more normal (Eadie & Doyle, 2004). Clinicians should be willing to help alaryngeal speakers pursue this goal by committing time to such endeavors.

STAGES OF LOSS

Alaryngeal speakers have more in common than trying to regain the ability to communicate verbally. Almost all of them have experienced a diagnosis of cancer and the loss of a defining part of themselves—their voice. They often share their immediate and long-term reactions during group therapy sessions, Nu-Voice Club discussions, and other support group meetings. Frequently, laryngectomized individuals are surprised and relieved to learn that other people experience similar feelings. It is comforting for them to realize they are not alone (see Chapters 15 and 26 in this text).

Feelings and behaviors associated with the loss of a larynx may be similar to those discussed by Kubler-Ross (1974). In her book, *Death and Dying,* she described a series of behaviors that were associated with different stages of loss and

exhibited by terminally ill cancer patients. These stages are (a) denial and isolation, (b) anger, (c) bargaining, (d) depression, and (e) acceptance. Not all individuals experience these behaviors or feelings in the given order. Also, people experience the stages for different amounts of time, so there may be short or long times
within or between any of them. It is likely that each person who is laryngectomized and members of his or her family move in and out of these various stages
long after the surgery. Clinicians should help the patients and families understand
that these behaviors are normal.

I believe that these behaviors can be applied to *any* loss, not just loss of life,
and I feel that the losses experienced by all alaryngeal speakers cause them to
demonstrate many of these behaviors. Kubler-Ross indicated that such behaviors
could be expected and considered normal reactions by anyone experiencing puz-
zlement, anguish, and pain associated with loss. Individuals who have undergone
laryngectomy have experienced a significant loss—that of their larynx. Regardless of the type of alaryngeal voice these individuals use, they demonstrate many
of the same acting-out behaviors. A sampling of such behaviors is described in
the following paragraphs.

Most laryngectomized individuals have been diagnosed with cancer and
will forever—either in the forefront or in the back of their minds—be fearful of
disease recurrence. Over time, this fear may lessen, but it will never totally go
away. Initially, the fear is so strong that one faithfully looks and feels for signs of
recurrence and approaches follow-up appointments with many questions that
often are never stated aloud. Most patients have *bargained* with someone or with
some superior being to let them be cancer-free before going to a follow-up appointment or hearing the exam results. After the first postoperative year, many
have *denied* symptoms that might indicate recurrence. Patients or spouses may
have noticed a lump, a lesion, some coughing up of blood, or something else that
was worrisome, but decided to assume a wait-and-see attitude. It is a difficult call
because no one wants to be an alarmist and no one wants to be embarrassed by
"wasting" a doctor's time when the findings might turn out to be of no significance. On the other hand, denial of symptoms may have serious consequences if
the individuals dwell for too long on whether and when to seek medical advice.
If they put off taking action, others may say they are indecisive. On the other
hand, if they take immediate action, they might be labeled as hypochondriacs.

Family and friends may expect individuals who are laryngectomized to
"bounce back" from surgery too quickly, and the patients' pride may not permit
them to admit fatigue. After discharge from the hospital, however, they are weak
and tired; often they need to *isolate* themselves and have time to consider the
"newness" of their condition and to plan some coping strategies. They need time
to adjust to the sense of loss of their voice, which they likely associate with their
personalities. Most of all they need to learn how to use a new voice and how to
regain control of their immediate surroundings. For example, one may experience feelings similar to those of another patient with whom I worked, a woman
who had amyotrophic lateral sclerosis. She said to me, "If I lose my speech, I'm
going to be erased as a person!" Most of those who are laryngectomized realize

that the best way to regain control of their environment is to learn an effective communication method. Because there are so many things to learn and consider all at once, alaryngeal speakers need time to think and take action, and many need to withdraw for some period of time.

Many of those who are laryngectomized experience feelings of *anger* related to a variety of questions: Why did this happen to them? Why is their alaryngeal speech less effective than someone else's? Why has a special friend or member of the family not accepted this new voice? Why did it take so long to get approved for disability or supplemental insurance? Although they may have a reason to feel angry, they often do not realize how often they express it. Spouses often indicate that their laryngectomized husbands or wives have a short fuse, that they become angry about things that never bothered them before surgery, and that they stay angry or sulk longer than they once did (Blood, Simpson, Dineen, Kaufmann, & Raimondi, 1993; Doyle, 1999). These observations support the loss that they feel and the consequences of that loss (Blood et al., 1994; see also Chapters 1 and 28 in this text).

Depression is also common for individuals following laryngectomy. Many feel that they have less control over their lives, or their vocational or social outlets have become more restrictive, or their communicative skills are less effective, or their life expectancy is threatened. All of these concerns are legitimate reasons for feeling depressed as a result of the voice handicap they experience (Schuster et al., 2004).

In spite of their grievous loss, those individuals who are well rehabilitated following laryngectomy reach the stage of *acceptance* and are able to resume a fulfilling lifestyle. At this point, they become satisfied with the selection of alaryngeal voice type and begin focusing on perfecting its use. Generally speaking, their communicative skills are sufficient to take back control of their lives. They are now in a position to think of someone else's concerns more than their own and to function on the behalf of others. They may find humor in the way listeners respond to their alaryngeal voice or turn the reaction into an educational experience. Many have a strong desire to help newly laryngectomized individuals and provide them with information and support.

SUMMARY

This chapter has addressed a variety of commonalities among alaryngeal speech methods. Topics have included selection of alaryngeal speech method, placement of speech aids, distractors and frustrations, and speech parameters. The treatment suggestions provided for each speech mode can be adapted for either individual or group therapy. Finally, the feelings and behaviors associated with the emotional impact of laryngectomy have been discussed. All of these concerns cross boundaries of alaryngeal speech method. By considering these factors collectively, clinicians will have better understanding of the consequences of laryngectomy and consider rehabilitation efforts in a broader context than previously.

REFERENCES

Beaudin, P. G., Doyle, P. C., & Eadie, T. L. (2004, May). *Psychophysical evaluation of pleasantness and acceptability for electrolaryngeal speech.* Paper presented at the Annual Conference of the Canadian Association of Speech–Language Pathologists and Audiologists, Ottawa, Ontario.

Beaudin, P. G., Meltzner, G., Doyle, P. C., & Hillman, R. E. (2004, May). *Paired-comparison evaluation of listener preference for electrolaryngeal sentence stimuli.* Paper presented at the Annual Conference of the Canadian Association of Speech–Language Pathologists and Audiologists, Ottawa, Ontario.

Blood, G. W., Simpson, K. C., Dineen, M., Kaufmann, S. M., & Riamondi, S. C. (1993). Spouses of individuals with laryngeal cancer: Caregiver strain and burden. *American Journal of Communication Disorders, 27,* 1–17.

Blood, G. W., Simpson, K. C., Riamondi, S. C., Dineen, M., Kaufmann, S. M., & Staggard, K. A. (1994). Social support of laryngeal cancer survivors: Voice and adjustment issues. *American Journal of Speech–Language Pathology and Audiology, 3,* 37–44.

Bosone, Z. T. (1999). Tracheoesophageal speech: Treatment considerations before and after surgery. In S. J. Salmon (Ed.), *Alaryngeal speech rehabilitation: For clinicians by clinicians* (2nd ed., pp. 105–150). Austin, TX: PRO-ED.

Clark, J. G. (1985). Alaryngeal speech intelligibility and the older listener. *Journal of Speech and Hearing Disorders, 50,* 60–65.

Clark, J. G., & Stemple, J. C. (1982). Assessment of three modes of alaryngeal speech with a synthetic sentence identification (SSI) task in varying message-to-competition ratios. *Journal of Speech and Hearing Research, 25,* 333–338.

Doyle, P. C. (1994). Comparative performance by esophageal, artificial laryngeal, and tracheoesophageal speakers. In P. C. Doyle (Ed.), *Foundations of voice and speech rehabilitation following laryngeal cancer* (pp. 225–245). San Diego: Singular.

Doyle, P. C. (1999). Postlaryngectomy speech rehabilitation: Contemporary concerns in clinical care. *Journal of Speech–Language Pathology and Audiology, 23,* 109–116.

Doyle, P. C., Danhauer, J. L., & Reed, C. G. (1988). Listeners' perceptions of consonants produced by esophageal and tracheoesophageal talkers. *Journal of Speech and Hearing Disorders, 53,* 400–407.

Doyle, P. C., & Haaf, R. G. (1989). Pre- and postvocalic consonant intelligibility in tracheoesophageal talkers. *Journal of Otolaryngology, 18,* 350–353.

Eadie, T. L., & Doyle, P. C. (2004). Auditory–perceptual scaling and quality of life in tracheoesophageal speakers. *Laryngoscope, 114,* 753–759.

Eksteen, E. C., Rieger, J., Nesbitt, M., & Seikaly, H. (2003). Comparison of voice characteristics following three different methods of treatment for laryngeal cancer. *Journal of Otolaryngology, 32,* 250–253.

Fagan, J. J., Lentin, R., Oyarzabal, M. F., Issacs, S., & Sellars, S. L. (2003). Tracheoesophageal speech in a developing world community. *Archives of Otolaryngology—Head and Neck Surgery, 128,* 50–53.

Gelman, J. (1995, November 20). Trends in alaryngeal speech: Use of artificial larynx, prosthetic-assisted speech on the rise. *Advance for Speech–Language Pathologists and Audiologists,* pp. 5–15.

Hillman, R. E., Walsh, M. L., Wolf, G. T., Fisher, S. G., & Hong, W. K. (1998). Functional outcomes following treatment for advanced laryngeal cancer: Part I—Voice preservation in advanced laryngeal cancer; Part II—Laryngectomy rehabilitation: The state of the art in the VA system. *Annals of Otology, Rhinology and Laryngology, 107*(5), 1–27.

Kubler-Ross, E. (1974). *On death and dying.* New York: Macmillan.

Merwin, G. E., Goldstein, L. P., & Rothman, H. B. (1985). A comparison of speech using artificial larynx and tracheoesophageal puncture with valve in the same speakers. *Laryngoscope, 95,* 730–773.

Pauloski, B. R. (1998). Acoustic and aerodynamic characteristics of tracheoesophageal voice. In E. D. Blom, M. I. Singer, & R. C. Hamaker (Eds.), *Tracheoesophageal voice restoration following total laryngectomy* (pp. 123–141). San Diego: Singular.

Robbins, J., Fisher, H. B., Blom, E. C., & Singer, M.I. (1984). A comparative acoustic study of normal, esophageal, and tracheoesophageal speech production. *Journal of Speech and Hearing Disorders, 49,* 202–210.

Sacco, P. R., Mann, M. B., & Schultz, M. C. (1967). Perceptual confusions among selected phonemes in esophageal speech. *Journal of the Indiana Speech and Hearing Association, 26,* 19–33.

Salmon, S. J. (1999a). Artificial larynx devices. In S. J. Salmon (Ed.), *Alaryngeal speech rehabilitation: For clinicians by clinicians* (pp. 79–104). Austin, TX: PRO-ED.

Salmon, S. J. (1999b). [Survey responses from laryngectomees concerning primary and back-up use of alaryngeal speech alternatives]. Unpublished raw data.

Schuster, M., Lohscheller, J., Hoppe, U., Kummer, P., Eysholdt, U., & Rosanowski, F. (2004). Voice handicap of laryngectomees with tracheoesophageal speech. *Folia Phoniatrica and Logopaedia, 56,* 62–67.

Shames, G. H., Font, J., & Matthews, J. (1963). Factors related to speech proficiency of the laryngectomized. *Journal of Speech and Hearing Disorders, 28,* 273–287.

Shipp, T. (1967). Frequency, duration, and perceptual measures in relation to judgments of alaryngeal speech acceptability. *Journal of Speech and Hearing Research, 10,* 417–427.

Singer, M. I., & Blom, E. D. (1980). An endoscopic technique for restoration of voice after laryngectomy. *Annals of Otology, Rhinology and Laryngology, 89,* 529–533.

Smith, B. E., Weinberg, B., & Horii, Y. (1980). Long time spectral and intensity characteristics of esophageal speech. *Journal of the Acoustical Society of America, 67,* 1781–1784.

Tikofsky, R. C. (1965). A comparison of the intelligibility of esophageal and normal speakers. *Folia Phoniatrica, 17,* 19–32.

van As, C. J., Koopmans-van Beinum, F. J., Pols, L. C., & Hilgers, F. J. (2003). Perceptual evaluation of tracheoesophageal speech by naive and experienced judges through the use of semantic differential scales. *Journal of Speech-Language-Hearing Research, 46,* 947–959.

Weinberg, B., & Westerhouse, J. (1971). A study of buccal speech. *Journal of Speech and Hearing Research, 14,* 652–658.

Weinberg, B., & Westerhouse, J. (1973). A study of pharyngeal speech. *Journal of Speech and Hearing Disorders, 38,* 111–118.

Williams, S. E., & Watson, J. B. (1987). Speaking proficiency variations in laryngectomees. *Laryngoscope, 97,* 737–739.

Chapter 4

Laryngectomy Speech Rehabilitation
A Review of Outcomes

Robert E. Hillman, Michael J. Walsh,
and James T. Heaton

Total laryngectomy results in a loss of ability to produce normal voice and speech, necessitating the use of rehabilitative approaches to restore voice and speech for oral communication. The purpose of this chapter is to review research that reports on the outcomes of speech rehabilitation approaches for those who have undergone total laryngectomy. The review examines the different modes of alaryngeal communication that are available to laryngectomy patients in terms of the prevalence of use, communication proficiency, and overall communication function. Much of the material in this chapter is based on an extension of a 1998 report in which we reviewed the state of the art in laryngectomy speech rehabilitation and described the results of a large prospective study that involved 148 total laryngectomy patients across 15 Veterans Administration (VA) hospitals (Hillman, Walsh, Wolf, Fisher, & Hong, 1998). The Hillman et al. study, which was part of a larger clinical trial of treatments for advanced laryngeal cancer, represented an unprecedented opportunity to collect data in a prospective, standardized fashion from a significantly large number of individuals who had undergone total laryngectomy for treatment of laryngeal cancer.

MODES OF ALARYNGEAL COMMUNICATION: PREVALENCE OF USE

There are currently three primary options for the voice and speech rehabilitation of laryngectomy patients: esophageal speech, use of an artificial larynx, and tracheoesophageal (TE) voice restoration. Occasionally, other surgical or surgical–prosthetic approaches have been described in the literature (see Shedd & Weinberg, 1980), but to date none of these approaches has gained widespread use. Results from studies that have examined the prevalence of use for each of the three most common modes of alaryngeal oral communication are summarized in the subsequent section.

Esophageal Speech

Early studies of voice rehabilitation in laryngectomy patients examined the acquisition of esophageal speech as the primary mode of alaryngeal speech. These early retrospective studies (Hunt, 1964; Johnson, 1960; King, Fowlks, & Peirson, 1968) reported relatively high acquisition rates for esophageal speech, ranging from 38% to 97%. In the 1980s, investigators generally reported lower rates of esophageal speech acquisition, ranging from 26% in a study by Gates, Ryan, Cooper, et al. (1982) to 12% in a VA population reported on by Schaefer and Johns (1982). A second arm of the Gates, Ryan, Cooper, et al. (1982) study revealed a 62% acquisition rate in patients who were studied retrospectively. These authors concluded that the higher acquisition rate for retrospective studies was artificially inflated by selection bias. More recent studies have also reported much lower rates of esophageal speech acquisition. For example, St. Guily et al. (1992) found that only 5% of their laryngectomy patients acquired esophageal speech. Similarly, in our study that prospectively tracked the speech rehabilitation outcomes of 148 total laryngectomy patients in the VA system (Hillman et al., 1998), we reported that no more

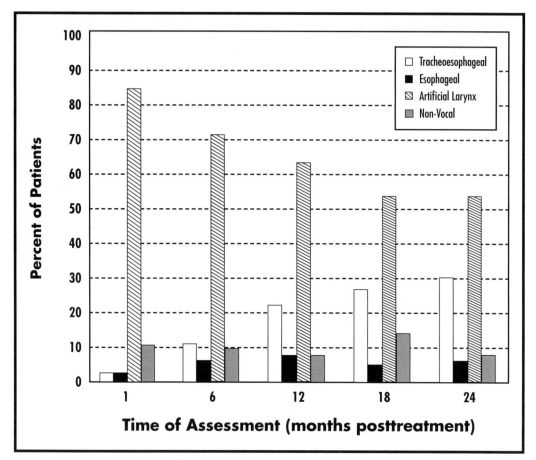

FIGURE 4.1. Percentage of total laryngectomy patients who reported using each of four modes of alaryngeal communication at 1, 6, 12, 18, and 24 months posttreatment. From "Functional Outcomes Following Treatment for Advanced Laryngeal Cancer. Part I—Voice Preservation in Advanced Laryngeal Cancer. Part II—Laryngectomy Rehabilitation: The State of the Art in the VA System." R. E. Hillman, M. J. Walsh, G. T. Wolf, S. G. Fisher, and W. K. Hong, 1998. *Annals of Otology, Rhinology and Laryngology, Supplement, 172,* pp. 1–27. Copyright 1998 by Annals Publishing Company. Reprinted with permission.

than 7% of the survivors developed usable esophageal speech at any point in time across the 2-year follow-up period (see Figure 4.1).

Various factors have been associated with successful acquisition of esophageal speech, including extent of surgery, positive attitude, psychosocial adjustment, frequency of speech therapy, and family support (Gates, Ryan, Cantu, & Hearne, 1982; Richardson, 1981; Richardson & Bourque, 1985; Volin, 1980; see also Chapter 19 in this text). Failure to acquire esophageal speech has been associated with lack of motivation, limited physical strength, postoperative radiotherapy, dysphagia, and limited speech therapy (Gates, Ryan, Cantu, & Hearne, 1982; Richardson & Bourque, 1985; Volin, 1980; see also Chapter 16 in this text). From a historical perspective, it is reasonable to assume that the apparent decrease in esophageal speech acquisition is at least partly associated with the emergence in the 1980s (Singer & Blom, 1980) of tracheoesophageal speech (see Chapter 17 in this text), and possibly to the increased acceptance of artificial electrolarynx use as a viable option.

Artificial Larynx Speech

In reports on the prevalence of artificial larynx use among those who are laryngectomized, the term *artificial larynx* is synonymous with *electrolarynx*, which describes a class of devices that are battery-powered buzzers (see Chapter 23 in this text). Previous reports of artificial larynx use among laryngectomy patients, like reports of esophageal speech use, have varied. Most past estimates of artificial larynx use ranged from 5% to 34% (Diedrich & Youngstrom, 1977; Gates, Ryan, Cooper, et al., 1982; Johnson, 1960; King et al., 1968; Kommers & Sullivan, 1979; Richardson & Bourque, 1985; Webster & Duguay, 1990). Until recently, only Gray and Konrad (1976) reported a markedly higher rate of 66% for artificial larynx use among these postlaryngectomy patients. In our prospective study of 148 total laryngectomy patients in the VA system (Hillman et al., 1998), we reported that artificial larynx use was the predominant mode of alaryngeal communication across follow-up. Most patients in that study were using an artificial larynx at 1 month post–cancer treatment (85%), and a majority (55%) were still using it as their primary means of communication as of the last scheduled assessment at 24 months posttreatment (see Figure 4.1). These results agree with other survey-based studies, which report more than half of those undergoing total laryngectomy end up using an electrolarynx (Carr, Schmidbauer, Majaess, & Smith, 2000; Culton & Gerwin, 1998).

     Ease of use, immediate postlaryngectomy voice production, and elimination of any delay in reacquiring verbal communication (Diedrich & Youngstrom, 1977; Martin, 1963) have been cited as some reasons for successful artificial larynx use (see also Chapter 22 in this text). Failure to successfully use an artificial larynx has been attributed to a variety of reasons, including dissatisfaction with its mechanical sound quality, loss of low-frequency components of the acoustic signal, low volume, reduced intelligibility, inconvenience of using one hand to hold the device, failure to encourage its use, and altered neck tissue properties (i.e., postsurgery tissue changes or postradiation fibrosis) which preclude the use of the most popular neck-type devices (Bennett & Weinberg, 1973; Merwin, Goldstein, & Rothman, 1985; Qi & Weinberg, 1991; Verdolini, Skinner, Patton, & Walker, 1985; Weiss, Yeni-Komshian, & Heinz, 1979; see also Chapter 22 in this text). For more details about the performance of current electrolaryngeal devices, see Chapter 23.

Tracheoesophageal Speech

Since its introduction in 1980 (Singer & Blom, 1980), the tracheoesophageal puncture (TEP) technique for postlaryngectomy voice restoration has gained

widespread popularity as the third major method of voice and speech rehabilitation for laryngectomy patients (Lopez, Kraybill, McElroy, & Guerra, 1987;
Webster & Duguay, 1990). Numerous single-institution, retrospective studies
have reported acquisition rates for TE speech (Juarbe, 1989). Early studies, which
focused on carefully selected groups of patients who underwent TEP as a sec-
ondary procedure, reported success rates ranging from 56% to 93% (Donegan,
Gluckman, & Singh, 1981; Singer, Blom, & Hamaker, 1981; Wood, Rusnov,
Tucker, & Levine, 1981). More recent studies focusing on TEP as a primary procedure (Hamaker, Singer, Blom, & Daniels, 1985; Maniglia, Lundy, Casiano, &
Swim, 1989) reported acquisition rates ranging from 30% to 93% (Kao, Mohr,
Kimmel, Getch, & Silverman, 1994; Lau, Wei, Ho, & Lam, 1988; Quer, Burgues-
Vila, & Garcia-Crespillo, 1992). In our prospective study of 148 laryngectomy
patients (Hillman et al., 1998), we noted that there was an increase in TE
speech acquisition across the 2-year follow-up period, with 2% using TE speech
at 1-month post–cancer treatment and 31% using TE speech at 24 months. The
noted increase in TE speech use across follow-up appeared to account primarily
for the concurrent decrease in artificial larynx use (see Figure 4.1).

Success with TE speech has been attributed to the relative ease of the surgical procedure and to the quality of speech, which is fluent, intelligible, and
spontaneously acquired with minimal speech therapy (Blom, Singer, & Hamaker,
1986; Doyle, 1994; Kao et al., 1994; Lau et al., 1988). Failure to acquire primary
or secondary TE speech has been associated with postoperative complications
such as mediastinitis, aspiration pneumonia, persistent pharyngocutaneous fistula,
stomal stenosis, salivary aspiration, cellulitis or infection, abscess, cervical spine
fracture, false tract creation, pharyngoesophageal stenosis, and pharyngospasm
(Andrews, Mickel, Hanson, Monahan, & Ward, 1987; Blom, Pauloski, & Hamaker,
1995; Izdebski, Reed, Ross, & Hilsinger, 1994; Maniglia et al., 1989; Silver, Gluckman, & Donegan, 1985; see also Chapter 21 in this text). Behavioral factors, such as
difficulty with digital occlusion, gagging, inadvertent prosthesis dislodgment with
fistula closure, aspiration of the prosthesis, lack of motivation, and failure to care for
the stoma or prosthesis (Izdebski et al., 1994; McConnel & Duck, 1986; Quer et al.,
1992), have also been implicated in the failure to acquire TE speech.

Two surveys of postlaryngectomy vocal rehabilitation practices among head
and neck surgeons (Lopez et al., 1987; Webster & Duguay, 1990) compared the
acquisition rate of TE speech with other forms of alaryngeal communication;
they found that TE speech acquisition among laryngectomy patients ranged from
30% to 38%. This acquisition rate is comparable to our study, which revealed a
31% TE acquisition rate by 2 years post–cancer treatment (Hillman et al., 1998).
Similar to earlier studies, these investigators reported a range of values for esophageal speech acquisition (38% to 49%) and artificial larynx use (21% to 48%).
They also reported that the mode of postlaryngectomy communication was unknown for 2% to 9% of the patients reviewed. In another survey study, Culton
and Gerwin (1998) examined the perceptions of experienced speech–language
pathologists with respect to the speech rehabilitation of laryngectomy patients
since the advent of contemporary TE voice restoration. Even though TE was
ranked as the most preferred alaryngeal speech option, and electrolarynx use was

considered the least preferred approach, the electrolarynx continued to be the most frequently used method according to speech–language pathologists surveyed. In a more recent survey of laryngectomy patients in Nova Scotia, Carr et al. (2000) reported that only 8.5% of patients were using TE speech as compared to 57% who were using an electrolarynx and 19% who were using esophageal speech.

Overall, there is a paucity of long-term follow-up information concerning the extent to which surviving laryngectomy patients continue to use any of the primary modes of alaryngeal communication (see Chapter 5 in this text). In a 5-year study in France that followed 270 patients who had initially received a TE voice prosthesis for postlaryngectomy speech rehabilitation, de Raucourt et al. (1998) reported that the success rate dropped from 81% at 1 year to 61% at 5 years. These results prompted de Raucourt et al. to conclude that, even though the TEP approach to voice restoration produces good initial results, maintaining it requires "extensive care" and the outcome may deteriorate with time. Gathering similar long-term follow-up information on all modes of alaryngeal communication is important for obtaining a more accurate sense of relative prevalence of use over time after laryngectomy.

Nonvocal Communication

A number of studies have reported on the prevalence of writing and nonvocal communication among individuals postlaryngectomy (i.e., those who do not develop or adopt one of the three main options for alaryngeal speech communication). Better than half of these studies (Blom et al., 1986; Clements, Rassekh, Seikaly, Hokanson, & Calhoun, 1997; Gates, Ryan, Cooper et al., 1982; Johnson, 1960; King et al., 1968; Kommers & Sullivan, 1979; Richardson & Bourque, 1985), including the prospective study by Gates, Ryan, Cooper, et al. (1982) reported nonvocal communication rates that ranged from 17% to 35%. The remaining studies (Ackerstaff, Hilgers, Aaronson, & Balm, 1994; Diedrich & Youngstrom, 1977; Gray & Konrad, 1976; Lopez et al., 1987) reported lower rates, ranging from 5% to 10%, which are closer to our reported findings (Hillman et al., 1998). In our study of functional outcomes postlaryngectomy, nonvocal communication was employed by relatively few patients across the 24-month follow-up period (ranging from 7% to 13% of patients), with 8% being nonvocal at the final assessment.

PROFICIENCY OF COMMUNICATION

Proficiency of postlaryngectomy communication has been reported (Beukelman, Cummings, Dobie, & Weymuller, 1980; Hoops & Noll, 1969; Williams & Watson, 1985) to be based on the temporal characteristics of the message and the efficient transfer of information from speaker to listener, as measured by the rate of speech and intelligibility, respectively. Results from studies that have examined reading rates and intelligibility for the different modes of alaryngeal speech are summarized in the following sections.

Reading Rate

A number of investigations have gathered specific data on the average speaking rates associated with the different modes of alaryngeal communication. Previously published speaking rates for all three modes of alaryngeal communication are slower than the rate of 173 words per minute (wpm) reported for normal laryngeal speakers (Robbins, Fisher, Blom, & Singer, 1984). The reported mean rate of speech for esophageal speakers has ranged from 99 wpm to 114 wpm (Hoops & Noll, 1969; Robbins et al., 1984), whereas higher rates of speech have been reported for male (127 wpm; Robbins et al., 1984) and female (138 wpm; Trudeau & Qi, 1990) TE speakers. Previously published data on the speaking rate of artificial larynx users are limited, but suggest that the rate may be slower than that of TE speakers and faster than that of esophageal speakers (Hyman, 1955; Merwin et al., 1985).

In our study (Hillman et al., 1998), esophageal speakers displayed a slower average reading rate at the final assessment than the other two groups of alaryngeal speakers (see Figure 4.2). An average rate of 98 wpm (121 syllables per minute) for esophageal speakers fell at the low end of the range of values previously reported for this group (Hoops & Noll, 1969; Robbins et al., 1984). The intermediate reading rate of 130 wpm (160.6 syllables per minute) was displayed by the artificial larynx users. At the final assessment, the TE speakers displayed an average oral reading rate of 155 wpm (191.6 syllables per minute). This rate approximated the average prelaryngectomy performance for the entire patient sample, and is somewhat faster than what has been reported in previous studies of oral reading rates for TE speakers using different reading material (Robbins et al., 1984; Trudeau & Qi, 1990). Our overall finding that artificial larynx users display average oral reading rates that are faster than esophageal speakers and slower than TE speakers is in general agreement with previous reports (Hyman, 1955; Merwin et al., 1985).

Intelligibility

Studies of average speech intelligibility (i.e., percentage of speech items correctly identified by the listener) have demonstrated that none of the three major modes of alaryngeal communication is 100% intelligible and that there is considerable variation in intelligibility data both within and across alaryngeal modes. One obvious source of the variation in intelligibility measurements across studies is the use of different types of stimulus materials (e.g., single words vs. contextual speech) and listening tasks (e.g., multiple choice vs. direct transcription). Results from studies of artificial larynx speech are quite variable, with reported intelligibility values ranging from 32% to 90% (Weiss & Basili, 1985; Weiss et al., 1979). In our study (Hillman et al., 1998), average intelligibility for artificial larynx users fell toward the upper end of this range, with a mean of 80.5% at the final assessment (see Figure 4.3).

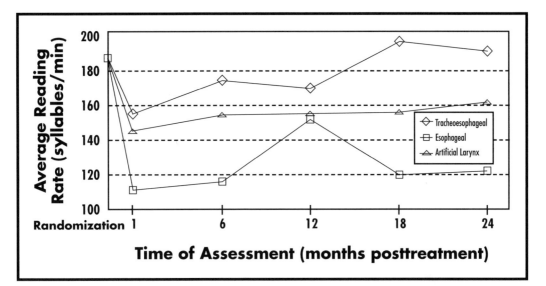

FIGURE 4.2. Average reading rate (syllables per minute) for each of three alaryngeal speaker groups at randomization and 1, 6, 12, 18, and 24 months posttreatment. From "Functional Outcomes Following Treatment for Advanced Laryngeal Cancer. Part I—Voice Preservation in Advanced Laryngeal Cancer. Part II—Laryngectomy Rehabilitation: The State of the Art in the VA System." R. E. Hillman, M. J. Walsh, G. T. Wolf, S. G. Fisher, and W. K. Hong, 1998. *Annals of Otology, Rhinology and Laryngology, Supplement, 172,* pp. 1–27. Copyright 1998 by Annals Publishing Company. Reprinted with permission.

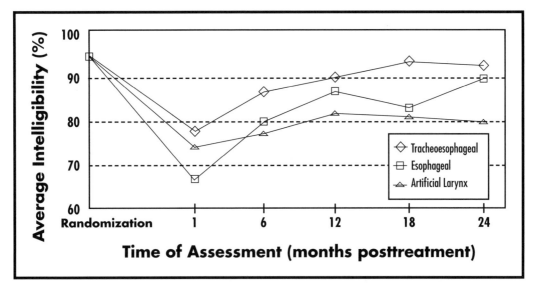

FIGURE 4.3. Average percentage of intelligibility for each of three alaryngeal speaker groups at randomization and 1, 6, 12, 18, and 24 months posttreatment. From "Functional Outcomes Following Treatment for Advanced Laryngeal Cancer. Part I—Voice Preservation in Advanced Laryngeal Cancer. Part II—Laryngectomy Rehabilitation: The State of the Art in the VA System." R. E. Hillman, M. J. Walsh, G. T. Wolf, S. G. Fisher, and W. K. Hong, 1998. *Annals of Otology, Rhinology and Laryngology, Supplement, 172,* pp. 1–27. Copyright 1998 by Annals Publishing Company. Reprinted with permission.

Investigations of the intelligibility of esophageal speech have reported values ranging from 49% to 96% (Blom et al., 1986; Doyle, Danhauer, & Reed, 1988; Horii & Weinberg, 1975; Hyman, 1955; Kalb & Carpenter, 1981; McCroskey & Mulligan, 1963; Pindzola & Cain, 1988). Again, the results from our study (Hillman et al., 1998) fell toward the upper end of this range, with the esophageal speakers displaying an average intelligibility of 90% by the end of the 2-year follow-up period (see Figure 4.3).

Intelligibility values for TE speakers have been reported to range from 65% to 93% (Blom et al., 1986; Doyle et al., 1988; Merwin et al., 1985; Pindzola & Cain, 1988; Tardy-Mitzell, Andrews, & Bowman, 1985) and have displayed a narrower range of variation, with scores that are skewed higher than the other two modes of alaryngeal communication. Once again, the TE speakers in our study (Hillman et al., 1998) ended up at the high end of this range, with a final average intelligibility score of 91.9% (see Figure 4.3). A limited number of studies have directly compared all three modes of alaryngeal speech (e.g., Blom et al., 1986) and found that the highest intelligibility scores were obtained for TE speech.

OVERALL COMMUNICATION FUNCTION

A variety of problems in communication common to all laryngectomy patients has been discussed in the literature, including concern about the sound quality of the voice (Wallen & Webb, 1975), difficulty communicating over the phone (Clements et al., 1997; Harwood & Rawlinson, 1983), and difficulty communicating in social situations (Clements et al., 1997; Harwood & Rawlinson, 1983). The overall level of communication function for alaryngeal speakers appears to be mode dependent and related to patient satisfaction with voice and listener acceptability (Beaudin, Meltzner, Hillman, & Doyle, 2003; Beaudin, Meltzner, Doyle, & Hillman, 2004; Eadie & Doyle, 2002, in press-a, in press-b; see also Chapter 21 in this text).

Satisfaction with voice, including phone use, was reported to be high in most patients who underwent surgical prosthetic voice restoration (i.e., TEP) (Ackerstaff et al., 1994; Clements et al., 1997; Silverman & Black, 1994). Clements et al. (1997) found that satisfaction with TE speech was higher than that for other modes of alaryngeal communication on a variety of satisfaction measures, including overall satisfaction with speech quality, phone use, limitations of interactions, and satisfaction with quality of life. Miani, Bertino, Bellomo, and Staffieri (1998) directly compared listener judgments of the voice and speech of esophageal versus TE speakers and reported that listeners judged TE voice to be significantly more "pleasant" and "acceptable" than esophageal voice.

Numerous studies of esophageal speakers have reported several speech-related problems, such as difficulty being understood or inability to speak, with these problems being exacerbated in social settings (Dhillon, Palmer, Pittam, & Shaw, 1982; Jones, Lund, Howard, Greenberg, & McCarthy, 1992; Natvig, 1983, 1984). As already discussed, even though artificial larynx use is quite common among laryngectomy patients, the resulting speech has been characterized as having an artificial, mechanical quality (Bennett & Weinberg, 1973; Qi & Weinberg, 1991). Clements et al. (1997) found that esophageal speakers reported a higher level of satisfaction with communication than did artificial larynx users on most of their measures, and that all three alaryngeal speaker groups reported higher satisfaction than did nonvocal communicators. Laryngectomy patients who were dissatisfied with their voices reported less frequent use of the telephone and anxiety about speaking with new listeners (Ackerstaff et al., 1994). Listeners have rated both esophageal speech and artificial larynx speech as less acceptable than the speech of individuals with normal larynxes (Bennett & Weinberg, 1973). Finally, although TE speech has been perceived by listeners to be superior to communication using either esophageal speech or artificial larynx speech, it has not been judged as comparable to normal speech (Williams & Watson, 1987).

In our study (Hillman et al., 1998), we assessed patients' overall level of communication functioning by having them complete a Communication Profile that was adapted from an instrument originally proposed by Logemann, Fisher, and Becker (1980). Respondents used a 5-point scale to express their agreement or disagreement with 24 statements about communication situations (e.g., "I avoid answering the telephone"). In general, a higher score is associated with a higher level of communication function. Results (reported in Figure 4.4) were essentially in line with what might have been predicted based on our findings for speech intelligibility, and also generally in agreement with previous reports dealing with communication satisfaction among alaryngeal speakers. The two groups that displayed the best recovery of intelligibility (i.e., TE and esophageal speakers) also showed the best recovery of communication functioning. The TE and esophageal speaker groups actually ended up at the final assessment with average Communication Profile scores that were slightly higher than (76.5 for TE) or comparable to (74.2 for esophageal) that for the entire patient sample prelaryngectomy (74.1). We also found that the artificial larynx users had lower average Communication Profile scores (69.2) than the other two alaryngeal speaker groups, and that the lowest scores were displayed by the nonvocal communication group (62.6). These results are in general agreement with previous research (Clements et al., 1997).

Even though esophageal speakers must talk at slower rates, their speech often is more intelligible than that produced by artificial larynx users. Thus, it seems quite reasonable that intelligibility probably contributes much more to overall communication functioning than does speech rate. It must also be acknowledged that the nonhuman, mechanical sound quality of currently available artificial larynxes (Bennett & Weinberg, 1973; Qi & Weinberg, 1991) probably contributed (at least to some extent) to the lower overall level of communication functioning that was displayed by electrolarynx users. This assumption is supported by a previous study in which artificial larynx users stated that their speech was a source of embarrassment to them (Shames, Font, & Matthews, 1963). Therefore, physical characteristics of the alaryngeal mode, as well as personal assessments of laryngeal communication, must be considered in postlaryngectomy outcomes.

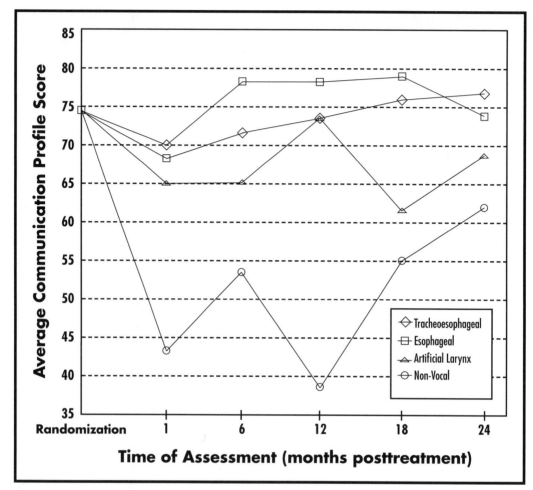

FIGURE 4.4. Average Communication Profile score for each of three alaryngeal speaker groups at randomization and 1, 6, 12, 18, and 24 months posttreatment. From "Functional Outcomes Following Treatment for Advanced Laryngeal Cancer. Part I—Voice Preservation in Advanced Laryngeal Cancer. Part II—Laryngectomy Rehabilitation: The State of the Art in the VA System." R. E. Hillman, M. J. Walsh, G. T. Wolf, S. G. Fisher, and W. K. Hong, 1998. *Annals of Otology, Rhinology and Laryngology, Supplement, 172,* pp. 1–27. Copyright 1998 by Annals Publishing Company. Reprinted with permission.

SUMMARY

This chapter has addressed the outcomes of speech rehabilitation in individuals undergoing total laryngectomy. A review of the literature reveals that TE speakers display the best overall communication proficiency and function, followed by esophageal speakers, artificial larynx users, and finally those patients who use nonvocal communication. Evidence suggests that fewer laryngectomy patients are currently acquiring esophageal speech than was the case in past decades. Even though TE speech has gained increased prominence, there still appears to be an important role for the artificial larynx in the speech rehabilitation of total laryngectomy patients.

REFERENCES

Ackerstaff, A. H., Hilgers, F. J., Aaronson, N. K., & Balm, A. J. (1994). Communication, functional disorders and lifestyle changes after total laryngectomy. *Clinical Otolaryngology, 19,* 295–300.

Andrews, J. C., Mickel, R. A., Hanson, D. G., Monahan, G. P., & Ward, P. H. (1987). Major complications following tracheoesophageal puncture for voice rehabilitation. *Laryngoscope, 97,* 562–567.

Beaudin, P. G., Meltzner, G., Hillman, R. E., & Doyle, P. C. (2003, May). A paired-comparison assessment of preference for the speech of a prototype electrolarynx. Paper presented at the Annual Meeting of the Canadian Association of Speech-Language Pathologists and Audiologists, St. John's, Newfoundland.

Beaudin, P. G., Meltzner, G. S., Doyle, P. C., & Hillman, R. E. (2004, May). Paired-comparison evaluation of listener preference for electrolaryngeal sentence stimuli. Paper presented at the Annual Conference of the Canadian Association of Speech-Language Pathologists and Audiologists. Ottawa, Ontario.

Bennett, S., & Weinberg, B. (1973). Acceptability ratings of normal, esophageal, and artificial larynx speech. *Journal of Speech and Hearing Research, 16,* 608–615.

Beukelman, D. R., Cummings, C. W., Dobie, R. A., & Weymuller, E. A., Jr. (1980). Objective assessment of laryngectomized patients with surgical reconstruction. *Archives of Otolaryngology, 106,* 715–718.

Blom, E. D., Pauloski, B. R., & Hamaker, R. C. (1995). Functional outcome after surgery for prevention of pharyngospasms in tracheoesophageal speakers: Part I. Speech characteristics. *Laryngoscope, 105,* 1093–1103.

Blom, E. D., Singer, M. I., & Hamaker, R. C. (1986). A prospective study of tracheoesophageal speech. *Archives of Otolaryngology—Head and Neck Surgery, 112,* 440–447.

Carr, M. M., Schmidbauer, J. A., Majaess, L., & Smith, R. L. (2000). Communication after laryngectomy: An assessment of quality of life. *Otolaryngology—Head and Neck Surgery, 122,* 39–43.

Clements, K. S., Rassekh, C. H., Seikaly, H., Hokanson, J. A., & Calhoun, K. H. (1997). Communication after laryngectomy: An assessment of patient satisfaction. *Archives of Otolaryngology—Head and Neck Surgery, 123,* 493–496.

Culton, G. L., & Gerwin, J. M. (1998). Current trends in laryngectomy rehabilitation: A survey of speech–language pathologists. *Otolaryngology—Head and Neck Surgery, 118,* 458–463.

de Raucourt, D., Rame, J. P., Daliphard, F., Le Pennec, D., Bequignon, A., & Luquet, A. (1998). Voice rehabilitation with a voice prosthesis: Study of 62 patients with 5 years follow-up. *Review of Laryngology, Otology, and Rhinology, 119*(5), 297–300.

Dhillon, R. S., Palmer, B.V., Pittam, M. R., & Shaw, H. J. (1982). Rehabilitation after major head and neck surgery—The patients' view. *Clinical Otolaryngology, 7*(5), 319–324.

Diedrich, W., & Youngstrom, K. (1977). *Alaryngeal speech.* Springfield, IL: Thomas.

Donegan, J. O., Gluckman, J. L., & Singh, J. (1981). Limitations of the Blom–Singer technique for voice restoration. *Annals of Otology, Rhinology and Laryngology, 90*(5, Pt. 1), 495–497.

Doyle, P. C. (1994). *Foundations of voice and speech rehabilitation following laryngectomy.* San Diego, CA: Singular.

Doyle, P. C., Danhauer, J. L., & Reed, C. G. (1988). Listeners' perceptions of consonants produced by esophageal and tracheoesophageal talkers. *Journal of Speech and Hearing Disorders, 53,* 400–407.

Eadie, T. L., & Doyle, P. C. (2002). DME and EAI scaling of naturalness and severity in tracheo-esophageal (TE) speakers. *Journal of Speech, Language, and Hearing Research, 45,* 1088–1096.

Eadie, T. L., & Doyle, P. C. (in press-a). Quality of life in male tracheoesophageal (TE) speakers. *Journal of Rehabilitation Research and Development.*

Eadie, T. L., & Doyle, P. C. (in press-b). Scaling of voice pleasantness and acceptability in tracheo-esophageal (TE) speakers. *Journal of Voice.*

Gates, G. A., Ryan, W., Cantu, E., & Hearne, E. (1982). Current status of laryngectomee rehabilitation: II. Causes of failure. *American Journal of Otolaryngology, 3*(1), 8–14.

Gates, G. A., Ryan, W., Cooper, J. C., Jr., Lawlis, G. F., Cantu, E., Hayashi, T., Lauder, E., Welch, R. W., & Hearne, E. (1982). Current status of laryngectomee rehabilitation: I. Results of therapy. *American Journal of Otolaryngology, 3*(1), 1–7.

Gray, S., & Konrad, H. R. (1976). Laryngectomy: Postsurgical rehabilitation of communication. *Archives of Physical Medicine and Rehabilitation, 57*(3), 140–142.

Hamaker, R. C., Singer, M. I., Blom, E. D., & Daniels, H. A. (1985). Primary voice restoration at laryngectomy. *Archives of Otolaryngology, 111,* 182–186.

Harwood, A. R., & Rawlinson, E. (1983). The quality of life of patients following treatment for laryngeal cancer. *International Journal of Radiation Oncology and Biological Physics, 9,* 335–338.

Hillman, R. E., Walsh, M. J., Wolf, G. T., Fisher, S. G., & Hong, W. K. (1998). Functional outcomes following treatment for advanced laryngeal cancer. Part I—Voice preservation in advanced laryngeal cancer; Part II—Laryngectomy rehabilitation: The state of the art in the VA System. *Annals of Otology, Rhinology and Laryngology, 172*(Suppl.), 1–27.

Hoops, H., & Noll, J. (1969). Relationship of selected acoustic variables to judgements of esophageal speech. *Journal of Communication Disorders, 2,* 1–13.

Horii, Y., & Weinberg, B. (1975). Intelligibility characteristics of superior esophageal speech presented under various levels of masking noise. *Journal of Speech and Hearing Research, 18,* 413–419.

Hunt, R. (1964). Rehabilitation of the laryngectomee. *Laryngoscope, 74,* 382–395.

Hyman, M. (1955). An experimental study of artificial larynx and esophageal speech. *Journal of Speech and Hearing Disorders, 20,* 291–299.

Izdebski, K., Reed, C. G., Ross, J. C., & Hilsinger, R. L., Jr. (1994). Problems with tracheoesophageal fistula voice restoration in totally laryngectomized patients: A review of 95 cases. *Archives of Otolaryngology—Head and Neck Surgery, 120,* 840–845.

Johnson, C. (1960). A survey of laryngectomee patients in Veterans Administration hospitals. *Archives of Otolaryngology, 72,* 768–773.

Jones, E., Lund, V. J., Howard, D. J., Greenberg, M. P., & McCarthy, M. (1992). Quality of life of patients treated surgically for head and neck cancer. *Journal of Laryngology and Otology, 106,* 238–242.

Juarbe, C. (1989). Overview of results with tracheoesophageal puncture after total laryngectomy. *Bolivian Association of Medical P R, 81*(11), 455–457.

Kalb, M. B., & Carpenter, M. A. (1981). Individual speaker influence on relative intelligibility of esophageal speech and artificial larynx speech. *Journal of Speech and Hearing Disorders, 46,* 77–80.

Kao, W. W., Mohr, R. M., Kimmel, C. A., Getch, C., & Silverman, C. (1994). The outcome and techniques of primary and secondary tracheoesophageal puncture. *Archives of Otolaryngology—Head and Neck Surgery, 120,* 301–307.

King, P. S., Fowlks, E. W., & Peirson, G. A. (1968). Rehabilitation and adaptation of laryngectomy patients. *American Journal of Physical Medicine, 47*(4), 192–203.

Kommers, M. S., & Sullivan, M. D. (1979). Wives' evaluation of problems related to laryngectomy. *Journal of Communication Disorders, 12,* 411–430.

Lau, W. F., Wei, W. I., Ho, C. M., & Lam, K. H. (1988). Immediate tracheoesophageal puncture for voice restoration in laryngopharyngeal resection. *American Journal of Surgery, 156*(4), 269–272.

Logemann, J., Fisher, H., & Becker, N. (1980). Northwestern Otolaryngology Communication Profile for Head and Neck Cancer Patients. In D. Shedd & B. Weinberg (Eds.), *Surgical and prosthetic approaches to speech rehabilitation* (pp. 283–294). Boston: Hall.

Lopez, M. J., Kraybill, W., McElroy, T. H., & Guerra, O. (1987). Voice rehabilitation practices among head and neck surgeons. *Annals of Otology, Rhinology and Laryngology, 96*(3, Pt. 1), 261–263.

Maniglia, A. J., Lundy, D. S., Casiano, R. C., & Swim, S. C. (1989). Speech restoration and complications of primary versus secondary tracheoesophageal puncture following total laryngectomy. *Laryngoscope, 99,* 489–491.

Martin, H. (1963). Rehabilitation of the laryngectomee. *Cancer, 16,* 823–841.

McConnel, F. M., & Duck, S. W. (1986). Indications for tracheoesophageal puncture speech rehabilitation. *Laryngoscope, 96,* 1065–1068.

McCroskey, R. L., & Mulligan, M. (1963). The relative intelligibility of esophageal speech and artificial-larynx speech. *Journal of Speech and Hearing Disorders, 28,* 37–41.

Merwin, G. E., Goldstein, L. P., & Rothman, H. B. (1985). A comparison of speech using artificial larynx and tracheoesophageal puncture with valve in the same speaker. *Laryngoscope, 95,* 730–734.

Miani, C., Bertino, G., Bellomo, A., & Staffieri, A. (1998). [Analysis of qualitative voice and speech quality judgments after total laryngectomy]. *Acta Otorhinolaryngologica Italia, 18*(3), 143–147.

Natvig, K. (1983). Study No. 1: Social, personal, and behavioral factors related to present mastery of the laryngectomy event. *Journal of Otolaryngology, 12,* 155–162.

Natvig, K. (1984). Laryngectomees in Norway: Study no. 5. Problems of everyday life. *Journal of Otolaryngology, 13,* 15–22.

Pindzola, R. H., & Cain, B. H. (1988). Acceptability ratings of tracheoesophageal speech. *Laryngoscope, 98,* 394–397.

Qi, Y. Y., & Weinberg, B. (1991). Low-frequency energy deficit in electrolaryngeal speech. *Journal of Speech and Hearing Research, 34,* 1250–1256.

Quer, M., Burgues-Vila, J., & Garcia-Crespillo, P. (1992). Primary tracheoesophageal puncture vs. esophageal speech. *Archives of Otolaryngology—Head and Neck Surgery, 118,* 188–190.

Richardson, J. L. (1981). Surgical and radiological effects upon the development of speech after total laryngectomy. *Annals of Otology, Rhinology and Laryngology, 90*(3, Pt. 1), 294–297.

Richardson, J., & Bourque, L. (1985). Communication after laryngectomy. *Journal of Psychosocial Oncology, 3,* 83–97.

Robbins, J., Fisher, H. B., Blom, E. D., & Singer, M. I. (1984). Selected acoustic features of tracheoesophageal, esophageal, and laryngeal speech. *Archives of Otolaryngology, 110,* 670–672.

Schaefer, S. D., & Johns, D. F. (1982). Attaining functional esophageal speech. *Archives of Otolaryngology, 108,* 647–649.

Shames, G., Font, J., & Matthews, J. (1963). Factors related to speech proficiency of the laryngectomized. *Journal of Speech and Hearing Disorders, 28,* 273–287.

Shedd, D. P., & Weinberg, B. (1980). *Surgical and prosthetic approaches to speech rehabilitation.* Boston: Hall.

Silver, F. M., Gluckman, J. L., & Donegan, J. O. (1985). Operative complications of tracheoesophageal puncture. *Laryngoscope, 95,* 1360–1362.

Silverman, A. H., & Black, M. J. (1994). Efficacy of primary tracheoesophageal puncture in laryngectomy rehabilitation. *Journal of Otolaryngology, 23,* 370–377.

Singer, M. I., & Blom, E. D. (1980). An endoscopic technique for restoration of voice after laryngectomy. *Annals of Otology, Rhinology and Laryngology, 89*(6, Pt. 1), 529–533.

Singer, M. I., Blom, E. D., & Hamaker, R. C. (1981). Further experience with voice restoration after total laryngectomy. *Annals of Otology, Rhinology and Laryngology, 90*(5, Pt. 1), 498–502.

St. Guily, J. L., Angelard, B., el-Bez, M., Julien, N., Debry, C., Fichaux, P., & Gondret, R. (1992). Postlaryngectomy voice restoration: A prospective study in 83 patients. *Archives of Otolaryngology—Head and Neck Surgery, 118,* 252–255.

Tardy-Mitzell, S., Andrews, M. L., & Bowman, S. A. (1985). Acceptability and intelligibility of tracheoesophageal speech. *Archives of Otolaryngology, 111,* 213–215.

Trudeau, M. D., & Qi, Y. Y. (1990). Acoustic characteristics of female tracheoesophageal speech. *Journal of Speech and Hearing Disorders, 55,* 244–250.

Verdolini, K., Skinner, M. W., Patton, T., & Walker, P. A. (1985). Effect of amplification on the intelligibility of speech produced with an electrolarynx. *Laryngoscope, 95,* 720–726.

Volin, R. A. (1980). Predicting failure to speak after laryngectomy. *Laryngoscope, 90*(10, Pt. 1), 1727–1736.

Wallen, V., & Webb, V. P. (1975). A survey of the background characteristics of 2,000 laryngectomees: A preliminary report. *Military Medicine, 140,* 532–534.

Webster, P. M., & Duguay, M. J. (1990). Surgeons' reported attitudes and practices regarding alaryngeal speech. *Annals of Otology, Rhinology and Laryngology, 99*(3, Pt. 1), 197–200.

Weiss, M. S., & Basili, A. G. (1985). Electrolaryngeal speech produced by laryngectomized subjects: Perceptual characteristics. *Journal of Speech and Hearing Research, 28,* 294–300.

Weiss, M. S., Yeni-Komshian, G. H., & Heinz, J. M. (1979). Acoustical and perceptual characteristics of speech produced with an electronic artificial larynx. *Journal of the Acoustical Society of America, 65*(5), 1298–1308.

Williams, S. E., & Watson, J. B. (1985). Differences in speaking proficiencies in three laryngectomee groups. *Archives of Otolaryngology, 111,* 216–219.

Williams, S. E., & Watson, J. B. (1987). Speaking proficiency variations according to method of alaryngeal voicing. *Laryngoscope, 97,* 737–739.

Wood, B. G., Rusnov, M. G., Tucker, H. M., & Levine, H. L. (1981). Tracheoesophageal puncture for alaryngeal voice restoration. *Annals of Otology, Rhinology and Laryngology, 90*(5, Pt. 1), 492–494.

Chapter 5

Rehabilitation for Laryngectomy and Long-Term Success of Alaryngeal Speakers

William J. Ryan

n 1985, Bailey proposed that the history of surgical treatment for laryngeal cancer could be segmented into three periods of approximately 40 years each. Bailey identified the first 40-year period, 1860 to 1900, as one of reluctant acceptance of the concept of conservation surgery; the second period, 1900 to 1940, as one of popularization and basic development; and the third period, 1940 to 1980, as being characterized by rapid development in medical science. Similarly, I have based this chapter on the premise that the history of postlaryngectomy rehabilitation can be divided conceptually into three distinct, yet not mutually exclusive, eras or periods. The first era was characterized predominately by concerns about postlaryngectomy survivability and encompasses a period from approximately the 1860s to the 1950s. The second era includes the dominance of interest in the acquisition of postlaryngectomy speech that characterized much of the work reported in the literature from the 1950s to the 1980s. The third era represents a gradual shift in attention toward the concept of what will be called successful, long-term, total rehabilitation that began during the late 1980s and continues today.

The purpose of this chapter is to discuss these three periods of postlaryngectomy rehabilitation. In doing so, special emphasis is placed on research that exemplifies the attention being paid during the third period to successful, long-term, total rehabilitation. Specifically, the chapter includes overviews of the eras related to survivability and speech acquisition, with the intent of providing a context for a more detailed discussion of the third era. Because the third era comprises a conceptual framework based on a retrospective view of the literature, it is rare to find individual studies that explicitly address "successful, long-term, total rehabilitation" as an entity. Rather, individual studies tend to focus on one or more aspects of postlaryngectomy rehabilitation that collectively seem to fall into the category assumed to result in successful, long-term, total rehabilitation. Hence, the findings of these studies are the major focus of the chapter.

SURVIVABILITY

From the late 1800s to the early 1950s, the primary objective of total laryngectomy was to remove the malignancy in such a way that the patient survived beyond the time that would be expected if the tumor had not been removed. In other words, the medical viewpoint was that "the disease was worse than the cure." Unfortunately, initial attempts at surgical extirpation of the larynx often failed to ensure survivability for more than a few weeks. Postoperative complications such as bacterial infections, hemorrhaging, and aspiration pneumonia often produced unacceptably high mortality rates. In fact, there was a period in the late 1800s during which it was argued by some that total laryngectomy, as it was performed then, should be abandoned because of the serious postoperative complications and low rates of survivability. Despite these arguments that "the cure was worse than the disease," some surgeons persisted in their efforts to remove the larynx while simultaneously creating an airway that was independent of the digestive tract. With the continued development and refinement of anesthetics, antibiotics, surgical instruments, and sophisticated surgical techniques, total laryngectomy gradually became accepted as the treatment of choice for laryngeal

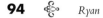

tumors that were not otherwise treatable with radiotherapy or conservative procedures such as cordectomy and laryngofissure. As a consequence, survivability gradually became less of an issue.

SPEECH ACQUISITION

By the early 1950s, concerns about survivability began to give way to the second era, during which speech acquisition and verbal communication emerged as the major challenge facing the person with a laryngectomy. The appearance of books devoted specifically to the topic of postlaryngectomy speech rehabilitation attested to its growing importance among clinicians and researchers (Damsté, 1958; DiCarlo, Amster, & Herer, 1955; Diedrich & Youngstrom, 1966; Gardner, 1971; Snidecor, 1962). Although postlaryngectomy speech communication had not been totally ignored during the first half of the 20th century, the 1950s and 1960s ushered in an era in which the major focus of postlaryngectomy rehabilitation became the production of intelligible alaryngeal speech. At that time, the primary modes of "pseudovoice" production consisted of esophageal voice (speech) and use of some type of pneumatic or electromechanical device (see Chapter 2 in this text). Much of the research and clinical work carried out during this era primarily addressed speech-related issues, including methods for impounding air into the esophagus (Damsté, 1958; Diedrich & Youngstrom, 1966); comparison of the intelligibility and acceptability of esophageal speech versus alaryngeal speech produced with an artificial larynx (e.g., Bennett & Weinberg, 1973; Hoops & Curtis, 1971; Hyman, 1955); descriptive studies of the preferred methods of postoperative communication (Horn, 1962); measurement of various acoustic and physiologic parameters associated with the production of esophageal speech (Berlin, 1963, 1965; Weinberg & Bennett, 1972); and technological refinements of artificial devices, especially those of the electromechanical type (Barney, 1958; Barney, Haworth, & Dunn, 1959).

Unfortunately, some of the findings from these early studies led to incorrect assumptions about the success rates of esophageal voice acquisition and, subsequently, to the view that the artificial larynx was a less than acceptable means of postlaryngectomy verbal communication (see Chapter 4 in this text). Some individuals who had undergone laryngectomy early in this era were actually forbidden by their physicians to use any type of artificial device until all efforts at esophageal voice acquisition had failed. Speech–language pathologists and laryngectomized individuals alike believed that they had "failed" if the laryngectomized person did not achieve "acceptable" esophageal voice.[1] By the same token, some individuals were informed about the existence of artificial larynxes but

---

[1]Terms such as *acceptable, satisfactory, and good* as they pertain to alaryngeal voice and speech have been defined in numerous ways across a wide variety of studies and, collectively, constitute a matter worthy of additional study. For the purposes of this chapter, however, use of *acceptable* and similar terms reflects the general intent of the author(s) cited without a detailed definition unless otherwise specified.

were never provided exposure to the devices (see Chapter 22 in this text). Sadly, this philosophy persisted overtly or subtly throughout the 1960s and 1970s, even though significant progress was made in understanding the process of alaryngeal speech communication during this period (e.g., the advancement of knowledge pertaining to speech acoustics, aerodynamic features, perceptual attributes, and intelligibility).

This confluence of the expectation for esophageal voice to be the primary means of alaryngeal communication, the lack of success in acquiring it for some individuals, and the increased understanding of the process of postlaryngectomy communication provided the impetus for what was to come in the ensuing decade. Clinicians and researchers continued to search for better ways to serve the communication needs of people with laryngectomies. The results of these efforts were instrumental in bringing about major changes in the decade of the 1980s.

In the early 1980s, a number of developments occurred that would create a significant change in attitudes toward the approaches to and management of postlaryngectomy speech acquisition. Clinical researchers such as Singer and Blom (1980) began reporting preliminary findings for their endoscopic tracheo-esophageal puncture (TEP) techniques, in which the use of a one-way valve allowed air from the lungs to pass into the upper esophagus while preventing esophageal food and liquids from entering the trachea. These surgical–prosthetic methods ensured that a continuous stream of pulmonary air was delivered to the esophageal air reservoir below the pharyngoesophageal segment, thereby producing a pseudovoice that was alleged to be much more acceptable, natural, and intelligible than that created by traditional esophageal or artificial larynx methods (Singer & Blom, 1980).

At about the same time, Gates, Ryan, and coworkers published a series of reports based on a prospective study of a large number of individuals who had undergone total laryngectomy (Gates, Ryan, Cantu, & Hearne, 1982; Gates, Ryan, Cooper et al., 1982; Gates, Ryan, & Lauder, 1982; Ryan, Gates, Cantu, & Hearne, 1982). The major objectives of this investigation were to accurately assess the impact of laryngectomy and to identify factors that promoted success or led to failure in postlaryngectomy rehabilitation. Of the many findings reported, some had significant impact on the way in which postlaryngectomy rehabilitation would be viewed in the future.

One of the most important results reported by this team of researchers was that, in contrast to earlier reports of approximately 60% success rates based on retrospective analyses (Hunt, 1964; King, Fowlks, & Peirson, 1968; Snidecor, 1975), less than one third of the laryngectomized group prospectively studied by Gates, Ryan, Cooper, et al. (1982; Ryan et al., 1982) used esophageal voice as the primary means of communication at 6 months postlaryngectomy. This finding, later confirmed by Schaefer and Johns (1982), led Gates, Ryan, Cooper, et al. (1982; Ryan et al., 1982) to argue that esophageal voice acquisition was not always a realistic expectation for the person with a laryngectomy, and that an alternative means of communication, such as the artificial larynx, should be viewed as an equally acceptable postlaryngectomy communication method (see Chapter 4 in this text). As an extension of this argument, and as had others before them

(Diedrich & Youngstrom, 1966), Gates, Ryan, Cantu, and Hearne (1982) suggested that "functional communication" should be the ultimate target of postlaryngectomy rehabilitation regardless of the method(s) used. Furthermore, Gates, Ryan, and Lauder (1982) emphasized the importance of reassessing a number of prevailing attitudes that were based on erroneous assumptions or incomplete data.[2]

Taken in the aggregate, the findings and recommendations reported by Gates, Ryan, Cooper, et al. (1982; Ryan et al., 1982) helped set the stage for a gradual shift in thinking about the impact of laryngectomy and the process of postlaryngectomy rehabilitation. In addition, the apparently low success rate of approximately 30% for esophageal voice acquisition reported by Gates, Ryan, Cooper, et al. (1982) and confirmed by Schaefer and Johns (1982) provided impetus for the rapidly emerging acceptance of surgical–prosthetic restoration of voice via the TEP technique (Singer & Blom, 1980).

In a prospective study based on the methodology used in the 1982 series by Gates and colleagues, Blom, Singer, and Hamaker (1986) reported that 94% of the individuals who underwent TEP achieved "good to superior" speech after surgery, and, at 1 year post-TEP, 83% continued to use their voice prostheses. Other researchers focused their attention on various aspects of tracheoesophageal (TE) speech, including acoustic characteristics (Baggs & Pine, 1983; Qi & Weinberg, 1991; Robbins, 1984; Robbins, Fisher, Blom, & Singer, 1984), aerodynamic parameters (Moon & Weinberg, 1987; Vuyk, Festin, Spoelstra, & Tiwari, 1987), perceptual features (Sedory, Hamlet, & Connor, 1989; Williams, Scanio, & Ritterman, 1989), and intelligibility (Tardy-Mitzell, Andrews, & Bowman, 1985). Overall, the findings of these and similar studies suggested that TE speech was a viable alternative for alaryngeal speakers who could not or chose not to use esophageal speech or an artificial device, although it is not problem free (Karlen & Maisel, 2001).

By the late 1980s, then, it had become generally accepted that postlaryngectomy speech acquisition in one or more of its three basic forms (artificial larynx, esophageal, and TE) was a realistic expectation for the majority of individuals undergoing surgical removal of the larynx. As a result, some clinicians and researchers began to focus less on concerns about speech acquisition and more on issues pertaining to overall rehabilitation success.

SUCCESSFUL TOTAL REHABILITATION

As survivability and speech acquisition have become less of a challenge, the third major era of postlaryngectomy rehabilitation, namely, successful total rehabilitation, has begun to evolve. Professionals who are interested in the overall well-

---

[2]See Gates, Ryan, and Lauder (1982) and Doyle (1994) for a detailed discussion of myths and erroneous attitudes that can have an adverse effect on postlaryngectomy rehabilitation.

being of laryngectomized individuals also recognize that speech acquisition is only part of a much more complex process (Doyle, 1994; Gilmore, 1994). Certainly, this is not a new concept to have surfaced in the 1990s. Relevant textbooks and articles published in the 1960s and 1970s acknowledged the need to consider the physical, psychological, and social sequelae of total laryngectomy (Diedrich & Youngstrom, 1966; Gardner, 1971; King et al., 1968; Snidecor, 1962). A review of the literature, however, clearly indicates a surge of interest since the late 1980s in one or more aspects of successful, long-term, total rehabilitation, such as postlaryngectomy communication satisfaction, the impact of laryngectomy on the life of the individual and members of his or her family, quality-of-life issues (Terrell et al., 2004), and the long-term success of those who have undergone TEP procedures (see Chapters 3, 24, and 26 in this text). Also, major changes brought about by surgical–prosthetic methods of voice restoration, technological advances in the design of artificial laryngeal devices (see Chapter 23 in this text), and evolving attitudes about postlaryngectomy rehabilitation since the mid-1980s make comparisons with earlier studies difficult. The remainder of this chapter, then, will be most concerned with a review of selected contributions made from the late 1980s to the present, contributions that seem to exemplify increased interest in the notion of successful, long-term, total rehabilitation.

What Defines Successful Long-Term Rehabilitation?

One of the most difficult tasks encountered when attempting to investigate levels of success achieved in addressing the overall needs of the laryngectomized person throughout his or her postoperative life, is defining what is meant by the terms *successful, long-term,* and *total rehabilitation.* For example, consider a person who has undergone a secondary surgical–prosthetic voice restoration procedure and after 1 week is producing speech that is highly intelligible, relatively pleasant sounding, and without related problems such as air leaking from the stoma. By most accounts, speech acquisition would be judged as "successful." But does success in this context mean the same thing to the physician or speech–language pathologist as it does to the person with a laryngectomy, to his or her spouse, or to other members of the family? Does the resulting voice meet the preoperative expectations of these individuals? Will the laryngectomized person still be using the voice prosthesis in 6 months, 1 year, or 10 years? What is this individual's status with regard to reentering the workforce, or resuming preoperative social activities, avocations, and sexual relations? How well does he or she cope with other anatomical and physiological changes brought about by surgical removal of the larynx? These are just some of the questions that must be considered when addressing the determinants of successful, long-term, total rehabilitation.

Merely demonstrating acceptable, pleasant-sounding speech a week after surgery, however, falls far short of establishing that successful, long-term, total rehabilitation has taken place. Although no one has yet created a composite picture of what constitutes successful, long-term, total rehabilitation, reports in the literature over the last decade have begun to acknowledge the "bigger picture" in which speech plays an important but not the only part. In addition to providing increased insight into and understanding of the magnitude of the problem, partial solutions at the clinical services delivery level, as well as thoughtful suggestions for additional research, have begun to emerge. Researchers have approached the study of successful, long-term, total rehabilitation from a number of perspectives, including the relationship between speaking proficiency and communication satisfaction, gender differences, overall adjustment to laryngeal cancer and surgery, the impact of laryngectomy on quality of life, consequences of voice preservation and conservation laryngectomy techniques, and long-term success of surgical–prosthetic voice restoration. I conclude the section with observations about the studies discussed and their relevance to clinical services. The remainder of this chapter is devoted to a review and discussion of these issues.

Communication Attitudes and Satisfaction

Williams and Watson (1988) examined one aspect of total rehabilitation in their study of the relationships among communication attitudes, voicing methods, and speaking proficiency in a group of individuals with laryngectomies and laryngeal speakers. They compared four groups of speakers—laryngeal ($n = 10$), esophageal ($n = 12$), electrolarynx ($n = 11$), and tracheoesophageal ($n = 10$)—using the *Inventory of Communication Attitudes* (originally developed by the second author in 1981, as cited in Williams & Watson, 1988) to assess communication attitudes of people who stutter. This tool is a self-report inventory of feelings, thoughts, and behaviors associated with 12 different types of speaking situations, such as asking for flight information when late for the plane, talking to a store clerk when others are waiting in line, and so on. Items were rated by the respondents on the following 7-point equal-appearing interval scales: Affective, Behavioral, Cognitive A, Cognitive B, and Frequency. For example, on the Affective scale, a rating of 1 meant "I definitely enjoy speaking in this situation," whereas a rating of 7 meant "I hate speaking in this situation."

Williams and Watson (1988) determined voicing proficiency by playing videotaped samples of each subject performing a variety of speech tasks, including counting to 25, reading 50 phonetically balanced words, reading 10 sentences, describing a picture, and conversing with the examiner. Nine judges watched and listened to the tapes under optimal listening conditions to obtain ratings of voicing proficiency. Again, a 7-point equal-appearing interval scale with *excellent* and *poor* at the end points was used to assess the level of communicative effectiveness for each participant in the study. Williams and Watson used discriminate analyses to determine whether respondents' communication attitudes, as expressed on the *Inventory of Communication Attitudes,* could be used to differentiate among groups of speakers.

Interestingly, the attitudes measured did not significantly differentiate between laryngeal and alaryngeal speakers. Williams and Watson (1988) attributed this finding to the heterogeneity of the communication attitudes expressed by the laryngeal group, which made it impossible to discriminate between them and the three alaryngeal groups. Attitudes measured, however, did differentiate in one way between esophageal speakers and those who used the electrolarynx: In situations demanding memorized or automatic speech, electrolarynx speakers expressed attitudes that were significantly more positive than those of esophageal speakers. Williams and Watson speculated that because voice initiation is typically more reliable when using an electrolarynx, esophageal speakers might feel less secure in these situations, thereby prompting poor attitudes regarding such situations.

Perhaps more important, Williams and Watson (1988) found no substantial relationship between attitudes toward communication and speaking proficiency for any of the groups. Williams and Watson noted that earlier studies (Amster et al., 1972; Bisi & Conley, 1965; DiBartolo, 1971; Salmon & Goldstein, 1978; Shames et al., 1963; all cited in Williams & Watson, 1988) suggested that motivation and various personality variables may be related to speaking proficiency in alaryngeal speakers. In their concluding comments, Williams and Watson stated, "Our research suggests, however, that communication attitudes of patients post-laryngectomy should not be used as prognostic indicators as they do not appear to be related to judgments of speaking proficiency" (p. 66).

Changes in postlaryngectomy communication satisfaction experienced by alaryngeal speakers and their spouses were also of interest to Oates, Lochert, and McMahon (1990). They, like Williams and Watson (1988), attempted to determine whether changes in communication satisfaction, if present, are related to alaryngeal speech proficiency. Twenty subjects (10 esophageal speakers and 10 speakers who used the Servox artificial larynx as their primary means of communication) were rated on separate 7-point equal-appearing interval scales of alaryngeal speech proficiency developed by Oates and O'Brien in 1987 (as cited in Oates et al., 1990). For the esophageal group, a value of 1 was assigned for individuals who exhibited only involuntary or no esophageal sound production, whereas a value of 7 was assigned to those who produced natural conversational speech in which only the esophageal sound source distinguished it from laryngeal speech. For the electrolarynx users, a value of 1 was assigned to those for whom there was no usable sound conduction through the neck tissue, whereas a value of 7 was assigned for production of natural conversational speech in which only the artificial larynx sound source limitations distinguished it from laryngeal speech. Two speech–language pathologists experienced in the rehabilitation of persons with laryngectomies provided the ratings from audiotape-recorded samples of the study participants reading the "Rainbow Passage" (Fairbanks, 1960).

In addition, each alaryngeal speaker and his or her spouse responded to preoperative and postoperative communication satisfaction questionnaires, also using a 7-point scale from 1 (*very dissatisfied*) to 7 (*very satisfied*). Sample items included the following: "When talking on the telephone to your wife," "When talking on the telephone to strangers," and "When talking with friends/family at a social gathering." For example, a participant might assign a rating of 7 (*very satisfied*) when asked prior to surgery about communication via telephone. The same question asked postoperatively might elicit a rating of 1 (*very dissatisfied*), thereby indicating a decrease in satisfaction for that specific communication setting. Not surprisingly, a significant decrease in postoperative communication satisfaction was noted for the alaryngeal speaking groups in all four of the situations under study: talking on the telephone, with spouse, with friends/family, and with strangers. Spouses exhibited a decrease in satisfaction only when their partners were communicating with friends and family members.

Like Williams and Watson (1988), Oates et al. (1990) found no significant relationship between alaryngeal speech proficiency (as measured on the 7-point voicing proficiency scale) and magnitude of postoperative communicative satisfaction (as measured on the communication satisfaction questionnaire). Also, they reported no significant difference in the change in communication satisfaction between esophageal and electrolarynx speakers, or for their respective spouses. Oates et al. concluded that factors other than speech proficiency probably account for the variance in postlaryngectomy communicative satisfaction. Indeed, they went on to state,

> The present study, for example, indicated that subjects with the highest degree of speech proficiency were among those least satisfied with alaryngeal communication. It may be that such speakers had high levels of achievement motivation and unrealistically high expectations of their communicative abilities after laryngectomy. If the determinants of communicative satisfaction can be established, speech–language pathologists and other professionals involved in laryngectomee rehabilitation will have targets for intervention to prevent the decrease in satisfaction as experienced by laryngectomees and their spouses in the present research. (p. 15)

The studies by Williams and Watson (1988) and Oates et al. (1990) are important in at least two respects. First, they represent a departure from the speech acquisition era of research mentioned earlier. Instead, they address the more inclusive topic of overall communication satisfaction. Second, the findings of these studies justify this departure from an emphasis on alaryngeal speech acquisition by providing evidence that the mode of alaryngeal speech acquisition, per se, might not be as important to alaryngeal speakers when compared to other factors that come into play during postlaryngectomy rehabilitation.

Gender and Counseling Issues

In recognition of the continuing increase in the female postlaryngectomy population, some researchers have begun to direct their attention to the special needs of women who have undergone total laryngectomy (Brown & Doyle, 1999; Doyle, 1997; Doyle & White, 2004; Eadie & Doyle, 2004; Salva & Kallail, 1989; Stack, 1994). Salva and Kallail (1989) reported on an investigation of the counseling needs of males and females who had undergone laryngectomy. They surveyed 120 laryngectomized individuals (58% male, 42% female) of various ages, geographic locations, educational levels, years since surgery, and methods of communication. Among their numerous findings, Salva and Kallail concluded that differences between female and male alaryngeal speakers fell into three distinct areas: feelings, informational needs, and lifestyle changes. For example, females reported more fear and anxiety and more feelings of embarrassment related to their mode of communication than did their male counterparts. Also, physicians were regarded as less helpful by the laryngectomized females than by the males. Most troublesome, however, is the finding that fully 40% of *all* participants in the study reported that they received no counseling prior to or following surgery. Salva and Kallail (1989) summarized their findings as follows:

> The results made it apparent that the counseling needs of laryngectomees were not met adequately by qualified professionals. Adequate counseling by qualified professionals must be available to laryngectomees and their spouses. In addition, differences in counseling needs were revealed between male and female laryngectomees. Sex differences must be understood and dealt with by all members of the rehabilitation team to rehabilitate effectively the laryngectomy patient. (p. 301)

The feminine viewpoint has also been discussed by Stack (1994). A laryngectomized person herself, Stack reported the results from a survey conducted in 1991. Forty-four laryngectomized women responded to a series of questions pertaining to personal data, demography, years since surgery, postoperative coping and adjustment, and mode of communication. The findings reported were in general agreement with those reported earlier by Salva and Kallail (1989). Interestingly, Stack had previously conducted a survey of a similar nature in 1978. According to her account in 1994, many of the same problems continued to exist for women in 1991 as compared to those reported in 1978, providing additional support for the previously noted recommendations by Salva and Kallail.

Doyle (1997) recognized the importance of acknowledging gender differences in an article dealing with treatment considerations following conservation laryngectomy. Doyle noted that although men may prefer a "rough" postoperative voice, a breathy postoperative voice may be preferred by some females because it is viewed as more socially acceptable. Doyle (1997) stated, "Thus, realistic and pragmatic considerations must override a desire for an 'improved' voice quality because the social penalties associated with some voice qualities, relative to speaker gender, may be real and substantial" (p. 32).

Brown and Doyle (1999) reviewed several issues that could have an impact on clinical practice for women who have been diagnosed and treated for laryngeal cancer. They suggested that parallels can be drawn between breast and laryngeal cancer, especially with regard to disfigurement stigmata and changes in body image. Brown and Doyle noted the need to expand the focus of existing rehabilitation programs to include multiple factors that might affect the treatment outcomes for a given individual. They stated,

Given the increasing incidence of women diagnosed with laryngeal cancer, the ability to evaluate the impact of the disease and treatment on the patient in general, and on women in particular, may offer insights into how to modify counselling and treatment programs. With such information at hand, it is suggested that an improved understanding of the female who is treated for laryngeal cancer will evolve and that our strategies for clinical care may be modified accordingly. (p. 59)

Again, as the reports by Salva and Kallail (1989), Stack (1994), Doyle (1997), and Brown and Doyle (1999) indicate, the overall impact of laryngectomy transcends concerns limited to speech acquisition alone and appears to be different in some ways for female alaryngeal speakers than for their male counterparts. The increased attention to these differences is further evidence of an effort to address successful total rehabilitation for people who have undergone laryngectomies. By the same token, other researchers have begun to examine issues pertaining to overall adjustment and coping behaviors manifested by laryngectomized individuals.

OVERALL ADJUSTMENT TO LARYNGECTOMY

Blood, Luther, and Stemple (1992) examined the relationships among types of voice restoration, length of survival, coping strategies, and overall adjustment to laryngeal cancer in a group of 41 (32 male, 9 female) alaryngeal speakers from southwestern Ohio and central Pennsylvania. This study also represented a substantial shift of attention from concern about speech acquisition to attempting to define and describe the overall impact of laryngeal cancer and subsequent laryngectomy on the individual patient. Blood et al. (1992) set out to describe how well people with laryngectomies adjust to and cope with cancer. They also attempted to determine if differences in coping and adjustment vary as a function of the type of alaryngeal voice used and the length of time since laryngectomy, and whether relationships exist between one's perception of his or her alaryngeal speech and one's adjustment and coping.

In general, Blood et al. (1992) found that the majority of the laryngectomized individuals studied were well adjusted to their cancer and to their laryngectomies. They had a tendency to use problem-focused coping strategies as opposed to wishful thinking and self-blame, and sought out support from family and friends. The amount of time that had passed since their laryngectomies was positively correlated to successful coping, adjustment, self-esteem, and general well-being. As noted by Blood et al. (1992), "Significant differences between recent and distant survivors showed that time does seem to heal" (p. 67).

An additional finding reported by Blood et al. (1992) has direct implications for professionals involved with overall or total rehabilitation of individuals with laryngectomies. They found no relationship between type of speech used and subsequent adjustment. Blood et al. (1992) stated,

The absence of a relationship between type of speech and adjustment is very encouraging. It seems important to reinforce the result that none of the three communication groups had superiority over the others. This is a good indication that whatever communication model is chosen does not interfere with overall adjustment, self-esteem, or general well-being. (p. 67)

The foregoing statement and findings reported by Blood et al. (1992) should dispel any remaining myths about the alleged superiority of certain modes of alaryngeal speech when compared to others. As noted earlier in this chapter, the preoccupation by some clinicians with acquisition of esophageal speech only was probably misguided and may have been, in fact, detrimental to the overall successful rehabilitation of some individuals. The comments and findings by Blood et al. should be welcomed as representing a more enlightened and contemporary view of the relative importance of mode of alaryngeal speech in the overall adjustment of people who have undergone laryngectomy.

Another aspect of overall adjustment to laryngectomy was addressed by Blood, Blood, Kaufmann, Raimondi, and Dineen (1995) They investigated life after laryngectomy for older and younger survivors of laryngeal cancer. Blood et al. were specifically interested in the potential relationships between age and adjustment styles, communication attributes, and functional capabilities in activities of daily living. Their study was designed to examine adjustment, communication, and functional independence in 62 laryngectomized males who ranged in age from 46 to 65 years of age (mean = 52 years) and 62 laryngectomized males who ranged in age from 66 to 82 years (mean = 73 years). The authors used standardized measurement scales including the *Psychosocial Adjustment to Illness Scale* (PAIS; Derogatis & Lopez, 1983, as cited in Blood et al., 1995) and the *Self-Evaluation of Communication Experiences after Laryngectomy* (SECEL; Blood, 1993) to assess such things as adjustment to cancer, functional capacities, the ability to live independently, communication needs, and perceived awkwardness in communication. Overall, their results suggest that older people with laryngectomies are as well or better adjusted to their cancer than are their younger counterparts. They also reported no age-related differences for communication traits and capacity for independent living, although 70% of their subjects, regardless of age, reported difficulties in their communication environment, attitudes, or both. Blood et al. (1995) noted,

Some of these problems included not getting the attention of their listener, difficulties in yelling or calling out to people, or trouble speaking on the telephone. These types of problems could be discussed with speech–language pathologists or other health care workers, and immediate solutions such as amplifiers, and nonverbal ways of getting attention could be offered. Other problems including frustration, depression, hesitation in meeting new people, or feeling left out of a group because of their speech may be addressed in voice therapy sessions, support group meetings, and psychological counseling sessions. (p. 44)

QUALITY OF LIFE

Perhaps as a partial outgrowth of the recent interest in overall adjustment to laryngectomy, the somewhat related issue of quality of life for laryngectomized individuals has also begun to receive increased attention. Quality of life (QOL) is a relatively new concept in the speech–pathology literature that represents the belief by some that there is more to the definition of postlaryngectomy rehabilitation success than simply surviving surgery and learning a new mode of communication (see Chapter 26 in this text). QOL is usually operationally defined by researchers on the basis of one or more measurements that purport to assess various aspects of postlaryngectomy life experience. DeSanto, Olsen, Perry, Rohe, and Keith (1995) examined their notion of QOL in three groups of individuals: total laryngectomy ($n = 111$), near-total laryngectomy ($n = 38$), and partial laryngectomy ($n = 23$). DeSanto et al. used the previously mentioned PAIS along with the *Mayo Clinic Postlaryngectomy Questionnaire* in an effort to determine the impact of surgery on areas of life experience, including health attitudes, work or school, relationship with spouse, sexuality, family relationships, hobbies and activities, and psychological status.

Somewhat surprisingly, individuals in the total and near-total laryngectomy groups had nearly the same perceptions about their QOL. This result suggests that voice is not a primary factor in determining QOL, because the total laryngectomy group used various forms of alaryngeal voice (including 50% who used an electrolarynx), whereas the near-total laryngectomy group used their own lung power and reconstructed, residual laryngeal tissue to produce voice. On the other hand, individuals in the partial laryngectomy group (no stoma) adjusted much better than those in the total or near-total groups (those individuals with a stoma) regardless of voice quality.

DeSanto et al. (1995) summarized their conclusions as follows:

1. Quality of life and quality of speech are not the same. Altered speech is consistent with a satisfactory quality of life.
2. Permanent tracheostomy seems to have a major influence on quality of life. Patients with a stoma but with lung-powered speech (near-total laryngectomy) report a quality of life very similar to that of patients who had total laryngectomy, many of whom communicate with an electrolarynx.
3. The measurement of quality of life is not standardized. More studies are needed. The goal of a standardized and acceptable measurement tool is realistic.
4. From this work, it is clear that the criteria used to measure success in cancer treatment, such as survival and function, are not sufficient. Understanding the full impact of what we do to patients is important. (p. 769)

Although the finding by DeSanto et al. (1995) of an apparent relationship between higher QOL ratings in the absence of a stoma is provocative, it should also be kept in mind that the groups comprising the respondents used in that study were substantially unequal in number. It is possible that the apparent relationship between absence of stoma and higher QOL ratings could be an artifact resulting from comparison of responses from only 23 individuals in the partial laryngec- tomy group with 149 responses from the combined total and near-total groups. Furthermore, the total laryngectomy ($n = 111$) and near-total laryngectomy ($n = 38$) groups consisted of both men and women, whereas the partial laryn- gectomy group ($n = 23$) included only men. Doyle's (1997) findings that showed a potential for gender bias, discussed earlier, should provide a note of caution in the interpretation of the findings by DeSanto et al. (1995).

Organ Preservation

If the findings of DeSanto et al. (1995) can be replicated, then nonsurgical treat- ment of laryngeal cancer, so that the patient has no stoma, might be a step toward enhancing the QOL for some laryngectomized individuals. Indeed, Orlikoff and Kraus (1996) indicated that increasing numbers of people with advanced laryn- geal carcinoma are choosing organ preservation or conservation treatments in- stead of the more traditional total laryngectomy (see Chapter 10 in this text). Un- fortunately, the improved ability to preserve the larynx even in advanced cases of laryngeal carcinoma may also result in the creation of voice problems specific to this population (see Chapter 11 in this text). As a result, the clinician may be less concerned about voice restoration, but may be faced with the equally challeng- ing task of voice rehabilitation (Doyle, 1997).

Because the long-term effects of organ-preservation treatments on voice and other functions are largely unknown, it is difficult to determine at this time what the successful management strategies might be. It is obvious, however, that simply opting for a nonsurgical treatment of advanced laryngeal cancer will not resolve all of the postoperative problems encountered by the person who under- goes total laryngectomy. In addition, the individual who chooses nonsurgical intervention still runs the risk of recurrence and subsequent salvage surgery (i.e., total laryngectomy) with all of its ramifications. As Orlikoff and Kraus (1996) pointed out,

> Clearly, an advanced cancer patient rendered severely dysphonic posttreat- ment may face greater communicative disturbance than the laryngectomized patient provided with effective voice restoration. Thus, it is the responsibility of physicians, voice specialists, and other health professionals to work in con- cert so that, ultimately, patients will not only present no evidence of disease, but no evidence of disability as well. (p. 51)

Although organ preservation and conservation treatments are in the early stages of development, they clearly represent a departure from earlier eras and provide yet another excellent example of a shift in thinking toward a more multi- dimensional view of overall successful rehabilitation of individuals diagnosed with cancer of the larynx. It can be anticipated that as nonsurgical treatments become more refined, they will have an increasing impact on the way in which people adjust to and cope with a diagnosis of laryngeal cancer.

Long-Term Effects of TE Fistulization

The notion of long-term, successful rehabilitation has also captured attention in the literature about the concern over the effects of the extended use of a TE prosthesis (see Chapters 17 and 18 in this text). Prior to the introduction of contemporary surgical–prosthetic voice restoration techniques (Singer & Blom, 1980), long-term success generally referred to survival rates and whether the laryngectomized person had acquired some type of alaryngeal speech that was "acceptable" for communication. There was no reason to suspect that, once learned, esophageal voice, use of an artificial larynx, or both would be abandoned over time unless there was evidence of recurrent disease.

In spite of widespread use of surgical–prosthetic voice restoration, however, it has become evident that TEP procedures are not without complications and that some individuals who have undergone TEP fail to continue to use TE speech as their primary means of communication (Bosone, 1994; Ho, Wei, Lain, & Lam, 1991; Jacobson, Franssen, Birt, Davidson, & Gilbert, 1997; Karlen & Maisel, 2001; see also Chapters 4 and 24 in this text). This observation has obvious implications for postlaryngectomy treatment planning and management, especially in view of some of the findings reported earlier in this chapter. In other words, if type of voice used is relatively unimportant with regard to postlaryngectomy coping, adjustment, and QOL (Blood et al., 1995; Blood et al., 1992) and if surgical–prosthetic voice restoration is found to have significant long-term failure rates, it could change clinicians' thinking about what is best for patients over the long run of their rehabilitation.

Fortunately, researchers have recognized this potential dilemma and have begun to examine success rates in an effort to determine criteria for candidacy, reduce postoperative failures, and ensure the successful and long-term use of TE speech. Cantu, Ryan, Tansey, and Johnson (1998) examined long-term success rates and predictors of success for 31 males and 5 females who had undergone either primary ($n = 22$) or secondary ($n = 14$) TEP. Cantu et al. were also interested in obtaining a preliminary measure of social (ecological) validity by comparing ratings of communicative effectiveness made by a speech–language pathologist with those made by the laryngectomized person or his or her significant other. Communication effectiveness was rated on a functional communication inventory similar to that proposed by Sarno (1969; as cited in Cantu et al., 1998).

Briefly, the functional communication inventory consists of a 5-point scale on which a value of 1 represents *no usable communication,* 3 represents *communication is moderately poorer from premorbid level,* and 5 indicates that *communication is at premorbid level.* Preliminary analysis of the functional communication ratings resulted in 23 participants receiving ratings of 4 or 5, and 13 participants receiving a rating of 1 or 2. Subsequently, participants with a rating of 4 or 5 were identified as being successful whereas those with ratings of 1 or 2 were identified as being unsuccessful.

Of importance to the present discussion, Cantu et al. (1998) found that approximately two thirds of the participants were judged to be successful at an average of approximately 4 years after their TE fistulization procedure. These data generally supported those reported by other investigators and confirmed the long-term nature of communication effectiveness in a majority of individuals undergoing surgical voice restoration. The findings also revealed, however, that a substantial proportion of individuals failed to achieve a long-term successful level of postoperative communication effectiveness, even though they may have achieved a level of speech success immediately following the TE fistulization procedure.

Interestingly, Cantu et al. (1998) also discovered that, in general, the speech–language pathologist and laryngectomized individual or significant other agreed when assessing postfistulization communication effectiveness as evidenced by their ratings on the functional communication inventory. However, in one third of the comparisons, there were discrepancies of at least one scale value, and the clinician almost always assigned the higher value (i.e., a rating that was more favorable). Cantu et al. speculated that the speech–language pathologist may be judging postoperative communication effectiveness based on experience and the immediate prelaryngectomy communication status, whereas the laryngectomized person or significant other might be using an idealized standard that would be difficult to achieve using TE voice production. Cantu et al. (1998) went on to state,

> Regardless of the underlying reasons for these discrepancies in judgment, clinicians should recognize that "success" according to a clinical standard may not necessarily be viewed at the same level or be based on the same standard from the vantage point of the patient or significant other. Accordingly, it might be necessary to place greater emphasis on establishing realistic postoperative expectations during preoperative counseling and education. (p. 16)

Not surprisingly, the comments of Cantu et al. (1998) are reminiscent of those made by others, including Salva and Kallail (1989), Oates et al. (1990), and Blood et al. (1992), mentioned earlier in this chapter. Consequently, "successful" postlaryngectomy rehabilitation is a complex phenomenon that encompasses far more than a single measure of acceptability of alaryngeal speech acquisition.

Observations

Although much has been learned about factors that may influence successful, long-term, total rehabilitation of the person with a laryngectomy, the reader should recognize that each study mentioned represents only one part of a complex picture, and that the results from any study can be affected by design limitations, small sample sizes, inadequate measurement instruments, and other pitfalls with which researchers are all too familiar. Nevertheless, some common themes have emerged that lend themselves to further discussion. The most troubling and pervasive finding was the direct and indirect evidence that pre- and postoperative counseling continues to be inadequate at best and totally absent at worst. In spite of approximately 50 years in which dozens of books and hundreds of articles have promoted and encouraged continuous counseling as part of successful management of laryngectomized individuals (Diedrich & Youngstrom, 1966; Doyle, 1994; Gardner, 1971; Gates, Ryan, Cantu, & Hearne, 1982; Keith & Darley, 1994; Salmon & Mount, 1991; Snidecor, 1962), researchers continue to report many instances of poor or inadequate counseling, even in the same studies that show the importance of good counseling in the overall adjustment of the laryngectomized person (Salva & Kallail, 1989; Stack, 1994).

Also, the findings of the studies reported herein have clearly confirmed that the type of alaryngeal speech and the proficiency with which it is used have little or no relationship to the overall adjustment of the patient with a laryngectomy. That is not to say that clinicians should abandon all efforts to provide each patient with the best possible postoperative voice; it merely suggests that preoccupation with speech type and skill may distract clinicians from other issues that can have a stronger influence on successful, long-term, total rehabilitation. It is not appropriate, then, to provide a person with an acceptable pseudovoice without a commitment to long-term follow-up in other important areas as well. Essentially, postlaryngectomy rehabilitation should be characterized by programs that emphasize a more holistic approach in which each individual is treated in the context of how laryngectomy specifically affects his or her life (see Chapter 6 in this text). For some individuals, that may mean long-term counseling and participation in a support group such as a local Lost Chord Club (see Chapters 25 and 26 in this text). For others, it could be something as simple as providing voice amplification in the work environment.

On a more positive note, it is encouraging to find that most laryngectomized individuals have adjusted well to their cancer and subsequent surgery (Blood et al., 1992). Moreover, the finding that older people with laryngectomies are as well adjusted as their younger counterparts, and that individuals more distant from their surgery have adjusted better than those who have had surgery more recently portends well for those concerned about the long-term nature of postlaryngectomy rehabilitation (Blood et al., 1995). Similarly, the relatively positive long-term success rates for surgical–prosthetic restoration of functional communication (Cantu et al., 1998) are encouraging for those who choose this form of speech rehabilitation. It should be remembered, however, that 20% to 30% of patients undergoing surgical–prosthetic voice restoration may not enjoy long-term success in the production of functional speech. This potential for a disparity between preoperative expectations and postoperative results should also be taken into account when counseling the laryngectomized person who is contemplating some type of TE fistulization procedure.

Largely through the efforts of Blood and coworkers (Blood et al., 1995; Blood et al., 1992), speech–language pathologists have better insight into the coping and adjustment problems confronting those who have undergone laryngectomy. Also, the field has reliable and valid measuring instruments that have direct clinical applications as screening tools and that can be used to collect useful data for research and cross-clinic comparisons. I am optimistic that future research will continue to enhance understanding of what constitutes successful, long-term, total rehabilitation for individuals with laryngectomies.

The speculation that the presence or absence of a stoma may be of major importance in determining overall quality of life for patients with laryngeal cancer, if confirmed through additional research, could have a substantial impact on clinicians' thinking about total rehabilitation of the individual. As noted by Orlikoff and Kraus (1996), methods are now available to treat even advanced laryngeal carcinoma without removal of the larynx. Given the apparent negative experiences associated with a tracheostoma, a shift may occur from traditional radical surgical treatment of laryngeal cancer to organ preservation or conservation therapies. If so, the clinical management of these individuals may have to begin addressing voice rehabilitation or conservation as opposed to voice restoration, although the long-term vocal effects of organ preservation methods are not well known. Presumably, however, there will be a need for continuing therapy and counseling regardless of the method chosen to control the cancer.

Overall, a number of changes in thinking about what comprises successful, total, rehabilitation of people with laryngeal cancer has occurred in recent years. Especially important is the understanding that total rehabilitation encompasses a great deal more than simply the restoration of speech. Clinicians can take some satisfaction from the findings that show apparent successful adjustment and good quality of life for a large majority of individuals with laryngectomy. A substantial number of individuals, however, continues to have difficulty coping with a diagnosis of cancer and adjusting to a life lived without a larynx (see Chapter 26 in this text). Ironically, although professionals already know how to help many laryngectomized individuals achieve a good quality of life and successful adjustment to their surgery, the professionals simply may not be doing it or may not have the time to do it in today's ever-changing managed care environment.

Good pre- and postoperative counseling and long-term follow-up have been consistently shown to be major factors in achieving successful, long-term rehabilitation for laryngectomized individuals (see Chapter 15 in this text). How to provide that counseling may be the next major challenge facing physicians, speech–language pathologists, and health care workers as they continue to pursue successful, long-term, total rehabilitation.

SUMMARY

This chapter was written from the position that the history of postlaryngectomy rehabilitation can be segmented into three eras: survivability, speech acquisition, and successful, long-term, total rehabilitation. Survivability and speech acquisition eras were reviewed briefly to provide a context for a more detailed discussion of selected studies that exemplify a recent trend toward concern about one or more aspects of successful, long-term, total rehabilitation. Areas of interest included communication satisfaction and its relationship to voicing proficiency, gender differences that may influence postlaryngectomy rehabilitation success, overall adjustment to laryngeal cancer and subsequent surgery, postlaryngectomy quality of life, consequences of voice preservation and conservation techniques, and long-term success of surgical–prosthetic voice restoration.

Although disparate in purpose and methodology, the studies reviewed have at least two common threads. First, they all represent a departure from an era in which speech acquisition was the primary focus of clinicians and researchers who were concerned about postlaryngectomy speech rehabilitation. Second, they all address aspects of postlaryngectomy rehabilitation that, when viewed collectively, provide a solid foundation for the continuing pursuit of successful, long-term, total rehabilitation for each individual who has undergone or will undergo treatment for cancer of the larynx. I feel optimistic that this era has only just begun and will ultimately bring with it a true understanding of what constitutes successful and total rehabilitation of people with laryngectomies.

REFERENCES

Baggs, T., & Pine, S. (1983). Acoustic characteristics: Tracheoesophageal speech. *Journal of Communication Disorders, 16,* 299–307.

Barney, H. L. (1958). A discussion of some technical aspects of speech aids for postlaryngectomized patients. *Annals of Otology, Rhinology and Laryngology, 67,* 558–570.

Barney, H. L., Haworth, F., & Dunn, H. (1959). An experimental transistorized artificial larynx. *Bell System Technical Journal, 38,* 1337–1356.

Bennett, S., & Weinberg, B. (1973). Acceptability ratings of normal, esophageal, and artificial larynx speech. *Journal of Speech and Hearing Research, 16,* 608–615.

Berlin, C. I. (1963). Clinical measurement of esophageal speech: I. Methodology and curves of skill acquisition. *Journal of Speech and Hearing Disorders, 28,* 42–51.

Berlin, C. I. (1965). Clinical measurement of esophageal speech: III. Performance of non–biased groups. *Journal of Speech and Hearing Disorders, 30,* 174–183.

Blom, E. D., Singer, M. I., & Hamaker, R. C. (1986). A prospective study of tracheoesophageal speech. *Archives of Otolarynogology—Head and Neck Surgery, 112,* 440–447.

Blood, G. W. (1993). Development and assessment of a scale addressing communication needs of patients with laryngectomies. *American Journal of Speech–Language Pathology, 2,* 82–90.

Blood, G. W., Blood, I. M., Kaufmann, S., Raimondi, S. C., & Dineen, M. (1995). A comparison of older and younger individuals living after the surgical treatment of laryngeal cancer. *Journal of Rehabilitation, 4,* 41–45.

Blood, G. W., Luther, A. R., & Stemple, J. C. (1992). Coping and adjustment in alaryngeal speakers. *American Journal of Speech–Language Pathology, 1,* 63–69.

Bosone, B. (1994). Tracheoesophageal fistulization/puncture for voice restoration: Presurgical considerations and troubleshooting procedures. In R. L. Keith & F. L. Darley (Eds.), *Laryngectomee rehabilitation* (pp. 359–381). Austin, TX: PRO-ED.

Brown, S. I., & Doyle, P. C. (1999). The woman who is laryngectomized: Parallels, perspectives, and reevaluation of practice. *Journal of Speech–Language Pathology and Audiology, 23,* 54–60.

Cantu, E., Ryan, W. J., Tansey, S., & Johnson, C. S. (1998). Tracheoesophageal speech: Predictors of success and social validity ratings. *American Journal of Otolaryngology, 19,* 12–17.

Damsté, P. H. (1958). *Oesophageal speech after laryngectomy.* Groningen, The Netherlands: Hoitsema.

DeSanto, L. W., Olsen, K. D., Perry, W. C., Rohe, D. E., & Keith, R. L. (1995). Quality of life after surgical treatment of cancer of the larynx. *Annals of Otology, Rhinology and Laryngology, 104,* 763–769.

DiCarlo, L. M., Amster, W., & Herer, G. (1955). *Speech after laryngectomy.* Syracuse, NY: Syracuse University Press.

Diedrich, W. M., & Youngstrom, K. A. (1966). *Alaryngeal speech.* Springfield, IL: Thomas.

Doyle, P. C. (1994). *Foundations of voice and speech rehabilitation following laryngeal cancer.* San Diego, CA: Singular.

Doyle, P. C. (1997). Voice refinement following conservation surgery for cancer of the larynx: A conceptual framework for treatment intervention. *American Journal of Speech–Language Pathology, 6,* 27–35.

Doyle, P. C., & White, H. D. (2004, May). *Use of the Rotterdam Symptom Checklist in laryngectomized men and women.* Paper presented at the Annual Conference of the Canadian Association of Speech–Language Pathologists and Audiologists, Ottawa, Ontario.

Eadie, T. L., & Doyle, P. C. (2004). Auditory–perceptual scaling and quality of life in tracheoesophageal speakers. *Laryngoscope, 114,* 753–759.

Fairbanks, G. (1960). *Voice and articulation handbook.* New York: Harper and Row.

Gardner, W. H. (1971). *Laryngectomee speech rehabilitation.* Springfield, IL: Thomas.

Gates, G. A., Ryan, W., Cantu, E., & Hearne, E. (1982). Current status of laryngectomee rehabilitation: II. Causes of failure. *American Journal of Otolaryngology, 3,* 8–14.

Gates, G. A., Ryan, W., Cooper, J. C., Lawliss, G. F., Cantu, E., Hayashi, T., Lauder, E., Welch, R. W., & Hearne, E. (1982). Current status of laryngectomee rehabilitation: I. Results of therapy. *American Journal of Otolaryngology, 3,* 1–7.

Gates, G. A., Ryan, W., & Lauder, E. (1982). Current status of laryngectomee rehabilitation: IV. Attitudes about laryngectomee rehabilitation should change. *American Journal of Otolaryngology, 3,* 97–103.

Gilmore, S. I. (1994). The physical, social, occupational, and psychological concomitants of laryngectomy. In R. L. Keith, & F. L. Darley (Eds.), *Laryngectomee rehabilitation* (pp. 395–486). Austin, TX: PRO-ED.

Ho, C. M., Wei, W. I., Lain, W. F., & Lam, K. H. (1991). Tracheostomal stenosis after immediate tracheoesophageal puncture. *Archives of Otolaryngology—Head and Neck Surgery, 117,* 662–665.

Hoops, H. R., & Curtis, J. F. (1971). Intelligibility of the esophageal speaker. *Archives of Otolaryngology, 93,* 300–303.

Horn, D. (1962). *Laryngectomy survey report.* New York: International Association of Laryngectomees.

Hunt, R. B. (1964). Rehabilitation of the laryngectomee. *Laryngoscope, 74,* 382–395.

Hyman, M. (1955). An experimental study of artificial larynx and esophageal speech. *Journal of Speech and Hearing Disorders, 20,* 291–299.

Jacobson, M. C., Franssen, E., Birt, B. D., Davidson, M. J., & Gilbert, R. W. (1997). Predicting post-laryngectomy voice outcome in an era of primary tracheoesophageal fistulization: A retrospective evaluation. *Journal of Otolaryngology, 26,* 171–179.

Karlen, R. G., & Maisel, R. H. (2001). Does primary tracheoesophageal puncture reduce complications after laryngectomy and improve patient communication? *American Journal of Otolaryngology, 22,* 324–328.

Keith, R. L., & Darley, F. L. (Eds.). (1994). *Laryngectomee rehabilitation* (3rd ed.). Austin, TX: PRO-ED.

King, P. S., Fowlks, E. W., & Peirson, G. A. (1968). Rehabilitation and adaptation of laryngectomy patients. *American Journal of Physical Medicine, 47,* 192–203.

Moon, J. B., & Weinberg, B. (1987). Aerodynamic and myoelastic contributions to tracheoesophageal voice production. *Journal of Speech and Hearing Research, 30,* 387–395.

Oates, J., Lochert, S., & McMahon, J. (1990). Change in communicative satisfaction experienced by laryngectomees and their spouses post-laryngectomy. *Australian Journal of Human Communication Disorders, 18,* 5–17.

Orlikoff, R. F., & Kraus, D. H. (1996). Dysphonia following nonsurgical management of advanced laryngeal carcinoma. *American Journal of Speech–Language Pathology, 5,* 47–52.

Qi, Y., & Weinberg, B. (1991). Spectral slope vowels produced by tracheoesophageal speakers. *Journal of Speech and Hearing Research, 34,* 243–247.

Robbins, J. (1984). Acoustic differentiation of laryngeal, esophageal, and tracheoesophageal speech. *Journal of Speech and Hearing Research, 27,* 577–585.

Robbins, J., Fisher, H., Blom, E., & Singer, M. (1984). A comparative acoustic study of normal, esophageal, and tracheoesophageal speech production. *Journal of Speech and Hearing Disorders, 49,* 202–210.

Ryan, W., Gates, G. A., Cantu, E., & Hearne, E. (1982). Current status of laryngectomee rehabilitation: III. Understanding esophageal speech. *American Journal of Otolaryngology, 3,* 91–96.

Salmon, S. J., & Goldstein, L. P. (1978). *The Artificial Larynx Handbook.* New York: Grune & Stratton.

Salmon, S. J., & Mount, K. H. (Eds.). (1991). *Alaryngeal speech rehabilitation: For clinicians by clinicians.* Austin, TX: PRO-ED.

Salva, C. T., & Kallail, K. J. (1989). An investigation of the counseling needs of male and female laryngectomees. *Journal of Communication Disorders, 22,* 291–304.

Schaefer, S., & Johns, D. (1982). Attaining esophageal speech. *Archives of Otolaryngology, 108,* 647–649.

Sedory, S. E., Hamlet, S. L., & Connor, N. P. (1989). Comparisons of perceptual and acoustic characteristics of tracheoesophageal and excellent esophageal speech. *Journal of Speech and Hearing Disorders, 54,* 209–214.

Singer, M. I., & Blom, E. D. (1980). An endoscopic technique for restoration of voice after laryngectomy. *Annals of Otology, Rhinology and Laryngology, 89,* 529–533.

Snidecor, J. C. (Ed.). (1962). *Speech rehabilitation of the laryngectomized.* Springfield, IL: Thomas.

Snidecor, J. C. (1975). Some scientific foundations for voice restoration. *Laryngoscope, 85,* 640–648.

Stack, F. M. (1994). The feminine viewpoint of being a laryngectomee. In R. L. Keith & F. L. Darley (Eds.), *Laryngectomee rehabilitation* (pp. 515–521). Austin, TX: PRO-ED.

Tardy-Mitzell, S., Andrews, M. L., & Bowman, S. A. (1985). Acceptability and intelligibility of tracheoesophageal speech. *Archives of Otolaryngology, 111,* 213–215.

Terrell, J. E., Ronis, D. L., Fowler, K. E., Bradford, C. R., Chepeha, D. B., Prince, M. E., Teknos, T. N., Wolf, G. T., & Duffy, S. A. (2004). Clinical predictors of quality of life in patients with head and neck cancer. *Archives of Otolaryngology—Head and Neck Surgery, 130,* 401–408.

Vuyk, H. D., Festin, J. M., Spoelstra, A. J. G., & Tiwari, R. M. (1987). Acoustic and aerodynamic parameters of speech after laryngectomy and the Staffieri procedure. *Clinical Otolaryngology, 12,* 421–428.

Weinberg, B., & Bennett, S. (1972). Selected acoustic characteristics of esophageal speech produced by female laryngectomees. *Journal of Speech and Hearing Research, 15,* 211–216.

Williams, S. E., Scanio, T. S., & Ritterman, S. R. (1989). Temporal and perceptual characteristics of tracheoesophageal voice. *Laryngoscope, 99,* 846–850.

Williams, S. E., & Watson, J. B. (1988). The relationship between communication attitudes, voicing methods, and speaking proficiency of laryngectomees. *Australian Journal of Human Communication Disorders, 16,* 57–69.

Chapter 6

The Perceptual Nature of Alaryngeal Voice and Speech

Philip C. Doyle and Tanya L. Eadie

Research addressing voice and speech production and perception following total laryngectomy has a long history in the speech pathology, speech science, and medical literature. In many instances this body of research has been descriptive and comparative (Doyle, 1994), with alaryngeal speech methods being evaluated relative to the inherent characteristics (broadly defined) of normal laryngeal voice and speech. This type of work has often led to comparisons of alaryngeal methods with the voice and speech of normal laryngeal speakers. Comparisons of this nature, however, may have served little purpose in understanding alaryngeal speech production.[1] By comparing methods of alaryngeal speech with one another, many researchers assumed that one method would emerge as "superior" to others, at least as it pertained to any given parameter or dimension under investigation. Nevertheless, attempts at defining the superiority of one alaryngeal method over that of another have fallen considerably short of this goal.

The purpose of this chapter is to address issues related to the productive and perceptual character of alaryngeal speech. By learning to better understand the types of signal changes that exist following total laryngectomy, and how the new voice source interacts with the postlaryngectomy vocal tract for any mode of alaryngeal speech, researchers may be able to anticipate the influence of these types of changes on the larger issue of "communication." Specifically, the collective attributes of alaryngeal voice and speech, rather than discrete parameters, are likely to provide a better index of speaker performance. Because performance is an essential component of communicating, professionals might be better served by examining postlaryngectomy voice and speech within a social context. In keeping with the theme of communicative performance and the necessary outgrowth that might be termed "communication effectiveness," a different type of descriptive perceptual information would seem to be urgently needed; that is, comprehensive perceptual judgments of alaryngeal speech provide the ultimate index of postlaryngectomy communication effectiveness or success as perceived by the listener in a communicative context. Thus, the most critical component of auditory–perceptual measures may be seen in the area of rehabilitation, which the World Health Organization (WHO, 2000) has termed "participation" in the *International Classification of Functioning, Disability and Health* (ICIDH–2).

Within the ICIDH–2 context, "participation" reflects one's involvement in life situations. Participation restrictions (formerly called "handicap") (WHO, 1980) may be experienced by an individual who has difficulty communicating, thereby limiting his or her involvement in societal activities. We address issues related to these difficulties through a brief review of basic information on productive elements of alaryngeal speech, along with a selective evaluation of perceptual studies

---

[1]Evaluation of speech intelligibility is likely to be the most justified type of comparison between methods of alaryngeal speech and that of normal "control" speakers. The type of stimuli used, however, may have significant influences on the objective intelligibility scores gathered. For example, the phonetic structure of standard word lists may have considerable influences on the intelligibility scores obtained for the same speaker or speaker group (Doyle & Glenn, 1988; Glenn & Doyle, 1989).

that have appeared in the literature over the past 40 years.[2] Our specific goal is to encourage and outline a path of continuing research into the perceptual characteristics of all methods of alaryngeal speech. Our goal is to provide an improved understanding of what best describes postlaryngectomy verbal communication in the context of judgments by listeners. By doing so, we hope to stimulate further study and the development of clinical tools that will assist in identifying strengths and weaknesses of each method of communication. Although no single alaryngeal speech method is perfect, some sets of strengths and weaknesses may be more acceptable to a given individual when specific communicative needs are considered.

The discussion to follow begins with an overview of information on what is known about specific aspects of alaryngeal speech. The discussion centers on parametric measures of the alaryngeal voice and speech signal. In large part, this information is related to physical measures of the vocal signal. Physical descriptions of alaryngeal speech provide a starting point from which more global descriptions of alaryngeal speech may emerge. Thus, although knowledge of isolated parameters or features is not unimportant, it is the collective attribute of the alaryngeal speech signal that most likely serves a listener's ability to judge the proficiency of an alaryngeal speaker. This link may provide a unique perspective from which an improved understanding of how listeners evaluate and judge alaryngeal speakers may be garnered.

THE NATURE OF ALARYNGEAL SPEECH

Information obtained from previous descriptive and comparative work on alaryngeal voice and speech has provided a substantial database from which professionals, as well as those individuals who undergo total laryngectomy, can benefit. Descriptive information obtained and reported to date provides a framework from which a simple comparison across alaryngeal methods can occur. The information gathered from this collective body of descriptive and comparative work has great potential value for determining the direct influence of surgical treatment, and possibly rehabilitation, on specific unidimensional measures of voice and speech (fundamental frequency, speech rate, etc.) or on the multidimensional character of the person's ability to verbally communicate. Using today's vernacular, this prior work has the capacity to serve as a frame of reference

---

[2]For our "selective" review, we include a group of publications that has been frequently referenced as "key" contributions relative to alaryngeal speech. Such a selective review carries with it the potential for bias by the authors. However, within this review we have attempted to identify areas of concern where continuing controversy exists for specific data pools, rather than controversy perceived solely by the present authors. As with all work published in the literature dealing with communication and its disorders, we must seek to identify concerns in the areas of both internal and external validity of findings. The reassessment of past work has the following goals: (a) identifying areas of inconsistency as they pertain to specific productive or perceptual dimensions for alaryngeal speech; (b) detecting the presence and or absence of "statistically" identified dimensions or features; and (c) identifying apparent statistical relationships between a given set of features. Such examination will help reveal new questions for empirical inquiry.

for determining one or more aspect(s) of postlaryngectomy outcomes for individuals who use alaryngeal speech (esophageal, tracheoesophageal, or artificial laryngeal methods of postlaryngectomy communication). Use of these types of measures as an index of rehabilitation outcome may, however, be poorly understood; that is, regardless of the mode used by a given individual, the essential nature of the alaryngeal voice and speech signal is not normal. In this regard, multidimensional aspects of the voice, such as issues of alaryngeal *voice quality,* may become primary to assessment, monitoring, and perhaps treatment design considerations for all methods of postlaryngectomy verbal communication (Beaudin, Doyle, & Eadie, 2004; Beaudin, Meltzner, Doyle, & Hillman, 2004).

The concern over what dimension may best describe the effectiveness, efficiency, or proficiency of alaryngeal speech has direct and tremendous impact on how clinicians and their patients must view all methods of alaryngeal speech. Unfortunately, the clinical application of traditional descriptive and comparative data presented in the literature has limited utility relative to alaryngeal speech. In essence, measures of particular physical parameters of the alaryngeal signal (e.g., frequency, loudness) and, perhaps more important, perceptual measures of psychophysical aspects of that same parameter, have been stripped of a contextual reference. Despite the rather substantial database obtained relative to physical and sometimes related psychophysical measures, little work has been pursued in relation to what perceptual measures (i.e., features or descriptors) best define a given type of alaryngeal voice and speech. Additionally, little is known about how these features correlate with one another and, ultimately, what perceptual characteristics may best serve as a clinical outcome measure for each type of alaryngeal speaker. The point to be stressed in this context pertains to how these measures merge to form a cohesive whole that will most likely characterize speaker proficiency.

THE IMPACT OF ALARYNGEAL VOICE AND SPEECH ON THE LISTENER

One could argue that the fundamental concern about the ultimate communicative impact of any method of alaryngeal speech production is directly manifested in how the listener makes judgments about the alaryngeal signal. The potential exists to perceptually scale "features" that have direct physical correlates in alaryngeal speech (e.g., pitch and frequency). In isolation, these types of discrete measures are not likely to have true rehabilitative value specific to alaryngeal methods of postlaryngectomy verbal communication. Stated differently, although perceptual "trees" do indeed comprise the "forest" of psychological (and most likely psychophysical) reality, we would like to suggest that successful postlaryngectomy rehabilitative outcomes specific to communication are best indexed by making judgments of the forest in a more naturalistic framework. Doing so is likely to have direct and critical bearing upon the individual from a social perspective, and hence may be the most valuable measure of each individual's postlaryngectomy and posttherapeutic performance. The concerns noted above necessarily have significant clinical importance for both the speech–language pathologist and those who will or have undergone total laryngectomy for cancer treatment. It also affects family members and other individuals within the social milieu of the person who lost his or her larynx to cancer.

DESCRIPTIVE ASPECTS OF ALARYNGEAL VOICE AND SPEECH

Much of the empirical work concerning alaryngeal speech to date has, for the most part, focused on evaluation and determination of the so-called objective measures of voice and speech relative to physical dimensions. Considerable information is available on all methods of alaryngeal speech, including esophageal, electrolaryngeal, and tracheoesophageal (TE) communication modes. A rich literature is available outlining postlaryngectomy alaryngeal speech measures in the frequency, intensity, and durational domains, with seminal reports in the literature providing classic contributions in this area (e.g., Blom, Singer, & Hamaker, 1986; Curry & Snidecor, 1961; Diedrich, 1968; Robbins, Fisher, Blom, & Singer, 1984; Weinberg & Bennett, 1972). Early research required professionals to seek information on what parametric decrements were observed and thus provide a means to determine "how good" a given alaryngeal speaker or given alaryngeal speaker group was in relation to other alaryngeal speakers or speaker groups. Not surprisingly, the findings of this broad body of work have repeatedly found that alaryngeal voice and speech differ significantly from that of the signal produced by the normal larynx. Although this finding is not unexpected to those familiar with postlaryngectomy voice, the multidimensional interaction of these changes at the level of listener perception, and upon communication, is less well understood.

Numerous factors have been inconsistently identified as potential "predictors" of alaryngeal speech success, yet definitive predictors have yet to emerge. As stated by Weinberg (1982), "Although significant relationships have been found between a sizable number of variables and speech proficiency, such data should not be interpreted to support the view that predictors for esophageal voice and speech have been established"(p. 29). Although Weinberg's statement relates specifically to esophageal speech, the same can be said for all other methods of alaryngeal voice and speech, including artificial laryngeal speech and TE speech. The critical communicative link between speaker and listener defines the efficiency of human communication, and for the purposes of the present discussion, this linkage best defines how any given alaryngeal signal is judged perceptually. Thus, information related to how the listener evaluates the alaryngeal speaker is of critical importance if therapy endeavors are to be optimized to effect the best performance or to reduce the societal penalty from a communicative perspective (Eadie & Doyle, 2004).

Descriptive information on alaryngeal voice and speech has proliferated in the literature, particularly over the past three decades. Information provided in the literature presents a comprehensive and rational basis for understanding a variety of changes that occur in the speech capacity of the alaryngeal system. Although an exhaustive summary of this information exceeds the needs of this chapter, it is important to acknowledge some of the trends. Physical measures of the alaryngeal signal are the most prominent in the literature; hence, summarizing such information is of value in the present context. Fundamental frequency, intensity, and durational measures of alaryngeal voice and speech form the largest body of descriptive information on postlaryngectomy communication. We provide selected summaries of information on these physical measures to identify the significant reductions in the speech of those who must acquire an alaryngeal mode of verbal communication. Rehabilitative outcomes specific to objective physical measures (frequency, intensity, and duration) are summarized first, followed by a discussion of global auditory–perceptual judgments (i. e., intelligibility, voice quality and acceptability) and multidimensional aspects of listener perception.

Fundamental Frequency

From a comparative standpoint, information on fundamental frequency gathered from esophageal, tracheoesophageal, and artificial laryngeal speakers, as well as from normal laryngeal speakers, is provided in Table 6.1. This summary clearly documents the changes associated with the physical dimension that corresponds to the perceptual identification of the speaker's pitch level. Individuals who rely on an intrinsic method of alaryngeal speech, either esophageal or TE, exhibit substantial reductions in the frequency domain compared to normal speakers. This change is directly related to the vibratory characteristics and inherent limitations of the upper esophageal or pharyngoesophageal segment used for voice generation in these alaryngeal methods. In esophageal speakers, this level of reduced fundamental frequency capability is related to the fact that the alaryngeal voice source is a rather fixed system in respect to its inability to be modified in any substantial fashion. Thus, some esophageal speakers may be restricted in their ability to substantially modulate frequency because they are unable to modify the structural characteristics of the sphincter that result in perceptually recognizable changes in pitch (Damsté, 1994; Salmon, 1994; Shanks, 1994a, 1994b; Snidecor & Curry, 1960; Weinberg & Bennett, 1972).

In contrast, although TE speakers use the same vibratory structure for alaryngeal voicing, these speakers are able to modulate fundamental frequency due to their direct access of the pulmonary system. Access to the substantial air volume of the lungs facilitates these speakers' abilities to achieve higher transpseudoglottal airflows, with subsequent changes in the duty cycle of the voicing source (Robbins et al., 1984).[3] Despite the increased airflows allowed by TE speech, limitations in attaining normal ranges for pitch are most obvious for female TE and esophageal speakers (Shanks, 1994c; Trudeau, 1994). For example,

---

[3]Trans-pseudoglottal refers to airflow across the upper esophageal sphincter or pharyngoesophageal segment. Although esophageal speakers also require such airflow across the sphincter, their ability to increase flow rates is reduced due to the limited volume of the esophageal reservoir during traditional esophageal speech production (see Chapter 21 in this text).

TABLE 6.1

Comparative Mean Values for Fundamental Frequency (F_o) Measures Obtained for Normal Laryngeal (L), Esophageal (E), Tracheoesophageal (TE), and Electrolaryngeal (EL) Male and Female Speakers

Study	Sample	Acoustical Measures (mean F_o)	Perceptual Measures
Weinberg & Bennett (1972)	15 female E 18 male E	Female: 87 Hz Male: 69 Hz	
Blood (1984)	10 male TE 10 male E 10 male L	*Oral Reading* TE: 88.3 Hz E: 64.6 Hz L: 120.8 Hz *Sustained Vowels* TE: 89.3 Hz E: 63.6 Hz L: 119.5 Hz	
Robbins, Fisher, Blom, & Singer (1984)	15 male TE 15 male E 15 male L	*Oral Reading* TE: 101.7 Hz E: 77.1 Hz L: 102.8 Hz	
Robbins et al. (1984)		*Sustained Vowels* TE: 82.8 Hz E: 65.3 Hz L: 103.4 Hz	
Williams & Watson (1985)	12 male TE 12 male E 12 male EL		*Pitch and Voice Quality* Informed Listeners: TE > E, EL E > EL Expert Listeners: ns diff pitch (TE, E, EL)
Trudeau & Qi (1990)	10 female TE	*Oral Reading* 108.6 Hz (77.7–147.4 Hz)	
Finizia, Dotevall, Lund-ström, & Lindström (1999)	12 male TE 12 male RT, with larynx 10 male L	*Oral Reading* 105.2 Hz; ns diff with RT, or L	

Note. ns diff = not significant difference; RT = radiation therapy.

Trudeau and Qi (1990) noted that 10 female TE speakers had a mean fundamental frequency of 108.6 Hz. This compares with expected means of 165 to 255 Hz for normal female laryngeal speakers (Fitch & Holbrook, 1970). In contrast, male TE speakers were found to have a mean fundamental frequency of 101.7 Hz during oral reading (Robbins et al., 1984). This value falls in the range normally expected for male laryngeal speakers (Fitch & Holbrook, 1970). The potential societal penalties for a lowered pitch in female alaryngeal speakers, therefore, might differentially impact issues such as self-acceptance, femininity, and rehabilitative success judged by others in a social context. Such differential gender-related effects remain a topic for further investigation.

Intensity

Information related to intensity and its perceptual correlate, loudness, as it pertains to alaryngeal speakers is found in Table 6.2. Similar to frequency effects, use of pulmonary air for speech subsequent to the TE puncture voice restoration

TABLE 6.2

Comparative Mean Values for Intensity (dB SPL) Measures Obtained for Normal Laryngeal (L), Esophageal (E), Tracheoesophageal (TE), and Electrolaryngeal (EL) Male Speakers

Study	Sample	Acoustical Measures (mean, dB SPL)	Perceptual Measures

Weinberg, Horii, & Smith (1980)	10 E
	5 L
		Oral Reading
		  E: 65.1 (61.9–69.0)
		  L: 74.5
		
		Modal Intensity Level
		  E: 67
		  L: 82	

Baggs & Pine (1983)	5 TE 4 E 5 L		TE, L; ns diff TE, L > E on relative intensity

Blood (1984)	10 TE
	10 E
	10 L
		Oral Reading
		  TE: 82
		  E: 70
		  L: 84	

Robbins, Fisher, Blom, & Singer (1984)	15 TE
	15 E
	15 L
		Oral Reading
		  TE: 79.4
		  E: 59.3
		  L: 69.3
		
		Sustained Vowels
		  TE: 88.1
		  E: 73.8
		  L: 76.9	

Williams & Watson (1985)	12 TE
	12 E
	12 EL
			Oral Reading
			Naive Listeners:
			  TE > EL
			Informed Listeners:
			  TE > E, EL; E > EL
			Expert Listeners:
			  ns diff (TE, E, EL)

Max, Steurs, & de Bruyn (1996)	10 TE
	10 E
		Maximum Intensity Level
		  E: 61.9
		  TE: 70.7	

Note. db SPL = decibels–sounds pressure level; ns diff = not significant difference.

procedure allows for acoustic speech characteristics that are more like those of normal speakers (e.g., Blood, 1984; Robbins et al., 1984). In fact, pressure-related factors (Searl, 2002), coupled with high airflow rates and neuromuscular and biomechanical constraints imposed by the nature of the source, may indicate why some researchers have found that on average TE speakers produce speech at levels 10 dB more intense than laryngeal speakers (e.g., Robbins et al., 1984). Intensity level (loudness) represents a relative weakness of esophageal speech. As highlighted by Van Riper and Emerick (1984, p. 399), the weakness of the sound produced has been listed among the most important disadvantages of esophageal speech. This may well contribute to a reduced intelligibility among esophageal speakers (see the later section titled "Intelligibility") at multiple levels (phonemic, word, etc.).

Durational Measures

Comparative and descriptive data relative to durational measures of alaryngeal speech are found in Table 6.3. TE speakers use pulmonary air and therefore speak at rates comparable to normal. Esophageal speakers' rates, however, are slower on average because of the time involved in insufflation and the capacity limits of the esophageal reservoir (Diedrich, 1968; Salmon, 1994). This same air charge is sufficient for only about 3 or 4 words (Pindzola & Cain, 1989; Snidecor & Curry, 1959, 1960). Contrasting with the internal mode of esophageal voice production, users of electrolaryngeal devices seem to speak at rates closer to normal speakers due to an entirely external power supply and vibrator source. One possible explanation for the slower rate of electrolaryngeal speech compared with laryngeal speech may be the associated tradeoff with articulatory precision. For example, Hillman, Walsh, Wolf, Fisher, and Hong (1998) found that speakers using electrolaryngeal speech had a rate of 130 words per minute (wpm), which is slower than that expected for normal laryngeal speakers (149.5–196.1 wpm).

Intelligibility

When speech intelligibility is compared across speakers using alaryngeal voice and speech production methods, most studies have found that the highest intelligibility scores were obtained for TE speech (e.g., Blom et al., 1986; Pindzola & Cain, 1988). These studies have also demonstrated, however, that none of the three major modes of alaryngeal communication is 100% intelligible, and that a great amount of variation exists across modes and particular users (see Table 6.4). There is no doubt that specific parameters feed into the ability to be understood by others, including, but not limited to, the features already outlined such as frequency–pitch, intensity–loudness, and rate. Aspects of voice quality, however, also potentially contribute to intelligibility ratings. For example, in a study that investigated laryngeal speakers diagnosed with amyotrophic lateral sclerosis, Southwood and Weismer (1993) found that voice–speech qualities

TABLE 6.3

Comparative Mean Values for Speaking Rate Obtained for Normal Laryngeal (L), Esophageal (E), Tracheoesophageal (TE), and Electrolaryngeal (EL) Male and Female Speakers

Study	Sample	Acoustical Measures	Perceptual Measures
Robbins, Fisher, Blom, & Singer (1984)	15 male TE 15 male E 15 male L	*Oral Reading* (wpm) TE: 127.5 E: 99.1 L: 172.8	
Pindzola & Cain (1989)	5 TE 5 E 15 L	*Oral Reading* (wpm) TE: 152.2 E: 93.8 L: 158.8	
Trudeau & Qi (1990)	10 female TE	*Oral Reading* (wpm) 138.03 (87.5–198.6)	
Hillman, Walsh, Wolf, Fisher, & Hong (1998)	21 (mostly male) TE 5 E 30 EL	*Oral Reading* Syllables/min TE: 191.6 E: 121.1 EL: 160.6 wpm (Normals, expect 149.5–196.1) TE: 155 E: 98 EL: 130	
Finizia, Dotevall, Lundström, & Lindström (1999)	12 male TE 12 male RT, with larynx 10 male L		*Inhalation Time* TE > RT, L ns diff in breathing pauses

Note. wpm = words per minute; RT = radiation therapy; ns diff = not significant difference.

such as naturalness, bizarreness, acceptability, and normalcy were dependent on a global rating of severity, as indexed by intelligibility scores. The multidimensional nature of such features remains a focus of alaryngeal communicators and a topic for further investigation. Such interactions will be discussed in a later section, "Interrelationships Among Physical and Perceptual Measures."

Voice Quality and Acceptability

Although voice–speech "acceptability" of TE speakers has been shown to be high (e.g., Tardy-Mitzell, Andrews, & Bowman, 1985; Trudeau, 1987), it must be emphasized that the voice quality of alaryngeal methods is clearly judged less acceptable and poorer than that of normal laryngeal speakers (see Table 6.5). Moreover, even when acoustical (so-called objective) measures such as frequency

TABLE 6.4

Comparative Mean Values for Intelligibility Measures (% Understood by Listeners) Obtained for Normal Laryngeal (L), Esophageal (E), Tracheoesophageal (TE), and Electrolaryngeal (EL) Male and Female Speakers

Study	Sample	Perceptual Measures

Williams & Watson (1985)	12 male TE
	12 male E
	12 male EL
		Naive Listeners:
		  TE, E > EL
		Informed Listeners:
		  TE > E, EL; E > EL
		Expert Listeners:
		  TE > E, EL

Weiss & Basili (1985)	2 EL	6 Experienced Listeners:[a] Western Electric: $M = 33\%$ (16%– 54%) Servox: $M = 36\%$ (19%–55%)

Doyle, Danhauer, & Reed (1988)	3 male E
	3 male TE
	1 male dual mode
	  communicator
		Stimuli: CVCVC
		  E: 56% (52%–62%)
		  TE: 65% (59%–72%)
		  Dual: 42% E; 71% TE (TE > E)

Pindzola & Cain (1988)	5 TE
	5 E
	5 L
		Stimuli: Words in a Multiple-choice
		  test (24 months postop.)
		  E: 83.12%
		  TE: 93.2%
		  L: 94.0%
		  (L, TE > E)

Hillman, Walsh, Wolf, Fisher, & Hong (1998)	(Mostly male)
	21 TE
	  5 E
	30 EL
		Stimuli: Phonetically balanced
		  word list
		  TE: 91.9% (±7.5)
		  E: 90.0% (±8.0)
		  EL: 80.5% (±12.0)

Finizia, Dotevall, Lundström, & Lindström (1999)	12 male TE
	12 male RT, with larynx
	10 male L
		Self-Assessment
		  TE < RT, L
		Other Listeners:
		  TE < RT, L

[a]Most common perceptual error for voiceless stops in initial position was for voiced cognate. When initial voiced stops were intended, intelligibility increased to higher levels (64%–90%).

perturbation (i.e., jitter) do not detect differences in speakers, there is a difference perceptually. Finizia, Dotevall, Lundström, and Lindström (1999) found that, according to assessments of voice quality and acceptability by both self and others, those speakers who had undergone a laryngectomy (TE speakers) were found to be perceptually poorer in voice quality and less acceptable than both normal speakers and those who had undergone radiation therapy instead of the surgical procedure. These ratings occurred despite the fact that the acoustic data showed no statistical difference between the individuals who had undergone radiation therapy and those who had undergone laryngectomy and used TE speech. This example serves to illustrate the following principle: Although alaryngeal modes of

TABLE 6.5

Comparative Values for Acoustical and Perceptual Voice Quality Measures Obtained for Normal Laryngeal (L), Esophageal (E), Tracheoesophageal (TE), and Electrolaryngeal (EL) Male and Female Speakers

Study	Sample	Acoustical Measures	Perceptual Measures
Clark & Stemple (1982)	1 L 1 TE 1 E 1 EL (Servox)		20 Listeners: *Most Pleasant* TE: 55% AL: 25% E: 20% *Least Pleasant* E: 60% AL: 20% TE: 20%

Robbins, Fisher, Blom, & Singer (1984)	15 male TE
	15 male E
	15 male L
		Jitter (Frequency perturbation)
		  M (Hz) Ratio
		  TE: 0.7 51.4
		  E: 4.1 182.5
		  L: 0.1 7.7
		Shimmer (Amplitude perturbation)
		  TE: 0.8 dB SPL
		  E: 1.9 dB SPL
		  L: 0.3 dB SPL	

van As, Hilgers, Verdonck-de Leeuw, & Koopmans-van Beinum (1998)	21 male TE (Servox) 20 male L	*NHR* *APQ* *sPPQ* TE: .505 17.2% 7.82% L: .168 7.10% 1.01% Significant difference for all acoustic measures (TE worse quality than L for all but mean F_o).	TE < L TE rated more ugly, unsteady, weak, dull, breathy, low, abnormal.
Finizia, Dotevall, Lundström, & Lindström (1999)	12 male TE 12 male RT, with larynx 10 male L	*Acoustics* *Frequency perturbation* L < RT, TE (no diff)	*Voice Quality and Acceptability* Self-Assessment: TE < L, RT Other Listeners: TE < L, RT

Note. NHR = noise to harmonics ratio; APQ = amplitude perturbation quotient; sPPQ = smoothed pitch period perturbation quotient; F_o = fundamental frequency; RT = radiation therapy.

communication have improved in the past few decades, alaryngeal speakers can still be identified as "different" from the normal laryngeal speaker (Eadie & Doyle, 2002, 2004; van As, Koopmans-van Beinum, Pols, & Hilgers, 2003). This perceived difference has implications for social interaction and adjustment of people who undergo laryngectomy and also targets an area for further research improvements in alaryngeal voice production development. Broad auditory–perceptual dimensions, such as voice quality and acceptability, also assume more of a social context than parameters such as pitch, loudness, or rate.

Interrelationships Among Physical and Perceptual Measures

The multidimensional nature of the alaryngeal signal represents the critical interaction between the sound source and the resonant capacity of the postlaryngectomy vocal tract; that is, the signal carries the emphasis of how the listener perceives alaryngeal speech, and it consequently mirrors how the listener makes judgments about the speaker. Shipp (1967) was the first investigator to seek information on potential relationships between frequency and durational measures and "acceptability" judgments by listeners. His work was based on acoustic measures and perceptual judgments of the second sentence of the "Rainbow Passage" (Fairbanks, 1960). One of Shipp's most prominent findings was that increased pitch levels demonstrated by a group of 33 esophageal speakers elicited better listener judgments for speech acceptability. Although this potential relationship had been noted in an earlier study by Snidecor and Curry (1960), no clear identification of this possible relationship existed before Shipp's (1967) report. Shipp also found that several other factors he studied revealed significant correlations. His data suggested that, in addition to mean fundamental frequency, measures of total duration, a respiratory noise rating, the percentage of periodic phonation, and the percentage of silence appeared to influence listener judgments. This study was the first to provide empirical support for the idea that potential relationships between specific measures, either physical or perceptual, may have influenced listener judgments at least for esophageal voice–speech signals.

At a minimum Shipp's (1967) study suggested that some factors correlated closely and that more widespread correlational relationships between multiple measures may be seen in esophageal speakers. The essential point of interest in this work is that all aspects of the alaryngeal signal should be viewed in a collective fashion rather than as distinct entities. Shipp's (1967) work led Hoops and Noll (1969) to undertake additional investigation on the potential relationship(s) between selected acoustic variables and listener judgments of speech proficiency in 22 esophageal speakers. Their findings indicated that measures of mean fundamental frequency, frequency variation, wave-to-wave variability (or degree of aperiodicity), and vocal intensity and its variation were not related to "communicative effectiveness."[4] Hoops and Noll did find, however, that speaking rate was related to judgments of speech proficiency for their group of speakers. In the

---

[4]In the framework of the Hoops and Noll (1969) article, the terms "speaking ability" (p. 2), "general communicative effectiveness" (p. 3), and "speech proficiency" (p. 11) appear to be used as synonyms. The authors did, however, explicitly seek to evaluate "general communicative effectiveness," and they appear to be the first authors to provide this dimension as an index of speaker performance. The composite mean rating of speaker effectiveness was judged to be an index of speaker ability. Because of the usage of this interchangeable terminology in their article, the reader is cautioned that other authors who use the terms "speaking ability" and "speech proficiency" may have defined these terms in a unique fashion. As such, care in defining potential distinctions between these, as well as other descriptive terms, in this chapter or within other articles or chapters is recommended.

speech pathology literature, speech rate has been suggested to correlate to a global feature termed speech "naturalness" (see Martin, Haroldson, & Triden, 1984). The somewhat contradictory findings between Shipp (1967) and Hoops and Noll (1969) provided the initial window into the unique and almost certainly complex nature of esophageal voice signals and the perception of these signals by listeners. This complex relationship also is likely to be found with TE and artificial laryngeal speakers. Interrelationships among perceptual attributes are also common in laryngeal speakers. The interactions are especially noted in the motor speech literature (e.g., Kent et al., 2000; Southwood & Weismer, 1993) and the vocal pathophysiology literature (e.g., Kreiman, Gerratt, & Berke, 1994; Wolfe & Ratusnik, 1988).

Despite Shipp's (1967) seminal work and subsequent investigation by Hoops and Noll (1969), only a handful of investigations have sought to provide further insights into the multidimensional nature of alaryngeal speech in the more than 30 years that have passed. Because of this, professionals are now at an empirical crossroads where clinical endeavors must seek to identify what truly constitutes "success" relative to rehabilitation outcome. Determining success of postlaryngectomy speech is not an easy task, and it requires clinicians to reassess how things have been done in the past and redefine the new criteria that may culminate in making each individual as successful as possible regardless of alaryngeal speech method chosen.

THE MULTIDIMENSIONAL STRUCTURE OF ALARYNGEAL SPEECH

As stated by Colton and Estill (1981), "When we try to define voice quality, we quickly become aware of the multiplicity of factors that contribute to its creation, variation, and perception" (p. 312). Although their statement was made in reference to laryngeal voice, there is no reason to think that this "multiplicity of factors" does not also exist for the quality of voice in those who use one of the various methods of alaryngeal speech (Beaudin, Doyle, & Eadie, 2004; Beaudin, Meltzner, et al., 2004; Eadie & Doyle, 2002, 2004; van As et al., 2003). Such definitions of voice quality are necessarily based on multidimensional constructs that distinctly affect judgments of that signal. Given that alaryngeal voice is characterized by a substantial number of parameters, the interaction among these variables must be delineated so that a comprehensive approach to rehabilitation is undertaken. Such rehabilitative efforts go well beyond that of voice and speech acquisition as a simple and sole metric of clinical "success" (see Chapter 5 in this text).

These productive factors collectively culminate as perceptually salient attributes of the alaryngeal speech signal, regardless of alaryngeal mode. Researchers, however, are just beginning to understand alaryngeal voice and speech at a perceptual level. Findings indicate that the frequency of alaryngeal voice, regardless of mode, is usually less than normal (see Table 6.1), that intensity may vary by method, and that durational features are linked to the driving alaryngeal sound source, whether intrinsically or extrinsically powered. To date, research efforts have not provided sufficient information as to why one method is preferred over another, or why this finding may be inconsistent from speaker to speaker. As further information becomes available, our understanding of alaryngeal speech and its impact on social communication will be enhanced.

Slavin and Ferrand (1995) sought to evaluate relative differences in the characteristics of "proficient" esophageal speech by undertaking factor and cluster analyses, from which four distinct profiles emerged based on acoustic measures. Data gathered from these analyses were interpreted to reflect "anatomical differences and physiologic strengths and weaknesses" (p. 1228). As such, this work provided a more enhanced characterization, one that was multidimensional, than that previously found in the literature. Despite this initial glimpse into a more comprehensive description of esophageal (and perhaps other methods of alaryngeal speech), however, Slavin and Ferrand (1995) stated, "Clearly, proficient esophageal speech is not predicated on one set of acoustic values. Even the most proficient esophageal speaker may speak with relatively high or low F_0, more or less rapidly, or with greater or lesser degrees of intensity" (p. 1230). Therefore, although attempts to describe alaryngeal modes of voice and speech in a multidimensional manner are considered to be of value, extreme care must be taken in generalizing such data within or across groups of speakers. For example, in Slavin and Ferrand's work, esophageal speakers were required to undergo a "stringent selection process" to confirm their speech proficiency. Only these speakers were assessed. As such, diversity that certainly exists among other esophageal speakers must be carefully considered in the context of acoustic descriptions of proficient speech production. In light of the work by Slavin and Ferrand (1995) and others (Hoops & Noll, 1969; Shipp, 1967), it is obvious that alaryngeal speaker proficiency is not dependent on one critical parameter. Rather, alaryngeal proficiency is likely based on the voice–speech signal as a whole. Findings such as these necessitate the use of "larger" (i.e., more global) descriptive features in auditory-perceptual evaluation of alaryngeal speech.

APPLICATION OF LARGER DESCRIPTIVE FEATURES IN THE PERCEPTUAL EVALUATION OF ALARYNGEAL SPEECH

Regardless of a listener's level of sophistication, alaryngeal speech clearly sounds very different from the normal voice and speech signal. By nature, voice and speech produced after the larynx is removed is termed *alaryngeal* because it does not rely on the larynx as a sound source. Thus, the voice and speech signal is quite distinct along parametric lines (e.g., frequency, intensity) when compared to the normal signal. This distinction is directly related to changes in how the alaryngeal speaker generates a "voice" signal and how that signal is modulated into "speech." These changes are well documented in numerous sources (e.g., Blom, Singer, & Hamaker, 1998; Diedrich & Youngstrom, 1966; Doyle, 1994; Eadie & Doyle,

2002, 2004; Snidecor, 1978; Weinberg, 1982). Much work has been done on defining the more "microacoustic" character of the alaryngeal voice signal. This includes work directed at assessing a clear characteristic of alaryngeal speech—the fact that it is indeed a noisy signal (Beaudin, Doyle, & Eadie, 2004; Beaudin, Meltzner, et al,, 2004; Robbins et al., 1984; Smith, Weinberg, Feth, & Horii, 1978). One of the issues that emerges from the observation of these changes in the physical structure and composition of the voice and speech signal in those who produce alaryngeal speech is that larger scale changes in how the listener perceives alaryngeal voice are consequently affected. It is not unreasonable to assume that each method will exhibit particular inherent patterns of performance, or that substantial variance will be exhibited within each group of speakers (although the degree of variance may be narrowed for some particular alaryngeal groups). This assumption raises a number of questions about the perceptual nature of alaryngeal speech and its impact on the listener and on communication and ultimately on how one defines rehabilitation success.[5]

FACTORS THAT CONTRIBUTE TO REHABILITATIVE SUCCESS

Perceptual evaluation of voice and voice disorders has gained considerable attention over the past decade (e.g., Kent, 1996; Kreiman, Gerratt, Kempster, Erman, & Berke, 1993). Although considerable attention has been directed toward disordered "laryngeal" voice, less attention has been directed at use of the many methods of alaryngeal communication. It is unlikely, however, that what has been found in relation to the disordered laryngeal voice will hold true for the alaryngeal voice. Much of the recent work addressing voice perception has indicated that numerous factors must be considered relative to interpreting data obtained. Factors such as listener experience, definitions of the feature under assessment, scale resolution, and interactions between the task and the listener, are critical elements to consider when perceptual questions are addressed (see Kreiman et al., 1993). Additionally, it might be suggested that multidimensional factors inherent in the alaryngeal speech signal must be considered of primary importance from the standpoint of rehabilitation outcomes. For example, the ultimate arbiter of alaryngeal speech "success" likely finds some component in the realm of how much the individual speaker is or, perhaps better stated, is not noticed as being "abnormal" or different from normal expectation (Eadie & Doyle, 2004).

---

[5]The possibility clearly exists that any given alaryngeal method may be a preferred mode of postlaryngectomy verbal communication by a given speaker despite specific information that shows that speaker to do better with another method. In this circumstance, the individual's choice must be respected, although the clinician is obliged to provide both clear and unbiased information to the individual about what differs for that person between given methods. Kalb and Carpenter (1981) have empirically documented the importance of individual speaker differences relative to alaryngeal speech.

Using Van Riper's (1978) classic definition of what constitutes a "speech" disorder—that speech is "abnormal when it deviates so far from the speech of other people that it calls attention to itself, interferes with communication, or causes the speaker or listener to be distressed" (p. 43)—and extrapolating it to considerations of "voice," one may see that the loss of the larynx, and resultant use of a non-normal voicing source, provides for the distinct likelihood that the speech signal will call attention to itself (Snidecor, 1978). These considerations extend beyond issues of speech intelligibility as a sole measure of alaryngeal speech success. Postlaryngectomy speech rehabilitation, therefore, must consider the tremendous impact that the gross abnormality of alaryngeal speech brings to the communicative situation. Considerations should include those factors that would exist relative to the listener and his or her perceptually biased attitudes toward the alaryngeal speaker, as well as the judgments and determinations made by the speaker him- or herself. A clear indicator of such overlapped concerns would be found in aspects of "preference" for a given alaryngeal speech mode (Green & Hults, 1982) and the "acceptability" of alaryngeal speech (e.g., Bennett & Weinberg, 1973; Doyle, Danhauer, & Reed, 1988; Eadie & Doyle, 2002; Hare, 2000; Niemi, 1999). These types of more global, comprehensive perceptual features would seem to be integral to any meaningful index of alaryngeal speech proficiency, but unfortunately this issue has received insufficient attention over the years. A line of research often overlooked is an attempt to determine whether refined (i.e., unidimensional) as opposed to global (i.e., multidimensional) assessment of alaryngeal voice and speech is most valuable for documenting postlaryngectomy "change in performance." These assessments must be performed relative to the social context of the speaker who uses alaryngeal methods (Doyle, 1994).

From a clinical point of view, the most important consideration of rehabilitation success would seem to correlate well with Van Riper's (1978) definition of a speech disorder. At face value it would appear that the "penalty" associated with alaryngeal speech would be minimized as the alaryngeal signal approaches characteristics of the normal signal. Questions of social penalty associated with an abnormal voice quality raise numerous concerns relative to the nature of the alaryngeal voice source (Eadie & Doyle, 2004). Specifically, varied considerations exist as a consequence of whether the alaryngeal source is intrinsic or extrinsic in nature. Intrinsic methods of alaryngeal speech involve use of existing anatomical structures—namely the pharyngoesophageal segment and associated musculature of the upper esophageal sphincter—as a voicing source (see Chapter 21 in this text). Intrinsic methods of alaryngeal voice production include esophageal and tracheoesophageal speech. In contrast, extrinsic methods rely on use of some external, supplementary voicing source, the best known of which would be the electrolarynx (see Chapters 4 and 22 in this text).[6] Distinctions in a voicing source of this nature will have direct influence on the perceptual judgments made by listeners regarding the character or attributes that exist in such signals. Hence,

---

[6]Pneumatic artificial laryngeal devices (e.g., the Tokyo device) would also be included in the category of extrinsic methods of alaryngeal speech.

comparisons across intrinsic and extrinsic methods have clear limitations from the standpoint of listener judgments at the present time (Beaudin, Doyle, & Eadie, 2004; Beaudin, Meltzner, et al., 2004).

In this respect, information about less dissimilar sources would appear to provide more representative indexes of the relative merits of any given method of alaryngeal speech. For example, early comparative work by Crouse (1962) indicated that when listeners were presented with esophageal and electrolaryngeal speech, esophageal speech was significantly preferred by both professional and nonprofessional listeners. Additionally, Crouse (1962) was the first to evaluate comparative judgments of audio-only and audiovisual samples. In determining preference for esophageal or electrolaryngeal speech in these presentation conditions, the issue of the visability of intrinsic (esophageal) versus extrinsic (electrolarynx) modes of alaryngeal speech production was raised by Crouse as a factor that must be considered. Additionally, stimulus type, mode of presentation (i.e., auditory, visual, both), and alaryngeal method are essential to consider if meaningful clinical applications of perceptual evaluation are to occur (Hubbard & Kushner, 1980). However, assessment of these factors does not exclude the value of direct comparisons of different alaryngeal methods; the critical issue herein lies in the ability to understand that the dissimilarity of the sources and the external validity of data interpretation will be judged and altered accordingly.

Within the realm of electrolaryngeal speech, numerous attempts to alter the electronic signal in an effort to optimize it (i.e., make the signal less mechanical) have been undertaken since the late 1970s (e.g., Everett, Mitchell, & Yanowitz, 1975; Galyas, Branderud, & McAllister, 1982; Sekey & Hanson, 1982; van Geel, 1982). Coincidental to many of these changes in source characteristics or the ability to manipulate the character of the source, has been an attempt to make electronic artificial laryngeal devices more discrete (Bailey, Everett, & Griffiths, 1976; Griffiths, Frederickson, & Bryce, 1976; Sekey & Hanson, 1982). Although additional changes have taken place over the past two decades, dramatic improvements are currently being pursued by the group at Massachusetts General Hospital, Massachusetts Eye and Ear Infirmary, Massachusetts Institute of Technology, and Harvard University (see Chapter 23 in this text). Contemporary researchers are advancing toward the goal of optimizing the electronic voicing signal via vocal tract modeling and online computerized optimization of the source from which speech is produced.

ATTRIBUTES OF ALARYNGEAL SPEECH

If one desires to comprehensively describe alaryngeal speech, considerable difficulty will be encountered. As with any voicing signal, whether normal or abnormal, judgments provided by listeners will be influenced by a number of factors. These factors will be influenced in most instances by the multidimensional nature of the signal of interest. Early efforts placed significant value on seeking to determine the potential importance of a variety of demographic factors, such as biographic and medical history, personality and social indexes, and communication and speech training on "speech proficiency" (Shames, Font, & Matthews, 1963). The findings of Shames et al. (1963) showed that when alaryngeal speakers are evaluated as a group, some factors are "significant" correlates, but the external validity of such findings is problematic. The fact of the matter is quite simple: Group designs have continuously fallen short of providing adequate predictors of what constitutes successful postlaryngectomy speech rehabilitation. The primary problem with group designs, regardless of how well intentioned, is that the long-term rehabilitative success of those who undergo total laryngectomy may be based substantially on variables that are intangible, in all but a few instances. The traditional index of performance within the descriptive or comparative domains is insufficient to categorize any true "population," and therefore has only limited application. This criticism does not discount the fact that this early work served (and continues to serve) a valuable purpose and remains an important point of reference for what occurs today. Beyond a plethora of studies of speech intelligibility over the years, however, little information is available on how listeners perceive the speech of the individual who is laryngectomized. Many composite factors and parameters affect the judgment of the listener in any given context.

As noted earlier in this chapter, one of the most significant concerns relative to judging alaryngeal speech is found in the fact that the signal is distinctly perceived as "non-normal," whether it be an intrinsic or extrinsic mode. This variation from normal has the potential to influence how the listener perceptually sorts components of the signal. Concerns related to listener experience, knowledge of abnormal voice in general and of alaryngeal voice in particular, as well as many other experiential determinants will bear directly upon auditory perceptual judgments. As a result, it is essential that work in the area of auditory–perceptual evaluation of alaryngeal speech is conducted, especially for those perceptual attributes that have yet undefined physical correlates (e.g., acceptability) (Eadie & Doyle, 2004).

REHABILITATIVE SUCCESS RELATIVE TO AUDITORY–PERCEPTUAL JUDGMENTS

Questions concerning how one best describes alaryngeal speech are valuable both perceptually (psychophysically) and clinically. Much information has been provided in the experimental literature over the past decade documenting that many factors influence perceptual judgments of disordered laryngeal voice and affect reliability (e.g., Kearns & Simmons, 1988; Kent, 1996; Kreiman & Gerratt, 1998; Kreiman et al., 1993; Kreiman, Gerratt, & Precoda, 1990). With alaryngeal speech, however, the listener is confronted with factors that will likely affect how he or she judges the sample.

The ultimate success or effectiveness of alaryngeal speech (and voice) has a long history in the literature dealing with postlaryngectomy communication (Diedrich & Youngstrom, 1966; Doyle, 1994; Snidecor, 1978). Early work was directed at identifying objectively measured physical parameters in an effort to describe, define, and differentiate alaryngeal modes from normal speech. Such work centered on issues that corresponded to frequency, intensity, and durational measures (Snidecor & Curry, 1960). Information of this type had value to both the clinician and the individual patient in that it provided some comparative index from which each patient's progress, or lack thereof, could be monitored and documented (see Berlin, 1963). The body of work was ultimately used to index the laryngectomized speaker using a predetermined anticipation of what came to be known as the "superior" speaker. The outcome of this early research effectively provided information that offered descriptive data that were in essence measures of maximum alaryngeal performance. Maximum performance measures have a long-standing and valuable use in communication sciences and disorders, but must also be carefully considered by those interpreting clinical data (Kent, Kent, & Rosenbek, 1987). For example, measures presented in the literature on the "superior esophageal speaker" actually offered only the top end of performance; no information on what was the typical clinical picture of performance across objective measures was available. This was problematic from several perspectives.

First, by not knowing what the average postlaryngectomy alaryngeal speaker could do (or not do), speech–language pathologists essentially did not know what to expect clinically, and whether perhaps what they observed was reasonable.[7] Second, many of these guidelines were used to direct therapy and monitor progress. Third, and perhaps most important, objective data in postlaryngectomy speech and voice rehabilitation fail to acknowledge changes in both resectioning and reconstruction surgical techniques. Surgical variation potentially has critical importance on the nature of the postlaryngectomy system relative to the physiologic output capacity of that system, regardless of alaryngeal mode. Thus, one must realize that parametric assessments and resulting data do not exist in an isolated fashion for the naive listener and perhaps even for the experienced or professional listener. The implications of this concern on how listeners judge the effectiveness of alaryngeal speech is, therefore, not unimportant.

TREES VERSUS FOREST: APPLICATIONS OF EXISTING PERCEPTUAL FEATURES TO ALARYNGEAL SPEECH

One of the most obvious questions when seeking to define or describe alaryngeal speech focuses on what is the "best" dimension or feature to use. The answer to this question is unknown; however, when efforts to answer this question are undertaken, some conceptual underpinning must drive the feature(s) chosen. For

---

[7]In the context of contemporary practice, what would be considered "reasonable" would not meet sufficient justification for either continuation or discharge from therapeutic intervention. Additionally, therapy for the alaryngeal speaker could easily be continued over many months, a likelihood that would probably be impossible in today's health care environment. This concern is not raised to argue current practice of clinical speech–language pathology services, but rather to provide a direct acknowledgment that early literature must be considered carefully in regard to the lack of limitations that clinicians currently experience on a daily basis. This observation solely points out that much of the superior data provided in the literature needs to be evaluated within the context of the current health care practices and environments.

example, specific features that are directly linked to physical processes may be addressed. In contrast, however, one may ultimately seek to describe the speech at a more global level. Which approach is best? That, too, is unknown, but it would seem logical that global measures likely correlate to larger issues of what type of penalty may be experienced by the speaker within the context of communicative acts. It may be that the degree or magnitude of difference from normal is what carries the greatest perceptual, and perhaps social, weight. The global feature is by nature a composite of many parameters that may have physical correlates, as well as many additive factors that influence the listener (e.g., pause time, stoma noise). Thus, aspects of acceptability, preference, naturalness, and so on, are quite global as perceptual dimensions.

Bennett and Weinberg (1973) were the first researchers to obtain comparative data on judgments of speech acceptability for normal, esophageal, and artificial larynx users (1 user of a transcervical electrolarynx and 3 who used pneumatic, reed-type devices powered by tracheal air). In their attempt to obtain information on acceptability, Bennett and Weinberg collected 18 speech samples from a group of speakers who were judged to be "highly proficient" by the investigators. Thirty-seven adult listeners were asked to provide equal-appearing interval scale judgments of each speaker's production of the second sentence of the "Rainbow Passage" (Fairbanks, 1960). The following definition of "speech acceptability" was provided to the listeners:

> In making your judgments about the speakers you are about to hear, give careful consideration to the attributes of pitch, rate, understandability, and voice quality. In other words, is the voice pleasing to listen to, or does it cause you some discomfort as a listener? (Bennett & Weinberg, 1973, p. 610)

The definition directly asks listeners to make a multidimensional judgment that concerns the speakers' communicative abilities.[8] The directions provided offer instructions to the listeners to make "forest" judgments despite the presence of many "trees." As such, it would seem plausible that judgments made would reflect the larger scale success of the speaker as a communicator.

Based on the listener judgments obtained, esophageal speakers and those using an artificial larynx were clearly distinguished from normal laryngeal speakers (Bennett & Weinberg, 1973). Furthermore, esophageal and artificial laryngeal users were judged less acceptable than normal laryngeal speakers. The data also indicated, however, that each alaryngeal method evaluated could also be distinguished on the basis of judgments of acceptability. Interestingly, electronic artificial larynx users were judged "less acceptable" in all instances when compared to the esophageal speakers, but one additional finding also emerged from this work. One of the speakers used in this study used a reed-type device called the Tokyo artificial larynx (Weinberg & Reikena, 1973). Listeners judged this speaker's performance

---

[8]The reader is referred to the definition of a speech disorder that was initially offered by Charles Van Riper (1978 or earlier editions) in various editions of his classic textbook *Speech Correction.*

on the feature of acceptability to be distinctly better than those of esophageal or electronic artificial larynx users, and to be equivalent to one of the normal speakers (although the normal mean rating was indeed higher). This finding is significant in relation to the fact that, when the alaryngeal speaker groups (esophageal and electrolarynx) studied by Bennett and Weinberg (1973) are considered, the Tokyo device permitted a much more natural communicative flow relative to prosodic aspects of speech. Thus, listeners appeared to have been sensitive to prosodic flow aspects inherent in the signal. This finding is also interesting when one considers that speech rate should in a general sense be similar for normal, Tokyo, and artificial larynx speakers. For the global measure of acceptability, however, something other than speech rate influenced the perceptual judgments.

Doyle (1996) reported that when pause time alone is manipulated in samples of esophageal and TE speech, the perceptual judgments of listeners change substantially. Specifically, Doyle manipulated these speech samples by introducing "esophageal" pause durations into TE samples, and TE pause durations into esophageal samples. Thus, through this temporal manipulation, an evaluation of how pause time influenced multiple perceptual features could be performed. The data revealed that as pause times became more like those of the normal speaker (i.e., unmodified TE samples and esophageal samples with TE pause times), listener judgments of several features became more favorable despite no direct change to the structural components of the voice signal. Although these data were preliminary, they raise considerable interest in how single aspects of the alaryngeal speech signal may influence larger (or smaller) auditory–perceptual aspects of the voice and speech of alaryngeal speakers.

One aspect of the speech signal that likely influenced judgments of electronic artificial larynx speech in the Bennett and Weinberg (1973) study was that this speech was indeed electronic in nature. Speech from artificial larynxes was clearly identified as less acceptable relative to the other alaryngeal modes evaluated. Overall, this work provided compelling evidence that listeners do sort many factors at the perceptual level when making assessments of alaryngeal speech. This work also provides information that should guide researchers to carefully consider the value of comparative work when substantial signal differences exist (e.g., electrolaryngeal vs. esophageal vs. pneumatic devices).

It is interesting that some of the terms used in Bennett and Weinberg's (1973) definition may have psychophysical reality. For example, aspects of "pitch rate" and "voice quality," along with the intelligibility of the sentence, required listener consideration. In addition to these features, it is of rehabilitative note that Bennett and Weinberg provided a secondary level of assessment that involved a feature centering on how "pleasing" the voice was to hear; this index specifically identifies that listeners must assess the speech signal in regard to their own judgments of discomfort. By doing so, aspects of the listener in a social context becomes a paramount consideration in how such speech signals are judged by listeners.

Although the global nature of speech acceptability that is provided in Bennett and Weinberg's (1973) study may be problematic for some to appreciate, such features or descriptors have the potential to demonstrate excellent sensitivity to the structure and composition of alaryngeal methods of speech production.

Consequently, judgments of features such as speech acceptability may hold great promise as a method for assessing speaker performance within the societal context. It should be easily seen that in this context, if the speaker is perceived as causing discomfort to the listener, the social penalty will erase any substantial and perhaps objectively measured abilities associated with intelligibility, speech rate, or other similar features that have so frequently been the subject of perceptual investigation.

SUMMARY

This chapter has provided information on the perceptual nature of alaryngeal voice and speech. Based on selected historical information found in the literature on postlaryngectomy speech production, the multidimensional nature of how perceptual judgments come to fruition is quite clear. Information presented has provided a framework from which both small- and large-scale aspects of one's speech ability may be evaluated. This information would seem to have direct importance to the rehabilitation process, not only from the perspective of expanding understanding of alaryngeal speech, but by increasing understanding about a larger interaction of multiple features on judgments of alaryngeal speech. To achieve more meaningful measures in those who use postlaryngectomy alaryngeal speech, clinicians must strive to avoid reductionist thinking in how to pursue measures gathered. If clinicians do not consider the multidimensional nature of the alaryngeal speech signal, they will continue to be mired in an inefficient process that has no consistent relationship to how well our patients eventually do. The data reviewed herein provide support for further research into the nature of alaryngeal speech and its impact on individuals who undergo total laryngectomy in the context of societal and human communication expectations. If such expectations can be better understood through the eyes of the communicative partner, clinicians and researchers may be better suited to organize and design meaningful measures of rehabilitation outcomes for those individuals who use any given method of alaryngeal speech. Without such consideration, professionals are likely to provide an unnecessary emphasis on isolated features that have no perceptual reality from the perspective of alaryngeal speech proficiency, acceptability, or effectiveness (Eadie & Doyle, 2004). Ultimately, clinicians' ability to define the success or failure of voice and speech rehabilitation following total laryngectomy will be insufficient at best. We hope that future auditory–perceptual work will embrace this philosophy in an attempt to further define the perceptual characteristics of alaryngeal speech and its influence on the listener.

REFERENCES

Baggs, T. W., & Pine, S. J. (1983). Acoustic characteristics of tracheoesophageal speech. *Journal of Communication Disorders, 16,* 299–307.

Bailey, B. J., Everett, R. L., &, Griffiths, C. M. (1976). An implanted electronic laryngeal prosthesis. *Annals of Otology, Rhinology and Laryngology, 85,* 472–483.

Beaudin, P. G., Doyle, P. C., & Eadie, T. L. (2004, May). *Psychophysical evaluation of pleasantness and acceptability for electrolaryngeal speech.* Paper presented at the Annual Conference of the Canadian Association of Speech–Language Pathologists and Audiologists, Ottawa, Ontario.

Beaudin, P. G., Meltzner, G., Doyle, P. C., & Hillman, R. E. (2004, May). *Paired-comparison evaluation of listener preference for electrolaryngeal sentence stimuli.* Paper presented at the Annual Conference of the Canadian Association of Speech–Language Pathologists and Audiologists, Ottawa, Ontario.

Bennett, S., & Weinberg, B. (1973). Acceptability ratings of normal, esophageal, and artificial larynx speech. *Journal of Speech and Hearing Research, 16,* 608–615.

Berlin, C. I. (1963). Clinical measurement of esophageal speech: I. Methodology and curves of speech acquisition. *Journal of Speech and Hearing Disorders, 28,* 42–51.

Blom, E., Singer, M., & Hamaker, R. (1986). A prospective study of tracheoesophageal speech. *Archives of Otolaryngology—Head and Neck Surgery, 112,* 440–447.

Blom, E. D., Singer, M. I., & Hamaker, R. C. (1998). *Tracheoesophageal voice restoration following total laryngectomy.* San Diego, CA: Singular.

Blood, G. W. (1984). Fundamental frequency and intensity measurements in laryngeal and alaryngeal speakers. *Journal of Communication Disorders, 17,* 319–324.

Clark, J. G., & Stemple, J. C. (1982). Assessment of three modes of alaryngeal speech with a synthetic sentence identification (SSI) task in varying message-to-competition ratio. *Journal of Speech and Hearing Research, 25,* 333–338.

Colton, R. H., & Estill, J. A. (1981). Elements of voice quality: Perceptual, acoustic, and physiologic aspects. In N. Lass (Ed.), *Speech and language: Vol. 5. Advances in basic research and practice* (pp. 311–403). New York: Academic Press.

Crouse, G. P. (1962). *An experimental study of esophageal and artificial laryngeal speech.* Unpublished master's thesis, Emory University, Atlanta, GA.

Curry, E. T., & Snidecor, J. C. (1961). Physical measurement and pitch perception in esophageal speech. *Laryngoscope, 71,* 415–424.

Damsté, P. H. (1994). Rehabilitation score-list of speech proficiency. In R. L. Keith & F. L. Darley (Eds.), *Laryngectomee rehabilitation* (3rd ed., pp. 219–234). Austin, TX: PRO-ED.

Diedrich, W. M. (1968). The mechanism of esophageal speech. *Annals of the New York Academy of Sciences, 155,* 303–317.

Diedrich, W. M., & Youngstrom, K. A. (1966). *Alaryngeal speech.* Springfield, IL: Thomas.

Doyle, P. C. (1994). *Foundations of voice and speech rehabilitation following laryngeal cancer.* San Diego, CA: Singular.

Doyle, P. C. (1996, November). *The influence of signal manipulation on the perception of esophageal and tracheoesophageal speech.* Paper presented at the annual convention of the American Speech-Language-Hearing Association, Seattle, WA.

Doyle, P. C., Danhauer, J. L., & Reed, C. G. (1988). Listeners' perceptions of consonants produced by esophageal and tracheoesophageal talkers. *Journal of Speech and Hearing Disorders, 53,* 400–407.

Doyle, P. C., & Glenn, K. L. (1988, May). *Comparison of three tests of speech intelligibility in evaluation of tracheoesophageal speech.* Paper presented at the annual meeting of the Canadian Association of Speech–Language Pathologists and Audiologists, Toronto, Ontario.

Eadie, T. L., & Doyle, P. C. (2002). Direct magnitude estimation and interval scaling of naturalness and severity in tracheoesophageal (TE) speakers. *Journal of Speech Language and Hearing Research, 45,* 1088–1096.

Eadie, T. L., & Doyle, P. C. (2004). Auditory–perceptual scaling and quality of life in tracheoesophageal speakers. *Laryngoscope, 114,* 753–759.

Everett, R. L., Mitchell, C., & Yanowitz, A. (1975). An electronic laryngeal prosthesis for production of natural sounding speech. *Proceedings of the Annual Conference of Engineering in Medicine and Biology, 17,* 202.

Fairbanks, G. (1960). *Voice and articulation handbook.* New York: Harper & Row.

Finizia, C., Dotevall, H., Lundström, E., & Lindström, J. (1999). Acoustic and perceptual evaluation of voice and speech quality. *Archives of Otolaryngology—Head and Neck Surgery, 125,* 157–163.

Fitch, J. L., & Holbrook, A. (1970). Modal fundamental frequency of young adults. *Archives of Otolaryngology, 92,* 382–397.

Galyas, K., Branderud, P., & McAllister, R. (1982). The "Intonator": Development of an electrolarynx with intonation control. In A. Sekey (Ed.), *Electroacoustic analysis and enhancement of alaryngeal speech* (pp. 184–189). Springfield, IL: Thomas.

Glenn, K. L., & Doyle, P. C. (1989, May). *The influence of phonetic composition on measures of alaryngeal speech intelligibility.* Paper presented at the annual meeting of the Canadian Association of Speech–Language Pathologists and Audiologists, Halifax, Nova Scotia.

Green, G., & Hults, M. (1982). Preferences for three types of alaryngeal speech. *Journal of Speech and Hearing Disorders, 47,* 141–145.

Griffiths, M. V., Frederickson, J. M., & Bryce, D. P. (1976). An implantable electro-magnetic sound source for speech production. *Archives of Otolaryngology, 102,* 676–682.

Hare, R. (2000). *A comparison of speech naturalness and voice quality in hemilaryngectomy, near-total laryngectomy, and tracheoesophageal speakers.* Unpublished master's thesis, University of Western Ontario, London, Ontario, Canada.

Hillman, R. E., Walsh, M. J., Wolf, G. T., Fisher, S. G., & Hong, W. K. (1998). Functional outcomes following treatment for advanced laryngeal cancer. *Annals of Otology, Rhinology and Laryngology, 107,* 2–27.

Hoops, H. R., & Noll, J. D. (1969). Relationship of selected acoustic variables to judgments of esophageal speech. *Journal of Communication Disorders, 2,* 1–13.

Hubbard, D. J., & Kushner, D. (1980). A comparison of speech intelligibility between esophageal and normal speakers via three modes of presentation. *Journal of Speech and Hearing Research, 23,* 909–916.

Kalb, M., & Carpenter, M. A. (1981). Individual speaker influence on relative intelligibility of esophageal speech and artificial larynx speech. *Journal of Speech and Hearing Disorders, 46,* 77–80.

Kearns, K. P., & Simmons, N. N. (1988). Interobserver reliability and perceptual ratings: More than meets the ear. *Journal of Speech and Hearing Research, 31,* 131–136.

Kent, R. D. (1996). Hearing and believing: Some limits to the auditory–perceptual assessment of speech and voice disorders. *American Journal of Speech–Language Pathology, 5,* 7–23.

Kent, R. D., Kent, J. F., Duffy, J. R., Thomas, J. E., Weismer, G., & Stuntebeck, S. (2000). Ataxic dysarthria. *Journal of Speech, Language, and Hearing Research, 43,* 1275–1289.

Kent, R. D., Kent, J. F., & Rosenbek, J. C. (1987). Maximum performance tests of speech production. *Journal of Speech and Hearing Disorders, 52,* 367–387.

Kreiman, J., & Gerratt, B. R. (1998). Validity of rating scale measures of voice quality. *Journal of the Acoustical Society of America, 104,* 1598–1608.

Kreiman, J., Gerratt, B. R., & Berke, G. S. (1994). The multidimensional nature of pathologic vocal quality. *Journal of the Acoustical Society of America, 95,* 1291–1302.

Kreiman, J., Gerratt, B. R., Kempster, G. B., Erman, A., & Berke, G. S. (1993). Perceptual evaluation of voice quality: Review, tutorial, and a framework for future research. *Journal of Speech and Hearing Research, 36,* 21–40.

Kreiman, J., Gerratt, B. R., & Precoda, K. (1990). Listener experience and perception of voice quality. *Journal of Speech and Hearing Research, 33,* 103–115.

Martin, R. R., Haroldson, S. K., & Triden, K. A. (1984). Stuttering and speech naturalness. *Journal of Speech and Hearing Disorders, 49,* 53–58.

Max, L., Steurs, W., & de Bruyn, W. (1996). Vocal capacities in esophageal and tracheoesophageal speakers. *Laryngoscope, 106,* 93–96.

Niemi, K. A. (1999). *An evaluation of tracheoesophageal speech acceptability using direct magnitude estimation.* Unpublished master's thesis, University of Western Ontario, London, Ontario, Canada.

Pindzola, R. H., & Cain, B. H. (1988). Acceptability ratings of tracheoesophageal speech. *Laryngoscope, 98,* 394–397.

Pindzola, R. H., & Cain, B. H. (1989). Duration and frequency characteristics of tracheoesophageal speech. *Annals of Otology, Rhinology and Laryngology, 98,* 960–964.

Robbins, J., Fisher, H. B., Blom, E. C., & Singer, M. I. (1984). A comparative acoustic study of normal, esophageal, and tracheoesophageal speech production. *Journal of Speech and Hearing Disorders, 49,* 202–210.

Salmon, S. J. (1994). Methods of air intake for esophageal speech and their associated problems. In R. L. Keith & F. L. Darley (Eds.), *Laryngectomee rehabilitation* (3rd ed., pp. 219–234). Austin, TX: PRO-ED.

Searl, J. P., (2002). Magnitude and variability of oral pressure in tracheoesophageal speech. *Folia Phoniatrica and Logopaedia, 54,* 312–328.

Sekey, A., & Hanson, R. (1982). Laryngectomee speech support system with prosodic control. In A. Sekey (Ed.), *Electroacoustic analysis and enhancement of alaryngeal speech* (pp. 166–183). Springfield, IL: Thomas.

Shames, G. H., Font, J., & Matthews, J. (1963). Factors related to speech proficiency of the laryngectomized. *Journal of Speech and Hearing Disorders, 28,* 273–287.

Shanks, J. (1994a). Developing esophageal communication. In R. L. Keith & F. L. Darley (Eds.), *Laryngectomee rehabilitation* (3rd ed., pp. 205–218). Austin, TX: PRO-ED.

Shanks, J. (1994b). Development of the feminine voice and refinement of esophageal voice. In R. L. Keith & F. L. Darley (Eds.), *Laryngectomee rehabilitation* (3rd ed., pp. 223–230). Austin, TX: PRO-ED.

Shanks, J. (1994c). Essentials for alaryngeal speech: Psychology and physiology. In R. L. Keith & F. L. Darley (Eds.), *Laryngectomee rehabilitation* (3rd ed., pp. 191–204). Austin, TX: PRO-ED.

Shipp, T. (1967). Frequency, duration, and perceptual measures in relation to judgments of alaryngeal speech acceptability. *Journal of Speech and Hearing Research, 10,* 417–427.

Slavin, D. C., & Ferrand, C. T. (1995). Factor analysis of proficient esophageal speech: Toward a multidimensional model. *Journal of Speech and Hearing Research, 38,* 1224–1231.

Smith, B. E., Weinberg, B., Feth, L. L., & Horii, Y. (1978). Vocal roughness and jitter characteristics of vowels produced by esophageal speakers. *Journal of Speech and Hearing Research, 21,* 240–249.

Snidecor, J. C. (Ed.). (1978). *Speech rehabilitation of the laryngectomized* (2nd ed.). Springfield, IL: Thomas.

Snidecor, J. C., & Curry, E. T. (1959). Temporal and pitch aspects of superior esophageal speech. *Annals of Otology, Rhinology & Laryngology, 68,* 1–14.

Snidecor, J. C., & Curry, E. T. (1960). How effectively can the laryngectomee expect to speak? *The Laryngoscope, 70,* 62–67.

Southwood, H., & Weismer, G. (1993). Listener judgments of the bizarreness, acceptability, naturalness, and normalcy of the dysarthria associated with amyotrophic lateral sclerosis. *Journal of Medical Speech–Language Pathology, 1,* 151–161.

Tardy-Mitzell, S., Andrews, M., & Bowman, S. A. (1985). Acceptability and intelligibility of tracheoesophageal speech. *Archives of Otolaryngology, 111,* 212–215.

Trudeau, M. D. (1987). A comparison of the speech acceptability of good and excellent esophageal and tracheoesophageal speakers. *Journal of Communication Disorders, 20,* 41–49.

Trudeau, M. D. (1994). The acoustical variability of tracheoesophageal speech. In R. L. Keith & F. L. Darley (Eds.), *Laryngectomee rehabilitation* (3rd ed., pp. 383–394). Austin, TX: PRO-ED.

Trudeau, M. D., & Qi, Y. (1990). Acoustic characteristics of female tracheoesophageal speech. *Journal of Speech and Hearing Disorders, 55,* 244–250.

van As, C. J., Hilgers, F. J. M., Verdonck-de Leeuw, I. M., & Koopmans-van Beinum, F. J. (1998). Acoustical analysis and perceptual evaluation of tracheoesophageal prosthetic voice. *Journal of Voice, 12,* 239–248.

van As, C. J., Koopmans-van Beinum, F. J., Pols, L. C., & Hilgers, F. J. (2003). Perceptual evaluation of tracheoesophageal speech by naive and experienced judges through use of semantic differential scales. *Journal of Speech–Language–Hearing Research, 46,* 947–959.

van Geel, R. C. (1982). Semi-automatic pitch control for an electrolarynx. In A. Sekey (Ed.), *Electroacoustic analysis and enhancement of alaryngeal speech* (pp. 190–197). Springfield, IL: Thomas.

Van Riper, C. (1978). *Speech correction: Principles and methods* (6th ed.). Englewood Cliffs, NJ: Prentice Hall.

Van Riper, C., & Emerick, L. L. (1984). *Speech correction: An introduction to speech pathology and audiology.* (7th ed.). Englewood Cliffs, NJ: Prentice Hall.

Weinberg, B. (1982). Speech after laryngectomy: An overview and review of acoustic and temporal characteristics of esophageal speech. In A. Sekey (Ed.), *Electroacoustic analysis and enhancement of alaryngeal speech* (pp. 5–48). Springfield, IL: Thomas.

Weinberg, B., & Bennett, S. (1972). Selected acoustic characteristics of esophageal speech produced by female laryngectomees. *Journal of Speech and Hearing Research, 15,* 211–216.

Weinberg, B., Horii, Y., & Smith, B. E. (1980). Long time spectral and intensity characteristics of esophageal speech. *Journal of the Acoustical Society of America, 67,* 1781–1784.

Weinberg, B., & Reikena, A. (1973). Speech produced with the Tokyo artificial larynx. *Journal of Speech and Hearing Disorders, 38,* 383–389.

Weiss, M. S., & Basili, A. B. (1985). Electrolaryngeal speech produced by laryngectomized subjects: Perceptual characteristics. *Journal of Speech and Hearing Research, 28,* 294–300.

Williams, S., & Watson, J. B. (1985). Differences in speaking proficiencies in three laryngectomy groups. *Archives of Otolaryngology, 111,* 216–219.

Wolfe, V. I., & Ratusnik, D. L. (1988). Acoustic and perceptual measurements of roughness influencing judgments of pitch. *Journal of Speech and Hearing Research, 30,* 230–240.

World Health Organization. (1980). *International classification of impairments, disabilities, and handicaps.* Geneva: Author.

World Health Organization. (2000). *International classification of functioning, disability and health.* [Pre-final draft, short version]. Geneva: Author.

PART II

Chapter 7

Evaluation of Individuals with Malignancy in the Upper Aerodigestive Tract

Howard B. Lampe and T. Wayne Matthews

The majority of cancers arising in the head and neck are squamous cell carcinomas developing from the mucosa lining in the upper aerodigestive tract. Salivary gland and thyroid gland malignancies are also encountered, along with a number of other rare malignancies (e.g., melanoma, sarcoma, and lymphoma) of the head and neck, but these are less likely to have an impact on speech and swallowing than are tumors arising from mucosal tissue (Medina & Weisman, 1998a, 1998b; Myers & Suen, 1996).

The clinical evaluation of a patient with a malignancy arising in the upper aerodigestive tract requires a complete history, physical examination, and review of appropriate imaging and other diagnostic investigations (e.g., electrocardiogram, pulmonary function test, audiological evaluation). At the time of patient presentation, the tumor may be causing physiologic or somatic changes, and the physician must attempt to understand the patient's premorbid function, as well as the potential impact of treatment on his or her posttherapy function. A proper and comprehensive assessment also includes evaluation of the patient's ability to manage his or her own care (self-care vs. assisted care) and any special therapy requirements (e.g., voice and speech therapy and physical therapy may require instruction vs. supervision). The purpose of this chapter is to provide an overview of the physician's evaluation so that a nonphysician health care professional who is involved as part of the treatment and rehabilitation team evaluating the patient can both understand the issues and contribute to his or her care and prognosis (Gallo, Sarno, Baroncelli, Bruschini, & Boddi, 2003). We address both pretherapy and posttherapy evaluation, including detection of recurrent cancer; this information should allow for the development of reasonable expectations for rehabilitation following treatment. We do not address, however, details concerning areas of medical care (e.g., cardiac status) that are unrelated to the main topic of this book; coverage of such issues can be found in other sources. Hence, the focus of the present chapter is specific to head and neck assessment, evaluation, treatment, and follow-up considerations in those with malignancies of the upper aerodigestive tract.

PRETREATMENT EVALUATION

History

The patient's ability and adequacy to verbally communicate and the primary language of communication should be established at the outset of the pretreatment evaluation. It also is important to know whether the patient can read and write in the primary language of each therapist involved. Family members may be able to assist with communication, but the team should clarify whether the patient agrees to this and whether the family member is willing and readily available for such purposes.[1] The ability of the patient to understand spoken instructions and

---

[1]We refer in this chapter to "the team," because multiple professionals (nurses, speech pathologists, audiologists, nutritionists, social workers, pastoral care workers, and others) are involved in comprehensive patient care.

to speak during the course of treatment may at times be inadequate without supplementation by reading or writing. In working with patients who cannot read and write, the team will encounter special challenges that must be considered. Additionally, many patients are temporarily without speech in the immediate postoperative period (due to tracheostomy), and therefore will benefit from using written communication or from pointing at words on a storyboard. Patients who are partially or totally illiterate or who do not speak the language of a caregiver may be required to use storyboards with pictures. These are best prepared preoperatively, and the patient can practice with them prior to treatment. The goal is to ensure that the patient will have some basic, functional method of communication in the immediate posttreatment period.

The patient's general medical condition can usually be ascertained by asking questions about his or her past medical history. When available, reports by the patient's other physicians, particularly the internist or family practitioner, should be reviewed. Special attention should be paid to preexisting health conditions that may influence treatment, recovery, and rehabilitation. The patient who is sedentary, either through habit or as the result of physical restriction from underlying cardiopulmonary disease, poses unique problems. The patient's ability—and motivation—to actively participate in rehabilitation may be limited in this circumstance. The physician and other team members should be careful not to impose their expectations on the patient. A patient who lives alone or is reclusive may not be as motivated to overcome the disability imposed by any treatment as is the patient who interacts with people every day through work, social, or other activities.

Reduced pulmonary function may be particularly important if the treatment will further compromise the patient's airway or ability to protect the airway. An adequate cough is essential to prevent significant complications from minor aspiration, which may become aspiration pneumonia in a patient whose pulmonary status is compromised. Pulmonary function testing may be helpful in further assessing and documenting compromised function. Similarly, underlying cardiac disease may limit the patient's active participation in postoperative rehabilitation. The presence of angina at rest or with minimal exertion leaves the patient little physical reserve for the extra activity and demands associated with the various therapies in the posttreatment period. Physical considerations of this nature also have the potential to influence psychological status.

The patient's mental state often is difficult to evaluate in a comprehensive manner. Depression, which is not uncommon in those diagnosed with cancer, seriously impairs the individual's ability to learn (Thomas, Mohan, Thomas, & Pandey, 2002). Dementia, as well as less severe impairments of cognitive functioning and memory, make learning new tasks very difficult and may have a significant impact on the rehabilitation process.

The patient's living arrangements are also important to consider. Not all patients have access to private telephones (allowing for confirmation of appointments for the tests and other services being arranged) or kitchen (special meal and food requirements) or bathroom (specialized equipment for care) facilities. The team should determine the availability of family members, friends, or other caregivers for immediate support at home (see Chapter 28 in this text). This information frequently may be difficult to obtain, and all members of the team should contribute to the overall understanding of the patient's situation.

Employment history, with particular attention to the specific demands of the patient's occupation (e.g., communication and physical requirements), always needs to be assessed and considered as part of treatment planning. The flexibility of the patient's work environment to adapt to potential changes caused by treatment should be explored, particularly when voice or speech is disrupted by treatment. In such instances, the potential economic impact must also be considered. Access to other professionals in the workplace may help in the transition back to employment.

Clinical Examination

The initial examination should include an overview of the patient's general physical appearance and condition. The presence of any signs of distress, either emotional or physical, should be noted. For example, the patient may be obviously depressed and crying or inappropriately euphoric, suggesting denial. The patient's general hygiene is often important as a predictor of his or her ability to cope with any form of therapy. It is difficult to instruct a patient in the proper care of a device requiring sterile handling if that person does not already wash daily. Active participation in recovery and rehabilitation requires the patient to manipulate various tools; some are as simple as a face cloth, but some individuals may have limited or no previous experience. The discovery of such limitations in advance of treatment allows the team to incorporate appropriate basic skills training in the treatment plan.

Examination of the patient's hearing should be undertaken, and when hearing loss is suspected, an audiogram should be obtained and reviewed. Assessment of hearing is most appropriate for those who are older. If not appropriately identified and managed, any significant hearing loss has the potential to seriously affect communication. The patient's hearing may require repeated evaluations during therapy, depending on what therapy is undertaken and its impact on hearing (e.g., radiotherapy may cause serous otitis, flap reconstructions may obstruct the external auditory canal).

The patient's face and general appearance of the head and neck should be evaluated and any structural asymmetry noted. Any muscle weakness, areas of erythema or ulceration, or previous evidence of treatment, including scars or lack of facial hair (secondary to radiotherapy) should be noted. Before examining the patient's neck, the physician should ask the patient if there are any areas of tenderness and apologize in advance for discomfort caused during the examination. The physician should gently palpate the neck to clarify the extent of disease, paying attention to any asymmetrical mass, noting the degree of firmness, and assessing whether the mass appears fixed to adjacent structures or is mobile within the neck. The neck acts as a biological filter for any cancer cells that may spread via the lymphatic system. The presence of lymph node involvement predicts a worse prognosis for the patient. The involvement of the neck requires that this region be included in any treatment plan and influences the patient's posttreatment function.

Cancer staging has evolved to allow for a mechanism of reporting on cases and allowing for comparison of treatment outcomes; it does not, however, dictate treatment (Maier, 1998; Union Internationale Contra Cancer, 1997). The TNM staging system is based on tumor (T), nodal involvement (N), and the presence of distant metastasis (M). The T category is based on a combination of tumor size, site, and tissue involvement (e.g., larger tumors, involving more than one site and invading adjacent structures, are rated higher), allowing a rating of 1 through 4. The N category describes nodal involvement, with specific focus on the number and volume of lymph nodes, as well as the presence of unilateral or bilateral involvement (e.g., increasing number and size are rated higher), allowing a rating of 0 through 3. Finally, the M category describes malignant involvement of distant sites (e.g., lung, bone, or brain), and the site is specified. (Table 13.1 in Chapter 13 lists all the TNM categories.) Higher stage tumors have a uniformly worse prognosis, but an individual patient's outcome cannot be accurately predicted. Clinical staging alone is not the only prognostic indicator. The tumor site, cell differentiation, and cell type all are important, as are many other factors that vary according to the tumor type.

The oral cavity is easily examined with a good light source and a tongue depressor. Again, the physician seeks to identify the presence of asymmetrical areas of fullness, erythema, ulceration, or obvious tumor. It is important to note the movement of the palate and tongue. Trismus (the inability of the patient to open his or her mouth) may make this evaluation difficult and should be noted. Trismus is a sign of tumor involving the muscles used in opening the jaw (i.e., pterygoid muscles) or soft tissue of the buccal space, which indicates deep infiltration and requires further investigation, such as via computerized tomography (CT) or magnetic resonance imaging (MRI) scans, to clarify the extent of tumor.

If available, diagnostic imaging studies should be reviewed. The CT and MRI allow the physician to better visualize many tumors and evaluate the full extent of the tumor and define its boundaries (Marchetta, Sako, & Badillo, 1964). The depth of tumor invasion, involvement of adjacent structures, and bone invasion may be evaluated, but no imaging study is tumor specific; only at the time of surgery can the definite extent of disease be properly evaluated and defined.

The oral cavity is normally symmetrical, so a tumor effect in the mouth may be obvious during an oral examination, but tumors involving the pharynx and tongue base may be less obvious to the examiner. The patient may indicate awareness of the mass effect(s) of a tumor by acknowledging "other" problems (e.g., ill-fitting dentures, a change in voice quality, or a reduction in speech intelligibility). Pain also is a common presenting symptom. The tumor may cause pain without specific stimulation, or may be affected by eating certain foods, such as those high in acid. Pain also may be referred to an area remote from the tumor site. This referred pain arises due to the common innervations of many sites in the head and neck from the same cranial nerve (e.g., the ear, tongue, tonsil, and pyriform sinus share innervations with the glossopharyngeal nerve). Patients with tumors involving the tongue, tonsil, and pharynx frequently have ear pain (referred otalgia). Pain may be referred to the neck, chest, or scalp depending on shared innervations and the tumor site.

As the tumor grows, it develops necrotic areas (e.g., areas of cell tissue death). These areas become infected secondarily, often causing a foul odor and may even lead to bleeding. These latter symptoms usually are associated with a more advanced tumor and make diagnosis easy but treatment more difficult. Post-treatment recovery and rehabilitative efforts also may be influenced in such circumstances.

Although larger tumors typically have more symptoms, a combination of tumor size, tumor location, and the patient's level of denial all combine to create the myriad symptoms the patient presents with during examination. The management of the tumor must be anticipated, and the resulting defect and disability will reflect a combination of the original extent of the tumor and the treatment chosen (Medina & Weisman, 1998a, 1998b). For example, if a tumor arising in the oral cavity requires resection of part of the tongue, the resulting defect is directly related to the tumor size and the reconstruction procedure, which may be as simple as primary closure for smaller tumors and as complex as free flap reconstruction for larger tumors (see Chapter 8 in this text).

In contrast to the oral cavity, the pharynx and larynx are not as easily evaluated. The presence of hoarseness may be associated with glottic cancers, but also with a myriad of benign diseases (e.g., laryngitis, polyps, nodules). Tumors not arising from the true vocal folds may not present with hoarseness or a change in voice quality until quite late, often secondary to impaired vocal fold movement; this is a sign of more advanced disease, where the arytenoid cartilage may be "fixed" due to tumor invasion or involvement of the recurrent laryngeal nerve. Pain may also be a presenting symptom and, again, may be referred to the ear or neck. Pain on swallowing is frequently associated with more advanced tumors involving the tongue base or pharynx (McGuirt, 1997). Unfortunately, many patients present with metastatic neck disease as the first sign or symptom of the underlying malignancy. The primary tumor is identified only after examination or diagnostic imaging studies.

When available, nasopharyngoscopy allows visualization of the larynx, but it often reveals a narrow field and one that is in two dimensions only. When combined with a careful review of appropriate imaging studies, a three-dimensional conceptualization of the tumor is often possible. Thus, multiple pieces of information may better define the extent of the tumor and influence treatment planning.

The resulting impact of therapy depends greatly on the extent of the tumor. Large-volume tumors involving adjacent structures require the removal of significant amounts of tissue and structures important to the patient's normal function. The treatment chosen attempts to balance a curative resection with preservation or reconstruction of structures removed. Unfortunately, the ability to manage such needs is not always easy, and essential tissue must be sacrificed for oncologic reasons. Although the initial treatment is intended to cure the patient, no treatment has a 100% cure rate. The proper medical management involves ongoing follow-up to detect a recurrent tumor early and allow for further treatment as appropriate.

POSTTREATMENT FOLLOW-UP

We cannot emphasize enough the importance of regular clinical follow-up. Regardless of the therapeutic modality chosen (surgery, radiation, or combined therapy), the patient who has had a tumor always has a significantly increased risk of exhibiting a second primary tumor or recurrence of the original tumor. Recurrent squamous cell carcinoma, regardless of the site, has certain characteristics. Recurrent tumor is frequently associated with pain at the primary site secondary to invasion into adjacent structures. Furthermore, recurrent tumor is usually associated with an area of ulceration, leukoplakia (white plaque), erythroplasia (red-colored inflammation), and most important, associated tissue induration (palpable hardness).

Unfortunately, it is beyond the scope of this chapter to provide a comprehensive overview of the myriad of signs and symptoms that can be associated with recurrence; however, several areas of concern deserve specific comment. Initially following treatment, many of the stages associated with healing are similar in appearance to recurrent tumor. For example, the healing ridge associated with the surgical scar is palpably indurated in a way similar to tumor. Following treatment, the physician will actively supervise the patient, and other health care personnel should avoid alarming the patient following any examination. When there is a question about a finding on examination, the treating physician should be asked whether the area of concern represents normal healing or a potential problem. Once the patient has completed the healing process, it is much easier to be alert to any unusual changes. These changes, which may include any of the signs and symptoms noted earlier, are frequently the first sign of recurrent tumor.

In a patient who has been doing well, and eating and swallowing without pain, any change in the symptom complex (e.g., decreased appetite, weight loss, or new areas of pain or discomfort) should alert the team to promptly review information carefully for possible recurrent tumor (Agrawal, deSilva, Buckley, & Schuller, 2004). In particular, palpable induration is a harbinger of recurrent tumor. The neck, which acts as a biological filter to tumor spread, frequently is the first site where recurrent tumor is detected. Palpable lymphadenopathy, particularly if painless and persistent for more than 6 weeks, is extremely suspicious. The most important point to be made is that all team members participating in a patient's management play a significant role in early detection of recurrent disease. In this regard, the use of simple, well-validated symptom checklists may be valuable (de Haes et al., 1996; de Haes, Van Knippenberg, & Neijt, 1990; Doyle & White, 2004; Stein et al., 2003; Thomas et al., 2002). With all team members attuned to changes, the appropriate diagnostic studies and biopsies may be arranged to allow for appropriate therapeutic intervention.

Follow-up is usually conducted daily in the initial postoperative period, then every 4 to 6 weeks for the next 2 years, decreasing to every 3 to 4 months for the next year, and then every 6 months for 1 year, and finally yearly after 5 years. The patient should understand that at any time a concern arises, he or she should make arrangements for earlier follow-up. A regular follow-up schedule is an important component of posttreatment monitoring following the diagnosis of malignant disease.

SUMMARY

This chapter has provided an overview of information related to the evaluation of the patient with a malignancy arising in the upper aerodigestive tract. A brief discussion of issues related to gathering history from the patient, details of the clinical examination, and posttreatment follow-up has been presented. Although information on the general signs and symptoms has been provided, the knowledge required to make a specific diagnosis has not been emphasized. This information is readily available in a variety of general otolaryngology textbooks.

The complex interaction of the patient's pretreatment condition and the effect of the tumor combines to create the morbidity requiring treatment and rehabilitation. The patient must be actively involved in his or her posttreatment rehabilitation. The extent to which the patient is able to participate actively in this process will help determine the appropriate rehabilitation and therapies to achieve the goals established over the rehabilitative process.

REFERENCES

Agrawal, A., deSilva, B. W., Buckley, B. M., & Schuller, D. E. (2004). Role of the physician versus the patient in the detection of recurrent disease following treatment for head and neck cancer. *Laryngoscope, 114,* 232–235.

de Haes, J. C. M., Olschewski, M., Fayers, P., Visser, M. R. M., Cull, A., Hopwood, P., & Sanderman, R. (1996). *The Rotterdam Symptom Checklist: A manual.* Groningen, The Netherlands: Northern Centre for Healthcare Research (NCH), University of Groningen.

de Haes, J. C. J. M., Van Knippenberg, F. C. E., & Neijt, J. P. (1990). Measuring psychological and physical distress in cancer patients: Structure and application of the Rotterdam Symptom Checklist. *British Journal of Cancer, 62,* 1034–1038.

Doyle, P. C., & White H. D. (2004, May). *Use of the Rotterdam Symptom Checklist in laryngectomized men and women.* Paper presented at the Annual Conference of the Canadian Association of Speech-Language Pathologists and Audiologists, Ottawa, Ontario.

Gallo, O., Sarno, A., Baroncelli, R., Bruschini, L., & Boddi, V. (2003). Multivariate analysis of prognostic factors in T3 N0 laryngeal carcinoma treated with total laryngectomy. *Otolaryngology —Head and Neck Surgery, 128,* 654–662.

Maier, H. (1998). Staging and prognosis of head and neck oncology. In A. S. Jones, D. E. Phillips, & F. J. Hilgers (Eds.), *Diseases of the head and neck, nose and throat.* New York: Oxford University Press.

Marchetta, F. C., Sako, K., & Badillo, J. (1964). Periosteal lymphatics of the mandible and intraoral carcinoma. *American Journal of Surgery, 108,* 505–507.

McGuirt, W. F. (1997). *Current concepts in laryngeal cancer: I. Otolaryngologic Clinics of North America.* Philadelphia: Saunders.

Medina, J. E., & Weisman, R. A. (1998a). *Management of the neck in head and neck cancer: Part I. Otolaryngologic Clinics of North America.* Philadelphia: Saunders.

Medina, J. E., & Weisman, R. A. (1998b). *Management of the neck in head and neck cancer: Part II. Otolaryngologic Clinics of North America.* Philadelphia: Saunders.

Myers, E. N., & Suen, J. Y. (1996). *Cancer of the head and neck* (3rd ed.). Philadelphia: Saunders.

Stein, K. D., Denniston, M., Baker, F., Dent, M., Hann, D. M., Bushhouse, S., & West, M. (2003). Validation of a modified Rotterdam Symptom Checklist for use with cancer patients in the United States. *Journal of Pain and Symptom Management, 26,* 975–989.

Thomas, B. C., Mohan, V. N., Thomas, I., & Pandey, M. (2002). Development of a distress inventory for cancer: Preliminary results. *Postgraduate Medicine, 48,* 16–20.

Union Internationale Contra Cancer. (1997). *TNM classification of malignant tumors* (5th ed.). L. H. Sobin & C. Wittekind (Eds.). New York: Wiley.

Chapter 8

Treatment Options in Oral Cancer

T. Wayne Matthews and
Howard B. Lampe

The selection of treatment for the individual diagnosed with cancer of the oral cavity is made on the basis of several generally accepted principles, as well as factors that are specific to the treating institutions and physicians. The decision is complicated by the great variability related to the subsite involved by malignant disease, the stage of the tumor, and the depth of tissue invasion and involvement of underlying structures. The stage of nodal metastases may influence the treatment of both the oral cavity tumor and regions of the neck. Patient age, health, expectations, and preferences must be taken into account in assessing each potential management approach as a possible treatment option. The available treatment facilities, physician experience, and physician preferences also play a role when more than one acceptable treatment option exists (e.g., radiotherapy vs. surgery vs. combined approaches to therapy).

Squamous cell carcinoma (SCCa) constitutes 95% of diagnosed malignancies in the oral cavity (Canadian Cancer Society, 1997). Although many of the treatment considerations also apply to less common cancers of the oral cavity, this chapter focuses specifically on oral cavity SCCa. Within this chapter, we address a variety of topics, including principles of treatment, radiotherapy, basic surgical procedures, and subsequent reconstructive options. Additionally, a variety of related concerns, including issues of short- and long-term treatment consequences, are presented.

PRINCIPLES OF TREATMENT

The primary goal of any cancer treatment is the full eradication of disease. Because distant metastases (i.e., malignant spread from the initial or primary site) are relatively uncommon in oral cancer without treatment failure, the elimination of the primary oral and cervical disease (locoregional control) is the first consideration in treatment. The basic therapeutic options for attaining locoregional control are radiotherapy and surgery, either alone or in combination. To date, the addition of chemotherapy concurrent with radiotherapy in patients with advanced disease remains experimental, although this approach appears promising in some patients (Ackerstaff et al., 2002; Cooper et al., 2004; El-Sayed & Nelson, 1996; Poole et al., 2001; Robbins, Doweck, Samant, Vieira, & Kumar, 2004; Robbins et al., 2000). Therapies aimed at reducing the possibility of distant metastases, such as chemotherapy before or after locoregional treatment, have not been shown to be efficacious (Bourhis et al., 1998; Browman, 1994). Because of this, the following discussion focuses on the two traditionally accepted treatment options in oral cancer: radiotherapy and surgery.

The likelihood of successful tumor control is the primary management issue that influences selection of surgery, radiotherapy, or combined surgery and radiotherapy. Another important consideration in treating oral cancer is the effect of the intervention on the patient's short- and long-term quality of life (see Chapter 28 in this text). Both surgery and radiotherapy have predictable acute and chronic morbidities that are associated with their use. The long-term morbidities largely relate to the treatment effect(s) on speech, swallowing, or both (see Chapters 13 and 14 in this text). The side effects of treatment depend on the treatment technique and the intensity of treatment. Surgical morbidity, however, can be significantly reduced through the appropriate application of various surgical reconstructive techniques.

In general, when two treatment options with equal probability of achieving locoregional control exist and the patient is felt to be capable of tolerating the expected acute morbidities associated with either option, the treatment modality with the lesser long-term morbidity is most often favored. Although the primary goal of any cancer treatment is the elimination of disease, in the treatment selection of oral or oropharyngeal tumors, maximal preservation of speech and deglutition is often the important secondary goal.

Maximizing functional outcome is an essential goal in the treatment of early-stage cancers of the oral cavity (i.e., Stage I and II disease—those tumors less than 4 cm in greatest dimension, and those confined to the oral cavity and without invasion of deep structures). In those clinical instances, a similarly high chance of disease control is possible with either single-modality treatment—surgery or radiotherapy (Fein, Mendenhall, Parsons, & McCarty, 1994). When the cancer is advanced in the mouth, neck, or both areas (i.e., Stage III and IV disease), treatment with a combination of surgery and radiotherapy is usually required for disease control (Fein et al., 1994). Unfortunately, such combined approaches to therapy also may result in increased acute and chronic morbidity, including the potential for impaired long-term speech and swallowing function and associated disability (Colangelo, Logemann, & Rademaker, 2000; Mady, Sader, Hoole, Zimmermann, & Horch, 2003). Where combined treatment is required, it is especially important for the surgeon to employ techniques that minimize the potential for such treatment morbidities as much as possible.

RADIOTHERAPY

External beam radiation treatment is a well-established and potentially curative therapy for head and neck cancers. Radiation therapy involves the application of high-energy, electromagnetic emissions to a specific tissue volume at a prescribed dose. Radiotherapy causes the production of unstable hydroxyl and oxygen radicals in the radiated tissue, which then leads to cell damage (Bristow & Hill, 1998). Either the damage created is repaired, or the cell dies. Like surgery, radiotherapy affects all tumor and normal cells found within the treatment volume (i.e., all cells located within the radiation field are subject to destruction). In contrast to surgery, in which a substantial margin of normal tissue around the malignancy must be resected to achieve disease control, radiation treatment affects cancerous and normal cells to different degrees by taking advantage of the greater ability of normal cells to repair the radiation damage (Wong & Hill, 1998).

A potential advantage of radiation treatment, therefore, is that it can often eradicate the tumor with less loss of normal tissue and less distortion of anatomy when compared to surgical excision. Furthermore, because of the aforementioned preferential effect on cancer cells, a larger volume of tissue can be treated with radiation with acceptable levels of morbidity as compared to surgery. Radiation also is less limiting in respect to concerns about the proximity of vital structures, such as the carotid artery or major nerves, when compared to surgery. The reason that radiation therapy has a distinct advantage in this situation is that, relative to surgery, tumor cells in close proximity to these structures can be treated and destroyed using radiation without unacceptable damage to these vital structures.

Radiotherapy does, however, have specific morbidities and limitations. Tumor cell kill is dependent on the partial pressure of oxygen in the tumor (Wong & Hill, 1998). Large tumors often expand beyond the limitations of their blood supplies and therefore are hypoxic (i. e., deficient in cell oxygen) or necrotic (i. e., exhibiting cell death), particularly in their geographic centers. This is one of the main factors that limits the ability of radiation treatment to successfully eliminate large tumors or necrotic masses. Such tumors often require surgical excision before or after radiation. Some cancer cells also seem to be inherently insensitive to lethal radiation damage; this may be related to their greater ability to repair irradiation damage and recover. Unfortunately, an assay does not yet exist that can predict the radiosensitivity of a patient's tumor prior to treatment.

Side Effects of Radiotherapy

The acute side effects of radiotherapy to the head and neck are related primarily to damage to epithelial structures such as the salivary glands, mucosa, and skin (Milas & Peters, 1999). Tissues with slower cell turnover, such as muscle, bone, blood vessels, and nerves, are generally less susceptible to the acute side effects of irradiation. Irradiation is a locoregional treatment and does not cause the acute systemic effects, such as nausea and vomiting, diffuse hair loss, immunosuppression, or organ failure, that are sometimes seen with systemic therapies such as chemotherapy (Rademaker et al., 2003; see also Chapter 10 in this text).

Radiation has a predictable impact on the function of the salivary glands. All salivary tissue within the treatment volume is affected. In treating oral and oropharyngeal cancers, the treatment field usually includes all of the major and minor salivary glands in the mouth and throat (see Chapter 13 in this text). Decreased salivary production begins early in treatment (Milas & Peters, 1999). Serous salivary cells are affected first and most severely, resulting in thicker, mucuslike saliva. The resulting xerostomia can exacerbate masticatory and swallowing problems during and after treatment (Gellrich et al., 2002; see also Chapter 14 in this text).

Acute mucositis is the most common cause of morbidity during or shortly after radiotherapy. Radiation mucositis presents as pain and tenderness of the mucosa within the radiation field. This usually includes most or all of the mucosa of the oropharynx, hypopharynx, larynx, and cervical esophagus. As with radiation dermatitis, the severity of the mucositis may vary from mild to severe, including erythema, edema, and ulceration. Mucositis may commonly result in dietary changes and weight loss. More severe forms can lead to dehydration or hoarseness. The condition usually starts after the irradiation begins and settles by about 4 weeks after the treatment is completed. Unusually severe cases can result in aspiration and pneumonia or even airway compromise. Supportive care may consist of systemic and topical analgesics, dietary counseling and alterations, and oral rinses. In severe cases, tube feeding may be required to allow completion of treatment (see Chapter 14 in this text).

Radiation dermatitis can cause local skin pain and tenderness in the treated area. This varies in severity from redness with intact skin to moist desquamation including epithelial loss. This complication can be painful, but it is often of limited duration and can usually be tolerated throughout treatment with appropriate supportive techniques.

The severity of the dermatitis or mucositis is related to the type of irradiation used, the radiation dose, and the length of time over which it is given, as well as the individual patient's inherent susceptibility to radiation damage (Milas & Peters, 1999). Continued smoking throughout treatment increases the chance of significant acute mucositis and is strongly discouraged. It is of utmost importance that radiation treatments are completed as prescribed; treatment interruption due to the acute effects of the treatment or patient noncompliance has a very negative impact on tumor response and locoregional cancer control (Milas & Peters, 1999; Parsons, Bova, & Million, 1980).

Chronic Effects of Radiotherapy

The chronic effects of irradiation to the head and neck determine the ultimate limitations of the treatment dose that can be delivered to patients with oral cancer. The chronic effects are related to direct tissue damage, as well as relative ischemia due to progressive sclerosis of the small vessels and capillaries in the radiated field. There is progressive scarring of the tissues, including muscle and fascia. The effects may not be noticeable for months after treatment and may progress for at least 18 months. Unfortunately, the long-term tissue changes subsequent to radiotherapy are permanent; this is the reason why a potentially curative dose can be administered to any given area of the body only once in a lifetime. The risks of severe long-term sequelae from radiotherapy are related to the volume of tissue treated, the total irradiation dosage, the dose per fraction of radiation given, and the individual patient's inherent vulnerability to these chronic tissue changes (McGregor & MacDonald, 1987; Milas & Peters, 1999). The potential chronic effects of radiation therapy following head and neck irradiation that are relevant to speech–language pathologists include scarring of the muscles and soft tissues lining the oral cavity and pharynx, xerostomia, and necrosis of the mandible (see Chapter 13 in this text).

Although radiation-induced fibrosis of the muscles of mastication and deglutition is probably always present to some extent after radiotherapy, clinically significant decreases in muscle strength and tissue elasticity are much less common. A minority of patients experience functional impairments, including trismus, decreased muscle strength, reduced coordination and elevation of both the tongue and soft palate, decreased pharyngeal propulsion, reduced laryngeal elevation, and esophageal stricture. When present, these impairments primarily affect chewing and swallowing. In rare and extreme cases, the disturbance of the pharyngeal phase of swallowing and laryngeal protection may even preclude safe oral feeding (see Chapter 14 in this text).

Xerostomia is a very common if not universal outcome following radiotherapy of the oral cavity and pharynx (Guchelaar, Vermes, & Meerwaldt, 1997). It is a sequelae of the acute and chronic effects of radiotherapy on salivary tissue. The severity of the dryness is variable. Irradiation of all of the salivary glands, increasing treatment dosages, and individual predisposition all affect the degree of reduced salivary production. Following curative doses of radiotherapy, the saliva is reduced in volume and increased in viscosity (Milas & Peters, 1999). The formation of a food bolus and pharyngeal transit of that bolus become more difficult, and as a consequence, additional fluids are often required with meals. The mouth becomes less capable of "self-cleaning," resulting in increased difficulty with oral hygiene. Alteration of the oral bacterial flora results in a pronounced susceptibility to caries in patients with teeth, and special preventative dental care is required (Harrison & Fass, 1990; Chapter 13 in this text). The management of radiation treatment–related xerostomia with salivary replacement has been of limited benefit to date. The use of a parasympathomimetic agent (pilocarpine) has been promising in its ability to reduce xerostomia in some patients (LeVeque, Montgomery, Potter, Zimmer et al., 1993; Chapter 10 in this text).

The blood supply to the mandible is primarily from the microcirculation of the periosteum. Following radiotherapy and the resulting sclerosis of these vessels, the lower jaw and the gingiva are relatively devascularized (Friedman, 1990). Radiation results in a reduced ability of the mandible to heal and resist infection. Even minor trauma can cause infection and irreparable damage to the mandible, including the risk of osteoradionecrosis, leading to exposed, dead bone and pathological fractures. Patients with remaining teeth are at risk of dental secondary osteoradionecrosis of the mandible and, therefore, require meticulous dental care before and after irradiation. Osteoradionecrosis of the mandible may require aggressive dental, medical, and surgical management, including advanced surgical reconstructive techniques (see Chapter 13 in this text).

Brachytherapy

Brachytherapy is a radiotherapy technique that, in carefully selected cases, can eliminate or reduce some of the undesirable consequences of external beam radiotherapy (Harrison, 1997). Brachytherapy involves the implantation of a radioactive source within the involved tissue. The radioactive material has a relatively short half-life and gives a predetermined dose of radiation to a small volume of tissue in a short time frame. The advantage is that the uninvolved oral and pharyngeal tissue is spared; consequently, xerostomia and fibrosis are largely avoided. The use of brachytherapy is limited by the size of the tumor, the proximity of the tumor to the mandible, the possible need for additional treatment of the neck, and the required expertise on the part of the radiation oncologist.

Modern radiotherapy techniques have evolved to allow the sophisticated planning and delivery of irradiation that has high curative potential with acceptable morbidity. Whether radiation therapy is used alone or combined with surgery, it plays a prominent role in the successful treatment of oral malignancies. Speech–language pathologists need to be cognizant of both the benefits and long-term consequences of radiotherapy in their patients treated for oral cancer using this modality.

SURGERY

Surgery can be the sole treatment for early-stage oral cancers, or part of a combined surgery–radiotherapy regimen for advanced tumors, or a "salvage" procedure after previous treatment has failed. The goal of surgery is the complete resection of all cancer. Intraoperative surgical judgment and frozen-section histological examination by a pathologist are required to determine the adequacy of the excision. Generally, a margin of 1 cm beyond the grossly involved tissue with intraoperative histological confirmation of the absence of tumor cells at the cut edges is sought (Baker, 1992). Some tissues such as periosteum are relatively tumor-resistant barriers that allow closer margins (Marchetta, Sako, & Badillo, 1964; Marchetta, Sako, & Camp, 1965; Marchetta, Sako, & Razack, 1977). Because of the necessity of achieving "clear margins," the volume resected is always considerably greater than the volume of tumor. Important structures such as dentition, sensory and motor nerves, and normal muscle and mucosa are often removed with the tumor. Scarring and fibrosis are inevitable after any operation. The loss of normal tissue and fibrosis can result in significant functional and cosmetic impairment postoperatively.

The functional anatomy of the oral cavity is complex. Some tissues and structures, such as the mandible, are largely supportive. Many are dynamic, such as the tongue, buccal units, and lips. Tissue "spacers" separate the dynamic muscular tissues from the mandible (and maxilla) and the floor of mouth and buccal mucosa. These spacer tissues are elastic and allow the dynamic elements to operate independently from the supportive structures. Because of this complexity, the consequences of surgery for oral cancers directly relate to the intraoral subsite resected, the type and amount of tissue lost, and the surgical techniques employed (Jacobsen, Franssen, Fliss, Birt, & Gilbert, 1995).

The loss of limited portions of the tongue is surprisingly well tolerated by most patients (Heller, Levy, & Sciubba, 1991). The extent of impairment is typically related to the volume of tongue resected (McConnel, Logemann, Rademaker, et al., 1994). Loss of the anterior tongue results in difficulties with sweeping food posteriorly and with bolus formation, as well as alteration of anterior speech sounds. The loss of the posterior oral tongue and tongue base can result in difficulty in bolus presentation to the pharynx and subsequent dysphagia and aspiration (see Chapter 14 in this text). Generally speaking, the postoperative disability resulting from surgery to the posterior oral cavity and oropharynx is more severe than that resulting from surgery to the anterior oral cavity (Ringstrom, Matthews, & Lampe, 1999).

In some instances, oral cancer may require removal of a partial thickness of bone without a loss in mandibular continuity (marginal mandibulectomy) or a complete loss of a segment of mandible with a gap between the remaining segments (segmental mandibulectomy). Following a marginal mandibulectomy, the primary disability is due to the loss of teeth, and subsequent difficulties in fitting dentures often occur because of the lowering of the height of the mandible. In contrast, segmental mandibular defects, if not reconstructed, cause more severe problems with mastication because of the loss in mandibular continuity (McGregor, 1993). Individuals who experience segmental mandibulectomy seldom can tolerate more than a soft diet. The remaining posterior segment of mandible tends to be pulled medially and superiorly by the pterygoid muscles, whereas the anterior segment drifts to the operated side and inferiorly because of the digastric muscles and scarring (Panje & Morris, 1992). Dysphagia due solely to the mandibular defect is not often seen. Cosmetic impairment is significant because of flattening of the mandibular contour and displacement of the residual mandibular fragments. Unreconstructed anterior mandibular resections that involve the arch of the mandible cause especially severe problems, often resulting in significant degrees of oral disability.

Loss of a portion of the maxilla results in loss of dentition and often a communication between the oral and nasal or paranasal cavities. Fortunately, most of these defects can be reconstructed successfully with special dental prostheses that can both separate the oral and nasal cavities and restore the dental arch. Prosthetic rehabilitation of partial maxillary defects limited to the hard palate need not lead to significant functional or cosmetic problems (Lapointe, Lampe, & Taylor, 1996; also see Chapter 13 in this text).

When soft tissues in the floor of mouth are removed (with or without partial glossectomy), the potential impairments in speech, deglutition, and swallowing are the result of tethering of the remaining normal tongue to the mandible (Imai & Michi, 1992; McGregor, 1993). In this circumstance, the remaining tongue may be rendered nonfunctional even when all or most of it remains intact. Similarly, if a significant amount of buccal tissue is lost and appropriate reconstruction is not performed, fibrosis and contracture leading to trismus may result.

Surgical Approaches

Surgical approaches to the oral cavity and oropharynx include transoral (through the mouth) excisions, elevation of cheek flaps, and mandibular osteotomies.

Small- to moderate-sized oral cancers can often be adequately resected and the defect reconstructed transorally without facial or cervical incisions (Baker, 1992; Shah, 1990). The feasibility of such a technique depends on the tumor size and location, involvement or proximity to the mandible, and the presence of teeth or trismus. Generally, an anterior tumor location, the absence of dentition or trismus, and a lack of deep involvement of the floor of the mouth favor a transoral approach. Lesions that abut the mandible can sometimes be removed transorally in conjunction with a marginal mandibulectomy. Tumors that deeply invade lateral tissues of the floor of mouth are sometimes removed with a combined transoral and transcervical approach in conjunction with a neck dissection. Figure 8.1 shows a tumor of the lateral tongue that could be removed by a transoral approach.

Resecting or reconstructing larger, more deeply invasive, or more posterior tumors often requires an approach through some form of transcervical or facial incision (Baker, 1992; Shah, 1990; Thawley & O'Leary, 1992). Incisions are placed in natural skin creases to minimize the long-term cosmetic impact of the surgical treatment. The most common incision involves a transverse incision in the middle third of the neck, which is then carried up the midline over the chin and through the lip. If the tumor is external to the mandible or if a mandibulectomy is necessary, the skin and soft tissue of the ipsilateral cheek are peeled posteriorly off the lateral surface of the mandible and a "cheek flap" is elevated (see Figure 8.2). If the tumor lies within the mandibular arch, a paramedian mandibulotomy (i.e., saw cut just anterior to the mental foramen) is performed (see Figure 8.3). This maneuver allows the ipsilateral jaw to swing open "like a book," providing excellent exposure. This can be extended posteriorly as far as the vallecula to gain access to the oropharynx. The extension of the incision along the floor of the mouth may precipitate injury to the lingual nerve. Transection of the hypoglossal nerve is not required by this approach but may occur because of direct tumor involvement. After the tumor has been adequately resected and any planned reconstruction completed, the floor of mouth incision is closed, the osteotomy is repaired using internal fixation techniques (see Figure 8.4), and the lip and external incisions are reapproximated. If no external tissue is resected and the mandible is intact or reconstructed, then the cosmetic deformity should be limited only to the external incisions.

RECONSTRUCTIVE OPTIONS

The long-term functional impact of oral cancer surgery can often be favorably affected by the selection and performance of appropriate reconstructive techniques. Whether to reconstruct and, if so, what method of reconstruction is most appropriate depend on many factors, including the location, area, depth, and composition of the tissue removed; the comorbidity associated with each technique; the patient's expectations; the surgeon's experience and preferences; and the facilities available. In the remainder of this chapter, we discuss the commonly considered techniques and their indications and limitations in order of increasing complexity.

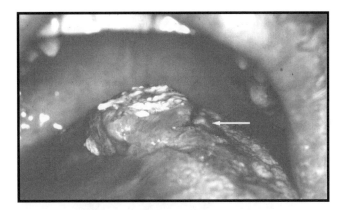

FIGURE 8.1. Squamous cell carcinoma of the lateral tongue (arrow). This cancer could be removed by a transoral approach. The choice of reconstruction would depend mostly upon tumor depth. In this case, a free radial forearm flap would be most appropriate.

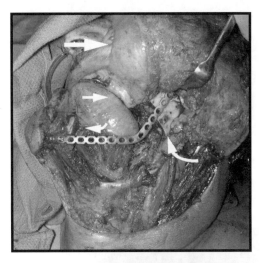

FIGURE 8.2. Cheek flap approach to a cancer involving the lateral floor of mouth and mandible which required a segmental resection of the mandible. The buccal mucosa and cheek (large straight arrow), hard palate (small straight arrow), and anterior and posterior segments (curved arrows) are identified. This defect is bridged with a reconstruction plate in preparation for final reconstruction with a free flap consisting of skin and bone, in this case a free fibula flap.

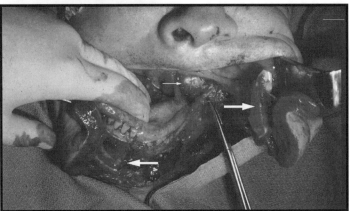

FIGURE 8.3. A paramedian osteotomy of the mandible to approach a tumor in the oropharynx (small straight arrow). Anterior and posterior segments of the mandible (large straight arrows) are identified.

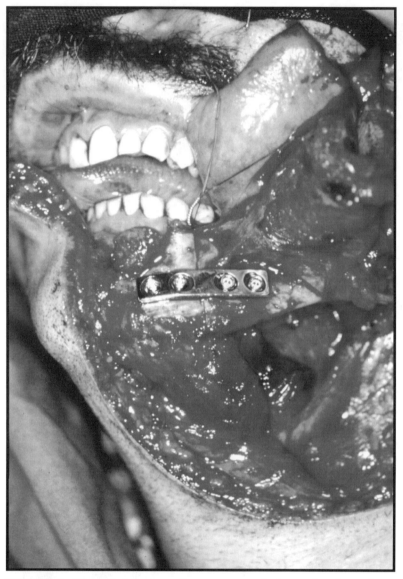

FIGURE 8.4. Closure of a paramedian osteotomy similar to that shown in Figure 8.3 using a plate.

Superficial Defects

Superficial defects of small to moderate area can be left open and allowed to heal by secondary intention. This is especially true for those defects involving the lateral tongue, hard palate, or retromandibular mucosa and, to a lesser extent, the buccal mucosa (Shah, 1990). This method is simple and fast and often causes less pain, swelling, and acute morbidity than direct surgical wound closure. Tracheotomy is usually avoided. Contraction of the soft tissue is inherent in the technique but typically does not cause long-term functional problems when it is applied to carefully selected defects. Healing takes place over 2 to 3 weeks and is promoted by appropriate oral hygiene. A fluid or semisolid diet is tolerated early in the postoperative course. This technique is commonly employed in conjunction with laser surgery for lateral tongue lesions not involving the floor of mouth.

Primary Closure

Primary closure refers to the direct approximation of the edges of the oral wound with sutures. This technique is most appropriately applied to defects of limited tissue surface area but of considerable depth. By definition there is 100% wound contracture. The primary closure method is useful for small- to moderate-sized defects of the tongue, especially if they are of greater depth (Shah, 1990). Primary closure of superficial tongue wounds causes more postoperative pain and swelling than healing by secondary intention. This closure method can be judiciously applied to small defects of the floor of mouth, retromolar trigone, or buccal mucosa, with good functional results. If applied to inappropriately large wounds, significant tongue tethering or trismus results (Imai & Michi, 1992). Primary wound closure is quick, simple, and reliable. It can provide satisfactory functional results in carefully selected cases.

Split-Thickness Skin Grafts

Split-thickness skin grafts consist of a shaving of skin (epidermis and the superficial dermis) for transfer to a wound location at another site. The donor area (usually the patient's thigh) heals by proliferation of the residual deep dermis and skin appendages. The graft is transferred to the recipient site, where it is held in close approximation to a clean wound. The thin graft, about .001 inch in thickness, survives initially by imbibing nutrients from the wound exudate and then from ingrowth of the microcirculation found in the wound bed. This process is dependent on the absence of shearing between the graft and the wound bed. Eventually, the graft becomes the new epithelium covering the wound. During this process, a partial contracture of the skin graft occurs, usually in the order of 50% of the original graft area (see Figure 8.5).

Skin grafting of oral wounds is most effective for defects of moderate to large area, but of limited thickness. The grafts themselves have no appreciable bulk for replacing muscle or other soft tissues. The technique is most applicable for superficial wounds of the floor of mouth, retromolar trigone, and buccal mucosa resulting from the excision of dysplasia, carcinoma in situ, or very superficially invasive cancers (Shah, 1990). Tissue shearing resulting from the constant movement of the tongue makes this method less reliable for tongue defects. Postoperative contracture is anticipated; therefore, to compensate for this shrinkage, the grafts are designed to be larger than the original defect. A bolster of dressing material is required to hold the graft firmly to the wound bed for 5 to 7 days postoperatively to ensure graft adhesion and survival. The bolster necessitates a

FIGURE 8.5. The final result of a superficial squamous cell carcinoma of the ventral tongue and floor of mouth resected via a transoral approach and reconstructed with a split-thickness skin graft. The area resected measured 4 cm in greatest dimension. Note that the mobility of the tongue has been maintained.

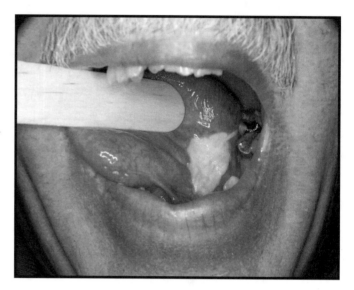

tracheotomy and nasogastric tube feeding during this time. Because of the long-term effect of radiotherapy on the microcirculation, skin grafting results are unpredictable when radiation treatment precedes surgery and is generally avoided in these patients.

Local Flaps

Local flaps consist of vascularized tissue that depends on a blood supply located near the surgical defect. The size and composition of the flap are determined by the local vascular anatomy. Local flaps for oral reconstruction may consist of mucosa, most often from the tongue, or skin, typically from the nasolabial area (DeSanto & Yarrington, 1983). Advantages include simplicity and the convenience of not having to operate at another body site, as well as good tissue texture matches with the oral mucosa. Disadvantages are that the flaps are small, can cause oral impairment when taken from another oral site, are limited in their ability to reach far from the pedicled bases, and often require two surgical stages to complete the reconstruction (McConnel, Teichgraeber, & Alder, 1987; see also Chapter 12 in this text). Thus, local flaps are most suitable for reconstructing small defects of the floor of mouth.

Regional Flaps

Regional flaps are similar in concept to local flaps, but they are generally based on larger vessels and are farther away from the oral cavity. The flaps tend to be larger and, therefore, are able to be translocated over larger distances and repair larger and thicker defects. Regional flaps may consist of skin and subcutaneous tissue, muscle with or without skin, and even bone. Regional flaps were the method of choice for major oral reconstruction from the 1960s through 1980s. The most commonly used regional flap in current oral reconstruction is the pectoralis major myocutaneous flap. This large flap consists of the pectoralis major muscle and usually the overlying chest skin (Serafin, 1996). The vascular supply is a branch of the axillary artery (the pectoral branch of the thoracoacromial artery), which is based below the lateral clavicle. The distal skin and muscle are passed under the upper chest skin into the neck and mouth for one-stage reconstruction of defects as large as total glossectomies. The flap is rather bulky in most people, especially heavy men and large-breasted women. This is a relatively simple and reliable reconstructive tool, but it can be hampered by the flap's thickness, limited arc of rotation, lack of a reliable bony component, and poor donor site cosmesis in women. It is most suitable for reconstruction of moderately large oropharyngeal defects and major losses of the oral tongue. It may limit residual tongue mobility to a degree in some patients because of thickness of the skin and soft tissue of the flap, and because of tethering at the attachment to the chest (McConnel et al., 1987). It is much less appropriate for the anterior floor of mouth or smaller and shallower defects at any intraoral site. In many centers, the regional flaps have been supplanted by the use of distant or free flaps.

Free Flap Procedures

The term *free flaps* is used to describe a large class of flaps that consists of a volume of tissue located outside of the head and neck, which is supplied by an identifiable named artery and its accompanying veins (the vascular pedicle). The tissue volume can be surgically isolated on the vascular pedicle and the blood vessels severed proximally, allowing the flap to be transferred to the oral defect. Once the flap is inserted in the oral defect, the artery and veins of the flap pedicle are anastomosed to arteries and veins in the neck to allow perfusion of the flap from the new recipient vessels. The revascularization of the flap requires the use of a microscope, micro-instruments, and microsutures. The success of the operation depends on maintenance of perfusion of this autologous "tissue transplant." Free flaps have the advantage of a large number of donor sites being available, which allows for the tailoring of the flap characteristics, such as composition (skin, muscle, bone), size, and bulk, to more closely mimic those of the resected tissue in the oral cavity. The limited reach associated with pedicled flaps does not apply to free flaps. The free flap technique is reliable in experienced hands. Disadvantages of free tissue reconstruction are the need for specialized equipment and skills, and the additional time and complexity of surgery. Free flap reconstruction has been a major advancement in the functional reconstruction of major intraoral defects following cancer surgery since the early 1980s.

The most widely used distant donor site for oral reconstruction consists of the skin, subcutaneous tissue, and fascia of the volar surface of the forearm based on the radial artery and its veins. This constitutes the *radial forearm flap* (Serafin, 1996). The moderately large area of thin and pliable skin available with the forearm flap makes it very suitable for reconstruction of the floor of mouth, buccal pouches, retromolar trigone, and oropharynx, and moderate-sized defects of the tongue (Jacobson et al., 1995).

When surgery is chosen as part of the treatment of an oral cancer, both the ablative approach and the reconstructive techniques used affect the outcome for the patient. Ablative surgery must be adequately extensive to eradicate the disease without unnecessarily sacrificing functional tissue. The reconstructive method is selected to achieve the best possible oral rehabilitation without imposing unjustified patient morbidity or surgical complexity (Doyle, Matthews, Ferri, & Lampe, 2000). Several widely varied ablative and reconstructive methods are available to realize these goals. Training, experience, and communication on the part of the surgeon and other health care providers are necessary to provide the best possible surgical outcome for patients with cancer of the oral cavity.

SUMMARY

The curative treatment of oral malignancies consists of surgery or radiotherapy alone or in combination. Treatment selection is complex. The primary objective of treatment must be the eradication of locoregional disease. Permanent elimination of disease in the head and neck, when it is achieved, usually results in so-called cure, as isolated distant recurrence is uncommon. Secondary considerations in making a treatment recommendation are the expected acute and chronic treatment morbidities. These are further influenced by the specific factors particular to each patient and tumor. Finally, patient and physician preferences are taken into account. A multidisciplinary team approach involving the relevant caregivers and the patient and family is necessary to reach the most appropriate decision and outcome.

REFERENCES

Ackerstaff, A. H., Tan, I. B., Rasch, C. R. N., Blam, A. J. M., Keus, R. B., Schornagel, J. H., & Hilgers, F. J. M. (2002). Quality-of-life assessment after supradose selective intra-arterial Cisplatin and concomitant radiation (RADPLAT) for inoperable stage IV head and neck squamous cell carcinoma. *Archives of Otolaryngology—Head and Neck Surgery, 128,* 1185–1190.

Baker, S. R. (1992). Malignant neoplasms of the oral cavity. In C. W. Cummings, J. M. Fredrickson, L. A. Harker, C. J. Krause, & D. E. Schuller (Eds.). *Otolaryngology—Head and neck surgery* (2nd ed., Vol. 2, pp. 1248–1321). St. Louis: Mosby Year Book.

Bourhis, J., Pignon, J. P., Designe, L., Luboinski, M., Guerin, S., & Doenge, C. (1998). Meta-analysis of chemotherapy in head and neck cancer (MACH-NC): (1) Locoregional treatment vs. same treatment + chemotherapy (CT). [Abstract]. *Proceedings of the American Society for Clinical Oncology, 17,* 382.

Bristow, R. G., & Hill, R. P. (1998). Cellular basis of radiotherapy. In I. Tannock (Ed.), *The basic science of oncology* (3rd ed., pp. 295–321). Toronto, Ontario, Canada: Pergamon Press.

Browman, G. P. (1994). Controversies in patient management: Evidence-based recommendations against neoadjuvant chemotherapy for routine management of patients with squamous cell head and neck cancer. *Cancer Investigation, 12,* 662–671.

Canadian Cancer Society. (1997). *Canadian cancer statistics, 1997* (10th anniversary ed.). Toronto, Ontario: National Cancer Institute of Canada, Statistics Canada, Provincial/Territorial Cancer Registries and Health Canada.

Colangelo, L., Logemann, J., & Rademaker, A. (2000). Tumor size and pre-treatment speech and swallowing in patients with resectable tumors. *Otolaryngology—Head and Neck Surgery, 122,* 653–662.

Cooper, J., Pajak, T., Forastiere, A., Jacobs, J., Campbell, B., Saxman, S., Kish, J., Kim, H., Cmelak, A., Rotman, M., Machtay, M., Ensley, J., Chao, C., Schultz, C., Lee, N., & Fu, K. (2004). Postoperative concurrent radiotherapy and chemotherapy for high-risk squamous-cell carcinoma of the head and neck. *New England Journal of Medicine, 350*(19), 1937–1944.

DeSanto, L. W., & Yarrington, C. T. (1983). Tongue flaps: Repair of oral and pharyngeal defects after resection for cancer. *Otolaryngology Clinics of North America, 16,* 343–351.

Doyle, P. C., Matthews, T. W., Ferri, C. L., & Lampe, H. (2000, July). *Vocal tract transmission characteristics following free radial forearm flap reconstruction for oral cancer.* Paper presented at the 5th International Conference on Head and Neck Cancer, San Francisco.

El-Sayed, S., & Nelson, N. (1996). Adjuvant and neoadjuvant chemotherapy in the management of squamous cell carcinoma in the head and neck region: A meta-analysis of prospective and randomized trials. *Journal of Clinical Oncology, 14,* 838–847.

Fein, D. A., Mendenhall, W. M., Parsons, J. T., & McCarty, P. J. (1994). Carcinoma of the oral tongue: A comparison of results and complications of treatment with radiotherapy and/or surgery. *Head and Neck, 16,* 358–365.

Friedman, R. B. (1990). Osteoradionecrosis: Causes and prevention. *NCI Monographs,* 145–149.

Gellrich, N. C., Schimming, R., Schramm, A., Schmalohr, D., Bremerich, A., & Kugler, J. (2002). Pain, function, and psychologic outcome before, during, and after intraoral tumor resection. *Journal of Oral and Maxillofacial Surgery, 60,* 772–777.

Guchelaar, H. J., Vermes, A., & Meerwaldt, J. H. (1997). Radiation-induced xerostomia: Pathophysiology, clinical course and supportive treatment. *Support Care Cancer 5,* 261–262.

Harrison, L. B. (1997). Applications of brachytherapy in head and neck cancer. *Seminars in Surgical Oncology, 13,* 177–184.

Harrison, L. B., & Fass, D. E. (1990). Radiation therapy for oral cavity cancer. *Dental Clinics of North America, 34,* 205–222.

Heller, K. S., Levy, J., & Sciubba, J. J. (1991). Speech patterns following partial glossectomy for small tumors of the tongue. *Head and Neck, 13,* 340–343.

Imai, S., & Michi, K. (1992). Articulatory function after resection of the tongue and floor of mouth: Palatometric and perceptual evaluation. *Journal of Speech and Hearing Research, 35,* 68–78.

Jacobson, M. C., Franssen, E., Fliss, D. M., Birt, B. D., & Gilbert, R. W. (1995). Free radial forearm flap in oral reconstruction: Functional outcome. *Archives of Otolaryngology—Head and Neck Surgery, 121,* 959–964.

Lapointe, H. J., Lampe, H. B., & Taylor, S. M. (1996). Comparison of maxillectomy patients with immediate versus delayed obturator prosthesis placement. *Journal of Otolaryngology, 117,* 218–220.

LeVeque, F., Montgomery, M., Potter, D., Zimmer, M., et al. (1993). A multicentre, randomized, double blinded, placebo controlled, dose-titration study of oral pilocarpine for treatment of radiation-induced xerostomia in head and neck cancer patients. *Clinical Journal of Oncology, 11,* 1124–1131.

Mady, K., Sader, R., Hoole, P. H., Zimmermann, A., & Horch, H. H. (2003). Speech evaluation and swallowing ability after intra-oral cancer. *Clinical Linguistics and Phonetics, 17,* 411–420.

Marchetta, F. C., Sako, K., & Badillo, J. (1964). Periosteal lymphatics of the mandible and intraoral carcinoma. *American Journal of Surgery, 108,* 505–507.

Marchetta, F. C., Sako, K., & Camp, F. (1965). Multiple malignancies in patients with head and neck cancer. *American Journal of Surgery, 110,* 537–541.

Marchetta, F. C., Sako, K., & Razack, M. S. (1977). Management of "localized" oral cancer. *American Journal of Surgery, 134,* 448–449.

McConnel, F. M. S., Logemann, J. A., Rademaker, A. W., et al. (1994). Surgical variables affecting postoperative swallowing efficiency in oral cancer patients: A pilot study. *Laryngoscope, 104,* 87–90.

McConnel, F. M. S., Teichgraeber, J. F., & Alder, R. K. (1987). A comparison of three methods of oral reconstruction. *Archives of Otolaryngology—Head and Neck Surgery, 113,* 496–500.

McGregor, I. A. (1993). The pursuit of function and cosmesis in managing oral cancer. *British Journal of Plastic Surgery, 46,* 22–31.

McGregor, I. A., & MacDonald, D. G. (1987). Spread of squamous cell carcinoma to the non-irradiated edentulous mandible: A preliminary report. *Head and Neck Surgery, 9,* 423–428.

Milas, L., & Peters, L. J. (1999). Biology of radiation therapy. In S. E. Thawley, W. R. Panje, J. G. Batsakis, & R. D. Lindberg (Eds.), *Comprehensive management of head and neck tumors* (2nd ed., Vol. 1, pp. 99–123). Philadelphia: Saunders.

Panje, W. R., & Morris, M. R. (1992). Oral cavity and oropharyngeal reconstruction. In C. W. Cummings, J. M. Fredrickson, L. A. Harker, C. J. Krause, & D. E. Schuller (Eds.), *Otolaryngology—Head and neck surgery* (2nd ed., Vol. 2, pp. 1479–1498), St. Louis: Mosby Year Book.

Parsons, J. T., Bova, F. J., & Million, R. R. (1980). A reevaluation of split-course technique for squamous cell carcinoma of the head and neck. *International Journal of Radiation Oncology and Biological Physics, 6,* 1645–1652.

Poole, M. E., Sailer, S. L., Rosenman, J. G., Tepper, J. E., Weissler, M. C., Shockley, W. W., Yarbrough, W. G., Pillsbury, H. C., Schell, M. J., & Bernard, S. A. (2001). Chemoradiation for locally advanced squamous cell carcinoma of the head and neck for organ preservation and palliation. *Archives of Otolaryngology—Head and Neck Surgery, 127,* 1446–1450.

Rademaker, A. W., Vonesh, E. F., Logemann, J. A., Pauloski, B. R., Liu, D., Lazarus, C. L., Newman, L. A., May, A. H., MacCracken, E., Gaziano, J., and Stachowiak, L. (2003). Eating ability in head and neck cancer patients after treatment with chemoradiation: A 12-month follow-up study accounting for dropout. *Head and Neck, 25,* 1034–1041.

Ringstrom, E., Matthews, T. W., & Lampe, H. B. (1999). The role of percutaneous gastrostomy tubes in the postoperative care of patients with cancer of the oral cavity and oropharynx. *Journal of Otolaryngology, 28,* 68–72.

Robbins, K. T., Doweck, I., Samant, S., Vieira, F., & Kumar, P. (2004). Factors predictive of local disease control after intra-arterial concomitant chemoradiation (RADPLAT). *Laryngoscope, 114,* 411–417.

Robbins, K. T., Kumar, P., Wong, F. S., Hartsell, W. F., Flick, P., Plamer, R., Weir, A. B., Neill, H. B., Murry, T., Ferguson, R., Hanchett, C., Vieira, F., Bush, A., & Howell, S. B. (2000). Targeted chemoradiation for advanced head and neck cancer: Analysis of 213 patients. *Head and Neck, 22,* 687–693.

Serafin, D. (1996). The pectoralis major muscle flap. In D. Serafin (Ed.), *Atlas of microsurgical composite tissue transplantation* (pp. 161–177). Philadelphia: Saunders.

Shah, J. P. (1990). The oral cavity and oropharynx. In J. P. Shah (Ed.), *Color atlas of head and neck surgery* (Vol. 2, pp. 9–58). Philadelphia: Saunders.

Thawley, S. E., & O'Leary, M. (1992). Malignant neoplasms of the oropharynx. In C. W. Cummings, J. M. Fredrickson, L. A. Harker, C. J. Krause, & D. E. Schuller (Eds.), *Otolaryngology—Head and Neck Surgery* (Vol. 2, pp. 1306–1354). St. Louis: Mosby Year Book.

Wong, C. S., & Hill, R. P. (1998). Experimental radiotherapy. In I. Tannock (Ed.), *The basic science of oncology* (3rd ed., pp. 322–349). Toronto, Ontario, Canada: Pergamon Press.

Chapter 9

Recent Advances in the Surgical Treatment of Laryngeal Cancer

Steven M. Zeitels

Laryngeal cancer was a rare disease in the 19th century, but its incidence increased dramatically in the 20th century due to the introduction of mass-produced cigarettes around 1910. Approximately 11,000 to 15,000 new cases of laryngeal cancer are diagnosed per year in the United States. Cure of the disease with surgery, radiotherapy, or both has appropriately been the primary treatment goal. Because there have not been substantial improvements in the cure rate through the last several decades, however, the emphasis of treatment developments has focused on functional preservation. The purpose of this chapter is to acquaint the reader with recent innovations in the surgical treatment of laryngeal cancer, which has primarily involved minimally invasive endoscopic techniques. Endoscopic resection of laryngeal cancer was first done over 100 years ago and was one of the first minimally invasive surgical oncological procedures (Fraenkel, 1886; Lynch, 1920). In addition, surgical–prosthetic voice restoration has assumed the foreground as a primary goal of function-enhancing treatment of patients who require a total laryngectomy (see Chapters 17 and 18 in this text).

VOCAL FOLD ATYPIA OR DYSPLASIA AND EARLY GLOTTIC CANCER

Disease Presentation

Premalignant changes to vocal fold epithelium in the form of atypia or dysplasia and early glottic cancer are primarily smoking-induced diseases. Lesions are frequently confined geographically to the superior ventricular surface of the vocal fold (Zeitels, 1993, 1995), allowing for complete preservation of layered microstructure on the medial valving surface of the glottis. Keratotic lesions of the vocal fold comprise most of the dysplastic glottic lesions identified by the laryngologist. Unfortunately, the magnitude and appearance of the keratosis does not belie the severity of the underlying cellular atypia or the presence of microinvasive carcinoma (Zeitels, 1995). Furthermore, selected biopsies do not accurately reflect the entire lesion. It is not unusual for varied severity of atypia to be present in the same high-power field despite uniform surface keratosis. Therefore, the entire lesion must be resected to ensure an accurate diagnosis (Zeitels, 1993, 1995). Erythroplasia (red lesions) is an infrequent finding and typically contains carcinoma in situ. Isolated ulceration of the musculomembranous vocal fold in an immunocompetent smoking host who does not have an infectious process typically reflects carcinoma.

Philosophy of Management

In that any adequate treatment for T1 glottic cancer (endoscopic excision, transcervical excision, radiation therapy) results in a cure rate of about 85% to 90% (Cragle & Brandenburg, 1993), a primary parameter by which the clinician should judge the success of a treatment is the resulting voice quality (see Table 13.1 in Chapter 13 for information on cancer staging). Recently, laryngologists have incorporated physiological principles of laryngeal sound production into the design of evaluating outcomes from oncological procedures. The surgeon, however, must not lose sight of the fact that a variety of circumstances might dictate a particular treatment approach (e.g., surgery vs. radiotherapy), and these must be considered (see Chapters 10 and 11 in this text).

A primary goal of the endoscopic management of T1 glottic cancer is to narrow the cancer-free margin to minimize patient morbidity, while at the same time not altering the cure rate. Phonomicrosurgical procedures can precisely accommodate the narrow deep resection margin of a T1 vocal fold cancer to the depth of invasion (invisible third dimension) (see Figures 9.1 and 9.2). A small amount of extra tissue excised with the deep margin can have a profound negative effect on the vocal outcome, while not necessarily improving the cure rate, especially for lesions that are confined to the epithelium or those that minimally invade the superficial lamina propria.

Zeitels and others have described the use of subepithelial infusion of saline and epinephrine into the superficial lamina propria, which has enhanced precise phonomicrosurgical resection of many vocal edge lesions (Hartig & Zeitels, 1998; Kass, Hillman, & Zeitels, 1996; Zeitels, 1995; Zeitels, Hillman, Franco, & Bunting, 2002; Zeitels & Vaughan, 1991b). Reinke's space infusion has helped to precisely determine the depth of invasion of T1 cancers before committing to the depth of the excision (Zeitels, 1995; Zeitels & Vaughan, 1991a, 1991b). In some individuals with T1 cancers, the infusion method has allowed for preservation of all of the vocal ligament and vocalis muscle, as well as part of the deep portion of the superficial lamina propria (Zeitels, 1994, 1995). We have had 1 microinvasive local failure in approximately 60 patients for whom this graded microsurgical approach was used (Zeitels, 1996a, 1996b), and that individual's cancer was controlled by means of a subsequent superficial endoscopic resection. The majority of those who have undergone phonomicrosurgical excision have been followed up for more than 3 years (Zeitels, 1995, 1996b).

Endoscopic excision of laryngeal cancer is associated with a very low complication rate; minor postoperative bleeding (Eckel & Thumfart, 1992; Koufman, 1986; Thomas, Olsen, Neel, DeSanto, & Suman, 1994; Vaughan, 1978) is rare, and granuloma formation is somewhat more frequent (Eckel & Thumfart, 1992; Koufman, 1986; Olsen, Thomas, DeSanto, & Suman, 1993; Thomas et al., 1994). An en block excisional biopsy provides an accurate diagnosis as well as an effective treatment (Davis, Kelley, & Hayes, 1991; Vaughan, 1978; Zeitels, Dailey, & Burns, 2004), and it does so with minimal morbidity. Whole-mount-section histological examination of resected specimens prevents overtreatment (i.e., too large an excision) or undertreatment (i.e., biopsy or resection without margins) of small glottic lesions. All treatment options (i.e., surgery and radiotherapy), including further transoral resections, are preserved after endoscopic excision.

Unlike radiotherapy, endoscopic resection treats only the lesion without ablating the remaining normal glottal tissue (see Figure 9.3). Postradiotherapy videostroboscopic exams suggest that both normal and cancerous tissues reflect fibrotic changes and impaired mucosal oscillation (Lehman, Bless, & Brandenburg, 1988; also see Chapter 10 in this text). The use of radiotherapy for early glottic

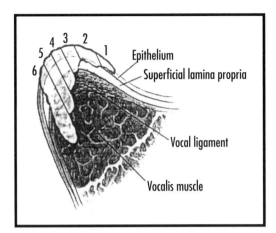

FIGURE 9.1. Diagram displaying how a surface vocal fold lesion may harbor a variety of invasion patterns. *Note.* From "Optimizing Voice in Conservation Surgery for Glottic Cancer," by G. Hartig and S. M. Zeitels, 1998, *Operative Techniques in Otolaryngology—Head and Neck Surgery (Phonosurgery Part 1), 9,* pp. 214–223. Copyright 1998 by Elsevier. Reprinted with permission.

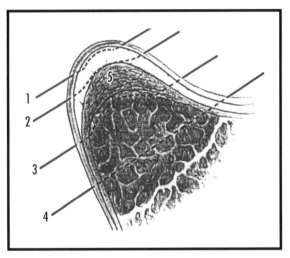

FIGURE 9.2. Coronal section of the vocal fold delineating the depth of potential resection margins for vocal fold atypia and cancer. *Note.* From "Optimizing Voice in Conservation Surgery for Glottic Cancer," by G. Hartig and S. M. Zeitels, 1998, *Operative Techniques in Otolaryngology— Head and Neck Surgery (Phonosurgery Part 1), 9,* pp. 214– 223. Copyright 1998 by Elsevier. Reprinted with permission.

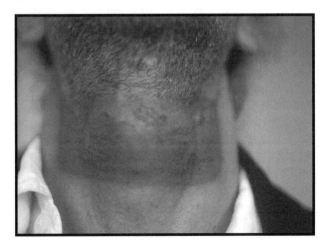

FIGURE 9.3. The appearance of the neck of an individual at the conclusion of radiation for a T1 glottic carcinoma. (Courtesy of Steven M. Zeitels.)

cancers precludes its further use for tumor recurrence or for new primary tumors and may even induce carcinogenesis in atypical epithelium (DeSanto, 1976; Hellquist, Lundgren, & Olafsson, 1982). Additionally, the cost of endoscopic excision is significantly less than open laryngeal surgery or radiation, both of which are typically preceded by a staging endoscopy (Cragle & Brandenburg, 1993; Myers, Wagner, & Johnson, 1993; Zeitels, 2004). Finally, the patient sustains the increased burden of time and travel commitments required by radiotherapy.

Disease in the Anterior Commissure

The anterior commissure tendon, or Broyle's ligament, is a confluence of the vocal ligament, the thyroepiglottic ligament, the conus elasticus, and the internal perichondrium of the thyroid alae (see Figures 9.4 and 9.5). There is a misconception that T1 cancers at the anterior commissure have a great predilection for understaging and that many of these lesions have occult invasion of the thyroid cartilage—T4 stage lesions (Kirchner, 1989; Kirchner & Carter, 1987; Pearson & Salassa, 2003). This misunderstanding occurs because the anatomy of the dense anterior commissure ligament is a less resilient tumor barrier than the adjacent thin thyroid perichondrium. Kirchner and Carter (1987) and Kirchner (1989) clearly demonstrated that T1a and T1b carcinomas rarely transgress Broyle's ligament to invade thyroid cartilage. Anterior commissure tumors that have thyroid cartilage invasion typically display cephalad surface invasion of the infrapetiole region of the supraglottis or caudal surface invasion of the subglottis (both T2 lesions by surface staging criteria); this is shown diagrammatically in Figure 9.5.

There have been divergent opinions as to whether cancer can be endoscopically eradicated from the anterior commissure. The proscriptions imposed by some surgeons are based primarily on the difficulty in obtaining adequate surgical exposure in this area (Wolfensberger & Dort, 1990). The actual limitation for a resection of an early cancer in the anterior commissure is the true extent of the disease (i.e., whether the cancer is invading cartilage) and the endoscopic exposure required to encompass the lesion. Davis, Jako, Hyams, and Shapshay (1982) from the Boston University group and later Koufman (1986) demonstrated that cancer could be removed from the anterior commissure; however, it required great skill to excise the lesion without vaporizing the specimen. With the exposure advantages of the patented (Zeitels, 1999c) triangular-shaped universal modular glottiscope (see Figure 9.6) with unique proximal and distal views (see Figure 9.7), Desloge and Zeitels (2000) demonstrated that curative resection of T1 glottic cancer was not problematic. Vaporizing cancer without clear en block resection margins is an inadequate surgical oncological technique. This factor, as well as underestimating the extent of disease, probably led to the reported failures by a number of previous investigators (Casiano, Cooper, Lundy, & Chandler, 1991; Krespi & Meltzer, 1989; Wetmore, Key, & Suen, 1986; Wolfensberger & Dort, 1990).

Because of the posttreatment failures reported in the literature cited previously, poor outcome of the cancer treatment was mistakenly attributed to the

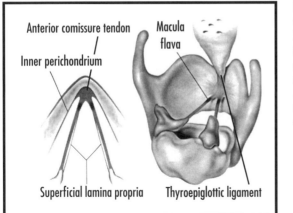

FIGURE 9.4. Diagrammatic representation of the anterior commissure tendon. *Note.* From "Optimizing Voice in Conservation Surgery for Glottic Cancer," by G. Hartig and S. M. Zeitels, 1998, *Operative Techniques in Otolaryngology—Head and Neck Surgery (Phonosurgery Part 1), 9,* pp. 214–223. Copyright 1998 by Elsevier. Reprinted with permission.

FIGURE 9.5. Diagrammatic representation of how cancer spreads around the anterior commissure tendon to invade the thyroid cartilage. *Note.* From "Optimizing Voice in Conservation Surgery for Glottic Cancer," by G. Hartig and S. M. Zeitels, 1998, *Operative Techniques in Otolaryngology—Head and Neck Surgery (Phonosurgery Part 1), 9,* pp. 214–223. Copyright 1998 by Elsevier. Reprinted with permission.

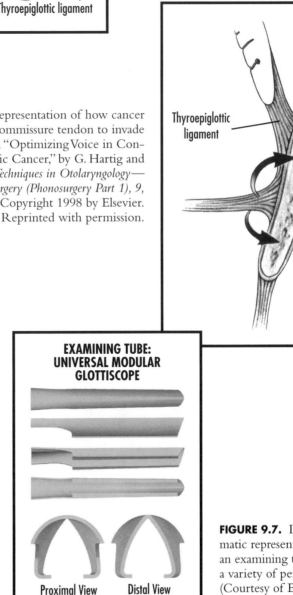

FIGURE 9.6. Zeitels universal modular glottiscope. (Courtesy of Endocraft LLC.)

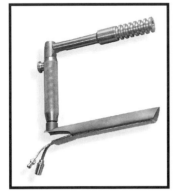

FIGURE 9.7. Diagrammatic representation of an examining tube from a variety of perspectives. (Courtesy of Endocraft LLC.)

biological behavior of the disease rather than the inadequate exposure and the compromised resection (Casiano et al., 1991; Krespi & Meltzer, 1989; Wetmore et al., 1986; Wolfensberger & Dort, 1990). Therefore, a procedure was designed to facilitate the diagnostic staging and treatment of early glottic cancer at the anterior commissure (Hartig & Zeitels, 1998; Zeitels, 1998). This procedure involves resecting the supraglottal tissue (infrapetiole region and anterior vestibular folds) cephalad to the anterior commissure tendon to determine whether limited anterior glottic cancer (AGC) had invaded the thyroid cartilage. A CO_2 laser resection of the uninvolved supraglottis is done in any case where the perimeter of the lesion cannot be visualized in its entirety (Desloge & Zeitels, 2000). This allows for positioning of the triangular glottiscope (Zeitels, 1999b) adjacent to the inner thyroid lamina above the AGC, thus facilitating clear resection of part or all of the anterior commissure tendon. There have been no resection failures (Desloge & Zeitels, 2000) in a limited number of cases (about 15) treated thus far. If the cancer is confined to the anterior commissure tendon and if resection of the tendon is not in the individual's best interest (i.e., poorer postoperative anticipated voice quality), radiation can commence promptly with confidence that there is true T1 stage disease.

If one accepts Kirchner's histopathological data regarding the invasion pattern of T1 glottic cancer (Kirchner, 1989; Kirchner & Carter, 1987), there is no reason to believe that an adequate soft-tissue resection of small-volume soft-tissue disease is not adequate treatment. This premise is further substantiated by a number of reports that did not find a correlation between anterior commissure involvement with T1 glottic cancer and failure of radiotherapy as a curative modality (Benninger, Gillen, Thieme, Jacobson, & Dragovich, 1994; Mendenhall, Parsons, Stringer, & Cassissi, 1994).

The extensive European experience reported by Eckel and Thumfart (1992), Rudert (1994a), and Steiner (1993) substantiates that glottic cancer in the anterior commissure can be removed transorally. The problem with any surgical approach to the anterior commissure (for true T1a, T1b, and T2 lesions) is that vocal quality is significantly impaired when these procedures disturb the structural integrity of both sides of the anterior commissure tendon. Lesions that invade cartilage are T4 by stage, require open partial laryngectomy, and are not suitable for endoscopic excision. An endoscopic exploration of the infrapetiole region of the supraglottis allows for definitive determination about whether a presumed T1 lesion has cartilage invasion, and therefore must be staged as a T4 lesion (Zeitels, 1998). This endoscopic procedure facilitates (a) precise staging without disarticulating Broyle's ligament, (b) commensurate management, and (c) optimal posttreatment voice quality.

Endoscopic Technique

The goal of endoscopic treatment of an isolated T1 lesion of the musculomembranous vocal fold is eradication of the disease with maximal preservation of the normal layered microstructure. This approach results in optimal postoperative voice quality without compromising oncological cure. There are four basic procedures that are based on the depth of excision (as depicted in Figure 9.2) (Zeitels, 1996b). These procedures are (a) dissection just deep to the epithelial basement membrane in the superficial aspect of the superficial lamina propria for atypical epithelium and microinvasive cancer; (b) dissection within the deep aspect of the superficial lamina propria for microinvasive cancer that is not attached to the vocal ligament (see Figure 9.8); (c) dissection between the deep lamina propria (vocal ligament) and the vocalis muscle for lesions that are attached to the ligament but do not penetrate through it (see Figure 9.9); and (d) dissection within the thyroarytenoid muscle for lesions penetrating the vocal ligament and invading the vocalis muscle. This approach can be fine-tuned further by performing partial resections of any of the layered microstructure. The specimen is always oriented for whole-mount histological analysis, and frozen-section margin assessment is employed selectively to verify a complete tumor excision (Zeitels, 1995, 1996b).

If dissection is performed within the superficial lamina propria (Reinke's space), cold instruments facilitate precise tangential dissection around the curving vocal fold. This allows for maximal preservation of the superficial lamina propria and for pliability of the regenerating epithelium (Zeitels, 1995, 1996a, 1996b). Dissection between the vocal ligament and the vocalis muscle can be performed equally well with cold instruments alone or with assistance of the CO_2 laser. Dissection within the muscle is performed most precisely with the CO_2 laser, which allows for improved visualization because of its hemostatic cutting properties.

In addition to improving preexcisional assessment of lesion depth, the subepithelial saline–epinephrine infusion into Reinke's space (see lamina propia in Figure 9.1) assists with the surgeon's technical execution of the surgery in a number of ways: (a) the infusion facilitates mucosal incisions by improving visualization of the lateral border of the lesion and by distending the superficial lamina propria so that the overlying epithelium is under tension; (b) the infusion also increases the depth of the superficial lamina propria, which facilitates a less traumatic dissection in this layer and leads to regenerated epithelium that is more flexible; (c) the epinephrine and hydrostatic pressure of the infusion vasoconstricts microvasculature in the superficial lamina propria, and this improves visualization and precise dissection; and (d) if the laser is used, the saline absorbs the thermal energy, which decreases heat-induced trauma to the normal vocal fold tissue.

Vocal Outcome After Endoscopic Resection of the Musculomembranous Region

Using ultra-narrow resection techniques along with laryngoplasty reconstructive methods (injection and transcervical medialization), normal conversational-level voices are usually achieved (Zeitels et al., 2002). The laryngologist can precisely

(text continues on p. 182)

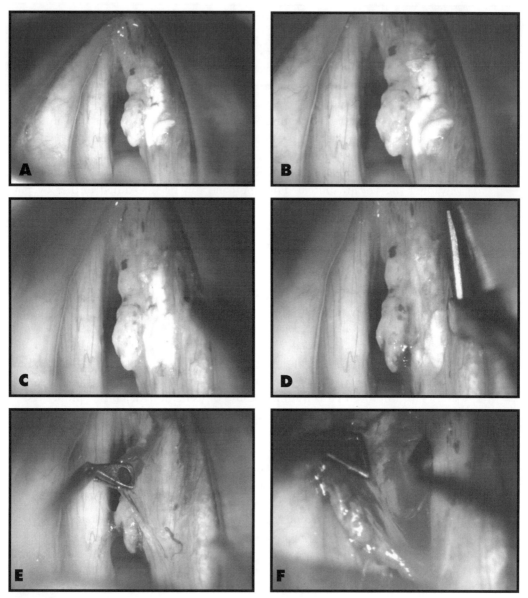

FIGURE 9.8. (A) A Shakespearean drama professor and actor with progressive hoarseness and a keratotic lesion of the right vocal fold. He had undergone a limited biopsy at another institution 3 years previously, which revealed severe atypia. The lesion was followed rather than removed for fear that the excision would lead to severe dysphonia. The appearance of the lesion deteriorated over time, and a presumed T1N0M0 (Stage I) was noted upon current presentation (magnification at 4×). (B) The lesion seen in Figure 9.8A at higher magnification (7×). (C) A subepithelial infusion is done; the specially designed needle is seen on the superior surface of the vocal fold (magnification at 7×). (D) An upturned scissor is used to perform an epithelial cordotomy, which serves as a perimeter margin (magnification at 7×). (E) The edge of the microflap is retracted medially with an angled forceps, which reveals normal superficial lamina propria. A left curved dissector is used to easily dissect the lesion from the residual normal superficial lamina propria (magnification at 7×). (F) The dissection is completed to the inferior margin of the lesion. The lesion is retracted and an upturned scissors is used to complete the resection (magnification at 7×). (Courtesy of Steven M. Zeitels.)

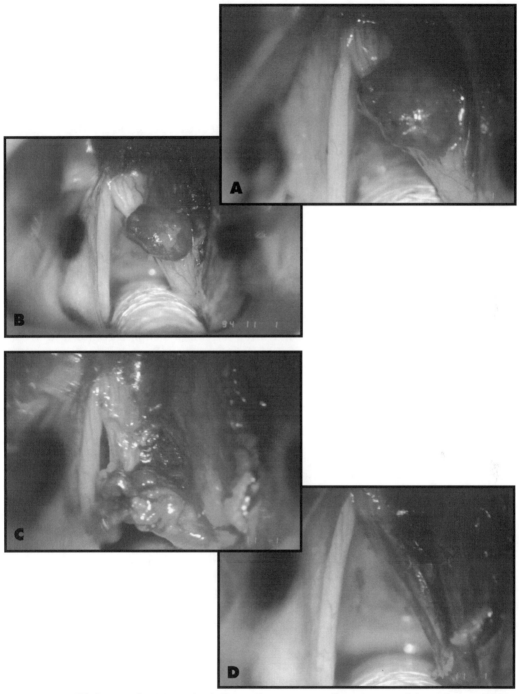

FIGURE 9.9. (A) An exophytic T1N0M0 (Stage I) squamous cell carcinoma of the right vocal fold (magnification at 7×). (B) The vestibular fold has been resected, which provides excellent exposure of the right vocal fold cancer (magnification at 7×). (C) The dissection is performed so that very little of the vocal muscle is disturbed and the vocal ligament is used as a margin (magnification at 7×). (D) The right vocal fold cancer has been resected en block with the vocal ligament as a margin. The right neocord is remarkably well contoured considering the extent of the resection (magnification at 7×). (Courtesy of Steven M. Zeitels.)

accommodate a microcontrolled excision to the three-dimensional characteristics of the vocal cord cancer. Unlike radiation, microlaryngeal excision avoids trauma to uninvolved tissue, such as the contralateral vocal fold, during treatment of a unilateral lesion (Lehman et al., 1988; see also Burns, Zeitels, & Dailey, 2004, and Chapter 10 in this text). It is expected that increasing the magnitude of the resection, especially its depth, leads to deteriorating vocal function (Burns et al., 2004; Doyle, 1997; Hirano, Hirade, & Kawasaki, 1985; McGuirt, Blalock, Koufman, & Feehs, 1992; Zeitels, 1996b). The graduated resection approach suggested by Hirano et al. (1985) and Koufman (1986) was developed further by Zeitels (1995, 1996a, 1996b).

The mucosal microflap technique that is useful for resection of epithelial atypia and microinvasive cancer can sometimes be confined to the superior surface of the vocal fold. After reepithelialization, typically the individual can comfortably increase subglottal driving pressures to achieve an objectively measured (via acoustical analysis) normal voice at conversational levels, as well as one that is judged improved perceptually. Maximal performance (dynamic range) tasks reveal some mild limitation of frequency variation, specifically a reduction in one's frequency range and in one's loudness capability. As a resection extends to the medial vocalizing surface of the vocal fold, there is further progression of vocal dysfunction (Zeitels, 1995). When the surgical dissection is confined to the superficial lamina propria in one vocal fold, perceptual assessment of the resulting voice is usually normal. Stroboscopy reveals mild impairment of mucosal-wave propagation with regard to both the amplitude and magnitude of vocal fold vibration wherever there has been dissection in the superficial lamina propria (Zeitels et al., 2002).

As the deep resection margin extends to include the vocalis muscle, there is further acoustic, aerodynamic, and stroboscopic impairment. When the superficial lamina propria is excised as a component of the cancer resection, the regenerated epithelial surface is adherent to the underlying body of the vocal cord (Davis, Hadley, & Smith, 2004; Zeitels, 1994, 1995; Zeitels et al., 2002); this results in unavoidable stiffness in the vibratory characteristics of the regenerated epithelium. We have not seen evidence that the pliable superficial lamina propria regenerates in the same manner that epithelium does after its removal; however, after a resection of the vocal fold epithelium and its underlying laminae propria, the healed neocord is usually smooth and straight and glottal closure is usually normal. Vocal limitations still may not be perceptible at conversational levels in some patients if glottal closure is complete. Obvious hoarseness, however, is usually observed when complete glottal closure does not occur because of tissue loss as a result of surgical excavation of the vocal edge (Zeitels, 1994, 1995; Zeitels et al., 2002). This defect can be reconstructed by endolaryngeal injection techniques (Burns et al., 2004) or transcervical laryngoplastic phonosurgical reconstruction (Desloge, Zeitels, Bunting, & Hillman, 1999; Zeitels, 1999a; Zeitels et al., 2002; Zeitels et al., 2001), which is described later in this chapter (see "Glottic Reconstruction and Voice Rehabilitation" in this chapter).

Mid-Sized Glottic Cancer: T2 and T3 Lesions

A primary objective in the surgical treatment of mid-sized glottic cancer is functional preservation and not necessarily organ preservation (Wolf et al., 1991). Glottic cancer is typically staged T2 because of impaired mobility or mucosal extension to the subglottis or supraglottis. Classical conservation surgical treatment for this disease is vertical partial laryngectomy, or hemilaryngectomy, which generally results in a local control and cure rate of about 75% to 80% (see Chapter 11 in this text). These procedures were championed by Leroux-Robert (1956), Som (1951), and Ogura and Biller (1969) during the mid-20th century. Most patients are decannulated after an initial perioperative tracheotomy. These procedures are described and illustrated in detail in a number of atlases (e.g., Silver, 1981a; Weinstein & Laccourreye, 2000) and are associated with alteration in both perceptual and acoustic characteristics of the vocal signal (Doyle, 1997; Doyle, Leeper, Houghton-Jones, Heeneman, & Martin, 1995; Leeper et al., 1993; Leeper, Heeneman, & Reynolds, 1990).

If the disease involves a majority of the glottis bilaterally, the musculomembranous glottis and lower supraglottis can be resected and reconstructed by means of a cricohyoidoepiglotticopexy (Majer & Reider, 1959). In recent years, this procedure has been refined and popularized (Laccourreye, Laccourreye, Menard, Weinstein, & Brasnu, 1990). Individuals who undergo cricohyoidoepiglotticopexy can typically be decannulated and will have a serviceable voice postsurgically. The sound source is provided by vibration of edematous superior arytenoid mucosa contacting the laryngeal surface of the residual epiglottis.

There has been growing support for resecting T2 and T3 lesions by means of CO_2 laser resection. Steiner (1984, 1993) advanced this initiative, and it has gained increased international acceptance. Recently, Zeitels et al. have reported on en block resection of mid-sized glottic cancer (Zeitels, Dailey, & Burns, 2004). The clear advantages of this approach are the lack of a tracheotomy and the accompanying shortened hospitalization. Furthermore, additional treatment options are preserved, including further endolaryngeal resections. Although these individuals are not usually reconstructed at the time of resection, phonosurgical reconstructive techniques (see next section) can be performed after epithelialization has occurred.

Although designed in the 1970s (Vaughan, 1978; Vaughan, Strong, & Jako, 1978), the CO_2 laser resection technique is difficult and is usually done by surgeons who are specially skilled. Endoscopic resection of T2 and T3 glottic cancer is not frequently taught in surgical training programs. Generally, radiation as a single-modality treatment will result in more local failures than partial laryngectomy and, therefore, will result in the need for more total laryngectomy procedures. When radiation is successful, however, this treatment generally results in better voice quality than that associated with open partial laryngectomy (see Chapter 11 in this text). It has not been clearly established whether the administration of neoadjuvant chemotherapy prior to radiation offers any survival advantage.

Glottic Reconstruction and Voice Rehabilitation

When a significant amount of vocalis muscle is removed as part of the deep surgical margin, the healed neocord is usually concave (see Figure 9.10A). The excavated neocord results in incomplete glottal closure during phonation (Zeitels et al., 2002). This leads to a stiff, leaking glottal valve and a dysphonic voice. As the depth of an excision leads to valvular incompetence of the glottis, there is an increase in (a) subglottal pressures and flows, (b) acoustical instability or perturbation (jitter and shimmer), and (c) compensatory supraglottal muscle strain patterns. Stroboscopy reveals no substantive mucosal-wave vibration, but rather mass motion of the stiff neocord body (Zeitels, 1995). Consequently, measurement of functional outcomes including assessment of voice is essential (Meleca, Dworkin, Kewson, Stachler, & Hill, 2003; Olthoff et al., 2003).

Once the neocord is healed, phonosurgical reconstruction may ensue if the vocal fold edge is excavated. Initially, this consists of microlaryngoscopic fat injection (see Figure 9.10; Burns et al., 2004; Zeitels et al., 2002). This may take one or two injections, based on how much tissue was initially resected and how much of the fat implant is resorbed. As necessary, a medialization laryngoplasty, an anterior commissure laryngoplasty, or both can be performed once there is adequate glottal tissue medial to the thyroid lamina. Gore-Tex has been ideal in this setting because it can be molded in vivo to conform to the abnormal postresection contours (Zeitels, 1999a; Zeitels, Jarboe, & Hillman, 2000). The advantage of the medialization is that it is done under local anesthesia with intravenous sedation, which allows for phonatory feedback during the procedure. The vocal outcome is often dependent on the flexibility of the normal layered microstructure of the uninvolved vocal fold.

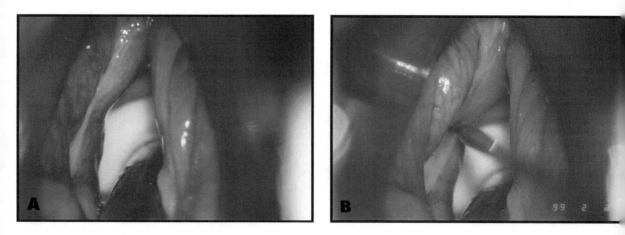

SUPRAGLOTTIC CANCER

Transcervical Horizontal Supraglottic Laryngectomy

Similar to hemilaryngectomy, open conservation surgery for supraglottic carcinoma was catalyzed in the mid-1900s (Alonso, 1947; Ogura, 1958; Ogura & Biller, 1969). In this procedure (Tucker, 1971; Tucker & Smith, 1962), the connective tissue compartment deep to the supraglottic mucosa is resected (upper paraglottic and preepiglottic spaces). The technical details of the resection are detailed in a number of textbooks (e.g., Laccourreye & Weinstein, 2000; Silver, 1981b). Generally, there has not been significant change in this procedure in recent decades. Unfortunately, no substantial randomized studies have compared radiation to supraglottic laryngectomy. Based on retrospective information, when disease is confined to the supraglottis, local control is about 80% with surgery and about 70% with radiation. The rate-limiting factor regarding survival in supraglottic cancer relates primarily to successful treatment of the neck.

The Philosophy of Endoscopic Resection

Endoscopic supraglottic surgery is done far less frequently than glottal surgery (Zeitels & Davis, 1994). The surgical field is typically much larger and, therefore, requires different laryngoscopes and hand instrumentation. A bivalved adjustable supraglottiscope was designed by Zeitels and Vaughan (1990) to facilitate

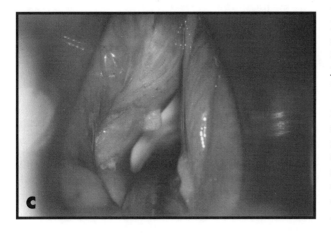

FIGURE 9.10. (A) Patient who has undergone phonomicrosurgical resection of a left T1a carcinoma and now has an excavated vocal fold in the musculo-membranous region (magnification at 4×). (B) A Brunings injection needle placed lateral to the concavity in the paraglottic space (magnification at 4×). (C) The vocal fold has been augmented with fat. A small amount of the graft is extruding from the puncture site and should be removed with cold instruments to avoid a granuloma. Note the new convexity of the vocal fold (magnification at 4×). (Courtesy of Steven M. Zeitels.)

endoscopic supraglottal surgery (Zeitels, Vaughan, & Domanowski, 1990). This instrument was a modification of Steiner's (1984) laryngoscope. A number of bi-valved spatula laryngoscopes that are suitable for performing supraglottal surgery are available from the major manufacturers. It is important for the surgeon to compare the distal distension strength prior to purchasing one. In principle, bi-valved laryngoscopes accommodate better to the large supraglottal surgical field and larger lesions that require increased hand-instrument angulation for tissue re-traction. Larger and sturdier hand instruments from the premicroscope era can still be purchased, or they can often be obtained from the mediastinoscopy set.

In addition to the aforementioned technical differences between endo-scopic supraglottal and glottal surgery, different functional issues are emphasized as well. If the airway is stable, the most common functional concern is preserva-tion of the voice in glottic surgery, but swallowing in supraglottal surgery (see Chapter 14 in this text). The microspot CO_2 laser is a very effective instrument for supraglottal surgery because thermal-induced fibrosis of residual supraglottal tissues results in beneficial cicatricial scarring and reestablishment of a competent supraglottic swallowing valve (Zeitels & Vaughan, 1990, 1991a; Zeitels, Vaughan, & Domanowski, 1990).

Background of Endoscopic Management

Direct laryngoscopic resection of supraglottic cancer dates back to the early 20th century. Jackson (1915) and Jackson and Jackson (1939) described the use of a tubular laryngoscope and a punch biopsy forceps for resecting suprahyoid epiglottic cancer. The lesion was resected by cutting around the lesion with the punch; if the tissue specimens within the punch were cancer free, the resection was considered curative. In 1941, by means of surgical diathermy, New and Dorton performed transoral ablation of several supraglottic carcinomas by em-ploying a Lynch suspension laryngoscope (Lynch, 1915, 1916), a modification of Killian's system (Killian, 1912, 1914). Vaughan (1978) was the first to describe mi-croscopically controlled CO_2 laser resection of supraglottic cancer. Subsequently, other Boston University trainees, including Davis and colleagues (Davis et al., 1982; Davis et al., 1991; Davis, Shapshay, Strong, & Hyams, 1983) and Zeitels and colleagues (Zeitels, Koufman, Davis, & Vaughan, 1994; Zeitels, Vaughan, Domanowski, Fuleihan, & Simpson, 1990), reported several series of CO_2 laser supraglottic cancer resections (Zeitels & Davis, 1994). When lesions were resected with frozen-section control of the margins and postoperative radiotherapy was administered, local failure resulting in total laryngectomy was a rare occurrence. Steiner (1984, 1988), Eckel and Thumfart (1992), and Rudert (1994b) also have been strong advocates of endoscopic management of supraglottic cancer.

These investigators, both in the United States and Germany, incorporated technological advancements in microlaryngeal surgery to expand Jackson's con-cepts. For a number of reasons, however, most surgeons in North America have not adopted the endoscopic excision approach despite its value and merit. First, most surgeons are not familiar with the details of the technique, and the endo-scopic approach represents a treatment paradigm shift. Second, larger lesions are technically difficult to resect if one is not familiar with the procedural details of the method. Furthermore, because teaching the technique is not effectively done in continuing education courses, large-scale teaching is not done. Finally, surgical resection of laryngeal cancer is declining at many centers because there has been a proliferation of organ-preservation protocols.

Curative Endoscopic Resection

Endoscopic resection of supraglottic cancer can be performed as a single-modal-ity treatment. Small lesions are excised during the staging endoscopy, and the re-section is both diagnostic and therapeutic (Zeitels, 1994). Therefore, any further treatment such as open surgery or radiation becomes superfluous and is not cost-effective. With endoscopic resection, there is no significant loss of laryngeal func-tion, most patients return to a normal diet within several days, and no patient has required artificial airway intervention.

Transoral excision of supraglottic cancer as a single-modality treatment is successful when lesions are selected for their small size and endoscopic accessibil-ity. Small-volume lesions that arise on the suprahyoid epiglottis, aryepiglottic fold, and vestibular fold are amenable to en block endoscopic resection because they are more perpendicular to the distal lumen of the laryngoscope. Specimen mar-gins are ideally established through multiple-section analysis of the en block re-sected specimen rather than by means of frozen sections from the patient. Deci-sions about postoperative radiotherapy and treatment of both sides of the neck should be based on the pathological assessment of the lesion. Controlling neck metastasis is critical if cure of supraglottic cancer is to be achieved (DeSanto, 1990; Desloge et al., 1999; Levendag et al., 1989; Lutz, Johnson, & Wagner, 1990). Consideration should be given to the volume of the cancer, the depth and loca-tion of its penetration, and the pattern of its invasion. Even small lesions of the aryepiglottic fold and vestibular fold will demonstrate early invasion of the para-glottic space, which places the neck at risk for occult metastasis. In contrast, early suprahyoid epiglottic carcinomas rarely invade the preepiglottic space and rarely metastasize to the neck if there is no occult tongue-base invasion (Zeitels & Vaughan, 1991a).

It is not clear whether radiation to the larynx is necessary if an adequate en-doscopic resection has been performed. Currently, the first multi-institutional study is being conducted to assess the reliability of endoscopic resection (without radiation) of any accessible supraglottic cancer. There are many T2 and T3 lesions in this series. The participants are Drs. Davis (University of Utah), DeSanto (Mayo Clinic), Gluckman (University of Cincinnati), Haughey (Washington Uni-versity), Hoffman (University of Iowa), Pearson (Mayo Clinic), Strome (Cleve-land Clinic), and Zeitels (Harvard University).

Endoscopic Resection Followed by Radiation Therapy

Transoral resection of larger supraglottic cancers followed by full-course radiotherapy to the primary site and both sides of the neck offers a more aggressive treatment approach for those individuals who otherwise would undergo radiotherapy as a sole treatment. The histopathologically controlled endoscopic resection results in a cancer-free field prior to the administration of full-course radiotherapy. This approach stresses laryngeal function preservation (airway, swallowing, and voice) rather than organ preservation (Wolf et al., 1991; see also Chapter 11 in this text).

These supraglottic endoscopic resections are considered excisional biopsies because margins are frequently close and the deep compartments (preepiglottic and paraglottic spaces) are not excised completely. These individuals have no clinical evidence of cancer when they commence radiotherapy. The success of obtaining clear margins in these excisional biopsies is based on the typical pattern of invasion that is broad and pushing with a pseudocapsule (Kirchner, 1989; Kirchner & Carter, 1987; Zeitels & Vaughan, 1991a). This pseudocapsule probably arises from the epiglottic perichondrium and the quadrangular membrane of the false vocal fold (Shapiro, Zeitels, & Fried, 1992; Zeitels & Vaughan, 1991a; Zeitels, Vaughan, & Domanowski, 1990).

Surgical Technique

Lesions that are larger in size and those arising on the infrahyoid epiglottis and upper false vocal fold are more difficult to resect transorally because they are visualized tangentially; that is, the lesion and the dissection plain are viewed at an angle (Rudert, 1994a; Steiner, 1993). Therefore, the surgeon must decide whether the neoplasm will be excised en block or in a piecemeal fashion. The philosophy of endoscopic en block excision maintains a more standard surgical oncological approach. Larger lesions, however, gradually fill the laryngoscope lumen as they are mobilized. This makes en block excision technically difficult. Some groups in Germany (Rudert, 1994a; Steiner, 1993) section the specimen and resect the tumor in a piecemeal fashion. There is little question that this makes the procedure technically easier. These investigators also maintain that transecting the lesion facilitates a precise assessment of the depth of invasion. They have not noted increased rates of local, regional, or distant failure.

Laryngeal Function After Endoscopic Excision

The airway and voice are not typically impaired by an endoscopic supraglottic resection. Often, however, the airway is improved when an exophytic lesion is excised. On occasion, a patient may require a late tracheotomy secondary to late stenosis from severe gastroesophageal reflux (Zeitels, 1994). Laryngeal protective sphincteric function may be impaired temporarily depending on the extent of the supraglottic tissues excised. No permanent swallowing impairment has occurred in patients who have otherwise normal swallowing mechanisms. Previous impairment in swallowing, such as that subsequent to stroke or previous head and neck surgery, is a relative contraindication to any partial laryngeal resection.

Limited resections of the suprahyoid epiglottis, aryepiglottic fold, or vestibular fold do not impair swallowing function because most of the sphincteric function of the supraglottis is unaffected. Additionally, the epiglottis is a vestigial organ in humans and often contains olfactory epithelium in mammals (Kirchner, 1986). More extensive resections of the supraglottis may predispose individuals to aspiration that may last from several days to 6 weeks depending on the magnitude of the resection. Although patients may require nasogastric feeding during this time, we have not observed occurrences of aspiration pneumonia during swallowing rehabilitation or from salivary soilage. Hospitalization from this procedure is usually 1 to 3 days.

The favorable swallowing rehabilitation after extensive transoral supraglottic resections occurs for several reasons (Zeitels, 1994, 1995). Most important, the superior laryngeal nerves are not disturbed proximal to the larynx. Therefore, the neosupraglottic region becomes fully sensate. Second, laryngeal elevation is not impaired due to either disturbance of the suprahyoid musculature or performance of a tracheotomy. Finally, because the supraglottic defect heals completely by secondary fibrosis and epithelialization, there is favorable cicatrization that results in a new supraglottic valve.

SUMMARY

There have been a number of advances in the surgical management of laryngeal cancer since the early 1990s. As in many surgical paradigms, these have centered around the evolution of minimally invasive techniques (endoscopic resection). Understandably, transoral resection of laryngeal cancer provides an effective treatment, with less morbidity and an enhanced functional outcome. This chapter was designed to familiarize the reader with the oncological and functional ramifications of this approach in the context of more standard treatment modalities (i.e., open surgery and radiotherapy). The management principles discussed herein should provide the foundation for understanding future innovative treatment methods that will occur based on a variety of new endoscopic surgical methods.

REFERENCES

Alonso, J. M. (1947). Conservation surgery of cancer of the larynx. *Transactions of the American Academy of Ophthalmology and Otolaryngology, 51,* 633–642.

Benninger, M., Gillen, J., Thieme, P., Jacobson, B., & Dragovich, J. (1994). Factors associated with recurrence and voice quality following radiation therapy for T1 and T2 glottic carcinomas. *Laryngoscope, 104,* 294–298.

Burns, J. A., Zeitels, S. M., & Dailey, S. H. (2004). Micro-stereo-laryngoscopic lipoinjection. *Laryngoscope, 114,* 1864–1867.

Casiano, R., Cooper, J. D., Lundy, D. S., & Chandler, J. R. (1991). Laser cordectomy for T1 glottic carcinoma: A 10-year experience and videostroboscopic findings. *Otolaryngology—Head and Neck Surgery, 104,* 831–837.

Cragle, S. P., & Brandenburg, J. H. (1993). Laser cordectomy or radiotherapy: Cure rates, communication, and cost. *Otolaryngology—Head and Neck Surgery, 108,* 648–653.

Davis, R. K., Hadley, K., & Smith, M. E. (2004). Endoscopic vertical partial laryngectomy. *Laryngoscope, 114,* 236–240.

Davis, R. K., Jako, G. J., Hyams, V. J., & Shapshay, S. M. (1982). The anatomic limitations of CO_2 laser cordectomy. *Laryngoscope, 92,* 980–984.

Davis, R. K., Kelley, S. M., & Hayes, J. (1991). Endoscopic CO_2 laser excisional biopsy of early supraglottic cancer. *Laryngoscope, 100,* 680–683.

Davis, R. K., Shapshay, S. M., Strong, S. M., & Hyams, V. J. (1983). Transoral partial supraglottic resection using the CO_2 laser. *Laryngoscope, 93,* 429–432.

DeSanto, L. W. (1976). *Selection of treatment for in situ and early invasive carcinoma of the glottis.* Workshops from the Centennial Conference on Laryngeal Cancer. New York: Appleton-Century-Crofts.

DeSanto, L. W. (1990). The "second" side of the neck in supraglottic cancer. *Otolaryngology—Head and Neck Surgery, 102,* 351–361.

Desloge, R. B., & Zeitels, S. M. (2000). Microsurgery at the anterior glottal commissure: Controversies and observations. *Annals of Otology, Rhinology and Laryngology, 109,* 385–392.

Desloge, R. B., Zeitels, S. M., Bunting, G., & Hillman, R. E. (1999, August). *Phonosurgical reconstruction subsequent to early glottic cancer resection.* Paper presented at the 30th Annual Symposium: Care of the Professional Voice, Philadelphia.

Doyle, P. C. (1997). Voice refinement following conservation surgery for cancer of the larynx: A conceptual framework for treatment intervention. *American Journal of Speech–Language Pathology, 6,* 27–35.

Doyle, P. C., Leeper, H. A., Houghton-Jones, C., Heeneman, H., & Martin, G. F. (1995). Perceptual characteristics of hemilaryngectomized and near-total laryngectomized male speakers. *Journal of Medical Speech–Language Pathology, 3,* 131–143.

Eckel, H., & Thumfart, W. F. (1992). Laser surgery for the treatment of larynx carcinomas: Indications, techniques, and preliminary results. *Annals of Otology, Rhinology and Laryngology, 101,* 113–118.

Fraenkel, B. (1886). First healing of a laryngeal cancer taken out through the natural passages. *Archives für Klinische Chirurgie, 12,* 283–286.

Hartig, G., & Zeitels, S. M. (1998). Optimizing voice in conservation surgery for glottic cancer. *Operative Techniques in Otolaryngology—Head and Neck Surgery (Phonosurgery Part 1), 9,* 214–223.

Hellquist, H., Lundgren, J., & Olafsson, J. (1982). Hyperplasia, keratosis, dysplasia and carcinoma in situ of the vocal cords—A follow-up study. *Clinical Otolaryngology, 7,* 11–27.

Hirano, M., Hirade, Y., & Kawasaki, H. (1985). Vocal function following carbon dioxide laser surgery for glottic carcinoma. *Annals of Otology, Rhinology and Laryngology, 94,* 232–235.

Jackson, C. (1915). Malignant disease of the epiglottis. In *Peroral endoscopy and laryngeal surgery* (pp. 438–439). St. Louis: Laryngoscope Co.

Jackson, C., & Jackson, C. L. (1939). Endoscopic removal of cancer of the epiglottis. In *Cancer of the larynx* (p. 52). Philadelphia: Saunders.

Kass, E. S., Hillman, R. E., & Zeitels, S. M. (1996). The submucosal infusion technique in pho-nomicrosurgery. *Annals of Otology, Rhinology and Laryngology, 105,* 341–347.

Killian, G. (1912). Die Schwebelaryngoskopie. *Archiv für Laryngologie und Rhinologie, 26,* 277–317.

Killian, G. (1914). Suspension laryngoscopy and its practical use. *Journal of Laryngology and Otology, 24,* 337–360.

Kirchner, J. A. (1986). *Pressman and Kellman's physiology of the larynx* [Monograph]. Washington DC: American Academy of Otolaryngology—Head and Neck Surgery Foundation.

Kirchner, J. A. (1989). What have whole organ sections contributed to the treatment of laryngeal cancer? *Annals of Otology, Rhinology and Laryngology, 98,* 661–667.

Kirchner, J. A., & Carter, D. (1987). Intralaryngeal barriers to the spread of cancer. *Acta Otolaryngo-logica (Stockholm), 103,* 503–513.

Koufman, J. A. (1986). The endoscopic management of early squamous carcinoma of the vocal cord with the carbon dioxide surgical laser: Clinical experience and a proposed subclassification. *Otolaryngology—Head and Neck Surgery, 95,* 531–537.

Krespi, Y., & Meltzer, C. J. (1989). Laser surgery for vocal cord carcinoma involving the anterior commissure. *Annals of Otology, Rhinology and Laryngology, 98,* 105–109.

Laccourreye, O., Laccourreye, H., Menard, M., Weinstein, G., & Brasnu, D. (1990). Vertical partial laryngectomies. *Annals of Otology, Rhinology and Laryngology, 99,* 421–426.

Laccourreye, O., & Weinstein, G. (2000). Supraglottic laryngectomy. In G. Weinstein, O. Laccourreye, D. Brasnu, & H. Laccourreye (Eds.), *Organ preservation surgery for laryngeal cancer* (pp. 107–125). San Diego: Singular.

Leeper, H. A., Doyle, P. C., Heeneman, H., Martin, G. F., Hoasjoe, D. K., & Wong, F. S. (1993). Acoustical characteristics of voice following hemilaryngectomy and near-total laryngec-tomy. *Journal of Medical Speech–Language Pathology, 1,* 89–94.

Leeper, H. A., Heeneman, H., & Reynolds, C. (1990). Vocal function following vertical partial lar-yngectomy: A preliminary investigation. *Journal of Otolaryngology, 19,* 62–67.

Lehman, J. J., Bless, D. M., & Brandenburg, J. H. (1988). An objective assessment of voice production after radiation therapy for Stage I squamous cell carcinoma of the glottis. *Otolaryngology—Head and Neck Surgery, 98,* 121–129.

Leroux-Robert, J. (1956). Indications for radical surgery, radiotherapy and combined surgery and radiotherapy for cancer of the larynx and hypopharynx. *Annals of Otology, Rhinology and Laryngology, 65,* 137–144.

Levendag, P., Sessions, R., Vikram, B., Strong, E. W., Shah, J. P., Spiro, R., & Gerrold, F. (1989). The problem of neck relapse in early stage supraglottic larynx cancer. *Cancer, 63,* 345–348.

Lutz, C. K., Johnson, J. T., & Wagner, R. L. (1990). Supraglottic cancer: Patterns of recurrence. *An-nals of Otology, Rhinology and Laryngology, 99,* 12–17.

Lynch, R. C. (1915). Suspension laryngoscopy and its accomplishments. *Annals of Otology, Rhinology and Laryngology, 24,* 429–446.

Lynch, R. C. (1916). A resume of my years work with suspension laryngoscopy. *Transactions of the American Laryngological Association, 38,* 158–175.

Lynch, R. C. (1920). Intrinsic carcinoma of the larynx, with a second report of the cases operated on by suspension and dissection. *Transactions of the American Laryngological Association, 40,* 119–126.

Majer, H., & Reider, W. (1959). Technique de laryngecomie permetant de conserver la permeabilite respiratoiré la cricohyoido-pexie. *Annales d'Oto-Laryngologie et de Chirurgie, 76,* 677–683.

McGuirt, W. F., Blalock, D., Koufman, J. A., & Feehs, R. S. (1992). Voice analysis of patients with endoscopically treated early laryngeal carcinoma. *Annals of Otology, Rhinology and Laryngology, 101,* 142–146.

Meleca, R. J., Dworkin, J. P., Kewson, D. T., Stachler, R. J., & Hill, S. L. (2003). Functional outcomes following nonsurgical treatment for advanced-stage laryngeal carcinoma. *Laryngoscope, 113,* 720–728.

Mendenhall, W., Parsons, J. T., Stringer, S. P., & Cassissi, N. J. (1994). Management of Tis, T1, T2 squamous cell carcinoma of the glottic larynx. *American Journal of Otolaryngology, 15,* 250–257.

Myers, E. N., Wagner, R. L., & Johnson, J. T. (1993). Microlaryngoscopic surgery for T1 glottic lesions: A cost effective option. *Annals of Otology, Rhinology and Laryngology, 103,* 28–30.

New, G. B., & Dorton, H. E. (1941). Suspension laryngoscopy in the treatment of malignant disease of the hypopharynx and larynx. *Mayo Clinic Proceedings, 16,* 411–416.

Ogura, J. H. (1958). Supraglottic subtotal laryngectomy and radical neck dissection for carcinoma of the epiglottis. *Laryngoscope, 68,* 983–1003.

Ogura, J. H., & Biller, H. (1969). Glottic reconstruction following extended fronto-lateral hemilaryngectomy. *Laryngoscope, 79,* 2181.

Olsen, K., Thomas, J.V., DeSanto, L. W., & Suman,V. J. (1993). Indications and results of cordectomy for early glottic carcinoma. *Otolaryngology—Head and Neck Surgery, 108,* 277–282.

Olthoff, A., Mrugalla, S., Laskawi, R., Frohlich, M., Stuermer, I., Kruse, E., Ambrosch, P., & Steiner, W. (2003). Assessment of irregular voices after total and laser surgical partial laryngectomy. *Archives of Otolaryngology—Head and Neck Surgery, 129,* 994–999.

Pearson, B. W., & Salassa, J. R. (2003). Transoral laser microresection for cancer of the larynx involving the anterior commissure. *Laryngoscope, 113,* 1104–1112.

Rudert, H. H. (1994a). Transoral CO_2-laser surgery of early glottic cancer (CIS-T2). In *Laryngeal cancer: Proceedings of the 2nd World Congress on Laryngeal Cancer.* Amsterdam: Elsevier.

Rudert, H. H. (1994b). Transoral CO_2-laser surgery in advanced supraglottic cancer. In *Laryngeal cancer: Proceedings of the 2nd World Congress on Laryngeal Cancer.* Amsterdam: Elsevier.

Shapiro, J., Zeitels, S. M., & Fried, M. F. (1992). Laser surgery for laryngeal cancer. *Operative Techniques in Otolaryngology—Head and Neck Surgery, 3,* 84–92.

Silver, C. E. (1981a). *Conservation surgery for glottic carcinoma.* New York: Churchill Livingstone.

Silver, C. E. (1981b). Supraglottic subtotal laryngectomy. In *Surgery for cancer of the larynx,* (pp. 127–137). New York: Churchill Livingstone.

Som, M. L. (1951). Hemilaryngectomy—A modified technique for cordal carcinoma with extension posteriorly. *Archives of Otolaryngology, 54,* 524.

Steiner, W. (1984). *Transoral microsurgical CO_2 laser resection of laryngeal carcinoma: Functional partial laryngectomy.* Berlin: Springer-Verlag.

Steiner, W. (1988). Experience in endoscopic laser surgery of malignant tumours of the upper aerodigestive tract. *Advances in Otorhinolaryngology, 39,* 135–144.

Steiner, W. (1993). Results of curative laser microsurgery of laryngeal carcinomas. *American Journal of Otolaryngology, 14,* 116–121.

Thomas, J., Olsen, K. D., Neel, H. B., DeSanto, L. W., & Suman,V. J. (1994). Recurrences after endoscopic management of early (T1) glottic cancer. *Laryngoscope, 104,* 1099–1104.

Tucker, G. F. (1971). *Human larynx coronal section atlas.* Washington, DC: Armed Forces Institute of Pathology.

Tucker, G. F., & Smith, H. R. (1962). A histological demonstration of the development of laryngeal connective tissue compartments. *Transactions of the American Academy of Ophthalmology and Otolaryngology, 82,* 308–318.

Vaughan, C. W. (1978). Transoral laryngeal surgery using the CO_2 laser: Laboratory experiments and clinical experience. *Laryngoscope, 88,* 1399–1420.

Vaughan, C. W., Strong, M. S., & Jako, G. J. (1978). Laryngeal carcinoma: Transoral treatment using the CO_2 laser. *American Journal of Surgery, 136,* 490–493.

Weinstein, G., & Laccourreye, O. (2000). Vertical partial laryngectomies. In G. Weinstein, O. Laccourreye, D. Brasnu, & H. Laccourreye (Eds.), (pp. 59–71). *Organ preservation surgery for laryngeal cancer*. San Diego: Singular.

Wetmore, S. J., Key, M., & Suen, J.Y. (1986). Laser therapy for T1 glottic carcinoma of the larynx. *Archives of Otolaryngology—Head and Neck Surgery, 112*, 853–855.

Wolf, G. T., Fisher, S. G., Hong, W. K., Hillman, R., Spaulding, M., Laramore, G. E., Endicott, J. W., McClatchey, K., & Henderson, W. G. (1991). Induction chemotherapy plus radiation compared with surgery plus radiation in patients with advanced laryngeal cancer. *New England Journal of Medicine, 324*, 1685–1690.

Wolfensberger, M., & Dort, J. C. (1990). Endoscopic laser surgery for early glottic carcinoma: A clinical and experimental study. *Laryngoscope, 100*, 1100–1105.

Zeitels, S. M. (1993). Microflap excisional biopsy for atypia and microinvasive glottic cancer. *Operative Techniques in Otolaryngology—Head and Neck Surgery (Phonosurgery edition), 4*, 218–222.

Zeitels, S. M. (Ed.). (1994). Transoral treatment of early glottic cancer. In *Laryngeal cancer: Proceedings of the 2nd World Congress on Laryngeal Cancer* (pp. 373–383). Amsterdam: Elsevier.

Zeitels, S. M. (1995). Premalignant epithelium and microinvasive cancer of the vocal fold: The evolution of phonomicrosurgical management. *Laryngoscope*, (Suppl. 67), 1–51.

Zeitels, S. M. (1996a). Laser versus cold instruments for microlaryngoscopic surgery. *Laryngoscope, 106*, 545–552.

Zeitels, S. M. (1996b). Phonomicrosurgical treatment of early glottic cancer and carcinoma in situ. *American Journal of Surgery, 172*, 704–709.

Zeitels, S. M. (1998). Infrapetiole exploration of the supraglottis for exposure of the anterior glottal commissure. *Journal of Voice, 12*, 117–122.

Zeitels, S. M. (1999a). Adduction arytenopexy with medialization laryngoplasty and crico-thyroid subluxation: A new approach to paralytic dysphonia. *Operative Techniques in Otolaryngology—Head and Neck Surgery, 10*, 9–16.

Zeitels, S. M. (1999b). A universal modular glottiscope system: The evolution of a century of design and technique for direct laryngoscopy. *Annals of Otology, Rhinology and Laryngology, 108* (Suppl. 179), 1–24.

Zeitels, S. M. (1999c). *U.S. Patent No. 5,893,830*. Washington, DC: U.S. Patent and Trademark Office.

Zeitels, S. M., (2004). Optimizing voice after endoscopic partial laryngectomy. *Otolaryngology Clinics of North America, 37*, 627–636.

Zeitels, S. M., Dailey, S. H., & Burns, J. A. (2004). Technique of en block laser endoscopic fronto-lateral laryngectomy for glottic cancer. *Laryngoscope, 114*, 175–180.

Zeitels, S. M., & Davis R. K. (Eds.). (1994). Cancer of the supraglottis: Endoscopic laser management. In *Laryngeal cancer: Proceedings of the 2nd World Congress on Laryngeal Cancer*. Amsterdam: Elsevier.

Zeitels, S. M., Hillman, R. E., Franco, R. A., & Bunting, G. (2002). Voice and treatment outcome from phonosurgical management of early glottic cancer. *Annals of Otology, Rhinology and Laryngology, 111*(Suppl. 190), 3–20.

Zeitels, S. M., Jarboe, J. K., & Franco, R. A. (2001). Phonological reconstuction of early glottic cancer. *Laryngoscope, 111*, 1862–1865.

Zeitels, S. M., Jarboe, J., & Hillman, R. E. (2000). *Goretex medialization for aerodynamic glottal incompetence*. Paper presented at the Voice Symposium, Philadelphia.

Zeitels, S. M., Koufman, J. A., Davis, R. K., & Vaughan, C. W. (1994). Endoscopic treatment of supraglottic and hypopharynx cancer. *Laryngoscope, 104*, 71–78.

Zeitels, S. M., & Vaughan, C. W. (1990). The adjustable supraglottiscope. *Otolaryngology—Head and Neck Surgery, 103*, 487–492.

Zeitels, S. M., & Vaughan, C. W. (1991a). Preepiglottic space invasion in "early" epiglottic cancer. *Annals of Otology, Rhinology and Laryngology, 100,* 789–792.

Zeitels, S. M., & Vaughan, C. W. (1991b). A submucosal vocal fold infusion needle. *Otolaryngology— Head and Neck Surgery, 105,* 478–479.

Zeitels, S. M., Vaughan, C. W., & Domanowski, G. F. (1990). Endoscopic management of early supraglottic cancer. *Annals of Otology, Rhinology and Laryngology, 99,* 951–956.

Zeitels, S. M., Vaughan, C. W., Domanowski, G. F., Fuleihan, N. F., & Simpson, G. T. (1990). Laser epiglottectomy: Endoscopic technique and indications. *Otolaryngology—Head and Neck Surgery, 103,* 337–343.

Chapter 10

Vocal Function Following Nonsurgical Treatment of Laryngeal Carcinoma

Robert F. Orlikoff

The development of laryngeal malignancy is a somewhat gradual, multi-stage process that appears to be tied predominantly to various environmental factors (and cofactors), such as smoking and immoderate alcohol consumption (American Cancer Society, 1999; Dorman & Lambie, 1994; Maier, Dietz, Gewelke, Heller, & Weidauer, 1994; Maier, Dietz, & Heller, 1992; Osteen, 1996; Wynder, Covey, Marbuchi, Johnson, & Muschinsky, 1976). Long-term exposure to these or other carcinogens (Maier, Dietz, & Heller, 1994; Muscat & Wynder, 1991; Welkoborsky & Mann, 1994) causes accumulated damage to the genetic code within the nucleus of a cell, which, in cancer of the larynx, is almost always found in the squamous epithelium of the laryngeal mucosa. In particular, carcinogenic agents induce DNA strands to break and to recombine in ways that cause certain genes to mutate into oncogenes. Oncogenes release the cell from the growth restraints normally placed upon it and cause the cell to change its size, shape, and function. The growth of cancer cells and their proliferation rate increase significantly and in an uncontrollable manner. Because the changes that have taken place within the cancer cell are tied to the cell's altered DNA (which directs the life cycle and reproduction of the cell), these changes are also passed on to the descendant cells arising from the original cancer cell. Unless these wayward cells succumb to the body's own immune system, they eventually aggregate (grow and cluster) until they form a distinct, palpable mass, or tumor.

As the proliferation of malignant cells continues, the tumor pushes outward from its boundaries, infiltrating and destroying the surrounding normal tissue. Small groups of cells may dislodge from the neoplasm and migrate, or *metastasize*, to distant sites, typically via the blood or lymphatic circulation. Following metastatic transfer, the cancer cells continue to multiply, forming secondary tumors in the newly affected organ. The qualities of tissue invasion and metastasis are characteristic of malignant disease. Untreated, local invasion at the primary disease site, regional incursion within the affected organ, or metastasis outside the site of primary disease will eventually disrupt the body's normal functions in ways that are incompatible with life.

As with all carcinomas, the treatment of laryngeal cancer is directed toward elimination of all malignant cells so as to preclude further tissue involvement and the threat of metastatic disease. Treatment may involve (a) surgically removing the tumor or (b) destroying the cancer cells through the introduction of various noxious stimuli (Armstrong & Gilbert, 2004; Corvo, Sanguineti, & Benasso, 1998; Kaplan, Johns, & Clark, 1984; Kelly et al., 1989; Laccourreye et al., 1996; Medini, Medini, Lee, Gapany, & Levitt, 1998a, 1998b; Pfister, Shaha, & Harrison, 1997; Rosier et al., 1998; Spector et al., 1999; Stewart, Brown, Palmer, & Cooper, 1975; Uno, Itami, Kotaka, & Toriyama, 1996; Wanebo et al., 1999). Ideally, treatment of a laryngeal tumor would spare all unaffected tissue while removing all risk of tumor recurrence or metastasis. In practice, however, laryngeal function may be severely compromised due not only to the destructive effects of malignant disease, but also to the fact that effective treatment, as described later, may require the sacrifice of a considerable amount of nearby healthy tissue (see Chapter 11 in this text). Thus, selecting the appropriate course of treatment requires consideration of the effect of intervention on both the duration and quality of the patient's survival (Bjordal, Kaasa, & Mastekaasa, 1994; Carrara-de-Angelis, Feher, Barros, Nishimoto, & Kowalski, 2003; DeSanto, Olsen, Perry, Rohe, &

Keith, 1995; Dickens, Cassisi, Million, & Bova, 1983; Doyle, 1997; Dropkin, 1989; Dworkin et al., 2003; Finizia & Bergman, 2001; Finizia, Hammerlid, Westin, & Lindstrom, 1998; Hammerlid et al., 1997; Harwood & Rawlinson, 1983; Hillman, Walsh, Wolf, Fisher, & Hong, 1998; Karnell, Funk, Tomblin, & Hoffman, 1999; List et al., 1996; McNeil, Weichselbaum, & Pauker, 1981; Morton, Davies, Baker, Baker, & Stell, 1984; Orlikoff & Kraus, 1996; Rathmell, Ash, Howes, & Nicholls, 1991; Shanks, 1995; Terrell, Fisher, & Wolf, 1998; Verdonck-de Leeuw et al., 1999; see also Chapter 28 in this text). The most successful treatment of laryngeal disease, therefore, will be the one that eradicates malignant disease while leaving the patient without significant vocal impairment. In most instances, this treatment will require the coordinated effort of oncologists and a cadre of allied health professionals, including the voice pathologist.

LARYNGEAL CARCINOMA AND VOICE PRODUCTION

The control and maintenance of phonation are known to be highly sensitive to the viscoelastic properties of the vocal fold mucosa (Berke & Gerratt, 1993; Hirano, 1977; Hirano & Kurita, 1986; Hiroto, 1966; Kakita, Hirano, & Ohmaru, 1981; see also Chapter 9 in this text). It is perhaps not surprising, then, that when tumor mass and tissue invasion involve one or both vocal folds, they result in nonuniformities in mucosal structure and biomechanics that can disrupt vibratory, and therefore glottal, dynamics. Disease-related glottal asymmetry and irregularities along the approximating vocal fold edges will also act to preclude a stable oscillatory pattern and may additionally hinder glottal closure. As a consequence, an excessive airflow rate and increased glottal air turbulence often accompany voice production. Such effects are clearly associated with phonatory inefficiency, if not with a readily perceptible vocal disorder that is characterized by a generally noisy and erratic acoustic product. Various studies have reported increased levels of frequency and amplitude perturbation, voice breaks, diplophonia, and restricted vocal flexibility that at times may be so severe as to lead to perceived monoloudness or monopitch during conversational speech (Doyle, 1997; Feijoo & Hernández, 1990; Hecker & Kreul, 1971; Koike, 1973; Koike, Takahashi, & Calcaterra, 1977; Kreul & Hecker, 1971; Lieberman, 1963; Ludlow, Coulter, & Gentges, 1983; Murry, 1978; Murry & Doherty, 1980; Murry & Singh, 1982; Orlikoff, Kraus, Budnick, Pfister, & Zelefsky, 1999; Orlikoff, Kraus, Harrison, Ho, & Gartner, 1997; Verdonck-de Leeuw & Koopmans-van Beinum, 1995).

In general, voice symptoms will evolve quicker and prove more debilitating when the primary malignant lesion occurs along the membranous portion of the vocal folds. By comparison, the earliest symptoms of supraglottic cancer are often vague and are more likely to become evident during swallowing than speaking (Karmody, 1983). Voice complaints, if they occur, typically develop later as the regional spread of the tumor involves the vocal folds. The rare subglottic tumor often becomes symptomatic quite late, when the progression of disease interferes with glottal function and causes breathing difficulty (dyspnea) or dysphonia. Although the vocal symptoms of these cancer patients may show certain overall similarities, the specific abnormalities observed have been found to be highly variable, even when patients with similar-stage disease and with apparently comparable tumor volume and location are compared. Thus, the details of any particular vocal assessment are notoriously difficult to predict; this is perhaps to be expected, in that it is well recognized that the ties that necessarily link vocal fold structure and biomechanics, vocal physiology, and the acoustic characteristics of the vocal signal are neither direct nor immutable. In the absence of any theory that may support it, any attempt to use acoustic indices of voice quality to distinguish benign from cancerous lesions, or for that matter between different stages of malignant laryngeal disease, is almost assuredly doomed to failure. When it comes to the management of these patients, the prudent clinician will remember that "laryngeal cancer" is a tissue diagnosis, not a voice disorder.

Although dysphonia may be among the earliest symptoms of laryngeal carcinoma (Dayal, 1981; Karmody, 1983; Osteen, 1996), it is surprising how long it takes for many speakers to recognize their voice changes as an indication of serious laryngeal disease. Usually, it is only after additional symptoms emerge—such as soreness, otalgia, dyspnea, stridor, persistent cough, and dysphagia—that patients seek medical advice and the tumor is detected (see Chapter 7 in this text). There are several reasons for this, but the following are perhaps most common and are particularly worthy of consideration from the perspective of the voice therapist.

- *Vocal symptoms are not unique to laryngeal carcinoma.* Clinical experience and the limited research that has been done indicate that the abnormal voice characteristics that evolve from malignant laryngeal disease do not have a unique acoustic–perceptual profile. The voice of the cancer patient may well sound hoarse in ways that are not unlike what most listeners would readily associate with the occasional cold, flu, or allergy, or with any number of "functional" voice disorders. Because tissue involvement is likely to lead to vocal inefficiency, it is quite likely that the speaker will find the need to adopt certain hyperfunctional compensatory behaviors. In the absence of a thorough medical examination, these behaviors may easily mislead some to conclude falsely that they are the cause of the vocal disorder.

- *Vocal symptoms tend to develop gradually.* Carcinogenesis is a slow process, and any resulting voice change likewise tends to develop gradually. Except in relatively rare circumstances (Sataloff, Hawkshaw, McCarter, & Spiegel, 1999), the abnormal voice characteristics do not attract immediate notice. Prior to malignancy, epithelial cells may enter a precancerous phase, known as *dysplasia.* Some cells will also enter the state of *carcinoma in situ,* whereby cancer cells are restricted to a specific microscopic site (Gillis, Incze, Strong, Vaughan, & Simpson, 1983). It may take decades for malignant disease to go through the entire process (American Cancer Society, 1999; Union Internationale Contra le Cancer, 1987) and to produce a tumor large enough to cause significant and consistent vocal symptoms.

- *The premorbid voices of laryngeal cancer patients are often noisy.* Those who develop laryngeal carcinoma are often heavy smokers for whom a rougher voice quality, some respiratory compromise, and so-called smoker's cough are common (Brindle & Morris, 1979; Mueller & Wilcox, 1980; Murphy & Doyle, 1987; Sorensen & Horii, 1982; Suen & Stern, 1995). Precancerous epithelial dysplasia involving keratosis (a scaly thickening of the surface epithelium) and leukoplakia (the presence of thick and irregular white "smoker's" patches), mucosal edema and irritation, and laryngoxerosis (abnormal dryness of the laryngeal mucous membrane) tied to smoking (Fuchs, 1989; Hirano & Sato, 1993) and excessive alcohol use (Niedzielska, Pruszewicz, & Swidzinski, 1994; Watanabe et al., 1994) can result in long-term voice changes to which the patient becomes largely habituated. Although acoustic indexes of voice quality (e.g., jitter, shimmer, signal-to-noise ratio) may be within normal limits for speakers of similar age and gender, these individuals tend to have fragile voices that are prone to breakdown even from usually innocuous environmental influences (Mendonca, 1975), such as those related to air quality or physical activity. Later vocal disruption due to the mechanical effects of the tumor, therefore, tends to be more quantitative than qualitative in nature.

- *Laryngeal carcinoma tends to develop relatively late in life.* Segre (1971, p. 223) called the voice "a mirror of age," and indeed presbylaryngis has been shown to adversely affect the quality of phonation (Benjamin, 1981; Bloch & Behrman, 2001; W. S. Brown, Morris, & Michel, 1989; Hagen, Lyons, & Nuss, 1996; Hollien & Shipp, 1972; Honjo & Isshiki, 1980; Kahane, 1980, 1990; Kahane & Beckford, 1991; Morsomme, Jamart, Boucquey, & Remacle, 1997; Orlikoff, 1990; Ramig & Ringel, 1983; Wilcox & Horii, 1980) in ways that are readily perceived by listeners (Linville & Fisher, 1985a; Ramig, Scherer, & Titze, 1985; Ryan & Burk, 1974; Shipp & Hollien, 1969; Xue & Mueller, 1997). For instance, it is known that typically within the third decade of life, men show evidence of endochondral ossification of the hyaline cartilages and calcification of the elastic cartilages of the larynx (Kahane, 1980). Accompanying histological changes, apparent by about age 40, in the muscular layer and in each of the mucosal layers of the vocal fold leads to a substantial loss of tissue compliance (Bach, Lederer, & Dinolt, 1941; Hirano, Kurita, & Nakashima, 1983; Honjo & Isshiki, 1980; Kahane, 1980, 1987; Roncallo, 1948) and an increase in biomechanical nonlinearity. These changes, along with an atrophic thinning of the vocal folds, alter vocal fold vibration and restrict the degree to which the biomechanical properties of the vocal folds can be adjusted or controlled (Baken, 1994; Ferreri, 1959; Hirano et al., 1983; Hommerich, 1972; Kahane, 1980; Mysak, 1959). Similar effects are known to occur in women as well, but these usually begin at a later age and not to the same extent (Biever & Bless, 1989; Higgins & Saxman, 1991; Hirano et al., 1983; Hirano, Kurita, & Sakaguchi, 1988; Kahane, 1987; Linville, 1987, 1988; Linville & Fisher, 1985a, 1985b; McGlone & Hollien, 1963; Stoicheff, 1981).

Malignant laryngeal lesions occur most often between the sixth and eighth decades of life and are more likely to develop in men than women. Thus, voice changes that accompany laryngeal disease may be confounded by, if not mistaken for, normal age-related involution. It is also worthy of note that normal age-related declines in the cardiovascular, musculoskeletal, respiratory, endocrine, immune, and central and peripheral nervous systems increase the older individual's vulnerability to a variety of ailments, including those that may contribute to, or detract attention from, vocal symptoms

(Behrman, Abramson, & Myssiorek, 2001; Chodzko-Zajko & Ringel, 1987; Cooper, 1970; Roberts-Thomson, Youngchaizud, Wittingham, & Makay, 1974; Rochet, 1991).

Because the majority of laryngeal cancer patients are older, the occupational demands on their voices may be less than they once were. Often the voice symptoms go unnoticed or are denied by the patients themselves. Instead, dysphonia is often recognized by friends, relatives, or coworkers, especially those who speak to the patient on occasion, but over extended intervals of time.

NONSURGICAL APPROACHES TO LARYNGEAL CANCER TREATMENT
Radiation Therapy

The use of high-energy ionizing radiation, such as X-rays and gamma rays, to destroy cancer cells has had a long history in medical practice. The use of radiation in treating laryngeal carcinoma can be traced to the earliest years of the 20th century (Lederman, 1975). Irradiation causes damage to the cancer cell DNA, which, if not lethal, nonetheless impairs its ability to reproduce. Although normal cells can be similarly affected, in general they have been found to be better able than malignant cells to repair DNA damage.

The dose absorbed from ionizing radiation is expressed in *Gray* (Gy). Until recently, dosage was measured in *rads* (an acronym for *rad*iation *a*bsorbed *d*ose; 1 Gy = 100 rads). For laryngeal carcinoma, the total dose typically varies between 50 and 80 Gy. To allow for better recovery of the normal tissue in the radiation field, the total amount of radiation is delivered in small doses called *fractions*. By using fractionation, a dose that is lethal to the tumor can still be delivered while minimizing the damage done to adjacent normal cells. Quite often a patient will receive a daily fraction of 2 Gy, 5 days per week. The total radiation dose will depend on several factors, including tumor volume, the radiosensitivity of the tumor (the susceptibility of the tumor to radiation effects), the dose per fraction, and the radiation tolerance of the nearby normal tissue (Morrison, 1971; Suwinski, Maciejewski, & Withers, 1998). The efficacy of modified radiotherapy (RT) schedules is currently being assessed (Mariya, Matsutani, Abe, & Nakaji, 1998; Saarilahti, Kajanti, Lehtonen, Hamalainen, & Joensuu, 1998; Skladowski, Tarnawski, Maciejewski, Wygoda, & Slosarek, 1999; Spector et al., 1999). These include hyperfractionation, whereby the patient receives multiple daily fractions so as to obtain a higher total dose, and accelerated hyperfractionation, whereby the patient receives multiple daily fractions to reach the prescribed total dose more quickly.

A large percentage of patients with early carcinoma of the vocal folds can expect excellent local tumor control and long-term survival when treated with either RT or surgery (DeSanto, 1982; Dickens et al., 1983; also see Chapter 9 in this text). Although McGuirt and his colleagues (1994) provide data to challenge the commonly held judgment that successful RT results in a voice superior to that of comparable patients treated endoscopically with a CO_2 surgical laser (Strong, 1975; Strong & Jako, 1972), laser incision may delay reepithelialization (Durkin, Duncavage, Toohill, Tieu, & Caya, 1986), leaving open the opportunity for permanent mucosal damage and localized scarring. Furthermore, although it is possible for the mucosa of the vocal fold to show negligible residual laser effects, Leonard, Gallia, and Charpied (1992) have suggested that laser incision can lead to substantial submucosal damage even when the surface epithelium appears normal. Hirano, Hirade, and Kawasaki (1985) found little difference in vocal function between postlaser and postirradiated patients who had presented with early glottic cancer, but noted a slightly greater incidence of residual hoarseness when treatment included microlaryngeal laser surgery. Casiano, Cooper, Lundy, and Chandler (1991) likewise reported that such dysphonia typically persists and seems to be tied to the extent of surgical resection. Thus, although RT is thought to result in a better voice quality and is at least as effective in disease management, while generally being less expensive than surgical procedures, radiation is now widely accepted as the treatment of choice for early vocal fold carcinoma (Becker, 1995; Dickens et al., 1983; Epstein, Lee, Kashima, & Johns, 1990; Foote, Buskirk, Grado, & Bonner, 1997; Lesnicar, Smid, & Zakotnik, 1996; Meleca, Dworkin, Kewson, Stachler, & Hill, 2003; Mendenhall, Amdur, Morris, & Hinerman, 2001; Mittal, Rao, Marks, & Ogura, 1983; Moose & Grevin, 1997; Pellitteri, Kennedy, Vrabec, Beller, & Hellstrom, 1991; Rydell, Schalén, Fex, & Elner, 1995; Tombolini et al., 1995). There are certainly exceptions, however, and disagreement among head and neck oncologists continues (Cragle & Brandenburg, 1993; Davis, 1997; Morris, Canonico, & Blank, 1994; Simpson, Postma, Stone, & Ossoff, 1997; Zeitels, 1996).

The treatment of advanced, resectable tumors of the larynx has been a subject of controversy for several years. Although patients with advanced disease are customarily treated with surgery, RT, or both, there has been considerable debate about whether the best oncologic approach is surgical resection of the entire gross tumor along with adequate margins to be followed by RT if needed, or, as is often elected in early-stage disease, definitive RT to be followed by surgical salvage if needed (Cummings, 1994; Hoffman, McCulloch, Gustin, & Karnell, 1997; Kaplan et al., 1984; Lo, Venkatesan, Matthews, & Rogers, 1998; Moose & Grevin, 1997). In practice, such decisions are typically predicated upon many factors, including tumor size, location, and the structures involved, as well as patient-specific considerations such as comorbidities (i.e., coexisting diseases and conditions) and expected tolerance for certain treatment modalities (Chen, Matson, Roberts, & Goepfert, 2001; Jørgensen, Godballe, Hansen, & Bastholt, 2002; Strome & Weinman, 2002).

Chemotherapy

In chemotherapy, certain chemicals or drugs known to have deleterious effects on malignant cells are therapeutically introduced (singly or in combination) into the patient's bloodstream. The cytotoxic (i.e., anticancer) drugs used in chemotherapy target rapidly growing and dividing cells by hindering their DNA, causing impairment of their ability to reproduce and the death of the cells. Because chemotherapy is a systemic approach, many healthy cells throughout the body may also be affected, in particular those cell types that tend to multiply quickly. These include hair follicles, the lining of the aerodigestive tract, cells in the reproductive system, and red and white blood cells forming in the bone marrow. As with radiation exposure, however, normal cells are better able than cancer cells to repair DNA damage.

The aim of chemotherapy differs depending on the type and stage of cancer, the primary site of disease, and the presence and location of secondary tumors. Chemotherapy may be used as the definitive treatment or as a supplement to other treatments in an effort to control tumor growth, to relieve certain tumor-related symptoms, or to destroy microscopic metastases. Although chemotherapy is not generally considered a curative modality in the management of laryngeal carcinoma, it can still elicit an impressive tumor response in many patients (Laccourreye et al., 1996; Pfister et al., 1997). As such, chemotherapy is often employed to improve local or regional control of disease when used in concert with primary surgery or RT and to serve a palliative role for those patients for whom no further surgical or radiation options are possible (Corvo et al., 1998; Nishioka et al., 1999; Pfister et al., 1997; Wanebo et al., 1999). Among the several chemotherapy agents used in those with advanced laryngeal cancer, the most common are cisplatin, 5-fluorouracil, methotrexate, carboplatin, vinblastine, bleomycin, and piclitaxel (also known as Taxol).

Chemotherapy is usually given as a course of several cycles of treatment, allowing a few weeks of rest between the administration of doses. Delivering a chemotherapy agent periodically allows time for the normal cells to repair any chemically induced damage and for the body to recover from any of a number of potential side effects. Also, because cells rest between reproductive divisions and chemotherapy agents are only effective when target cells are actively dividing, the delivery of protracted doses will affect a greater number of cancer cells.

When a course of chemotherapy is used as part of an overall treatment plan, it may be given prior to (*induction* or *neoadjuvant*), at the same time as (*concomitant*), or following (*adjuvant*) surgery or RT. It has been observed that previously untreated tumors that respond to chemotherapy also tend to be responsive to radiation, whereas chemoresistive tumors are most likely to be resistant to RT (Bosl, Strong, Harrison, & Pfister, 1991; Ensley et al., 1984; Pfister et al., 1991). Induction chemotherapy has accordingly become a common element in so-called larynx preservation therapy that uses definitive RT to treat advanced laryngeal carcinomas that would otherwise call for radical surgery, including total laryngectomy. Typically, patients who show a poor tumor response to high-dose induction chemotherapy are referred for surgery, whereas those who show a good chemoresponse go on to receive RT as their primary treatment (Brockstein, 2003; Corvo et al., 1998; Cox, 1998; Fu, 1997; Kraus et al., 1995; Lefebvre, 1998; Leon et al., 2001; Schenone et al., 1997; Stupp & Vokes, 1995; Wheeler & Spencer, 1995). In addition to predicting the effectiveness of RT, successful induction chemotherapy debulks the tumor, making it easier to treat with RT alone (Arcangeli et al., 1983; Department of Veteran Affairs Laryngeal Cancer Study Group, 1991; Jørgensen, Hansen, & Bastholt, 1994; Lo et al., 1998).

VOCAL CONSEQUENCES OF LARYNGEAL RADIATION AND CHEMOTHERAPY

By eradicating or significantly reducing the size of a vocal fold tumor, both chemotherapy and RT can lead to substantial phonatory improvement (Hoyt, Lettinga, Leopold, & Fisher, 1992; Karim, Snow, Siek, & Njo, 1983; Miller, Harrison, Solomon, & Sessions, 1990; Orlikoff et al., 1999; Orlikoff et al., 1997; Orr, Hamilton, & Glennie, 1972; Stoicheff, Ciampi, Passi, & Fredrickson, 1983). Although chemoradiation may be effective in managing disease, it is also well recognized that as a single treatment modality, radiotherapy itself can have short-term, long-term, or latent effects on laryngeal structure and vocal function (Berger, Freeman, Briant, Berry, & Noyek, 1984; Clerf, 1927; Fung et al., 2001; Harwood & Tiere, 1979; Kelly et al., 1989; Mendonca, 1975; Nishioka et al., 1999; Robbins, 2000; Robbins, Doweck, Samant, Vieira, & Kumar, 2004; Robbins et al., 2000; Verdonck-de Leeuw, 1998; Werner-Kukuk, von Leden, & Yanagihara, 1968; Zuppinger, 1951).

THE LARYNX AND THE VOCAL TRACT

Although the complications of chemotherapy are often gastrointestinal in nature—nausea and diarrhea are commonly reported side effects—several of the chemotherapy agents used to treat head and neck cancer may cause dryness (xerostomia and laryngoxerosis) and irritation of the mucous membranes of the airway in some patients. Sores may develop in the mouth (stomatitis) and pharynx (mucositis), with the lining of the oral cavity and pharynx becoming sensitive and prone to bleeding. A reduction in white blood cell production will make the patient more susceptible to infection, whereas anemia may cause the patient to fatigue easily. The development of a white and filmy thrush fungus (candidiasis) in the mouth, and often including the larynx, is a common sequela of chemotherapy (see Chapter 8 in this text). Although this side effect has not yet been studied systematically, clinical experience suggests that such infections can, by themselves, lead to substantial phonatory symptoms. The severity of several drug-induced problems can often be lessened during and after treatment with medication and when appropriate countermeasures are taken. Typically, these symptoms resolve once a course of chemotherapy is completed, but late side effects are also possible. The specific effects vary on an individual basis, by chemotherapy regimen, and by the drug or drug combinations used in treatment.

Radiation exposure can lead to multiple effects on the larynx and vocal tract. Some of these may resolve within a few months following RT, whereas others can persist indefinitely. It is also possible for some tissue changes to occur several years (if not decades) after completing treatment (e.g., Berger et al., 1984).

Although the specific laryngeal effects of laryngeal irradiation are not completely understood, many of the attendant tissue changes have also been associated with normal aging, continued smoking, and excessive alcohol intake (e.g., Fuchs, 1989; Hirano & Sato, 1993; Kahane, 1990; Watanabe et al., 1994).

In particular, late complications of radiation are known to include scarring and atrophy of the laryngeal muscles and mucosa, necrosis of laryngeal cartilage, and fibrosis of the lamina propria. Significant fibrosis of the neck is also common, which often serves to restrict laryngeal, lingual, and mandibular movement. Radiation may also induce accelerated ossification of the cartilaginous framework of the larynx (Dyess, Carter, Kirchner, & Baron, 1987), which can be expected to further restrict vocal flexibility. The vocal folds of postirradiated patients often show evidence of chronic edema, erythema (inflammatory redness), telangiectasis (engorgement of blood vessels), and keratosis. Another notable side effect is the damage done to both salivary and mucous glands, which results in a lack of lubrication in the larynx. Vocal fold edema and dryness may be exacerbated by other drying agents, such as caffeine, alcohol, and antihistamines, as well as by irritants such as gastroesophageal reflux, cigarette smoking, and airborne particulate matter. The saliva of these patients tends to be opaque, and its consistency is often quite thick and sticky. These patients commonly complain of excess phlegm production, but this may be an impression left by the relative difficulty they experience when trying to clear this more viscous type of secretion. Given these effects, it is not surprising that patients may present with an irritative, sometimes uncontrollable, dry cough (Mendonca, 1975; Zuppinger, 1951).

The vibratory edge of irradiated vocal folds is often irregular, due to the residual effects of malignant disease, postbiopsy scarring, and the myriad of possible radiation-induced changes noted earlier. Some investigators have noted bowing of the vocal folds, but the most common observations have been a general reduction in the amplitude of the mucosal wave, a failure of a portion of one or both vocal folds to vibrate, incomplete glottal closure, and a decreased vocal fold–contact interval (Dworkin & Aref, 1997; Lehman, Bless, & Brandenburg, 1988; Mendonca, 1975; Orlikoff et al., 1999; Verdonck-de Leeuw, 1998; Werner-Kukuk et al., 1968).

PHYSIOLOGIC AND ACOUSTIC VOICE CHARACTERISTICS

Although various structural and biomechanical changes have been associated with nonsurgical treatment of laryngeal carcinoma for some time, specific evidence regarding posttreatment vocal function has been slow to accumulate. Table 10.1 includes a list of studies that have objectively assessed the pre- and posttreatment voices of cancer patients using a variety of acoustic voice measures derived from the speech signal or by addressing voice physiology directly via measures of vibratory behavior, vocal aerodynamics, or both. As can be seen, most of these investigations have been conducted relatively recently as instrumentation has become more common in clinical practice. Any conclusions stemming from these

(text continues on p. 209)

TABLE 10.1

Studies of the Physiologic or Acoustic Voice Characteristics of Laryngeal Cancer Patients Before, During, and Following Radiotherapy (RT)[a]

Study	Patients	Age (years)	Disease Staging	Total Dose (GY)/RT Schedule[b]	Time of Voice Assessment	Objective Voice Measures[c]
Werner-Kukuk, von Leden, & Yanagihara (1968)	1 male	77	?	61.7/29	PreRT, During, PostRT: 4 mos	Spectrogram MPT, Airflow, Glottal area
Murry, Bone, & Von Essen (1974)	1 male	49	T1	58/29	PreRT, During, PostRT: 2 mos	F_o, MPFR, Airflow, P_{io}
Stoicheff (1975)	22 male	50–69	?	?	Post RT	SF_o
Colton, Sagerman, Chung, Yu, & Reed (1978)	5 male	65 (mean)	T1	60–66/6–7 weeks	PreRT, During, PostRT: 1–13 mos	LTAS
Lehman, Bless, & Brandenburg (1988)	20 male	55–80	T1	66/33	PostRT: 1–7 yrs	Jitter, Shimmer, SNR, MPFR, dB IL, MPT, Airflow, Estimated P_s
Harrison et al. (1990)	18 male	45–84	T1 T2	66/33 66–70/33–35	PreRT, During, PostRT: 1, 2, 3, 6, & 9 mos	Spectrogram, %Voicing
Benninger, Gillen, Thieme, Jacobson, & Dragovich (1994)	51 male, female	43–81	T1, T2	60–70/6–8 weeks	PostRT: 2 yrs+	F_o, MPFR, Jitter, Shimmer, SNR
Hoyt, Lettinga, Leopold, & Fisher (1992)	10 male	62 (median)	T1, T2	65/37	PreRT, PostRT: 6 mos	F_o, Jitter, %Voicing
Ott, Klingholz, Willich, & Kastenbauer (1992)	13 male, female	63 (mean)	T1, T2	?	PostRT: 1–8 yrs	SNR
Heeneman, Leeper, Hawkins, & Nordick (1994)	37 male 8 female	37–85 45–75	T1a	60/?	PreRT, PostRT: 0, 3, 6, 9, & 12 mos	F_o, MPFR, Jitter, Shimmer, SNR, MPT
Hirano, Mori, & Iwashita (1994)	34 male, female	?	Tis, T1a, T1b	60/?	PreRT, PostRT	MPFR, dB SPL range, Jitter, Shimmer, NNE, MPT, Airflow

(continues)

TABLE 10.1 *Continued.*

Studies of the Physiologic or Acoustic Voice Characteristics of Laryngeal Cancer Patients Before, During, and Following Radiotherapy (RT)[a]

Study	Patients	Age (years)	Disease Staging	Total Dose (GY)/RT Schedule[b]	Time of Voice Assessment	Objective Voice Measures[c]
McGuirt et al. (1994)	13 male	?	T1	63/28	PostRT: 6+ mos	Spectrogram, F_o, dB IL, Jitter, %Voicing, MPT, Estimated LAR
Rydell, Schalén, Fex, & Elner (1995)	18 male	43–77	T1a	64/32	PreRT, PostRT: 3 mos & 2 yrs	F_o, Jitter, Shimmer, HNR, Spectral noise
Woodson et al. (1996)	5 male 4 female	41–62 48–58	T3, T4	68–74/7–8 weeks	PostRT: 2–12 mos	Jitter, Shimmer, HNR, F_o–SD, Estimated LAR
Aref, Dworkin, Devi, Denton, & Fontanesi (1997)	12 male	?	T1	59.4–70/28–35	PostRT: 3 mos–7 yrs	F_o, Jitter, Shimmer, HNR, Airflow, Estimated P_s and LAR
Dagli, Mahieu, & Festen (1997)	16 male 4 female	43–86 57–87	T1a, T1b	57.5–70/ 23–35	PostRT: 1–13 yrs	F_o, Jitter, Shimmer, NNE, MPT, dB IL range
Dworkin & Aref (1997)	8 male 2 female	42–81 76	T1	66–70/ 29–35	PostRT: 1–7 yrs	F_o, Jitter, Shimmer, HNR, MPT, dB SPL, Airflow, Estimated P_s and LAR
Verdonck-de Leeuw (1998)	60 male	47–81	T1a, T1b	66/33 60/25–30	PreRT, PostRT: 6 mos & 2–10 yrs	F_o, Jitter, Shimmer, VRP, MPT, PQ, Spectral measures, Voice onset duration
Dworkin et al. (1999)	7 male 2 female	41–79	T1	67–70/ 20–22.5	PreRT, PostRT: 6 mos– 2 yrs 9 mos	Jitter, Shimmer, HNR, MPT, Airflow, Estimated P_s and LAR
Finizia, Dotevall, Lundström, & Lindström (1999)	12 male	49–73	T1, T2, T3, T4	62–68/ 26–34	PostRT: 6 mos–4yrs+	F_o, Jitter, MPT

(continues)

TABLE 10.1 *Continued.*

Studies of the Physiologic or Acoustic Voice Characteristics of Laryngeal Cancer Patients Before, During, and Following Radiotherapy (RT)[a]

Study	Patients	Age (years)	Disease Staging	Total Dose (GY)/RT Schedule[b]	Time of Voice Assessment	Objective Voice Measures[c]
Orlikoff, Kraus, Budnick, Pfister, & Zelefsky (1999)	9 male 3 female	45–75 42–72	T2, T3, T4	66–70/ 8 weeks	PreRT, PostRT: 1–2 mos	Jitter, Shimmer, NHR, MPT, MPFR, SPL range EGG, Airflow, Estimated LAR
Hocevar-Boltežar, Žargi, & Honocodeevar-Boltežar (2000)	44 male 6 female	20–86	T1, T2	61–68/?	PostRT: 1–10 yrs	Jitter, Shimmer, NHR
Behrman, Abramson, & Myssiorek (2001)	16 male 4 female	62–86 64–73	T1	66/33	PostRT: 1–12 yrs	Spectrography, VRP
Fung et al. (2001)	13 male	45–75	T1a	61/25	PostRT: >1 yr	Jitter, Shimmer, NNE, HNR, F$_o$, MPFR, MPT, Spectral measures, Airflow, vocal DDK

Note. mos = months; yrs = years; MPT = maximum phonation time; F$_o$ = vocal fundamental frequency; MPFR = maximum phonational frequency range; P$_{io}$ = intraoral pressure; SF$_o$ = speaking fundamental frequency; LTAS = long-term average spectrum; SNR = signal-to-noise ratio; dB IL = intensity level; P$_s$ = subglottic pressure; dB SPL = sound pressure level; NNE = normalized noise energy; LAR = laryngeal airway resistance; HNR (or NHR) = harmonics-to-noise ratio; F$_o$-SD = standard deviation of fundamental frequency; VRP = voice range profile (phonetogram); PQ = phonation quotient; EGG = electroglottogram; DDK = diadochokinetic rate.

[a] Patients with advanced stage disease (generally T3 and T4) are likely to have received induction or concomitant chemotherapy (see sources for details).

[b] Total RT dose/number of fractions (or duration of RT).

[c] See sources for specific measurement techniques and procedures.

studies, however, can only be considered preliminary given (a) the relatively small numbers of patients assessed; (b) the wide variation in disease stage, tumor location, and tumor volume characteristics of the patients' disease; (c) the differences in disease classification used (see, e.g., Ferlito, 1993; Ferlito et al., 1996); (d) differences in treatment schedules; (e) differences in voice measures selected for study; (f) discrepancies in measurement procedure; and perhaps most important, (g) inconsistencies regarding when the voices were assessed following treatment. These studies are also largely confounded by the fact that vocal function following treatment relates both to the reversal of the mechanical effects of the tumor and to the superimposed effects of the chemical agent or ionizing radiation used to eradicate the disease.

Nonetheless, for most patients, following either chemoradiation or RT alone, acoustic measures suggest improved vocal stability, as reflected by substantially decreased short-term frequency (jitter) and intensity (shimmer) perturbation and reduced turbulent noise. Better vocal capability and flexibility are often signaled by an expanded dynamic range (in sound pressure level), an expanded maximum phonational frequency range, and a more normal pitch sigma (i.e., the standard deviation of speaking fundamental frequency). Perhaps the most significant and consistent effect, however, is a drop in mean phonatory airflow toward more normal levels during and immediately following treatment (Hirano, Mori, & Iwashita, 1994; Murry, Bone, & Von Essen, 1974; Orlikoff et al., 1999; Werner-Kukuk et al., 1968). Although patients typically show improvement in many acoustic indexes of voice quality and in several measures of vocal physiology, it appears that relatively few improve to the point where they are indistinguishable from their age- and gender-matched peers (Aref, Dworkin, Devi, Denton, & Fontanesi, 1997; Dagli, Mahieu, & Festen, 1997; Dworkin & Aref, 1997; Dworkin et al., 1999; Hocevar-Boltežar, Žargi, & Honocodeevar-Boltežar, 2000; Karim et al., 1983; Lehman et al., 1988; Orlikoff et al., 1999; Stoicheff, 1975; Stoicheff et al., 1983; Verdonck-de Leeuw & Koopmans-van Beinum, 1995; Woodson et al., 1996). In addition, postirradiated patients appear to routinely adopt a higher subglottal driving pressure and to require greater vocal effort when speaking, even at conversational levels in relatively quiet speaking environments. Such changes are thought to be tied to the common complaints of voice strain, odynophonia, and vocal fatigue, as well as to the adoption of various compensatory behaviors that may ultimately prove to be vocally debilitating (Colton, Sagerman, Chung, Yu, & Reed, 1978; Harrison et al., 1990; Hoyt et al., 1992; Miller et al., 1990; Murry et al., 1974; Orlikoff et al., 1999; Orr et al., 1972; Stoicheff, 1975; Woodson et al., 1996).

Thus, although it is often difficult to compare and interpret the results obtained from various studies, it does appear safe to conclude that there are acute chemoradiation effects on both voice production and the vocal end product. The latent effects and the persistence of common early effects, however, are still mostly uncertain and remain a matter of some debate. What is clearly needed are comprehensive longitudinal studies of patients without vocal complaint who receive RT for localized supraglottic lesions, thereby allowing the study of radiation effects on healthy and anatomically normal vocal folds. In this way, those phonatory changes due to regression of the malignant mass may be disambiguated from those tied to radiation-induced alterations of periglottal structure.

PERCEIVED VOICE ATTRIBUTES

The voices of untreated laryngeal cancer patients have been described as breathy, tense, strained, and raspy (Benninger, Gillen, Thieme, Jacobson, & Dragovich, 1994; de Leeuw, 1991; Murry et al., 1974; Rydell et al., 1995; Stoicheff et al., 1983), whereas following RT or combined modality treatment, voices are often found to be far more variable and difficult to classify. Although many postirradiated voices reportedly sound normal or near-normal, others have been characterized as being particularly rough or in some way hoarse. As such, many published reports rely solely on unidimensional listener or patient rating scales of perceived voice quality or voice satisfaction. The results of such efforts can be described as equivocal at best. The inconsistency of these findings is compounded by the fact that the opinions of clinicians and other listeners regarding the normalcy or aesthetic quality of posttreatment voices are often at odds with those of the patients themselves, who are often quite pleased with their vocal outcome (e.g., Morgan, Robinson, Marsh, & Bradley, 1988; see also Chapter 6 in this text). It may be surmised that these patients, faced with the prospect of losing their larynx, are grateful for any quasi-natural and intelligible voice following organ-preservation treatment or that their perceptions are colored by the dramatic quality improvement such management can provide (Harrison et al., 1990; Hoyt et al., 1992; Llewellyn-Thomas et al., 1984; Miller et al., 1990). Some patients, in fact, claim that their voice is better after medical treatment than it was before the onset of the disease. This, in part, may be due to a cessation (or reduction) of smoking and alcohol use, or perhaps to a course of voice therapy and subsequent improvement in vocal and physical hygiene. Although many of the factors outlined earlier (premorbid status, speaker age, etc.) can forestall the early identification of tumor-based voice symptoms, these factors also may confuse appraisal of posttreatment change. Nevertheless, a significant group of patients find more fault with their voices following treatment than naive or trained listeners. There may be many reasons for such discrepancies; however, Woodson and her colleagues (1996) are probably correct in asserting that cancer patients will typically consider both the perceived quality of their voices and the perceived effort it takes for them to speak when making posttreatment voice judgments.

     It is also worthy of note that substantial sensorineural hearing loss can result from the use of some chemotherapy agents, such as cisplatin, especially when given in the high doses typical of many larynx preservation therapies (R. L. Brown, Nuss, Patterson, & Irey, 1983; Kopelman, Budnick, Sessions, Kramer, & Wong, 1988; Orlikoff et al., 1999). However, the extent to which treatment-related hearing changes may affect voice perception and vocal rehabilitation is not known.

MANAGING POSTTREATMENT VOICE SYMPTOMS

Voice outcome following radiotherapy can be significantly improved when patients cease smoking before beginning treatment and when less aggressive surgical procedures are used for diagnosis (Benninger et al., 1994; Karim et al., 1983; Verdonck-de Leeuw, 1998; Verdonck-de Leeuw et al., 1999). The avoidance of drying agents and other irritants will be vocally beneficial, as will proper management of gastroesophageal reflux, if present. Although post-RT patients are more likely to be troubled by reduced lubrication of the vocal fold mucosa than by inadequate tissue hydration, many patients nonetheless report at least short-term vocal improvement with fluid intake. Warm liquids, in particular, seem to be helpful, as are beverages that, unless restricted for medical reasons, include citrus and honey. Of course, alcohol and caffeinated drinks are best avoided.

Voice therapy has also been found to be an effective addition to chemoradiotherapy when it is provided to the patient to facilitate voice rehabilitation while minimizing the deleterious vocal effects stemming from treatment (Dworkin & Aref, 1997; Fex & Henriksson, 1970; Lehman et al., 1988; Olthoff et al., 2003; Sapir, 1994; Stoicheff, 1975). The details of voice therapy must necessarily follow from specific physiologic needs identified by the clinician, as well as from the communicative disability identified by the patient. Given the variety of symptoms possible, it is difficult to specify global therapeutic strategies, but clearly a large number of patients will benefit from techniques designed to maximize ventilatory support for speech, to improve voice frequency and intensity control and flexibility, and to renovate those vocal behaviors that are found to be maladaptive or inefficient or that require an undue amount of effort (Doyle, 1997; Orlikoff & Kraus, 1996). While not neglecting the patient's expectations regarding voice quality, the clinician must nonetheless place particular emphasis on improving the ease and effectiveness of voice production.

SUMMARY

Advancements in theory, technique, and technology have led to new options for treating laryngeal cancer. Many of these treatment approaches seek to provide local control and disease-free survival while avoiding the need for surgery and the functional deficits that typically accompany excision and resection. Unfortunately, organ-preservation treatments that employ radiotherapy or chemotherapy may also engender structural and biomechanical changes that can significantly affect vocal function. This chapter has addressed the nature of these nonsurgical approaches and has highlighted several patient-, disease-, and treatment-related factors that contribute both to the highly variable vocal symptoms that present following treatment and to the disparity between patients regarding voice satisfaction, disability, and handicap. Clearly, management options will continue to expand, and greater numbers of laryngeal cancer patients will be treated nonsurgically. Further investigation of posttreatment vocal impairment will help foster newer approaches that effectively treat the disease while minimizing deleterious iatrogenic vocal effects and leading to efficacious therapeutic strategies to resolve residual dysphonia.

REFERENCES

American Cancer Society. (1999). *Cancer facts and figures—1999*. Atlanta, GA: American Cancer Society.

Arcangeli, G., Nervi, C., Righini, R., Creton, G., Mirri, M. A., & Guerra, A. (1983). Combined radiation and drugs: The effect of intra-arterial chemotherapy followed by radiotherapy in head and neck cancer. *Radiotherapy and Oncology, 1,* 101–107.

Aref, A., Dworkin, J., Devi, S., Denton, L., & Fontanesi, J. (1997). Objective evaluation of the quality of voice following radiation therapy for T1 glottic cancer. *Radiotherapy and Oncology, 45,* 149–153.

Armstrong, T., & Gilbert, M. R. (2004). Central nervous system toxicity from cancer treatment. *Current Oncology Reports, 6,* 11–19.

Bach, A. C., Lederer, R. L., & Dinolt, R. (1941). Senile changes in the laryngeal musculature. *Archives of Otolaryngology, 34,* 47–56.

Baken, R. J. (1994). The aged voice: A new hypothesis. *Voice, 3,* 57–73.

Becker, A. (1995). Vergleichbare Stimmfunktion nach Laserresektion oder Bestrahlung von T1-Karzinomen der Stimmlippen [Comparative voice results after laser resection or irradiation of T1 vocal fold carcinoma]. *Strahlentherapie und Onkologie, 171,* 241–242.

Behrman, A., Abramson, A. L., & Myssiorek, D. (2001). A comparison of radiation-induced and presbylaryngeal dysphonia. *Otolaryngology—Head and Neck Surgery, 125,* 193–200.

Benjamin, B. J. (1981). Frequency variability in the aged voice. *Journal of Gerontology, 36,* 722–726.

Benninger, M. S., Gillen, J., Thieme, P., Jacobson, B., & Dragovich, J. (1994). Factors associated with recurrence and voice quality following radiation therapy for T1 and T2 glottic carcinomas. *Laryngoscope, 104,* 294–298.

Berger, G., Freeman, J. L., Briant, T. D., Berry, M., & Noyek, A. M. (1984). Late post radiation necrosis and fibrosis of the larynx. *Journal of Otolaryngology, 13,* 160–164.

Berke, G. S., & Gerratt, B. R. (1993). Laryngeal biomechanics: An overview of mucosal wave mechanics. *Journal of Voice, 7,* 123–128.

Biever, D. M., & Bless, D. M. (1989). Vibratory characteristics of the vocal folds in young adult and geriatric women. *Journal of Voice, 3,* 120–131.

Bjordal, K., Kaasa, S., & Mastekaasa, A. (1994). Quality-of-life in patients treated for head and neck cancer: A follow-up study 7 to 11 years after radiotherapy. *International Journal of Oncology, Biology, Physics, 28,* 847–856.

Bloch, I., & Behrman, A. (2001). Quantitative analysis of videostroboscopic images in presbylarynges. *Laryngoscope, 111,* 2022–2027.

Bosl, G. J., Strong, E. W., Harrison, L. B., & Pfister, D. G. (1991). Chemotherapy and the management of locally advanced squamous carcinoma of the head and neck: Role in larynx preservation. In V. T. Devita, S. Hellman, & S. A. Rosenberg (Eds.), *Important advances in oncology* (pp. 191–203). Philadelphia: Lippincott.

Brindle, B. R., & Morris, H. L. (1979). Prevalence of voice quality deviations in the normal adult population. *Journal of Communication Disorders, 12,* 439–445.

Brockstein, B. (2003). Organ preservation for advanced head and neck cancer treated with concomitant chemoradiation. *Cancer Treatment Research, 114,* 235–248.

Brown, R. L., Nuss, R. C., Patterson, R., & Irey, J. (1983). Audiometric monitoring of *cis*-Platinum ototoxicity. *Gynecologic Oncology, 16,* 254–262.

Brown, W. S., Jr., Morris, R. J., & Michel, J. F. (1989). Vocal jitter in young adult and aged female voices. *Journal of Voice, 3,* 113–119.

Carrara-de-Angelis, E., Feher, O., Barros, A. P., Nishimoto, I. N., & Kowalski, L. P. (2003). Voice and swallowing in patients enrolled in a larynx preservation trial. *Archives of Otolaryngology—Head and Neck Surgery, 129,* 733–738.

Casiano, R. R., Cooper, J. D., Lundy, D. S., & Chandler, J. R. (1991). Laser cordectomy for T1 glottic carcinoma: A 10-year experience and videostroboscopic findings. *Otolaryngology—Head and Neck Surgery, 104,* 831–837.

Chen, A. Y., Matson, L. K., Roberts, D., & Goepfert, H. (2001). The significance of comorbidity in advanced laryngeal cancer. *Head & Neck, 23,* 566–572.

Chodzko-Zajko, W. J., & Ringel, R. L. (1987). Physiological aspects of aging. *Journal of Voice, 1,* 18–26.

Clerf, L. H. (1927). Laryngeal complications of irradiation. *Archives of Otolaryngology, 6,* 338–345.

Colton, R. H., Sagerman, R. H., Chung, C. T., Yu, Y. W., & Reed, G. F. (1978). Voice change after radiotherapy: Some preliminary results. *Radiology, 127,* 821–824.

Cooper, M. (1970). Voice problems of the geriatric patient. *Geriatrics, 25,* 107–110.

Corvo, R., Sanguineti, G., & Benasso, M. (1998). Biological and clinical implications for multimodality treatment in patients affected by squamous cell carcinoma of the head and neck. *Tumori, 84,* 217–222.

Cox, J. D. (1998). Chemoradiation for malignant epithelial tumors. *Cancer Radiotherapie, 2,* 7–11.

Cragle, S. P., & Brandenburg, J. H. (1993). Laser cordectomy or radiotherapy: Cure rates, communication, and cost. *Otolaryngology—Head and Neck Surgery, 108,* 648–654.

Cummings, B. J. (1994). Definitive radiation therapy for glottic cancer. In R. Smee & G. P. Bridger (Eds.), *Laryngeal cancer* (pp. 9–13). Amsterdam: Elsevier Science.

Dagli, A. S., Mahieu, H. F., & Festen, J. M. (1997). Quantitative analysis of voice quality in early glottic laryngeal carcinomas treated with radiotherapy. *European Archives of Otorhinolaryngology, 254,* 78–80.

Davis, R. K. (1997). Endoscopic surgical management of glottic laryngeal cancer. *Otolaryngologic Clinics of North America, 30,* 79–86.

Dayal, V. S. (1981). *Clinical otolaryngology.* Philadelphia: Lippincott.

de Leeuw, I. M. (1991). Perceptual evaluation of voice quality before and after radiotherapy of patients with early glottic cancer and of normal speakers. *Proceedings of the Institute of Phonetic Science Amsterdam, 15,* 109–120.

Department of Veteran Affairs Laryngeal Cancer Study Group. (1991). Induction chemotherapy plus radiation compared with surgery plus radiation in patients with advanced laryngeal cancer. *New England Journal of Medicine, 324,* 1685–1690.

DeSanto, L. W. (1982). The options in early laryngeal carcinoma. *New England Journal of Medicine, 306,* 910–912.

DeSanto, L. W., Olsen, K. D., Perry, W. C., Rohe, D. E., & Keith, R. L. (1995). Quality of life after surgical treatment of cancer of the larynx. *Annals of Otology, Rhinology and Laryngology, 104,* 763–769.

Dickens, W. J., Cassisi, N. J., Million, R. R., & Bova, F. J. (1983). Treatment of early vocal cord carcinoma: A comparison of apples and apples. *Laryngoscope, 93,* 216–219.

Dorman, E. B., & Lambie, N. K. (1994). Dysplasia and carcinoma-in-situ of the larynx. In R. Smee & G. P. Bridger (Eds.), *Laryngeal cancer* (pp. 276–281). Amsterdam: Elsevier Science.

Doyle, P. C. (1997). Voice refinement following conservation surgery for cancer of the larynx: A conceptual framework for treatment intervention. *American Journal of Speech-Language Pathology, 6*(3), 27–35.

Dropkin, M. J. (1989). Coping with disfigurement and dysfunction after head and neck cancer surgery: A conceptual framework. *Seminars in Oncology Nursing, 5,* 213–219.

Durkin, G. E., Duncavage, J. A., Toohill, R. J., Tieu, T. M., & Caya, J. G. (1986). Wound healing of true vocal cord squamous epithelium after CO_2 laser ablation and cup forceps stripping. *Otolaryngology—Head and Neck Surgery, 95,* 273–277.

Dworkin, J. P., & Aref, A. (1997). Voice laboratory measures following radiation therapy for T1N0 glottic carcinoma. *Journal of Medical Speech–Language Pathology, 5,* 59–74.

Dworkin, J. P., Meleca, R. J., Abkarian, G. G., Stachler, R. J., Aref, A., & Garfield, I. (1999). Phonation subsystem outcomes following radiation therapy for T1 glottic carcinoma: A prospective voice laboratory investigation. *Journal of Medical Speech–Language Pathology, 7,* 181–193.

Dworkin, J. P., Meleca, R. J., Zacharek, M. A., Stachler, R. J., Pasha, R., Abkarian, G. G., Culatta, R. A., & Jacobs, J. R. (2003). Voice and deglutition functions after the supracricoid and total laryngectomy procedures for advanced stage laryngeal carcinoma. *Otolaryngology—Head and Neck Surgery, 129,* 311–320.

Dyess, C. L., Carter, D., Kirchner, J. A., & Baron, R. E. (1987). A morphometric comparison of the changes in the laryngeal skeleton associated with invasion by tumor and by external-beam radiation. *Cancer, 59,* 1117–1122.

Ensley, J. F., Jacobs, J. R., Weaver, A., Kinzie, J., Crissman, J., Kish, J. A., Cummings, G., & Al-Sarraf, M. (1984). Correlation between response to cisplatinum-combination chemotherapy and subsequent radiotherapy in previously untreated patients with advanced squamous cell cancers of the head and neck. *Cancer, 54,* 811–814.

Epstein, B. E., Lee, D. J., Kashima, H., & Johns, M. E. (1990). Stage T1 glottic carcinoma: Results of radiation therapy or laser excision. *Radiology, 175,* 567–570.

Feijoo, S., & Hernández, C. (1990). Short-term stability measures for the evaluation of vocal quality. *Journal of Speech and Hearing Research, 33,* 324–334.

Ferlito, A. (1993). The World Health Organization's revised classification of tumors of the larynx, hypopharynx, and trachea. *Annals of Otology, Rhinology and Laryngology, 102,* 666–669.

Ferlito, A., Carbone, A., DeSanto, L. W., Barnes, L., Rinaldo, A., D'Angelo, L., & Devaney, K. O. (1996). "Early" cancer of the larynx: The concept as defined by clinicians, pathologists, and biologists. *Annals of Otology, Rhinology and Laryngology, 105,* 245–250.

Ferreri, G. (1959). Senescence of the larynx. *Italian General Review of Oto-Rhino-Laryngology, 1,* 640–709.

Fex, S., & Henriksson, B. (1970). Phoniatric treatment combined with radiotherapy of laryngeal cancer for the avoidance of radiation damage. *Acta Otolaryngologica, 263,* 128–129.

Finizia, C., & Bergman, B. (2001). Health-related quality of life in patients with laryngeal cancer: A post-treatment comparison of different modes of communication. *Laryngoscope, 111,* 918–923.

Finizia, C., Dotevall, H., Lundström, E., & Lindström, J. (1999). Acoustic and perceptual evaluation of voice and speech quality: A study of patients with laryngeal cancer treated with laryngectomy vs. irradiation. *Archives of Otolaryngology—Head and Neck Surgery, 125,* 157–163.

Finizia, C., Hammerlid, E., Westin, T., & Lindström, J. (1998). Quality of life and voice in patients with laryngeal carcinoma: A posttreatment comparison of laryngectomy (salvage surgery) versus radiotherapy. *Laryngoscope, 108,* 1566–1573.

Foote, R. L., Buskirk, S. J., Grado, G. L., & Bonner, J. A. (1997). Has radiotherapy become too expensive to be considered a treatment option for early glottic cancer? *Head and Neck, 19,* 692–700.

Fu, K. K. (1997). Combined-modality therapy for head and neck cancer. *Oncology, 11,* 1781–1790.

Fuchs, B. (1989). Zur Pathogenese und Klinik des Reinke-Odems: Langzeitstudien [Pathogenesis and clinical aspects of Reinke edema: Long-term studies]. *HNO, 37,* 490–495.

Fung, K., Yoo, J., Leeper, H. A., Hawkins, S., Heeneman, H., Doyle, P. C., & Venkatesan, V. M. (2001). Vocal function following radiation for non-laryngeal versus laryngeal tumors of the head and neck. *Laryngoscope, 111,* 1920–1924.

Gillis, T. M., Ince, J., Strong, M. S., Vaughan, C. W., & Simpson, G. T. (1983). Natural history and management of keratosis, atypia, carcinoma-in-situ, and microinvasive cancer of the larynx. *American Journal of Surgery, 146,* 512–526.

Hagen, P., Lyons, G. D., & Nuss, D. W. (1996). Dysphonia in the elderly: Diagnosis and management of age-related voice changes. *Southern Medical Journal, 89,* 204–207.

Hammerlid, E., Bjordal, K., Ahlner-Elmqvist, M., Jannert, M., Kaasa, S., Sullivan, M., et al. (1997). Prospective, longitudinal quality-of-life study of patients with head and neck cancer: A feasibility study including the EORTC QLQ-C30. *Otolaryngology—Head and Neck Surgery, 116,* 666–673.

Harrison, L. B., Solomon, B., Miller, S., Fass, D. E., Armstrong, J., & Sessions, R. B. (1990). Prospective computer-assisted voice analysis for patients with early stage glottic cancer: A preliminary report of the functional result of laryngeal irradiation. *International Journal of Radiation Oncology, Biology, Physics, 19,* 123–127.

Harwood, A. R., & Rawlinson, E. (1983). The quality of life of patients following treatment for laryngeal cancer. *International Journal of Radiation Oncology, Biology, Physics, 9,* 335–338.

Harwood, A. R, & Tiere, A. (1979). Radiation of early glottic carcinoma II. *International Journal of Radiation Oncology, Biology, Physics, 5,* 477–482.

Hecker, M. H. L., & Kreul, E. J. (1971). Descriptions of the speech of patients with cancer of the vocal folds: Part I. Measures of fundamental frequency. *Journal of the Acoustical Society of America, 49,* 1275–1282.

Heeneman, H., Leeper, H. A., Hawkins, S., & Nordick, K. A. (1994). Vocal function following radiotherapy for early (T₁) laryngeal cancer: A prospective study. In R. Smee & G. P. Bridger (Eds.), *Laryngeal cancer* (pp. 355–359). Amsterdam: Elsevier Science.

Higgins, M. B., & Saxman, J. H. (1991). A comparison of selected phonatory behaviors of healthy aged and young adults. *Journal of Speech and Hearing Research, 34,* 1000–1010.

Hillman, R. E., Walsh, M. J., Wolf, G. T., Fisher, S. G., & Hong, W. K. (1998). Functional outcomes following treatment for advanced laryngeal cancer. *Annals of Otology, Rhinology and Laryngology, 107*(Suppl. 172), 2–27.

Hirano, M. (1977). Structure and vibratory behavior of the vocal folds. In M. Sawashima & F. S. Cooper (Eds.), *Dynamic aspects of speech production* (pp. 13–30). Tokyo, Japan: University of Tokyo Press.

Hirano, M., Hirade, Y., & Kawasaki, H. (1985). Vocal function following carbon dioxide laser surgery for glottic carcinoma. *Annals of Otology, Rhinology and Laryngology, 94,* 232–235.

Hirano, M., & Kurita, S. (1986). Histological structure of the vocal fold and its normal and pathological variations. In J. A. Kirchner (Ed.), *Vocal fold histopathology: A symposium* (pp. 17–24). San Diego, CA: College-Hill Press.

Hirano, M., Kurita, S., & Nakashima, T. (1983). Growth, development and aging of human vocal folds. In D. M. Bless & J. H. Abbs (Eds.), *Vocal fold physiology: Contemporary research and clinical issues* (pp. 22–43). San Diego, CA: College-Hill Press.

Hirano, M., Kurita, S., & Sakaguchi, S. (1988). Vocal fold tissue of a 104-year-old lady. *Annual Bulletin of the Research Institute of Logopedics and Phoniatrics, 22,* 1–5.

Hirano, M., Mori, K., & Iwashita, H. (1994). Voice in laryngeal cancer. In R. Smee & G. P. Bridger (Eds.), *Laryngeal cancer* (pp. 54–64). Amsterdam: Elsevier Science.

Hirano, M., & Sato, K. (1993). Laser surgery for epithelial hyperplasia of the vocal fold. *Annals of Otology, Rhinology and Laryngology, 102,* 85–91.

Hiroto, I. (1966). Pathophysiology of the larynx from the viewpoint of the vocal mechanism. *Practica Otologica Kyoto, 59,* 229–292.

Hocevar-Boltežar, I., Žargi, M., & Honocodeevar-Boltežar, I. (2000). Voice quality after radiation therapy for early glottic cancer. *Archives of Otolaryngology—Head and Neck Surgery, 126,* 1097–1100.

Hoffman, H. T., McCulloch, T., Gustin, D., & Karnell, L. H. (1997). Organ preservation therapy for advanced laryngeal carcinoma. *Otolaryngologic Clinics of North America, 30,* 113–130.

Hollien, H., & Shipp, T. (1972). Speaking fundamental frequency and chronologic age in males. *Journal of Speech and Hearing Research, 15,* 155–159.

Hommerich, K. W. (1972). Der alternde Larynx: Morphologische Aspekte [The aging larynx: Morphological aspects]. *HNO, 20,* 115–120.

Honjo, I., & Isshiki, N. (1980). Laryngoscopic and voice characteristics of aged persons. *Archives of Otolaryngology, 106,* 149–150.

Hoyt, D. J., Lettinga, J. W., Leopold, K. A., & Fisher, S. R. (1992). The effect of head and neck radiation therapy on voice quality. *Laryngoscope, 102,* 477–480.

Jørgensen, K., Godballe, C., Hansen, O., & Bastholt, L. (2002). Cancer of the larynx—Treatment results after primary radiotherapy with salvage surgery in a series of 1005 patients. *Acta Oncologica, 41,* 69–76.

Jørgensen, K., Hansen, O., & Bastholt, L. (1994). Organ preservation after primary irradiation of cancer of the larynx. In R. Smee & G. P. Bridger (Eds.), *Laryngeal cancer* (pp. 539–543). Amsterdam: Elsevier Science.

Kahane, J. C. (1980). Age related histological changes in the human male and female laryngeal cartilages: Biological and functional implications. In V. Lawrence & B. Weinberg (Eds.), *Transcripts of the ninth symposium: Care of the professional voice* (Part 1, pp. 11–20). New York: The Voice Foundation.

Kahane, J. C. (1987). Connective tissue changes in the larynx and their effects on voice. *Journal of Voice, 1,* 27–30.

Kahane, J. C. (1990). Age–related changes in the peripheral speech mechanism: Structural and physiological changes. *ASHA Reports, 19,* 75–87.

Kahane, J. C., & Beckford, N. S. (1991). The aging larynx and voice. In D. N. Ripich (Ed.), *Handbook of geriatric communication disorders* (pp. 165–186). Austin, TX: PRO-ED.

Kakita, Y., Hirano, M., & Ohmaru, K. (1981). Physical properties of the vocal fold tissue: Measurement on excised larynges. In K. N. Stevens & M. Hirano (Eds.), *Vocal fold physiology* (pp. 377–396). Tokyo, Japan: University of Tokyo Press.

Kaplan, M. J., Johns, M. E., & Clark, D. A. (1984). Glottic carcinoma: The roles of surgery and irradiation. *Cancer, 53,* 2641–2648.

Karim, A. B. M. F., Snow, G. B., Siek, H. T. H., & Njo, K. H. (1983). The quality of voice in patients irradiated for laryngeal carcinoma. *Cancer, 51,* 47–49.

Karmody, C. S. (1983). *Textbook of otolaryngology.* Philadelphia: Lea & Febiger.

Karnell, L. H., Funk, G. F., Tomblin, J. B., & Hoffman, H. T. (1999). Quality of life measurements of speech in the head and neck cancer patient population. *Head and Neck, 21,* 229–238.

Kelly, M. D., Hahn, S. S., Spaulding, C. A., Kersh, C. R., Constable, W. C., & Cantrell, R. W. (1989). Definitive radiotherapy in the management of Stage I and II carcinomas of the glottis. *Annals of Otology, Rhinology and Laryngology, 98,* 235–239.

Koike, Y. (1973). Application of some acoustic measures for the evaluation of laryngeal dysfunction. *Studia Phonologica, 7,* 17–23.

Koike, Y., Takahashi, H., & Calcaterra, T. C. (1977). Acoustic measures for detecting laryngeal pathology. *Acta Otolaryngologica, 84,* 105–117.

Kopelman, J., Budnick, A. S., Sessions, R. B., Kramer, M. B., & Wong, G. Y. (1988). Ototoxicity of high-dose cisplatin by bolus administration in patients with advanced cancers and normal hearing. *Laryngoscope, 98,* 858–864.

Kraus, D. H., Pfister, D. G, Harrison, L. B., Spiro, R. H., Strong, E. W., Zelefsky, M., Bosl, G. J., & Shah, J. P. (1995). Salvage laryngectomy for unsuccessful larynx preservation therapy. *Annals of Otology, Rhinology and Laryngology, 104,* 936–941.

Kreul, E. J., & Hecker, M. H. L. (1971). Descriptions of the speech of patients with cancer of the vocal folds: Part II. Judgments of age and voice quality. *Journal of the Acoustical Society of America, 49,* 1283–1287.

Laccourreye, O., Brasnu, D., Bassot, V., Menard, M., Khayat, D., & Laccourreye, H. (1996). Cisplatin-fluorouracil exclusive chemotherapy for T1-T3N0 glottic squamous cell carcinoma complete clinical responders: Five-year results. *Journal of Clinical Oncology, 14,* 2331–2336.

Lederman, M. (1975). History of radiotherapy in the treatment of cancer of the larynx, 1896–1939. *Laryngoscope, 85,* 333–353.

Lefebvre, J. L. (1998). Larynx preservation: The discussion is not closed. *Otolaryngology—Head and Neck Surgery, 118,* 389–393.

Lehman, J. J., Bless, D. M., & Brandenburg, J. H. (1988). An objective assessment of voice production after radiation therapy for Stage I squamous cell carcinoma of the glottis. *Otolaryngology—Head and Neck Surgery, 98,* 121–129.

Leon, X., Quer, M., Orus, C., Lopez, M., Gras, J. R., & Vega, M. (2001). Results of salvage surgery for local or regional recurrence after larynx preservation with induction chemotherapy and radiotherapy. *Head & Neck, 23,* 733–738.

Leonard, R. J., Gallia, L. J., & Charpied, G. (1992). Recovery of vocal fold mucosa from laser incision. *Journal of Voice, 6,* 286–291.

Lesnicar, H., Smid, L., & Zakotnik, B. (1996). Early glottic cancer: The influence of primary treatment on voice preservation. *International Journal of Radiation Oncology, Biology, Physics, 36,* 1025–1032.

Lieberman, P. (1963). Some acoustic measures of the fundamental periodicity of normal and pathologic larynges. *Journal of the Acoustical Society of America, 35,* 344–353.

Linville, S. E. (1987). Maximum phonational frequency range capabilities of women's voices with advancing age. *Folia Phoniatrica, 39,* 297–301.

Linville, S. E. (1988). Intraspeaker variability in fundamental frequency stability: An age-related phenomenon? *Journal of the Acoustical Society of America, 83,* 741–745.

Linville, S. E., & Fisher, H. B. (1985a). Acoustic characteristics of perceived versus actual vocal age in controlled phonation by adult females. *Journal of the Acoustical Society of America, 78,* 40–48.

Linville, S. E., & Fisher, H. B. (1985b). Acoustic characteristics of women's voices with advancing age. *Journal of Gerontology, 40,* 324–330.

List, M. A., Ritter-Sterr, C. A., Baker, T. M., Colangelo, L. A., Matz, G., Pauloski, B. R., & Logemann, J. A. (1996). Longitudinal assessment of quality of life in laryngeal cancer patients. *Head and Neck, 18,* 1–10.

Llewellyn-Thomas, H. A., Sutherland, H. J., Hogg, S. A., Ciampi, A., Harwood, A. R., Keane, T. J., Till, J. E., & Boyd, N. F. (1984). Linear analogue self-assessment of voice quality in laryngeal cancer. *Journal of Chronic Disorders, 37,* 917–924.

Lo, S. M., Venkatesan, V., Matthews, T. W., & Rogers, J. (1998). Tumour volume: Implications in T2/T3 glottic/supraglottic squamous cell carcinoma. *Journal of Otolaryngology, 27,* 247–251.

Ludlow, C., Coulter, D., & Gentges, F. (1983). The differential sensitivity of frequency perturbation to laryngeal neoplasms and neuropathologies. In D. M. Bless & J. H. Abbs (Eds.), *Vocal fold physiology: Contemporary research and clinical issues* (pp. 381–392). San Diego, CA: College-Hill Press.

Maier, H., Dietz, A., Gewelke, U., Heller, W. D., & Weidauer, H. (1994). Tobacco and alcohol and the risk of head and neck cancer. *Clinical Investigation, 70,* 320–327.

Maier, H., Dietz, A., & Heller, W. D. (1992). Occupational factors—Indoor air pollution and laryngeal cancer. In R. Smee & G. P. Bridger (Eds.), *Laryngeal cancer* (pp. 117–121). Amsterdam: Elsevier Science.

Mariya, Y., Matsutani, H., Abe, Y., & Nakaji, S. (1998). Enhanced regeneration response of laryngeal and hypopharyngeal mucosa with accelerated hyperfractionated radiation therapy for glottic cancers. *Radiation Medicine, 16,* 469–472.

McGlone, R., & Hollien, H. (1963). Vocal pitch characteristics of aged women. *Journal of Speech and Hearing Research, 6,* 165–170.

McGuirt, W. F., Koufman, J. A., Blalock, D., Feehs, R. S., Hilliard, A., Grevin, K., & Randall, M. (1994). Comparative voice results after laser resection or irradiation of T1 vocal cord carcinoma. *Archives of Otolaryngology—Head and Neck Surgery, 120,* 951–955.

McNeil, B. J., Weichselbaum, R., & Pauker, S. G. (1981). Speech and survival: Tradeoffs between quality and quantity of life in laryngeal cancer. *New England Journal of Medicine, 305,* 982–987.

Medini, E., Medini, I., Lee, C. K., Gapany, M., & Levitt, S. H. (1998a). The role of radiotherapy in the management of carcinoma in situ of the glottic larynx. *American Journal of Clinical Oncology, 21,* 298–301.

Medini, E., Medini, I., Lee, C. K., Gapany, M., & Levitt, S. H. (1998b). Curative radiotherapy for stage II–III squamous cell carcinoma of the glottic larynx. *American Journal of Clinical Oncology, 21,* 302–305.

Meleca, R. J., Dworkin, J. P., Kewson, D. T., Stachler, R. J., & Hill, S. L. (2003). Functional outcomes following nonsurgical treatment for advanced-stage laryngeal carcinoma. *Laryngoscope, 113,* 720–728.

Mendenhall, W. M., Amdur, R. J., Morris, C. G., & Hinerman, R. W. (2001). T1–T2N0 squamous cell carcinoma of the glottic larynx treated with radiation therapy. *Journal of Clinical Oncology, 19,* 4029–4036.

Mendonca, D. R. (1975). State of the patient after successful irradiation for laryngeal cancer. *Laryngoscope, 85,* 534–539.

Miller, S., Harrison, L. B., Solomon, B., & Sessions, R. B. (1990). Vocal changes in patients undergoing radiation therapy for glottic carcinoma. *Laryngoscope, 100,* 603–606.

Mittal, B., Rao, D. V., Marks, J. E., & Ogura, J. H. (1983). Comparative cost analysis of hemilaryngectomy and irradiation for early glottic carcinoma. *International Journal of Radiation Oncology, Biology, Physics, 9,* 407–408.

Moose, B. D., & Grevin, K. M. (1997). Definitive radiation management for carcinoma of the glottic larynx. *Otolaryngologic Clinics of North America, 30,* 131–143.

Morgan, D. A. L., Robinson, H. F., Marsh, L., & Bradley, P. J. (1988). Vocal quality 10 years after radiotherapy for early glottic cancer. *Clinical Radiology, 39,* 295–296.

Morris, M. R., Canonico, D., & Blank, C. (1994). A critical review of radiotherapy in the management of T1 glottic carcinoma. *American Journal of Otolaryngology, 15,* 276–280.

Morrison, R. (1971). Review article—Radiation therapy in diseases of the larynx. *British Journal of Radiology, 44,* 489–504.

Morsomme, D., Jamart, J., Boucquey, D., & Remacle, M. (1997). Presbyphonia: Voice differences between the sexes in the elderly—Comparison by maximum phonation time, phonation quotient and spectral analysis. *Logopedics Phoniatrics Vocology, 22,* 9–14.

Morton, R. P., Davies, A. D. M., Baker, J., Baker, G. A., & Stell, P. M. (1984). Quality of life in treated head and neck cancer patients: A preliminary report. *Clinical Otolaryngology, 9,* 181–185.

Mueller, P. B., & Wilcox, J. C. (1980). Effects of marijuana smoking on vocal pitch and quality. *Ear, Nose and Throat Journal, 59,* 506–509.

Murphy, C. H., & Doyle, P. C. (1987). The effects of cigarette smoking on voice-fundamental frequency. *Otolaryngology—Head and Neck Surgery, 97,* 376–380.

Murry, T. (1978). Speaking fundamental frequency characteristics associated with voice pathologies. *Journal of Speech and Hearing Disorders, 43,* 374–379.

Murry, T., Bone, R. C., & Von Essen, C. (1974). Changes in voice production during radiotherapy for laryngeal cancer. *Journal of Speech and Hearing Disorders, 39,* 194–201.

Murry, T., & Doherty, E. T. (1980). Selected acoustic characteristics of pathologic and normal speakers. *Journal of Speech and Hearing Research, 23,* 361–369.

Murry, T., & Singh, S. (1982). Acoustic and perceptual features of laryngeal cancer. In A. Sekey (Ed.), *Electroacoustic analysis and enhancement of alaryngeal speech* (pp. 119–134). Springfield, IL: Thomas.

Muscat, J. E., & Wynder, E. L. (1991). Tobacco, alcohol, asbestos, and occupational risk factors for laryngeal disease. *Cancer, 69,* 2244–2251.

Mysak, E. D. (1959). Pitch and duration characteristics of older males. *Journal of Speech and Hearing Research, 2,* 46–54.

Niedzielska, G., Pruszewicz, A., & Swidzinski, P. (1994). Acoustic evaluation of voice in individuals with alcohol addiction. *Folia Phoniatrica et Logopaedica, 46,* 115–122.

Nishioka, T., Shirato, H., Fukuda, S., Arimoto, T., Kamada, T., Furuta, Y., Nishino, S., Hosokawa, Y., Kitahara, T., Kagei, K., Inuyama, Y., & Miyasaka, K. (1999). A phase II study of concomitant chemoradiotherapy for laryngeal carcinoma using carboplatin. *Oncology, 56,* 36–42.

Olthoff, A., Mrugalla, S., Laskawi, R., Frohlich, M., Stuermer, I., Kruse, E., Ambrosch, P., & Steiner, W. (2003). Assessment of irregular voices after total and laser surgical partial laryngectomy. *Archives of Otolaryngology—Head and Neck Surgery, 129,* 994–999.

Orlikoff, R. F. (1990). The relationship of age and cardiovascular health to certain acoustic characteristics of male voices. *Journal of Speech and Hearing Research, 33,* 450–457.

Orlikoff, R. F., & Kraus, D. H. (1996). Dysphonia following nonsurgical management of advanced laryngeal carcinoma. *American Journal of Speech–Language Pathology, 5*(3), 47–52.

Orlikoff, R. F., Kraus, D. H., Budnick, A. S., Pfister, D. G., & Zelefsky, M. J. (1999). Vocal function following successful chemoradiation treatment for advanced laryngeal cancer: Preliminary results. *Phonoscope, 2,* 67–77.

Orlikoff, R. F., Kraus, D. H., Harrison, L. B., Ho, M. L., & Gartner, C. J. (1997). Vocal fundamental frequency measures as a reflection of tumor response to chemotherapy in patients with advanced laryngeal cancer. *Journal of Voice, 11,* 33–39.

Orr, N. M., Hamilton, M. D., & Glennie, J. M. (1972). Variations in voice quality with laryngeal tumours and radiotherapy of the larynx. *British Journal of Disorders of Communication, 7,* 135–140.

Osteen, R. T. (Ed.). (1996). *Cancer manual* (9th ed.). Atlanta, GA: American Cancer Society.

Ott, S., Klingholz, F., Willich, N., & Kastenbauer, E. (1992). Die bestimmung der qualität der sprechstimme nach therapie von T1- und T2- stimmlippenkarzinomen [Assessing the quality of the speaking voice after therapy for T1 and T2 vocal fold cancer]. *Laryngorhinootologie, 71,* 236–241.

Pellitteri, P. K., Kennedy, T. L., Vrabec, D. P., Beller, D., & Hellstrom, M. (1991). Radiotherapy, the mainstay in the treatment of early glottic carcinoma. *Archives of Otolaryngology—Head and Neck Surgery, 117,* 297–301.

Pfister, D. G., Shaha, A. R., & Harrison, L. B. (1997). The role of chemotherapy in the curative treatment of head and neck cancer. *Surgical Oncology Clinics of North America, 6,* 749–768.

Pfister, D. G., Strong, E. W., Harrison, L. B., Haines, I. E., Pfister, D. A., Sessions, R., Spiro, R., Shah, J., Gerold, F., McLure, T., Vikram, B., Fass, D., Armstrong, J., & Bosl, G. J. (1991). Larynx preservation with combined chemotherapy and radiation therapy in advanced but resectable head and neck cancer. *Journal of Clinical Oncology, 9,* 850–859.

Ramig, L. A., & Ringel, R. L. (1983). Effects of physiological aging on selected acoustic characteristics of voice. *Journal of Speech and Hearing Research, 26,* 22–30.

Ramig, L. A., Scherer, R. C., & Titze, I. R. (1985). Acoustic correlates of aging. *Research and Recording Center Research Report, 1,* 257–277.

Rathmell, A. J., Ash, D. V., Howes, M., & Nicholls, J. (1991). Assessing quality of life in patients treated for advanced head and neck cancer. *Clinical Oncology, 3,* 10–16.

Robbins, K. T. (2000). The evolving role of combined modality therapy in head and neck cancer. *Archives of Otolaryngology—Head and Neck Surgery, 126,* 265–269.

Robbins, K. T., Doweck, I., Samant, S., Vieira, F., & Kumar, P. (2004). Factors predictive of local disease control after intra-arterial concomitant chemoradiation (RADPLAT). *Laryngoscope, 114,* 411–417.

Robbins, K. T., Kumar, P., Wong, F. S., Hartsell, W. F., Flick, P., Palmer, R., Weir, A. B., Neill, H. B., Murry, T., Ferguson, R., Hanchett, C., Vieira, F., Bush, A., & Howell, S. B. (2000). Targeted chemoradiation for advanced head and neck cancer: Analysis of 213 patients. *Head and Neck, 22,* 687–693.

Roberts-Thomson, I. C., Youngchaizud, U., Wittingham, S., & Makay, I. R. (1974). Aging, immune response, and mortality. *Lancet, 2,* 368–370.

Rochet, A. P. (1991). Aging and the respiratory system. In D. N. Ripich (Ed.), *Handbook of geriatric communication disorders* (pp. 145–163). Austin, TX: PRO-ED.

Roncallo, P. (1948). Researches about ossification and conformation of the thyroid cartilage in men. *Acta Otolaryngologica, 36,* 110–134.

Rosier, J. F., Gregoire, V., Counoy, H., Octave-Prignot, M., Rombaut, P., Scalliet, P., Vanderlinden, F., & Hamoir, M. (1998). Comparison of external radiotherapy, laser microsurgery and partial laryngectomy for the treatment of T1N0M0 glottic carcinomas: A retrospective evaluation. *Radiotherapy and Oncology, 48,* 175–183.

Ryan, W., & Burk, K. (1974). Perceptual and acoustic correlates of aging in the speech of males. *Journal of Communication Disorders, 7,* 181–192.

Rydell, R., Schalén, L., Fex, S., & Elner, Å. (1995). Voice evaluation before and after laser excision vs. radiotherapy of T1A glottic carcinoma. *Acta Otolaryngologica, 115,* 560–565.

Saarilahti, K., Kajanti, M., Lehtonen, H., Hamalainen, T., & Joensuu, H. (1998). Repopulation during radical radiotherapy for T1 glottic cancer. *Radiotherapy and Oncology, 47,* 155–159.

Sapir, S. (1994). Medical, surgical, and behavioral approaches to vocal therapeutics. *Current Opinion in Otolaryngology—Head and Neck Surgery, 2,* 247–251.

Sataloff, R. T., Hawkshaw, M. J., McCarter, A. A., & Spiegel, J. R. (1999). Vocal fold cancer presenting as sudden dysphonia in the absence of risk factors. *Ear, Nose and Throat Journal, 78,* 148.

Schenone, G., Bussi, M., Magnano, M., De Stefani, A., Cavalot, A., Rosso, S., Merlano, M., & Cortesina, G. (1997). La chemioterapia nei carcinomi della testa e del collo [Chemotherapy of head and neck carcinomas]. *Acta Otorhinolaryngologica Italica, 17,* 124–135.

Segre, R. (1971). Senescence of the voice. *Eye, Ear, Nose, and Throat Monthly, 50,* 223–227.

Shanks, J. C. (1995). Coping with laryngeal cancer. *Seminars in Speech and Language, 16,* 180–190.

Shipp, T., & Hollien, H. (1969). Perception of the aging male voice. *Journal of Speech and Hearing Research, 12,* 703–710.

Simpson, C. B., Postma, G. N., Stone, R. E., & Ossoff, R. H. (1997). Speech outcomes after laryngeal cancer management. *Otolaryngologic Clinics of North America, 30,* 189–205.

Skladowski, K., Tarnawski, R., Maciejewski, B., Wygoda, A., & Slosarek, K. (1999). Clinical radiobiology of glottic T1 squamous cell carcinoma. *International Journal of Radiation Oncology, Biology, Physics, 43,* 101–106.

Sorensen, D., & Horii, Y. (1982). Cigarette smoking and voice fundamental frequency. *Journal of Communication Disorders, 15,* 135–144.

Spector, J. G., Sessions, D. G., Chao, K. S., Hanson, J. M., Simpson, J. R., & Perez, C. A. (1999). Management of stage II (T2N0M0) glottic carcinoma by radiotherapy and conservation surgery. *Head and Neck, 21,* 116–123.

Stewart, J. G., Brown, J. R., Palmer, M. K., & Cooper, A. (1975). The management of glottic carcinoma by primary irradiation with surgery in reserve. *Laryngoscope, 85,* 1477–1484.

Stoicheff, M. L. (1975). Voice following radiotherapy. *Laryngoscope, 85,* 608–618.

Stoicheff, M. L. (1981). Speaking fundamental frequency characteristics and phonational frequency ranges of non-smoking female adults. *Journal of Speech and Hearing Research, 24,* 437–441.

Stoicheff, M. L., Ciampi, A., Passi, J. E., & Fredrickson, J. M. (1983). The irradiated larynx and voice: A perceptual study. *Journal of Speech and Hearing Research, 26,* 482–485.

Strome, S. E., & Weinman, E. C. (2002). Advanced larynx cancer. *Current Treatment Options in Oncology, 3,* 11–20.

Strong, M. S. (1975). Laser excision of carcinoma of the larynx. *Laryngoscope, 85,* 1286–1289.

Strong, M. S., & Jako, G. J. (1972). Laser surgery in the larynx—Early clinical experience with continuous CO_2 laser. *Annals of Otology, Rhinology and Laryngology, 81,* 791–798.

Stupp, R., & Vokes, E. E. (1995). Fortschritte in der Therapie von Kopf- und Halstumoren: 1. Teil: Chemotherapie [Advances in the treatment of head and neck tumors: 1. Chemotherapy]. *Strahlentherapie und Onkologie, 171,* 12–17.

Suen, J. Y., & Stern, S. J. (1995). Premalignant lesions of the larynx. In J. S. Rubin, R. T. Sataloff, G. S. Korovin, & W. J. Gould (Eds.), *Diagnosis and treatment of voice disorders* (pp. 152–160). New York: Igaku-Shoin.

Suwinski, R., Maciejewski, B., & Withers, H. R. (1998). Dose-response relationship for elective neck irradiation of head and neck cancer—Facts and controversies. *Neoplasma, 45,* 107–112.

Terrell, J. E., Fisher, S. G., & Wolf, G. T. (1998). Long-term quality of life after treatment of laryngeal cancer: The Veterans Affairs Laryngeal Cancer Study Group. *Archives of Otolaryngology—Head and Neck Surgery, 124,* 964–971.

Tombolini, V., Zurio, A., Cavaceppi, P. Sarro, A., Guidi, C., Osti, M. F., Vitturini, A., & Banelli, E. (1995). Radiotherapy for T1 carcinoma of the glottis. *Tumori, 81,* 414–418.

Union Internationale Contra le Cancer. (1987). *Manual of clinical oncology* (4th ed.). New York: Springer-Verlag.

Uno, T., Itami, J., Kotaka, K., & Toriyama, M. (1996). Radical radiotherapy for T3 laryngeal cancers. *Strahlentherapie und Onkologie, 172,* 422–426.

Verdonck-de Leeuw, I. M. (1998). *Voice characteristics following radiotherapy: The development of a protocol.* Amsterdam: University of Amsterdam.

Verdonck-de Leeuw, I. M., Keus, R. B., Hilgers, F. J., Koopmans-van Beinum, F. J., Greven, A. J., de Jong, J. M., Vreeburg, G., & Bartelink, H. (1999). Consequences of voice impairment in daily life for patients following radiotherapy for early glottic cancer: Voice quality, vocal function, and vocal performance. *International Journal of Oncology, Biology, Physics, 44,* 1071–1078.

Verdonck-de Leeuw, I. M., & Koopmans-van Beinum, F. J. (1995). Voice quality before and after radiotherapy: Acoustical, clinical, and perceptual pitch measures. *Proceedings of the Institute of Phonetic Sciences Amsterdam, 19,* 1–9.

Wanebo, H. J., Chougule, P., Ready, N., Koness, R. J., Akerley, W., McRae, R., Nigri, P., Leone, L., Webber, B., & Safran, H. (1999). Preoperative paclitaxel, carboplatin, and radiation therapy in advanced head and neck cancer (Stage III and IV). *Seminars in Radiation Oncology, 9,* 77–84.

Watanabe, H., Shin, T., Matsuo, H., Okuno, F., Tsuji, T., Matsuoka, M., Fukaura, J., & Matsunaga, H. (1994). Studies on vocal fold injection and changes in pitch associated with alcohol intake. *Journal of Voice, 8,* 340–346.

Welkoborsky, H. J., & Mann, W. J. (1994). Multistep malignancy analysis in premalignant lesions and early stage cancer of the larynx. In R. Smee & G. P. Bridger (Eds.), *Laryngeal cancer* (pp. 282–288). Amsterdam: Elsevier Science.

Werner-Kukuk, E., von Leden, H., & Yanagihara, N. (1968). The effects of radiation therapy on laryngeal function. *Journal of Laryngology and Otology, 82,* 1–15.

Wheeler, R. H., & Spencer, S. (1995). Cisplatin plus radiation therapy. *Journal of Infusional Chemotherapy, 5,* 61–66.

Wilcox, K. A., & Horii, Y. (1980). Age and changes in vocal jitter. *Journal of Gerontology, 35,* 194–198.

Woodson, G. E., Rosen, C. A., Murry, T., Madasu, R., Wong, F., Hengesteg, A., & Robbins, K. T. (1996). Assessing vocal function after chemoradiation for advanced laryngeal carcinoma. *Archives of Otolaryngology—Head and Neck Surgery, 122,* 858–864.

Wynder, E. L., Covey, L. S., Marbuchi, K., Johnson, J., & Muschinsky, M. (1976). Environmental factors in cancer of the larynx: A second look. *Cancer, 38,* 1591–1601.

Xue, A., & Mueller, P. B. (1997). Acoustic and perceptual characteristics of the voice of sedentary and physically active elderly speakers. *Logopedics Phoniatrics Vocology, 22,* 51–60.

Zeitels, S. M. (1996). Phonomicrosurgical treatment of early glottic cancer and carcinoma in situ. *American Journal of Surgery, 172,* 704–709.

Zuppinger, A. (1951). Biological problems in X-ray therapy of intrinsic and extrinsic tumours of the larynx. *Clinical Radiology, 2,* 20–23.

Chapter 11

Recent Advances in Conservation Laryngectomy Procedures

Gail B. Kempster

The goal of any intervention in patients with laryngeal cancer is, first and foremost, cure of the disease. To this end, the primary treatment approaches of surgery and radiation therapy, sometimes in conjunction with chemotherapy, are used (see Chapter 10 in this text). Unfortunately, no prospective, randomized study directly compares outcomes between surgery and radiation therapy used as primary treatments (Lefebvre, 1998). Patients with early cancers of the larynx (i.e., Stages I and II; see Chapter 13) usually can be treated successfully with either radiation therapy or surgery. Which treatment a patient receives is related to a variety of factors, including the patient's tumor characteristics, geographic location, and premorbid health status (see Chapter 7 in this text). Patients with later stage disease (Stages III and IV) may be (a) treated surgically, often followed by radiation, or (b) treated with a protocol involving chemotherapy followed by either surgery or radiation treatment, depending on the response of the patient to chemotherapy. Under this type of protocol, a good response to chemotherapy is considered to be a good predictor of a favorable response to radiation treatment. Surgical salvage may follow radiation therapy should the disease recur (see Hoffman, McCulloch, Gustin, & Karnell, 1997; Jørgensen, Godballe, Hansen, & Bastholt, 2002).

For many decades, certain glottic and supraglottic laryngeal cancers have been treated with surgical approaches in which only part of the laryngeal complex is removed (e.g., Silver, 1981; Sinard, Netterville, Garrett, & Ossoff, 1996). Such techniques have been designed to maintain the expectation of cure while allowing for voice production without a permanent tracheostomy. Additionally, conservative surgical approaches aim to allow for adequate swallowing function without a permanent gastrostomy (Weinstein & Laccourreye, 2000b). These surgical approaches include supraglottic laryngectomy, vertical partial laryngectomy, surpacricoid laryngectomy with reconstruction, and near-total laryngectomy. Some authors refer to these techniques as organ-preservation surgeries in that the biological functions of the larynx, especially airway protection, are maintained despite the loss of several constituent parts of the larynx. *Conservation laryngectomy,* as used in this chapter, refers to the notion that at least part of the larynx is retained; this laryngeal remnant, along with any surgical reconstruction that is performed, functions as a phonatory source and allows for protection of the airway when swallowing.

The purpose of this chapter is to present current information about the common laryngeal conservation procedures of supraglottic laryngectomy and vertical partial laryngectomy. The somewhat less common procedures of near-total laryngectomy and supracricoid laryngectomy with reconstruction are also discussed. Existing data involving voice and swallowing outcomes following these procedures are reviewed. Because, as Lefebvre (1998) noted, "There are no precise or comparative data on the quality of larynx function after various types of treatment" (p. 390), the information presented reflects the variety of outcomes reported in the literature.

SUPRAGLOTTIC LARYNGECTOMY

The supraglottic laryngectomy (SGL) procedure is sometimes referred to as a subtotal horizontal laryngectomy. Although Ogura is the best known American surgeon whose work helped define and popularize the SGL procedure, he was likely influenced by Alonzo's reports from South America in the 1940s (Lawson & Biller, 1985). The one-stage SGL was introduced in the United States by Ogura in 1958. Earlier work by Pressman and his colleagues (Pressman, Dowdy, & Libby, 1956) determined that distinct anatomic boundaries exist in the supraglottis (Myers & Alvi, 1996). Pressman et al. demonstrated that dye injected into the supraglottis travels only as far inferiorly as the inferior border of the false vocal folds, despite the absence of an identifiable anatomic barrier within the body of the ventricle. Such a barrier does appear to exist, however, in the form of the anterior commissure tendon (Sinard et al., 1996). Tucker and Smith (1982) showed that the anterior commissure tendon is part of an avascular zone forming a kind of anatomic boundary between the glottis and supraglottis. The supraglottic area includes the epiglottis, the preepiglottic space, the laryngeal aspects of the aryepiglottic folds, the arytenoids, and the false vocal folds. The hyoid bone and the valleculae are considered part of the oropharynx.

That an anatomic boundary exists undoubtedly is related to the embryologic development of the larynx. Frasier (1909) determined that the supraglottic laryngeal structures arise from branchial arches III and IV, whereas the subglottis derives from arch VI. These different embryologic roots suggest that the larynx can be divided into "compartments": supraglottis, glottis, and subglottis (Lawson & Biller, 1985). The vascular and lymphatic systems of the larynx maintain this compartmentalization. Pressman et al.'s (1956) work demonstrated that lymphatic flow from the epiglottis is to the false vocal folds and ends abruptly along the inferior border of the false folds. Only with massive injections of dye does penetration inferior to the ventricle occur (Sinard et al., 1996).

As with any conservation laryngeal procedure, proper patient selection for an SGL is essential; the extent of the tumor and nodal metastasis can significantly affect cure with SGL (Myers & Alvi, 1996). Cure rates for patients who undergo an SGL and who are without lymph node involvement are reported to be as high as 85% (Ogura & Biller, 1969); however, when lymph nodes are involved, survival rates drop. If primary radiotherapy is used as the treatment of choice, survival rates drop to a range of 30% to 76% (Lawson & Biller, 1985; Lefebvre, 1998). One feature clearly affecting survival is the presence of cancer in the lymph nodes. Even in cases of combined therapy (i.e., when radiation therapy either precedes or follows surgery), the cure rates are similar to those of patients who receive surgery alone. Thus, some surgeons see little value in combining radiotherapy and SGL unless lymph nodes are involved (DeSanto, 1998). In a retrospective study, Vermund et al. (1998) indicated that "primary radiation therapy may be as effective as primary surgery for patients with advanced squamous cell carcinoma when no fixed or bilateral metastatic neck nodes are present" (p. 173). Although combined treatment modalities remain fairly common in the United States, at least two studies (as cited in DeSanto, 1998) have suggested that there is no significant benefit to combining surgery and radiation therapy in patients with a supraglottic tumor.

In a standard supraglottic laryngectomy, the surgeon makes a transverse cut of the thyroid cartilage above the level of the anterior commissure and resects the laryngeal tissue from the ventricle up to and including the hyoid bone and preepiglottic space. Often a cricopharyngeal myotomy is performed, theoretically to aid postoperative swallowing function. Many surgeons also prefer to suspend the remaining laryngeal tissue from the mandible via a suspension stitch; this is thought to rotate the anterior commissure up and forward to protect the airway and prevent aspiration (DeSanto, 1998).

This standard SGL surgery can be modifed, depending on the extent of a patient's tumor and the skill of the surgeon. Often a tumor may extend up and into the base of the tongue, so that part of the tongue base must also be resected. Problems arise, however, when the hypoglossal nerves are threatened. If part of the tongue base and one hypoglossal nerve are sacrificed, the patient will have difficulty swallowing (see Chapter 14 in this text); the postoperative course will likely be lengthy and complicated before the patient can resume a normal diet. It is not possible to swallow safely if both hypoglossal nerves and the supraglottic larynx are resected (DeSanto, 1998). If both hypoglossal nerves are resected, the tongue lacks motor control of the bolus during the oral and early pharyngeal stages of swallowing. Despite the protection provided by the true vocal folds, premature spillage of the bolus is a common outcome, resulting in aspiration prior to the onset of the swallow (see Chapter 14 in this text).

DeSanto (1998) suggested that supraglottic cancer should always be considered a midline disease: "If one side of the neck contains metastatic cancer, the other side also can contain cancer" (p. 1732). He recommended simultaneous bilateral neck dissections in all cases where one side of the neck is positive for cancer. His work also suggests, however, that if one side of the neck is negative, the other is likely to be negative as well. Levendag et al. (1989) also concluded that "both sides of the neck should be operated on in patients with supraglottic cancer" (as reported in Myers & Alvi, 1996, p. 562). Thus, it is evident that the staging of the neck becomes a critical variable in the survival of patients with supraglottic cancers. With small tumors and clinically negative nodes, neck dissections are not routinely performed in many centers. Evidence suggests, however, that bilateral neck dissections should be performed when any positive nodes are found, even if only on one side. Some authors currently are promoting bilateral neck dissections in almost every case. The probability of the risk of metastasis has been reported as high as 40%, even in cases of N0 cancers (i.e., no positive neck nodes present) (Thawley & Sessions, 1987).

Patients who receive an SGL frequently experience difficulty swallowing and a high risk of aspiration. Several authors (DeSanto, 1998; Lawson & Biller, 1985; Sinard et al., 1996) reported that aspiration and other swallowing problems occur up to 4 months following SGL. Thus, many patients leave the hospital unable to swallow normally and, therefore, with a feeding tube in place. Decannulation is usually postponed until the patient is eating safely by mouth. Should the

SGL procedure extend into the tongue base, even greater swallowing problems can be expected. Rademaker and colleagues (1993) found that patients who had such extended surgeries experienced up to about a 1-year delay in achieving normal dietary intake. In rare cases, a patient who experiences intractable aspiration then has to have the SGL converted to a total laryngectomy to eliminate the threat of chronic aspiration.

Few data-based studies of voice quality following SGL exist. In general, patients have an adequate, functional postoperative voice, although the quality can be described as hoarse. It is likely that the loss of significant supraglottal tissue would affect the overall quality of a patient's voice, if only in the resonance characteristics of voice output; however, this possibility has not been investigated using objective measures.

VERTICAL PARTIAL LARYNGECTOMY

Most early glottic tumors arise from the membranous vocal folds (Bailey, 1985). Bailey (1998) reported that "several published series of patients have shown that vertical partial laryngectomy and hemilaryngectomy offer better cure rates than radiation alone" (p. 1713). In a standard hemilaryngectomy, exactly one vertical half of the larynx is removed, yet this procedure is seldom performed (Bailey, 1985). Rather, vertical partial laryngectomy (VPL), sometimes called fronto-lateral laryngectomy, is a more commonly performed conservation laryngectomy procedure. This type of surgery is the standard procedure for carcinoma of the vocal fold where the fold remains mobile and the thyroid cartilage has not been invaded. If the vocal fold is fixed, a total laryngectomy is the surgery preferred by most surgeons. Due to the anatomy of this region, if the vocal fold remains mobile but the tumor has encroached upon the anterior commissure, an "extended" modification of the standard surgery can be performed (Davis, Hadley, & Smith, 2004; see also Chapter 9 in this text). The anterior commissure tendon attaches to the anterior commissure at midline. Because there is no perichrondrial layer at this point, the area is more susceptible to tumor invasion. Submucosal spread of cancer may occur despite a normal-appearing mucosa. In cases where the anterior commissure is vulnerable, surgeons extend the VPL to include the anterior portion of the true vocal fold on the contralateral side (Bailey, 1985, 1998).

With a standard VPL, the strap muscles are retracted and the thyroid cartilage is cut at or near midline contralateral to the tumor. The cricoid cartilage remains untouched, unless the tumor extends into the subglottic region. The entire true vocal fold, ventricle, and ventricular fold with the vocal process of the arytenoid on the side of the tumor are removed. The epiglottis remains in place. Should the tumor on the true vocal fold extend posteriorly as far as the vocal process, the entire arytenoid may be resected. The decision to perform this procedure is often determined based on histological information available during surgery.

The remaining vocal fold is sutured anteriorly to the perichondrium of the thyroid cartilage, which is then used to close the larynx anteriorly. Often a flap or a graft is positioned to add bulk in the area of the defect to reduce the possibility of aspiration. Reconstruction of the surgical defect is attempted using a bipedicle muscle flap from the sternohyoid, sternothyroid, thyrohyoid, or ventricular muscles (Bailey, 1998; Biacabe, Crevier-Buchman, Hans, Laccourreye, & Brasnu, 1999). Such flaps are positioned to allow the intact vocal fold to close against the reconstructed area and allow for vibration of tissue bilaterally for voice production. The suprahyoid muscles remain intact, at least unilaterally, allowing the larynx to be able to move up and forward under the tongue base. Because of this and the continued retroversion of the epiglottis during swallowing, the risk of aspiration is lower in VPL patients than in SGL patients.

Various modifications of the standard VPL have been described. A number of surgeons have described their preferences for resection and reconstruction (see Weinstein & Laccourreye, 2000b). In extended VPL where the tumor has crossed the anterior commissure, the resection of the contralateral vocal fold is extended. It is possible to remove all of the laryngeal tissue at the level of the vocal folds except for one arytenoid and the posterior commissure. In these cases, bilateral bipedicle muscle flaps are used to reconstruct a voicing source. In other cases, small lesions just in the area of the anterior commissure may be resected while retaining both arytenoid cartilages. When tumors are located in the area of the anterior commissure, it has been found that radiation therapy is not as effective as surgery. A VPL has been found to be an effective procedure when performed after radiation therapy failure, without a significant increase in costs or complications (DiNardo, Kaylie, & Isaacson, 1999).

As stated previously, those individuals who have received a vertical partial laryngectomy generally experience fewer swallowing problems than those who receive a supraglottic laryngectomy. Consequently, as a group these individuals resume a normal diet much earlier than do those who undergo SGL, with a median time of approximately 1 month reported following VPL (Rademaker et al., 1993).

The voices of patients who have undergone a VPL are not normal. They have been described as "rough" with variable "breathiness" (Doyle, 1997; Doyle, Leeper, Houghton-Jones, Heeneman, & Martin, 1995; Keith, Leeper, & Doyle, 1995). The voicing source is thought to consist of the combination of glottic and supraglottic tissue remnants following VPL surgery (Blaugrund et al., 1984). For Blaugrund et al.'s (1984) patients in whom the arytenoid cartilages were saved, the postoperative vocal frequency range was wider and the aerodynamic measures were more variable than for their patients who had had one arytenoid resected. More recently, those patients whose glottis had been reconstructed with a false vocal fold mucosal flap have been found to have slightly improved harmonics-to-noise ratios and fewer voice breaks compared to VPL patients without such a reconstruction (Biacabe et al., 1999). Biacabe et al. noted, however, that the vocal parameters of both groups of patients continued to improve in the months and years following surgery. They suggested the "existence of compensatory mechanisms coming into play postoperatively" (Biacabe et al., 1999, p. 703; see also Doyle, 1997).

NEAR-TOTAL LARYNGECTOMY

The near-total laryngectomy (NTL) was first reported by Pearson, Woods, and Hartman in 1980. The premise behind this procedure is to allow for voice production by means of a mucosal shunt from the trachea to the pharynx. The airway, however, is too narrow for adequate respiration, so a permanent tracheostoma is created. Pearson and colleagues do not classify the NTL as a conservation procedure, because neither true vocal fold vibration nor respiration without a stoma results following surgery (Pearson, DeSanto, Olsen, & Salassa, 1998). A discussion of this procedure is included in this chapter, however, because the NTL continues to be performed at a number of medical centers throughout the world. Although this procedure was viewed with some skepticism early on, it has gained in acceptance more recently as the outcomes from a number of patient series have been reported.

In the NTL, the entire vertical half of the larynx is removed, along with the anterior two thirds of the contralateral larynx, including the hyoid bone, the epiglottis, and the preepiglottic space. A segment of one arytenoid cartilage and enough cricoid cartilage to maintain a functional cricoarytenoid joint remain. It is important that innervated portions of the posterior cricoarytenoid, lateral cricoarytenoid, interarytenoid, thyroarytenoid, and cricothyroid muscles stay intact to maintain what might be considered a "dynamic" segment of tissue to help prevent aspiration. The surgical closure is different in this procedure than in an extended vertical partial laryngectomy. In the NTL, an epithelialized mucosal shunt is fashioned from an intact strip of laryngeal mucosa remaining in the area. The shunt is formed to connect the airway to the hypopharynx; however, it is too narrow for adequate respiration, so the patient has a permanent tracheostoma. Manual occlusion of the stoma is required to divert air from the lungs through the shunt into the pharynx for speech (Blaugrund et al., 1984).

Pearson et al. (1998) believe that the NTL procedure is an acceptable alternative for a patient with a supraglottic carcinoma for whom the risks of a supraglottic laryngectomy may be too great. The NTL also may serve as a good option for those patients who might be inappropriate candidates for the long-term responsibilities associated with use of a tracheoesophageal voice prosthesis (Gavilan, Herranz, Prim, & Rabanal, 1996; Premalatha, Shenoy, & Amantha, 1994; Spriano, Pellini, Romano, Muscatello, & Roselli, 2002).

The outcomes of patients who receive a near-total laryngectomy have been compared most often to patients who use a voice prosthesis following total laryngectomy. Gavilan et al. (1996) reported a high rate of fistulas, which require extended healing time. Because the mucosal shunt is a direct conduit to the trachea, it is not surprising that aspiration is reported as an occasional problem. In most reported series of patients, at least some degree of aspiration is a complication. Pearson et al. (1998) reported a significant degree of aspiration in 9% of 225 patients. In a few patients the aspiration is significant enough that the NTL must be converted to a total laryngectomy.

The exact phonatory source in NTL is unclear and may vary from patient to patient; in most cases it is likely the shunt itself that is set into vibration for voice. Leeper et al. (1993) suggested that the shunt is a highly individualized source for voice production; therefore, the voices of NTL speakers are likely to be highly variable (Hanamitsu, Kataoka, Takeuchi, & Kitajima, 1999). Most but not all NTL patients are able to produce voice adequately postoperatively. Pearson et al. (1998) reported a speech acquisition rate of 85%, whereas Hanamitsu et al. (1999) reported that 82% of their patients were able to produce voice. Acoustically, NTL voices have been found to be more acceptable than esophageal voices, but not quite as acceptable as tracheoesophageal (TE) puncture voices using a TE voice prosthesis (Premalatha et al., 1994). Fundamental frequency has been found to be higher and more variable than normal (Hoasjoe, Martin, Doyle, & Wong, 1992; Keith et al., 1995), although not all investigators have reported this pattern. Increased jitter and shimmer and shorter maximum phonation times are common findings (Doyle et al., 1995; Hoasjoe et al., 1992; Keith et al., 1995; Leeper et al., 1993).

SUPRACRICOID PARTIAL LARYNGECTOMY WITH RECONSTRUCTION

To conserve function in more advanced cases of supraglottic cancer, a supracricoid partial laryngectomy (SCPL) may also be performed, followed by reconstruction of the area by cricohyoidopexy (CHP) or cricohyoidoepiglottopexy (CHEP). In CHP the epiglottis is resected and the cricoid cartilage is sutured to the hyoid bone (Weinstein & Laccourreye, 2000a). When the epiglottis can be preserved, the CHEP procedure can be used whereby the cricoid is sutured to both the epiglottis and the hyoid. These techniques have been popular in Europe and are beginning to receive attention in the United States. An SCPL with either CHP or CHEP reconstruction allows for voice production without a permanent tracheostoma and enough protection of the airway so that a gastrostomy is not needed (Brasnu, 2003).

In an SCPL with either CHEP or CHP reconstruction, both true and false vocal folds, the ventricles, the paraglottic spaces, and the thyroid cartilage are resected. Only one functional cricoarytenoid unit with the recurrent laryngeal nerve and internal superior laryngeal nerve is preserved. The preservation of the recurrent laryngeal nerve is important to maintain some ability to rotate the arytenoid on the cricoid. This movement helps to close the airway to prevent aspiration. The internal branch of the superior laryngeal nerve is important for sensation to precipitate reflexive coughing. Often, even some of the noninvolved vocal fold is sacrificed, so that the arytenoid is able to function properly postoperatively (Weinstein et al., 2002). During the reconstruction, the arytenoid is repositioned anteriorly to create a narrow, T-shaped laryngeal lumen. It is thought that the horizontal bar of the T serves as the phonatory glottis, whereas the vertical part is more important in respiration; however, this notion has not been verified. It is important for the surgeon to align the anterior border of the cricoid with the hyoid bone and not to rotate the laryngeal skeleton in order to prevent aspiration. A cricopharyngeal myotomy may be performed as well, as a theoretical aid for postoperative swallowing function. (See Weinstein, Laccourreye, Brasnu, & Laccourreye, 2000, for a full discussion of these procedures.)

A report on a series of 124 patients who underwent SCPL with CHP revealed that normal swallowing without a permanent gastrostomy occurred within 1 year in 91% of these patients (Naudo et al., 1997). All but 1 patient was decannulated. Three patients required a permanent gastrostomy, and 3 others underwent a completion laryngectomy. Naudo et al. indicated that a cricopharyngeal myotomy was apparently not helpful in improving their patients' swallowing or in reducing the incidence of aspiration. Although complications were described in a follow-up publication (Naudo et al., 1998), the voice quality of the patients was not discussed in regard to outcomes (De Vincentiis, Minni, Gallo, & DiNardo, 1998).

An acoustic analysis of the voices of patients who received the SCPL with CHEP procedure was reported by Crevier-Buchman et al. (1998). In this series of 12 patients, vocal parameters, including jitter, shimmer, harmonics-to-noise ratio, and perceived quality, were compared pre- and postoperatively. The postoperative voices were judged to be rougher and had more jitter, shimmer, noise, and voiceless periods than preoperative voices. Furthermore, these parameters did not change to a significant degree between 6 and 18 months postoperatively.

SUMMARY

This chapter has reviewed information on a variety of conservation laryngectomy procedures. Included in this discussion was information on supraglottic laryngectomy, vertical partial laryngectomy (hemilaryngectomy), near-total laryngectomy, and supracricoid partial laryngectomy with reconstruction. It is apparent that surgeons are increasingly choosing from a variety of conservation laryngectomy approaches for appropriate patients. The future is likely to bring continued innovation in the evolution of such surgical techniques for the resection of laryngeal tumors and the reconstruction of the protective and phonatory functions of this important organ. A large number of questions regarding the functional results of conservation surgeries remains, however. Although data regarding morbidity and mortality are generally available, many quantitative measures of postoperative voice quality, swallowing function, and patient satisfaction are lacking. It is hoped that as more patients undergo these surgeries, more specific and objective data about their surgical outcomes, as well as postoperative vocal function outcomes, will be made available.

REFERENCES

Bailey, B. J. (1985). Glottic carcinoma. In B. Bailey & H. Biller (Eds.), *Surgery of the larynx* (pp. 257–278). Philadelphia: Saunders.

Bailey, B. J. (1998). Early glottic carcinoma. In B. Bailey (Ed.), *Head and neck surgery—Otolaryngology* (2nd ed., pp. 1703–1724). Philadelphia: Lippincott-Raven.

Biacabe, B., Crevier-Buchman, L., Hans, S., Laccourreye, O., & Brasnu, D. (1999). Vocal function after vertical partial laryngectomy with glottic reconstruction by false vocal fold flap: Durational and frequency measures. *Laryngoscope, 109,* 698–704.

Blaugrund, S. M., Meltzer, J., Gould, W. J., Bloch, C., Haji, T., & Baer, T. (1984). Voice analysis of the partially ablated larynx. *Annals of Otology, Rhinology and Laryngology, 93,* 311–317.

Brasnu, D. F. (2003). Supracricoid partial laryngectomy with cricohyoidopexy in the management of laryngeal carcinoma. *World Journal of Surgery, 27,* 817–823.

Crevier-Buchman, L., Laccourreye, O., Wuyts, F. L., Monfrais-Pfauwadel, M., Pillot, C., & Brasnu, D. (1998). Comparison and evolution of perceptual and acoustic characteristics of voice after supracricoid partial laryngectomy with cricohyoidoepiglottopexy. *Acta Otolaryngologica, 118,* 594–599.

Davis, R. K., Hadley, K., & Smith, M. E. (2004). Endoscopic vertical partial laryngectomy. *Laryngoscope, 114,* 236–240.

DeSanto, L. W. (1998). Supraglottic laryngectomy. In *Head and neck surgery—otolaryngology* (2nd ed., pp. 1725–1738). Philadelphia: Lippincott-Raven.

De Vincentiis, M., Minni, A., Gallo, A., & DiNardo, A. (1998). Supracricoid partial laryngectomies: Oncologic and functional results. *Head and Neck, 20,* 504–509.

DiNardo, L. J., Kaylie, D. M., & Isaacson, J. (1999). Current treatment practices for early laryngeal carcinoma. *Otolaryngology—Head and Neck Surgery, 120,* 30–37.

Doyle, P. C. (1997). Voice refinement following conservation surgery for cancer of the larynx: A conceptual framework for treatment intervention. *American Journal of Speech–Language Pathology, 6,* 27–35.

Doyle, P. C., Leeper, H. A., Houghton-Jones, C., Heeneman, H., & Martin, G. F. (1995). Perceptual characteristics of hemilaryngectomized and near-total laryngectomized male speakers. *Journal of Medical Speech–Language Pathology, 3,* 131–143.

Frasier, E. J. (1909). The development of the larynx. *Journal of Anatomy and Physiology, 44,* 156–191.

Gavilan, J., Herranz, J., Prim, P., & Rabanal, I. (1996). Speech results and complications of near-total laryngectomy. *Annals of Otology, Rhinology and Laryngology, 105,* 729–733.

Hanamitsu, M., Kataoka, H., Takeuchi, E., & Kitajima, K. (1999). Comparative study of vocal function after near-total laryngectomy. *Laryngoscope, 109,* 1320–1323.

Hoasjoe, D. K., Martin, G. F., Doyle, P. C., & Wong, F. S. (1992). A comparative acoustic analysis of voice production by near-total laryngectomy and normal laryngeal speakers. *The Journal of Otolaryngology, 21,* 39–43.

Hoffman, H. T., McCulloch, T., Gustin, D., & Karnell, L. H. (1997). Organ preservation therapy for advanced-stage laryngeal carcinoma. In W. F. McGuirt (Ed.), *The Otolaryngologic Clinics of North America: Current concepts in laryngeal cancer I* (Vol. 30, No. 1, pp. 113–130). Philadelphia: Saunders.

Jørgensen, K., Godballe, C., Hansen, O., & Bastholt, L. (2002). Cancer of the larynx: Treatment results after primary radiotherapy with salvage surgery in a series of 1005 patients. *Acta Oncologica, 41,* 69–76.

Keith, R. L., Leeper, H. A., & Doyle, P. C. (1995). Microanalytic acoustical voice characteristics of near-total laryngectomy. *Otolaryngology—Head and Neck Surgery, 113,* 689–694.

Lawson, W., & Biller, H. F. (1985). Supraglottic cancer. In B. J. Bailey & H .F. Biller (Eds.), *Surgery of the larynx* (pp. 243–255). Philadelphia: Saunders.

Leeper, H. A., Doyle, P. C., Heeneman, H., Martin, G. F., Hoasjoe, D. K., & Wong, F. S. (1993). Acoustical characteristics of voice following hemilaryngectomy and near-total laryngectomy. *Journal of Medical Speech–Language Pathology, 1*(2), 89–94.

Lefebvre, J. (1998). Larynx preservation: The discussion is not closed. *Otolaryngology—Head and Neck Surgery, 118,* 389–393.

Levendag, P., Sessions, R., Vikram, B., Strong, E. W., Shah, J. P., Spiro, R., & Gerold, F. (1989). The problem of neck relapse in early stage supraglottic larynx cancer. *Cancer, 63,* 345–348.

Myers, E. N., & Alvi, A. (1996). Management of carcinoma of the supraglottic larynx: Evolution, current concepts, and future trends. *Laryngoscope, 106,* 559–567.

Naudo, P., Laccourreye, O., Weinstein, G., Hans, S., Laccourreye, H., & Brasnu, D. (1997). Functional outcome and prognosis factors after supracricoid partial laryngectomy with crico-hyoidopexy. *Annals of Otology, Rhinology and Laryngology, 106,* 291–296.

Naudo, P., Laccourreye, O., Weinstein, G., Jouffre, V., Laccourreye, H., & Brasnu, D. (1998). Complications and functional outcome after supracricoid partial laryngectomy with crico-hyoidoepiglottopexy. *Otolaryngology—Head and Neck Surgery, 118,* 124–129.

Ogura, J. H. (1958). Supraglottic subtotal laryngectomy and radical neck dissection for carcinoma of the epiglottis. *Laryngoscope, 68,* 983–1003.

Ogura, J. H., & Biller, H. F. (1969). Conservative surgery in cancer of the head and neck. *Otolaryngologic Clinics of North America, 3,* 641–665.

Pearson, B. W., DeSanto, L. W., Olsen, K. D., & Salassa, J. R. (1998). Results of near-total laryngectomy. *Annals of Otology, Rhinology and Laryngology, 107,* 820–825.

Pearson, B. W., Woods, R. D., & Hartman, D. E. (1980). Extended hemilaryngectomy for T3 glottic carcinoma with preservation of speech and swallowing. *Laryngoscope, 90,* 1950–1961.

Premalatha, B. S., Shenoy, A. M., & Amantha, N. (1994). Speech evaluation after near total laryngectomy and total laryngectomy: A comparative acoustic analysis. *Indian Journal of Cancer, 31,* 244–249.

Pressman, J. J., Dowdy, A., & Libby, R. (1956). Further studies upon the submucosal compartments and lymphatics of the larynx by the injection of dyes and radioisotopes. *Annals of Otology, Rhinology and Laryngology, 65,* 963–980.

Rademaker, A. W., Logemann, J. A., Pauloski, B. R., Bowman, J. B., Lazarus, C. L., Sisson, G. A., Milianti, F. J., Graner, D., Cook, B. S., Collins, S. L., Stein, D. W., Beery, Q. C., Johnson, J. T., & Baker, T. M. (1993). Recovery of postoperative swallowing in patients undergoing partial laryngectomy. *Head and Neck, 15,* 325–334.

Silver, C. E. (1981). *Surgery for cancer of the larynx and related disorders.* New York: Churchill-Livingstone.

Sinard, R. J., Netterville, J. L., Garrett, C. G., & Ossoff, R. H. (1996). Cancer of the larynx. In E. N. Myers & J. Y. Suen (Eds.), *Cancer of the head and neck* (pp. 381–421). Philadelphia: Saunders.

Spriano, G., Pellini, R., Romano, G., Muscatello, L., & Roselli, R. (2002). Supracricoid partial laryngectomy as salvage surgery after radiation failure. *Head and Neck, 24,* 759–765.

Thawley, S. E., & Sessions, D. G. (1987). In S. E. Thawley, V. R. Panje, R. D. Batsakis, et al. (Eds.), *Comprehensive management of head and neck tumors* (pp. 959–990). Philadelphia: Saunders.

Tucker, G. F., & Smith, H. R. (1982). A histological demonstration of the development of laryngeal connective tissue compartments. *Transactions of the American Academy of Ophthalmology and Otolaryngology, 66,* 308–318.

Vermund, H., Boysen, M., Evensen, J. F., Jacobsen, A. B., Natvig, K., Tausjo, J., Wiley, A. L., & Winther, F. (1998). Recurrence after different primary treatment for cancer of the supra-glottic larynx. *Acta Oncologica, 37*(2), 167–173.

Weinstein, G. S., & Laccourreye, O. (2000a). Organ preservation surgery of the larynx: A new paradigm. In G. S. Weinstein, O. Laccourreye, D. Brasnu, & H. Laccourreye (Eds.), *Organ preservation surgery for laryngeal cancer* (pp. 1–8). San Diego: Singular.

Weinstein, G. S., & Laccourreye, O. (2000b). Vertical partial laryngectomies. In G. S. Weinstein, O. Laccourreye, D. Brasnu, & H. Laccourreye (Eds.), *Organ preservation surgery for laryngeal cancer* (pp. 59–72). San Diego: Singular.

Weinstein, G. S., Laccourreye, O., Brasnu, D., & Laccourreye, H. (Eds.). (2000). *Organ preservation surgery for laryngeal cancer.* San Diego: Singular.

Weinstein, G. S., Laccourreye, O., Ruiz, C., Dooley, P., Chalian, A., & Mirza, N. (2002). Larynx preservation with supracricoid partial laryngectomy with circohyoidepiglottopexy: Correlation of videostroboscopic findings and voice parameters. *Annals of Otology, Rhinology and Laryngology, 111,* 107.

Chapter 12

Surgical Reconstruction Following Total Laryngectomy with Extended or Total Pharyngectomy

Daniel G. Deschler

The treatment of each individual's laryngeal cancer is determined based on a variety of factors, including issues of tumor location and size as assessed by the otolaryngologist. In many situations, standard methods of nonsurgical or surgical treatment are common. Some tumors, however, may involve larger, more extended physical regions in the aerodigestive tract, requiring more significant methods of surgical management and subsequent surgical reconstruction. More extended surgical procedures and reconstruction are needed when the larynx, pharynx, and esophagus are involved by disease. Because procedures of this nature go beyond "simple" laryngectomy, it is important for clinicians from a variety of disciplines, particularly those in the area of voice and speech pathology, to understand the elements of such extended surgical methods. Therefore, this chapter examines surgical reconstruction after extended total laryngectomy with partial or total pharyngectomy, as well as laryngopharyngoesophagectomy. Specific attention is paid to the evolution of reconstruction for these challenging surgical defects, as well as information related to state-of-the-art methods (Deschler & Gray, 2004). Issues related to postoperative speech and swallowing rehabilitation are also addressed.

EXTENDED LARYNGECTOMY AND SURGICAL RECONSTRUCTION

The surgical management of laryngeal cancer often involves removal of the entire larynx. When this is completed, the surgical defect consists of the anterior pharyngeal wall from the tongue base to the cervical esophagus (see Figure 12.1). This defect must be reconstructed to allow for successful deglutition. The creation of a swallowing conduit between the oropharynx and the cervical esophagus results in the creation of a neopharynx. After standard laryngectomy, the neopharynx is created from available tissues after the removal of the tumor (Dedo, 1990). This primarily includes the mucosa from the posterior and lateral pharyngeal walls and from the remaining piriform sinuses. Below the mucosa is a layer of pharyngeal constrictor muscle, which is incorporated into the closure of the defect to provide support and muscle tone (see Figure 12.2).

In cases with more advanced cancers, a significant portion of tissue adjacent to the larynx may require removal. This may include so much pharyngeal tissue as to preclude successful creation of a functional neopharynx from the available tissues after the tumor resection. In this situation, viable tissues must be brought into the surgical field to augment the creation of the neopharynx. In more severe cases, no available tissue is left between the oropharynx and the cervical esophagus to allow creation of the neopharynx; this procedure is termed a *total laryngopharyngectomy* (see Figure 12.3). In such cases, sufficient tissue must be brought from elsewhere in the body to create a swallowing conduit that allows successful deglutition. In the most severe instance, the entire larynx, pharynx, and esophagus must be removed because of advanced disease—this is called a *laryngopharyngoesophagectomy*. In these cases, the surgical defect requires replacement of the entire swallowing conduit from the oropharynx to the stomach.

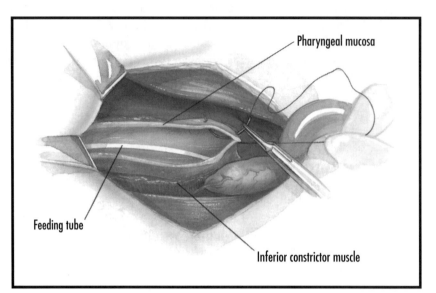

FIGURE 12.1. Defect following standard total laryngectomy. Base of tongue is at right, and trachea is at left. *Note.* From *Surgery of the Larynx and Trachea*, by H. H. Dedo, 1990, Philadelphia: Decker. Copyright 1990 by H. H. Dedo. Reprinted with permission.

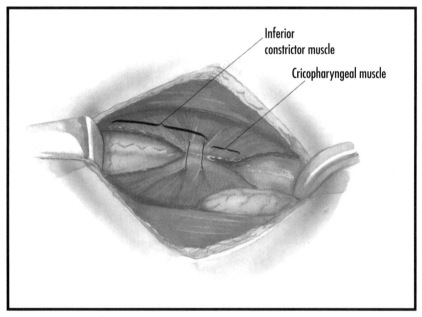

FIGURE 12.2. Muscle closure with standard laryngectomy. *Note.* From *Surgery of the Larynx and Trachea*, by H. H. Dedo, 1990, Philadelphia: Decker. Copyright 1990 by H. H. Dedo. Reprinted with permission.

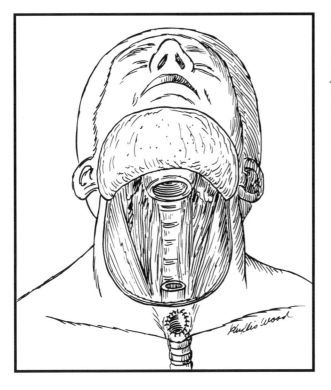

FIGURE 12.3. Defect following total laryngopharyngectomy with absence of a conduit from the oropharynx to the esophagus. *Note.* From *Otolaryngology—Head and Neck Surgery* (3rd ed.), by C. Cummings et al., 1998, St. Louis, MO: Mosby. Copyright 1998 by Mosby. Reprinted with permission.

In the past, after removal of the entire larynx and pharynx, the resulting anatomic defect was significant. Before the advent of modern reconstructive techniques, postoperative patients were left with an orostoma, which drained secretions from the oral cavity and oropharynx, as well as a separate esophagostoma located in the lower neck, which provided the entrance to the esophagus (see Figure 12.4). Anterior to this was the tracheostoma, which allowed for breathing. Following removal of the larynx and pharynx, the resultant postoperative defect was quite debilitating. Specifically, patients had no control of secretions draining from the superior stoma and required nutritional supplementation through a tube placed in the esophagostoma or through a separate gastrostomy site.

To avoid this undesirable postoperative state and, therefore, successfully reconstruct the laryngopharyngectomy defect, viable tissue from the patient must be formed into a tube connecting the orostoma and the esophagostoma. Such a conduit should allow nutritional support, as well as protection of the tracheostoma from unnecessary secretion. Once the successful reconstruction of the neopharynx has been completed to allow deglutition, issues related to postlaryngectomy speech rehabilitation can be addressed.

Cervical Rotation Flaps

The first major advance in the reconstruction of the neopharynx after total laryngopharyngectomy occurred in the 1940s with the procedure described by

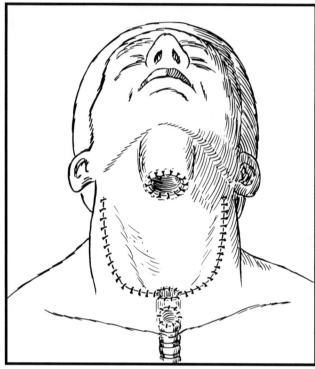

Wookey (1942). This procedure involved the creation of a stable orostoma, esophagostoma, and tracheostoma at the time of the primary tumor resection. Once sufficient healing had taken place, usually 6 to 8 weeks postoperatively, efforts were made to reconstruct the neopharynx. This first involved rolling skin flaps from the central neck toward the midline, creating a tube (see Figure 12.5). Available skin from the neck or chest was then moved to cover the rolled skin flaps. The procedure required many stages, and the complication rates were significant (Missotten, 1983; Wookey, 1942). Complications included pharyngocutaneous fistula, skin flap loss, carotid exposure, and nonhealing cervical wounds. The mortality rate with this procedure was approximately 7%, and complications occurred in nearly 94% of all patients who underwent such a reconstruction. An average of three procedures was needed to achieve successful closure, if attainable. The average hospital stay ranged from 6 to 16 weeks.

The limiting factor with this early reconstructive technique was that the skin flaps, which were rolled into the tube, had a very tenuous blood supply and could not be lifted widely from the tissues deep to them. Efforts to do so often resulted in skin flap loss and fistula formation. Another significant limitation in such a reconstruction was that most patients with disease of such severity to require a total laryngopharyngectomy often received extensive radiation therapy as an adjuvant measure to achieve cure. Radiation therapy significantly decreased the capillary vascularity of the tissues within the neck that were to be used for this reconstruction. For these reasons, the Wookey procedure had serious limitations, but presented the best reconstructive option available at the time.

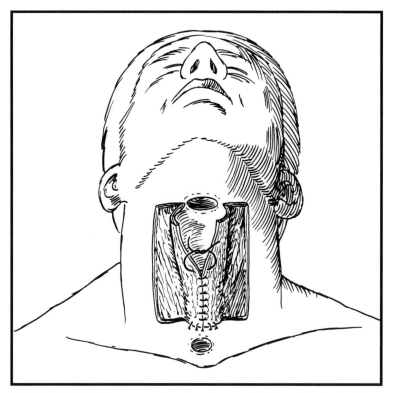

FIGURE 12.5. Wookey procedure for closure of defect with local skin flaps. *Note.* From *Otolaryngology—Head and Neck Surgery* (3rd ed.), by C. Cummings et al., 1998, St. Louis, MO: Mosby. Copyright 1998 by Mosby. Reprinted with permission.

The Deltopectoral Flap

The next major advance in postlaryngopharyngectomy reconstruction occurred in the 1960s with the introduction of the deltopectoral (DP) flap, as described by Bakamjian (Missotten, 1983). The deltopectoral flap is a flap of skin and underlying fatty tissue taken from the upper chest and shoulder. This flap of skin differs from the flaps described in the Wookey procedure because it has an artery and vein that run along the undersurface of the flap, providing a robust blood supply. This vascular pedicle originates from the internal mammary artery via the first and second intercostal perforators as they exit the thorax near the sternum. Consequently, when the DP flap is left attached medially based on this vascular pedicle, it can be lifted from the shoulder region and upper chest and rotated into the upper neck.

To reconstruct the pharynx using the DP flap, the distal part of the flap is rolled into a tube connecting it to the oropharynx and base of tongue. The skin is rolled into a partial tube, which exits at the superior chest (see Figure 12.6A). The skin at this point is attached to the esophagus. The neck wounds are now closed, and a skin graft is placed over the defect on the shoulder and chest (see Figure 12.6B).

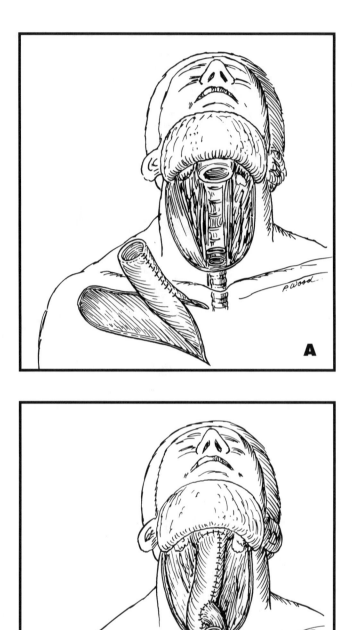

FIGURE 12.6. Deltopectoral flap closure as described by Bakamjian. (A) Tube is created and then (B) attached completely to the oropharynx and partially to the esophagus, allowing secretions to drain on the chest. Closure is completed at a later stage. *Note.* From *Otolaryngology—Head and Neck Surgery* (3rd ed.), by C. Cummings et al., 1998, St. Louis, MO: Mosby. Copyright 1998 by Mosby. Reprinted with permission.

After the first stage of the DP flap reconstruction, secretions from the oral cavity drain through the skin tube and onto the chest for a period of 3 to 6 weeks as the skin flap establishes a new blood supply from the surrounding tissues in the neck. When this 3- to 6-week period has passed, the inferior portion of the skin flap is divided from its attachment to the chest. The skin flap in the neck is rolled into a complete tube and attached to the esophagus completely. The chest and neck wounds are closed. At this point, there exists a skin-lined tube, which runs from the oropharynx to the upper esophagus.

Advantages of this form of reconstruction include (a) the improved vascularity of the skin that is being brought into the wound because it has its own vascular pedicle and (b) the fact that the skin, which is being brought in for reconstruction, has not been previously subjected to radiation therapy and has an improved vascularity compared with skin flaps taken from the radiated neck. Although the DP flap was an improvement over the Wookey procedure, the DP flap still had a high complication rate, well over 50%. An average of three separate, staged procedures were required to achieve complete closure. Hospital stays were still lengthy at 8 to 16 weeks. As a result, further advances were still required to satisfactorily achieve the goals of reconstruction in the individual who had undergone laryngopharyngectomy.

The Gastric Pull-up Procedure

The previously described efforts to reconstruct the neopharynx with cervical rotation flaps and the deltopectoral flap involved the use of skin flaps rolled into tubes to reconstruct a swallowing conduit. Another approach, first used in the 1960s and early 1970s, involves the mobilization of the stomach through the thorax into the neck to provide neopharyngeal reconstruction (Missotten, 1983). This procedure is referred to as the gastric pull-up operation as it involves pulling the stomach up through the chest into the neck. In this procedure a separate operation in the abdomen is required to mobilize the stomach and maintain a stable blood supply to it. Initially, an operation through the chest is likewise required to remove the entire esophagus and to guide the stomach into the neck. Eventually, it was found to be safe to bluntly complete the dissection through the center of the chest along the path of the esophagus. This dissection can be completed through the abdominal incision, and no chest incision is needed. With the dissection completed, the stomach is brought up into the neck. The body of the stomach is then incised and attached to the opening at the oropharynx (see Figure 12.7). This procedure necessitates the removal of the entire esophagus because the esophagus cannot be dissected from the thorax without severing its blood supply. The body of the stomach is used for the upper connection as it has a longer reach into the neck than the gastroesophageal (GE) junction. The GE junction is oversewn. With the stomach pulled up into the neck through the chest, the pyloric sphincter is incised and weakened to allow successful emptying of the stomach. Without easy emptying, food and secretions pool in the stomach and are easily regurgitated. Conversely, if emptying is too rapid, the intestinal dysfunction known as dumping occurs.

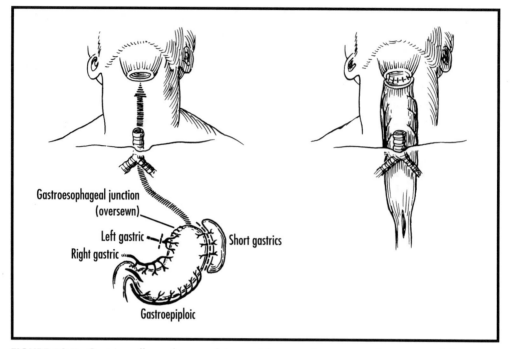

FIGURE 12.7. Gastric pull-up closure of the total laryngopharyngoesophagectomy defect. *Note.* From *Otolaryngology—Head and Neck Surgery* (3rd ed.), by C. Cummings et al., 1998, St. Louis, MO: Mosby. Copyright 1998 by Mosby. Reprinted with permission.

The gastric pull-up operation likewise provided a significant advance in reconstruction and remains the primary reconstruction method today, when advanced disease requires removal of the entire larynx, pharynx, and esophagus. For reconstruction of only the neopharyngeal segment, however, the procedure has limitations in that postoperative mortality rates can be as high as 10% and complication rates are in the 30% to 50% range (Missotten, 1983; Shah, Shemen, Spiro, & Strong, 1984). The procedure necessitates an abdominal operation, which may have further complications and can severely limit rehabilitation. The flap failure rate is relatively low at 3%, but eventual rehabilitation after surgery may be limited by issues of gastric dumping and regurgitation, which are specific to this reconstructive method.

The Pectoralis Major Flap

In the late 1970s, the pectoralis major flap was introduced for head and neck reconstruction (Baek, Lawson, & Biller, 1981). This procedure provided a significant advancement for reconstruction of numerous head and neck defects, including the neopharyngeal defect (Schuller, 1985; Shah et al., 1984). The pectoralis major flap is a myocutaneous pedicled flap, which by definition includes tissue composed of both muscle and skin. The blood supply to the pectoralis muscle is supplied by the pectoral artery and vein, which run on the undersurface of the

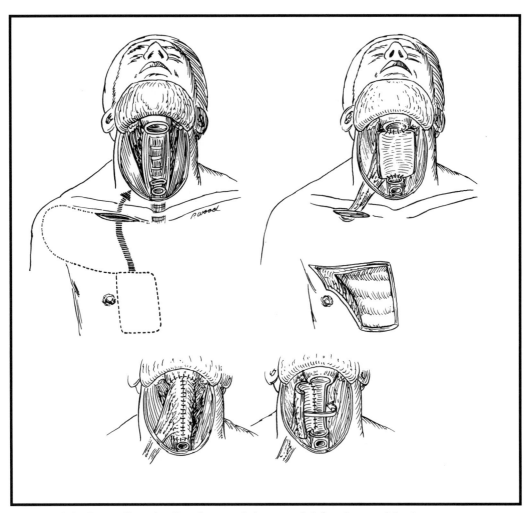

FIGURE 12.8. Pectoralis major flap closure of pharyngeal defect. Lower right demonstrates use of the flap for a partial defect of the pharynx. *Note.* From *Otolaryngology—Head and Neck Surgery* (3rd ed.), by C. Cummings et al., 1998, St. Louis, MO: Mosby. Copyright 1998 by Mosby. Reprinted with permission.

muscle. Perforating vessels then go through the muscle to supply blood and oxygen to the overlying skin. The pectoral vessels originate just lateral to the midpoint of the clavicle; therefore, this segment of tissue can be elevated from inferior to superior, maintaining its attachment at the clavicle and the integrity of its vascular pedicle, which allows for rotation of robust vascularized tissue into the head and neck defect. In situations where the entire neopharynx has been removed, a sufficient skin island is harvested on the chest and rolled into a tube. The tube is then attached at the superior oropharyngeal defect and inferiorly at the esophagus (see Figure 12.8). The neck and chest incisions are closed. The new conduit connecting the oropharynx to the esophagus is created in a single procedure, a significant advantage over the previously described skin flap procedures, which required multiple stages.

The pectoralis major flap is a highly reliable reconstructive method, with a failure rate ranging from 1% to 2% (Schuller, 1985). The flap can be used to reconstruct a complete pharyngeal defect as described previously or to provide closure of a partial defect as in the setting of an extended laryngectomy with partial pharyngectomy. With a partial pharyngectomy, a strip of mucosa and muscle remains posterior to the defect. There is not sufficient residual tissue to be tubed upon itself, so some further surgical reconstruction is required. In this case, the pectoralis major skin flap is sewn to the remaining strip of mucosa and muscle and provides closure of 270 to 300 degrees of the 360 degrees required for complete creation of a tube.

The postoperative fistula rate for pectoralis major flap reconstructions ranges from 10% to 20% (Schuller, 1985). Greater than 70% of those individuals reconstructed with the pectoralis major flap are able to maintain successful oral feeding. The flap is limited, however, when the defect is complete and circumferential, having lower success rates and higher fistula rates. The flap is best suited for reconstruction of partial defects (Schuller, 1985).

The Jejunal Free Flap

The previously described reconstructive techniques are all referred to as pedicled flap techniques, meaning that the vascular supply to the flap comes from a defined vascular pedicle, which remains attached at its origin. In the deltopectoral flap, the pedicle comes from the first and second intercostal perforators derived from the internal mammary artery; in the pectoralis major flap, the pectoral vessels form the pedicle; and in the gastric pull-up technique, the gastroepiploic vessels provide the blood supply. All these flap techniques are limited by the fact that in order to maintain good blood supply and hence the viability of the flap, the vascular pedicle must remain attached and not be compromised by kinking or severe stretching. For this reason, the point of rotation from which the pedicle originates limits any pedicled flap technique.

In the early 1980s, the technique of free tissue transfer with microvascular anastomosis demonstrated increasing success for the reconstruction of head and neck defects. In this technique, referred to as free flap reconstruction, a portion of tissue with an identifiable vascular pedicle, consisting of an artery and vein of sufficient size, is mobilized from elsewhere in the body. The tissue flap is then brought into the head and neck region and used for reconstruction. The artery supplying blood to this tissue and the vein draining the blood are connected to available vessels within the head and neck region. The arteries are usually reconnected (re-anastomosed) to available branches of the external carotid system, while the vein is attached to branches of the internal or external jugular system. In this manner, the free flap tissue is completely freed from its previous attachments and mobilized into the head and neck region, and a stable blood supply is reestablished.

As the neopharyngeal defect after laryngopharyngectomy involves the absence of a stable tube for swallowing, it stands to reason that a portion of intestine would provide a favorable reconstructive structure (i.e., because it is mucosally lined). The jejunal portion of the small intestine is sufficiently long and

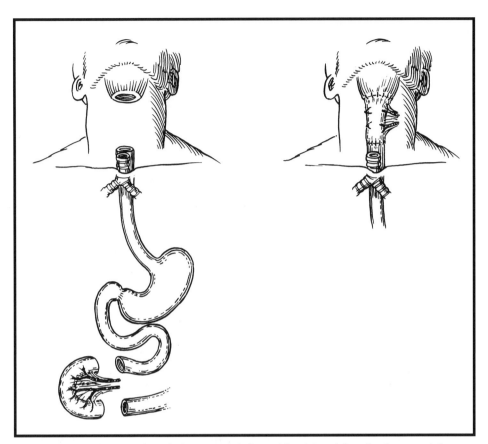

FIGURE 12.9. Closure of total pharyngeal defect with a jejunal free flap harvested from the abdomen with the blood vessels reattached in the neck. *Note.* From *Otolaryngology—Head and Neck Surgery* (3rd ed.), by C. Cummings et al., 1998, St. Louis, MO: Mosby. Copyright 1998 by Mosby. Reprinted with permission.

possesses a satisfactory blood supply in its mesentery to allow its harvest. A tube of sufficient length for reconstruction from the oropharynx to the esophagus is easily provided, with minimal to no impairment of the remaining bowel.

Interestingly, the jejunal free flap was first described for neopharyngeal reconstruction in 1959 by Seidenberg, Rosenak, Hurwitt, and Som. Four successful animal experiments were presented, and one successful transfer of the jejunum into the neck of a human was described. The technique did not gain immediate acceptance, however, and it was not until the 1980s that the jejunal free flap became the favored reconstructive method after total laryngopharyngectomy (Coleman et al., 1987; de Vries et al., 1989; Flynn, Banis, & Acland, 1989).

In the jejunal free flap technique, the abdomen is opened and a portion of jejunum with a favorable artery and vein within its mesentery is identified. This portion is harvested from the abdomen, and the two remaining ends of small intestine are reattached. The jejunal segment is then brought into the head and neck region and connected to the oropharynx superiorly and the esophagus inferiorly (see Figure 12.9). The artery supplying blood to the flap and the vein draining blood from it are reanastomosed in the neck. The wounds are closed in the standard manner in this one-stage procedure. The initially reported success rates with the jejunal free flap were somewhat limited by flap survival, with approximately a 10% flap loss rate (Coleman et al., 1987; de Vries et al., 1989); however, this rate is improved in later studies. A review of over 900 cases since 1975 demonstrated a graft failure rate of 7.5%. The fistula rate was noted to be 17%, with a stenosis rate of 9%.

One advantage to the jejunal free flap technique is that the tissue flap is already in the form of a tube, avoiding the long suture line needed to create a tube. Another advantage is that the jejunum produces its own lubricating secretions from the mucosa, which may aid deglutition. In contrast, a disadvantage to this technique is that the jejunum maintains independent peristaltic activity; this can adversely affect successful deglutition, as it may be discoordinate with the oral phase of swallowing. Even though the flap is placed in an isoperistaltic (with the flow of normal peristalsis) manner, peristalsis may occur at a time that blocks bolus transfer from the oral phase of swallowing. Finally, the harvest of the jejunal free flap requires a separate abdominal procedure, which subsequently may increase postoperative recovery time, especially in elderly patients and those with extensive comorbid conditions.

The Radial Forearm Free Flap

Another versatile free flap reconstructive technique is the radial forearm fasciocutaneous free flap (Souter & McGregor, 1986). This flap consists of the skin and subcutaneous tissues overlying the radial artery on the volar surface of the forearm. The vascular supply to this flap is dependable and the tissue is quite pliable which allows it to be tubed easily for neopharyngeal reconstruction. The radial forearm flap was first described for neopharyngeal reconstruction in the 1980s and has become a popular and dependable technique (Anthony, Singer, & Mathes, 1994; Harii et al., 1985).

In the radial forearm free flap technique, the skin overlying the volar surface of the forearm is elevated based on the radial artery and vein. The surgeon harvests a flap 7 to 9 cm wide and long enough to reach from the esophagus to the superior portion of the pharyngeal defect in the specific patient. This skin is then rolled on itself, creating a tube. This tube is attached superiorly at the oropharynx and inferiorly at the esophagus. To avoid stenosis, which is prone to occur with circular scars, the attachment to the esophagus is modified to make the opening wider and avoid a pure circle. This is done by insetting a dart of skin tissue into the esophagus (see Figure 12.10). The radial artery and the cephalic vein are reconnected in the neck. This technique provides a one-stage construction. The defect site on the arm is covered with a split-thickness skin graft from the thigh. The arm is then splinted for 5 to 9 days, allowing the skin graft to take. The donor site morbidity is minimal and usually limited to cosmetic changes on the arm from the appearance of the skin graft.

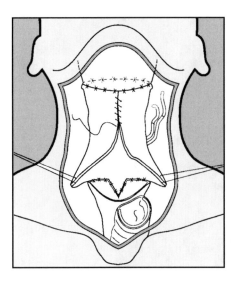

FIGURE 12.10. Radial forearm free flap closure of defect, demonstrating the modification of esophageal attachment to prevent stenosis. From *Otolaryngology—Head and Neck Surgery* (3rd ed.), by C. Cummings et al., 1998, St. Louis, MO: Mosby. Copyright 1998 by Mosby. Reprinted with permission.

A review of 108 radial forearm free flap reconstructions of the neopharynx in the literature revealed that graft failure rate was exceedingly low, 1% (Deschler, 1999). The pharyngeal fistula rate was noted to be higher than that with the jejunal free flap, at approximately 30%. The stenosis rates were also noted to be higher than the jejunal free flaps, nearing 20%. An advantage of the radial forearm free flap technique is that a separate abdominal procedure is not required. The radial forearm flap can be harvested at the same time as the tumor resection is completed, and the donor site morbidity is minimal.

The Lateral Thigh Free Flap

Another free tissue transfer technique that provides sufficient skin for neopharyngeal reconstruction is the lateral thigh free flap. This flap was first described in 1983 by Baek, but was popularized for neopharyngeal reconstruction by Hayden in the late 1980s (Hayden & Deschler, 1999). The lateral thigh free flap provides a large amount of tissue from the lateral thigh region based on an artery from the deep profunda femoris system in the leg and its associated vein. Donor site morbidity with this flap is minimal as the wound can usually be closed with sufficient tissue available at the donor site. This flap also provides a greater amount of tissue than can be harvested with the radial forearm flap, making it better suited for more extensive defects.

The lateral thigh free flap is harvested from the lateral thigh, and the donor site is closed. The flap is brought into the neck region and formed into a tube, which is attached superiorly to the oropharynx and inferiorly at the esophagus (see Figure 12.11). A portion of the flap is then brought into the neck to allow monitoring of its viability. This is referred to as a skin marker segment (see Figure 12.12). Should the marker segment demonstrate any evidence of impaired blood supply, this would indicate that the larger portion of the flap,

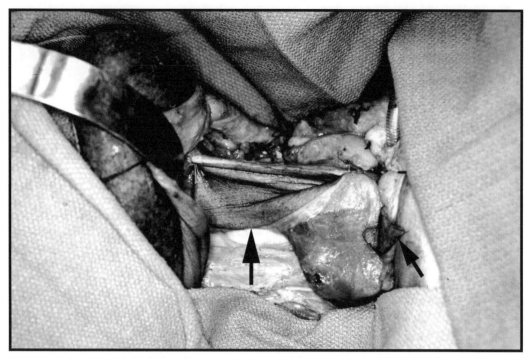

FIGURE 12.11. Lateral thigh free flap reconstruction with retractor placed at base of tongue. Large arrow demonstrates the flap being rolled into a tube and the small arrow shows the separate skin marker island.

which cannot be seen as it is buried under the neck skin, is having a similar problem. If compromise of the blood supply occurs, the patient is returned to the operating room and the microvascular connections are examined to assess for any thrombus or need of revision. Vascular compromise can occur any time within the first week, but most often happens within the first 48 hours postoperatively. Monitoring and revision allow for higher success rates using free tissue transfer. In a series of over 40 lateral thigh reconstructions of the neopharynx, a failure rate of 2% was noted, with similarly low fistula stenosis rates (Baek, 1983).

Other authors have described alternative skin free flaps for neopharyngeal reconstruction. These include the ulnar flap as described by Li et al. (1998). This flap is based on the ulnar artery and cephalic vein. Reconstruction with this flap is nearly identical to the radial forearm technique other than the arterial pedicle. The tensor fascia lata flap has been described by Endo and Nakayama (1995) for neopharyngeal reconstruction using skin from the upper lateral thigh and an underlying cuff of tensor fascia lata muscle.

Tissue Overview

The previous description of the reconstructive techniques for the neopharynx is based on a historical review. Another useful approach for understanding the ef-

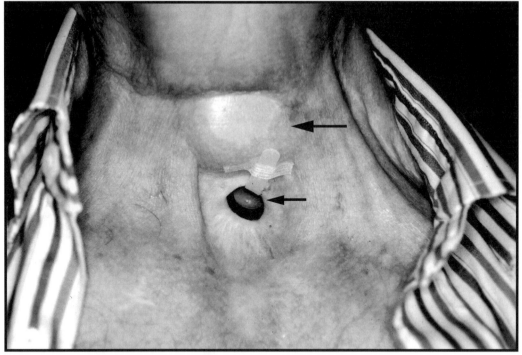

FIGURE 12.12. Postoperative photograph of patient following total laryngopharyngectomy with lateral thigh free flap reconstruction. Large arrow demonstrates skin marker segment incorporated into neck incisions, and small arrow shows functioning tracheoesophageal voice prosthesis.

fects and potential success of different reconstructive techniques is to classify each technique by the specific type of tissue it provides for reconstruction. In this way, issues such as deglutition and eventual speech rehabilitation can be analyzed in a more thorough and appropriate fashion. Classifying the techniques by type of tissue permits distinction of two main groups. First, there are those techniques that provide enteric tissue with secretory mucosa and a thin layer of underlying muscle. The gastric pull-up and the jejunal free flap are the two primary examples in this class. The reconstructed swallowing conduit during a barium swallow is shown in Figure 12.13. The next group consists of those techniques that provide skin tissue for lining the conduit. This skin is rolled into a tube to recreate the neopharyngeal conduit. A skin-lined tube will not have a secretory component or an underlying muscular layer to affect its function. The Wookey procedure, deltopectoral flap, pectoralis major flap, radial forearm flap, lateral thigh flap, and other skin-free flaps make up this group. The structure of this type of system is shown endoscopically in Figure 12.14.

Regarding deglutition, the two groups have some basic differences that do affect function. The skin flaps lack lubrication because they are not secretory. Intuitively, this might be considered a detriment, but usually there is sufficient salivary pooling within the skin-lined neopharynx to provide adequate lubrication. The skin flaps likewise lack muscle for peristalsis; however, this is actually an

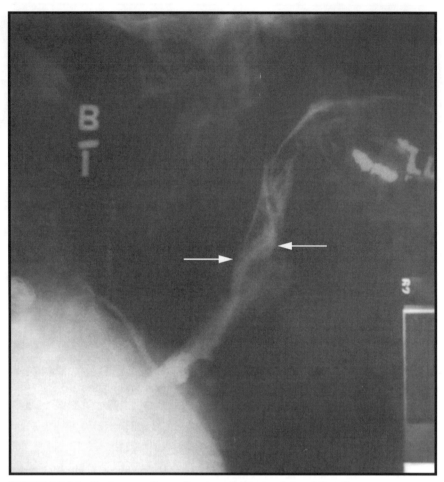

FIGURE 12.13. Barium swallow of patient following jejunal free flap reconstruction. Arrows demonstrate swallowing conduit.

advantage. The peristalsis that occurs with jejunal free flaps and to some extent with gastric pull-up flaps is more problematic than helpful. Such peristalsis is not specifically coordinated with the other stages of swallowing and can lead to restricted function.

In contrast, a distinct advantage to use of the mucosal enteric flaps is that they are already in the form of a tube and do not require the long suture line to create a tube. For this reason, the fistula rates are less than those noted with skin flaps. A lower fistula rate also provides for a lower eventual stenosis rate. Limiting both these complications increases the likelihood of successful reconstruction.

SPEECH

The available techniques for speech rehabilitation of individuals who undergo reconstruction of the neopharynx after laryngectomy with partial or total pharyn-

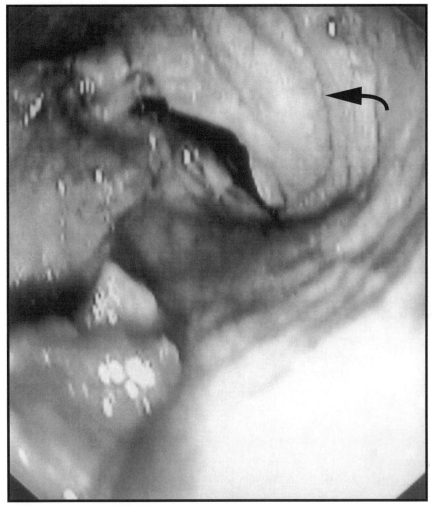

FIGURE 12.14. Endoscopic photograph of the skin-lined tube provided by a radial forearm flap reconstruction. View is from oropharynx, with the esophageal lumen noted at center. Arrow demonstrates the skin lining.

gectomy are the same as those of patients after standard laryngectomy. Use of an electrolarynx may be somewhat limited because of the extra tissue brought into the neck with the tissue flaps. Esophageal speech can also be limited in patients who undergo neopharyngeal reconstruction. Dividing reconstruction methods by tissue type is especially useful in analyzing speech rehabilitation. Traditional esophageal speech has been shown to be poorer in reconstructed patients. This is likely due to several factors. One is the absence of any sphincteric function at the upper esophagus, which acts to control airflow from the esophageal air reservoir. Another limitation is that the creation of a stable vibratory segment, which is critical to esophageal speech production, may be hampered by the altered anatomy that occurs in neopharyngeal reconstruction. Thick tissue such as skin often requires higher airflow rates to create a vibratory segment, which cannot be adequately provided from the esophageal air reservoir.

The tracheoesophageal puncture (TEP) technique of voice restoration as described by Blom and Singer (see Blom, Singer, & Hamaker, 1998; Singer, 2004; Singer, Blom, & Hamaker, 1983; see also Chapter 17 in this text) has been successfully employed in all the reconstructive methods reviewed herein (Cumberworth, O'Flynn, Perry, Bleach, & Cheesman, 1992; Hamaker, Singer, Blom, & Daniels, 1985; Juarbe et al., 1989; Maniglia, Leder, Goodwin, Sawyer, & Sasaki, 1989; Medina, Nance, Burns, & Overton, 1987; Wenig, Keller, Levy, Mullooly, & Abramson, 1989). Again, successful speech rehabilitation using the TEP technique requires the creation of a stable vibratory segment. This stability is more easily achieved with the TEP technique than with standard esophageal speech as the pulmonary reservoir is much greater and can provide a greater, stronger, and more continuous airflow to this vibratory segment (Deschler, Doherty, Reed, & Singer, 1999). Greater airflow is necessary to create vibration in the neopharynx that is reconstructed from jejunal or skin flaps.

The first study addressing overall function in individuals undergoing reconstruction after laryngopharyngectomy demonstrated exceedingly poor speech rehabilitation for the reconstructed group (Schechter, Baker, & Gilbert, 1987). Further analysis of individuals in this study demonstrated that no patients used tracheoesophageal voice restoration or any method other than the electrolarynx for speech production.

Medina et al. (1987) compared the voice of 10 patients reconstructed with various techniques (deltopectoral flaps, pectoralis major flaps, gastric pull-ups) to that of standard TEP speakers. The quantitative analysis demonstrated similar fundamental frequencies for the two groups but lower intensity values for the reconstructed group. No statistically significant differences were noted. Based on subjective, auditory–perceptual analysis of voice quality, the reconstructed group was described as having a low pitch with a soft and wet quality (see Chapter 6 in this text). Later studies confirmed these findings (Cumberworth et al., 1992; Juarbe et al., 1989; Maniglia et al., 1989).

A flaw in these studies was that the patient groups were either very small or consisted of different reconstruction types, which provided different tissues for the reconstruction and very different neopharyngeal segments. Mendelsohn, Morris, and Gallagher (1993) compared the speech of 7 patients with free jejunal reconstructions to the tracheoesophageal speech of 22 standard laryngectomy patients. They found no statistically significant differences in fundamental frequency or intensity levels, but significant differences for the subjective parameters. Reconstructed patients had impaired intelligibility, low voice, and less intonation. Wilson, Bruce-Lockhart, Johnson, and Rhys Evans (1994) described their experience with 9 patients after jejunal free flap reconstruction and reported that 8 had good voice. This study had no comparison group or statistical analysis.

Deschler, Doherty, Reed, Anthony, and Singer (1994) reported their experience with 6 patients after radial forearm flap reconstruction of the neopharynx and compared tracheoesophageal voice restoration in these patients with that of

5 standard laryngectomy controls who used TEP speech. No statistically significant differences were found in the objective parameters of fundamental frequency and intensity levels; however, a trend toward decreased stability of the vibratory segment was found in the patients with the radial forearm flap reconstructions. A rigorous subjective analysis was then completed over multiple parameters, including communicative effectiveness, general intelligibility, effective use of pitch and intensity, pleasantness, speaking rate, wetness, fluency, and number of words correct from a word list. These parameters were evaluated by both trained and naive listeners and subjected to statistical analysis. This study demonstrated that the reconstructed patients had significantly poorer function for all of the parameters when compared to the control patients. Although the reconstructed patients demonstrated poorer function, all had functional speech, which was intelligible enough to undergo rigorous analysis. This demonstrated that TEP speech is consistently attainable after radial forearm flap reconstruction of the neopharynx, although it is of a lesser quality when compared to standard TEP speakers.

The same research group (Deschler, Doherty, Reed, & Singer, 1998) studied patients who underwent pectoralis major flap reconstruction of the neopharynx and compared their speech to that of control TEP speakers. Again, no statistically significant differences between intensity levels and fundamental frequency were noted, yet the reconstructed patients had significantly poorer function for all 10 subjective parameters.

Limitations of each of the two reconstructive types discussed in this chapter—enteric flaps and skin flaps—can be inferred from review of the studies discussed. The "wet" speech, which characterizes jejunal free flap reconstructions (Mendelsohn et al., 1993; Wilson et al., 1994), is likely due to excess mucus production by the mucosa of the jejunum. A further problem can be noted with the speech production in jejunal free flap patients if there is redundancy of the reconstructed segment. This redundancy can impede airflow and the creation of a stable voicing segment.

The low voice associated with gastric pull-up reconstructions (Maniglia et al., 1989) can be related to the increased width of the tube provided by the stomach. In this case, the large conduit formed by the stomach may not allow the creation of opposing vibratory tissues or only provide voice with a low pitch. Such patients often benefit by applying gentle pressure to the neck above the puncture site, which can narrow this lumen and allow better vibration.

In contrast, the wet voice described with radial forearm flap reconstructions is not secondary to secretions produced by the lining of the neopharynx, but may be related to the pooling of secretions within this segment. The skin lining the neopharynx is thicker and bulkier than the mucosa lining the neopharynx in a standard laryngectomy patient. For this reason, a greater aerodynamic force may be required to create a vibratory region within this segment or adjacent to it. Similarly, there is no underlying muscle to provide muscular tone similar to that after standard laryngectomy closure. Such lack of muscle can affect issues such as intelligibility, effective use of pitch, and effective use of intensity. The limitations in speech rehabilitation in those individuals reconstructed with radial forearm free flap are understandable in the context of the specific tissue that this reconstructive technique provides.

SUMMARY

This chapter has addressed the issues related to the reconstruction of the neopharyngeal segment after extended laryngectomy with near-total or total pharyngectomy. Such reconstruction has undergone a positive evolution in the last 50 years. Current surgical techniques of free tissue transfer provide two excellent options for reconstruction after laryngopharyngectomy: the jejunal free flap and the radial forearm free flap. The technique of the pectoralis major flap is still useful for partial pharyngectomy defects, and the gastric pull-up technique remains the primary reconstructive method after total laryngopharyngoesophagectomy. An understanding of the tissues provided by each reconstructive method allows for greater comprehension of the limitations in deglutition and speech that patients may encounter after such extensive reconstructions (Robb & Lewin, 2003; Ward, Bishop, Frisby, & Stevens, 2002). Similarly, this knowledge can guide rehabilitation to achieve the highest possible function with each reconstructive method. The strengths and limitations of differing reconstructive methods can be compared and contrasted, allowing the selection of the optimum reconstruction for the individual patient.

REFERENCES

Anthony, J. P., Singer, M. I., & Mathes, S. J. (1994). Pharyngoesophageal reconstruction using the tubed free radial forearm flap. *Clinics in Plastic Surgery, 21,* 137–147.

Baek, S. M. (1983). Two new cutaneous free flaps: The medial and lateral thigh flap. *Plastic and Reconstructive Surgery, 71,* 354–363.

Baek, S. M., Lawson, W., & Biller H. F. (1981). Reconstruction of hypopharynx and cervical esophagus with pectoralis major island myocutaneous flap. *Annals of Plastic Surgery, 7,* 18–24.

Blom, E. D., Singer, M. I., & Hamaker, R. C. (1998). *Tracheoesophageal voice restoration following total laryngectomy.* San Diego: Singular.

Coleman, J. J., Searles, J. M., Hester, T. R., Nahai, F., Zubowicz, V., McConnel, F. M. S., & Jurkiewicz, M. J. (1987). Ten years experience with the free jejunal autograft. *American Journal of Surgery, 154,* 394–398.

Cumberworth, V. L., O'Flynn, P. O., Perry, A., Bleach, N. R., & Cheesman, A. D. (1992). Surgical voice restoration after laryngopharyngectomy with free radial forearm flap repair using a Blom-Singer prosthesis. *Journal of the Royal Society of Medicine, 85,* 760–761.

Cummings, C., Fredrickson, J. M., Harker, L. A., Krause, C. J., Schuller, D. E. , & Richardson, M. A. (1998). *Otolaryngology—head and neck surgery* (3rd ed.). St. Louis, MO: Mosby.

Dedo, H. H. (1990). *Surgery of the larynx and trachea.* Philadelphia: Decker.

Deschler, D. G. (1999, September). *Pharyngoesophageal reconstruction: State-of-the-art.* Paper presented at the American Academy of Otolaryngology—Head and Neck Surgery Foundation, New Orleans.

Deschler, D. G., Doherty, E. T., Reed, C. G., Anthony, J. P., & Singer, M. I. (1994). Tracheoesophageal voice following tubed free radial forearm flap reconstruction of the neopharynx. *Annals of Otology, Rhinology and Laryngology, 103,* 929–936.

Deschler, D. G., Doherty, E. T., Reed, C. G., & Singer, M. I. (1998). Quantitative and qualitative analysis of tracheoesophageal voice after pectoralis major flap reconstruction of the neopharynx. *Otolaryngology—Head and Neck Surgery, 118,* 771–776.

Deschler, D. G., Doherty, E. T., Reed, C. G., & Singer, M. I. (1999). Effects of sound pressure levels on fundamental frequency in tracheoesophageal speakers. *Otolaryngology—Head and Neck Surgery, 121,* 23–26.

Deschler, D. G., & Gray, S. T. (2004). Tracheoesophageal speech following laryngopharyngectomy and pharyngeal reconstruction. *Otolaryngology Clinics of North America, 37*(3), 567–583.

de Vries, E. J., Stein, D. W., Johnson, J. T., Wagner, R. L., Schusterman, M. A., Myers, E. N., Shestak, K., Jones, N. F., & Williams, S. (1989). Hypopharyngeal reconstruction: A comparison of two alternatives. *Laryngoscope, 99,* 614–617.

Endo, T., & Nakayama, Y. (1995). Pharyngoesophageal reconstruction with a tensor fasciae latae free flap. *Plastic and Reconstructive Surgery, 95,* 400–405.

Flynn, M. B., Banis, J., & Acland, R. (1989). Reconstruction with free bowel autografts after pharyngoesophageal or laryngopharyngoesophageal resection. *American Journal of Surgery, 158,* 333–336.

Hamaker, R. C., Singer, M. I., Blom, E. D., & Daniels, H. A. (1985). Primary voice restoration at laryngectomy. *Archives of Otolaryngology, 111,* 182–186.

Harii, K., Ebihara, S., Ono, I., Saito, H., Terui, S., & Takato, T. (1985). Pharyngoesophageal reconstruction using a fabricated forearm free flap. *Plastic and Reconstructive Surgery, 75,* 463–474.

Hayden, R. E., & Deschler, D. G. (1999). Lateral thigh free flap for head and neck reconstruction. *Laryngoscope, 109,* 1490–1494.

Juarbe, C., Shemen, L., Wang, R., Anand, V., Eberle, R., Sirovatka, A., Malanaphy, K., & Klatsky, I. (1989). Tracheoesophageal puncture for voice restoration after extended laryngopharyngectomy. *Archives of Otolaryngology—Head and Neck Surgery, 115,* 356–359.

Li, K. K., Salibian, A. H., Allison, G. R., Krugman, M. E., Armstrong, W., Wong, B., & Kelly, T. (1998). Pharyngoesophageal reconstruction with the ulnar forearm flap. *Archives of Otolaryngology—Head and Neck Surgery, 124,* 1146–1151.

Maniglia, A. J., Leder, S. B., Goodwin, W. J., Sawyer, R., & Sasaki, C. T. (1989). Tracheogastric puncture for vocal rehabilitation following total pharyngolaryngoesophagectomy. *Head & Neck, 11,* 524–527.

Medina, J. E., Nance, A., Burns, L., & Overton, R. (1987). Voice restoration after total laryngopharyngectomy and cervical esophagectomy using the duckbill prosthesis. *American Journal of Surgery, 154,* 407–410.

Mendelsohn, M., Morris, M., & Gallagher, R. (1993). A comparative study of speech after total laryngectomy and total laryngopharyngectomy. *Archives of Otolaryngology—Head and Neck Surgery, 119,* 508–510.

Missotten, F. E. (1983). Review: Historical review of pharyngo-oesophageal reconstructions after resection for carcinoma of pharynx and cervical oesophagus. *Clinical Otolaryngology and Allied Sciences, 8,* 345–362.

Robb, G. L., & Lewin, J. S. (2003). Speech and swallow outcomes in reconstructions of the pharynx and cervical esophagus. *Head & Neck, 25,* 232–244.

Schechter, G. L., Baker, J. W., & Gilbert, D. A. (1987). Functional evaluation of pharyngoesophageal reconstructive techniques. *Archives of Otolaryngology—Head and Neck Surgery, 113,* 40–44.

Schuller, D. E. (1985). Reconstructive options for pharyngeal and/or cervical esophageal defects. *Archives of Otolaryngology, 111,* 193–197

Seidenberg, B., Rosenak, S. S., Hurwitt, E. S., & Som, M. L. (1959). Immediate reconstruction of the cervical esophagus by a revascularized isolated jejunal segment. *American Journal of Surgery, 149,* 162–171.

Shah, J. P., Shemen, L., Spiro, R. H., & Strong, E. W. (1984). Selecting variants in pharyngeal reconstruction. *Annals of Otology, Rhinology and Laryngology, 93,* 318–321.

Singer, M. I., (2004). The development of successful tracheoesophageal voice restoration. *Otolaryngology Clinics of North America, 37,* 507–517.

Singer, M. I., Blom, E. D., & Hamaker, R. C. (1983). Voice rehabilitation after total laryngectomy. *Journal of Otolaryngology, 12,* 329–334.

Souter, D. S., & McGregor, I. A. (1986). The radial forearm flap in intraoral reconstruction: The experience of 60 consecutive cases. *Plastic and Reconstructive Surgery, 78,* 1–8.

Ward, E. C., Bishop, B., Frisby, J., & Stevens, M. (2002). Swallowing outcomes following laryngectomy and pharyngolaryngectomy. *Archives of Otolaryngology—Head and Neck Surgery, 128,* 181–186.

Wenig, B. L., Keller, A. J., Levy, J., Mullooly, V., & Abramson, A. L. (1989). Voice restoration after laryngopharyngoesophagectomy. *Otolaryngology—Head and Neck Surgery, 101,* 11–13.

Wilson, P. S., Bruce-Lockhart, F. J., Johnson, A. P., & Rhys Evans, P. H. (1994). Speech restoration following total laryngo-pharyngectomy with free jejunal repair. *Clinical Otolaryngology & Allied Sciences, 19,* 145–148.

Wookey, H. (1942). The surgical treatment of carcinoma of the pharynx and upper esophagus. *Surgery, Gynecology, and Obstetrics, 75,* 449–506.

Chapter 13

Maxillofacial Rehabilitation for Oral Cancer

Surgical, Prosthodontic, and Communication Aspects of Management

Herbert A. Leeper, David G. Gratton, Henry J. Lapointe, and J. E. A. Armstrong

Note. Herbert A. Leeper passed away on May 24, 2001.

ral cancer and its treatment has substantial and often dramatic influ-
...logical function from a variety of per-
...ges may be observed in a variety of
...often manifested in some degree of
...speech. Although changes that occur
...ictures treated, these changes require
...s rehabilitative efforts. When ablative
...bined, multidisciplinary approach to
...al treated for oral cancer is essential.
...uss and promote a team approach for
...cer affecting speech, mastication, and
...rous related issues, including aspects of
...ase, as well as the surgical, oncological,
...nent aspects of rehabilitation.

ence of Oral Cancer

(HNSCCa) may be defined as a malig-
...he mouth, nasal cavity, pharynx, or lar-
...ange of clinical, histological, and biologi-
...3). Worldwide, cancers of the head and
...all cancers in males (220,000 new cases
...s (90,000 new cases annually; Franceschi,
...ntario, the annual incidence of new cases
...00 in males and 4 per 100,000 in females

Etiology

Certain factors have been noted to significantly increase the risk of head and neck squamous cell carcinoma. Of primary importance is exposure to tobacco, whether from smoking or use of other products such as snuff or chewing to-bacco. Heavy use of alcohol has also been noted as a risk factor in the development of head and neck cancer. The combination of heavy smoking and drinking increases the risk of development of oral squamous cell carcinoma to 15 times that of those who neither smoke nor drink (Batsakis, 1979). Certain nutritional deficiencies, such as Plummer-Vinson syndrome (iron-deficiency anemia), also have been shown to increase risk (Shafer et al., 1983). Other risk factors include exposure to ionizing radiation and occupational exposure to carcinogens in nickel refining, woodworking, leather working, the asbestos industry, and rubber making (Cann, Fried, & Rothman, 1985). Oral submucous fibrosis, a disorder of the oral epithelium associated with the chewing of betel nut, is seen commonly in the Indian subcontinent and is associated with a higher risk of development of squamous cell carcinoma (Hardie, 1987). The phenomenon of field cancerization (the development of multiple primary foci of cancer in a given anatomical area) has been implicated in patients with synchronous or metachronous primary disease (Davis, 1985); this likely occurs as a function of widespread upper aerodigestive tract exposure to carcinogenic agents such as tobacco and alcohol (Shafer et al., 1983).

CLINICAL BEHAVIOR OF HEAD AND NECK SQUAMOUS CELL CARCINOMA

Although much of the variation in the clinical behavior of HNSCCa is a function of the anatomical location, further variation is dependent on the underlying biological behavior of the lesion. Typically, HNSCCa initially appears as an ulceration or thickening of the mucosa. With time, the lesion enlarges and invades underlying or adjacent tissues. The symptoms produced by this invasion often prompt the patient to seek attention. Typical symptoms include pain, loosening of teeth or dentures, hoarseness, or problems associated with obstruction such as dysphagia or dyspnea (see Chapter 7 in this text). Generally, an associated area of induration or firmness to the tissue occurs secondary to both the invasion of the underlying tissue and a fibrous overgrowth response induced by the tumor. As the lesion expands and invades, it may fix underlying muscular structures (tongue or floor of mouth) or interfere with neural structures, resulting in pain, paresthesia, or paralysis (Tiecke, 1965). Given time, HNSCCa is capable of metastatic spread. In the majority of cases (71%), metastasis are found in the adjacent lymphatic drainage of the neck. Less commonly (22%), metastases are found systemically, typically in the lung (Tiecke, 1965).

CLINICAL STAGING

Because of the clinical presentation of HNSCCa and the implications for prognosis and treatment, a clinical staging system was devised to allow clinicians in different locations to more meaningfully compare tumors and the results of therapeutic intervention. This staging system is based on the patient's preoperative clinical presentation (Ho, Zahurak, & Koch, 2004) and is not influenced by information gathered from pathological examination of excised tissue. This standard tumor, node, and metastasis (TNM) system is based on tumor size, the absence or presence and extent of local nodal spread, and the absence or presence of distant metastasis. The TNM classification system is summarized in Table 13.1 (Hermanek, Hutter, Sobin, Wagner, & Wittekind, 1997). TNM classification is combined to produce a composite clinical stage (see Table 13.2), which is of prognostic value (Hermanek et al., 1997).

Generally, prognosis is better for individuals with smaller, more localized lesions at the time of diagnosis. For oral squamous cell carcinoma, the 5-year survival rate has been reported to be 63% for localized disease (TXN0M0), com-

TABLE 13.1
Definition of TNM Categories for Head and Neck Squamous Cell Cancer

T: Tumor Classification for the Oral Cavity

   TX: primary tumor cannot be assessed

   T0: no evidence of primary tumor

   Tis: carcinoma in situ

   T1: tumor 2 cm or less in greater dimension

   T2: tumor greater than 2 cm, but not greater than 4 cm in greatest dimension

   T3: tumor greater than 4 cm in greatest dimension

   T4: massive tumor greater than 4 cm in diameter with deep invasion to involve antrum, pterygoid muscles, root of tongue, or skin of neck

N: Cervical Lymph Node Classification

   NX: regional lymph nodes cannot be assessed

   N0: no regional lymph node metastasis

   N1: metastasis in single ipsilateral lymph node 3 cm or less in greatest dimension

   N2: metastasis in a single ipsilateral lymph node, more than 3 cm, but not more than 6 cm in greatest dimension, or in bilateral or contralateral lymph nodes, none more than 6 cm in greatest dimension

   N2a: metastasis in a single ipsilateral lymph node, more than 3 cm, but not more than 6 cm in greatest dimension

   N2b: metastasis in multiple ipsilateral lymph nodes, none more than 6 cm in greatest dimension

   N2c: metastasis in bilateral or contralateral lymph nodes, none more than 6 cm in greatest dimension

   N3: metastasis in a lymph node more than 6 cm in greatest dimension

M: Metastasis Classification

   MX: presence of distant metastasis cannot be assessed

   M0: no distant metastasis

   M1: distant metastasis

Note. From *TNM Classification of Malignant Tumors* (4th ed.), by P. Hermanek, R.V. P. Hutter, L. H. Sobin, G. Wagner, and C. Wittekind, 1997, Indianapolis, IN: Wiley. Copyright 1997 by John Wiley & Sons. Reprinted with permission.

pared to 30% for those with regional spread (TXNXM0) and 17% for those with distant spread (TXNXMX) (Elwood & Gallagher, 1985). HNSCCa is graded histologically primarily on the basis of degree of differentiation (i.e., well, moderately, or poorly differentiated). Although the concept is controversial, Shafer et al. (1983) suggested that variation in the histological appearance of the cancerous tissues reflects biological activity, with poorly differentiated tumors growing more aggressively and having an increased tendency for nodal or systemic metastasis.

TABLE 13.2

Summary of Stage of Disease Groupings

	Tumor	Node	Metastasis
Stage 0:	Tis	N0	M0
Stage I:	T1	N0	M0
Stage II:	T2	N0	M0
Stage III:	T3	N0	M0
	T1 or T2 or T3	N1	M0
Stage IV:	T4	N0 or N1	M0
	T1 or T2 or T3 or T4	N2 or N3	M0
	T1 or T2 or T3 or T4	N0 or N1 or N2 or N3	M1

Note. From *TNM Classification of Malignant Tumors* (4th ed.), by P. Hermanek, R. V. P. Hutter, L. H. Sobin, G. Wagner, and C. Wittekind, 1997, Indianapolis, IN: Wiley. Copyright 1997 by John Wiley & Sons. Reprinted with permission.

LIMITATIONS OF CURRENT THERAPEUTIC MODALITIES

Most head and neck cancers are treated by surgery, radiotherapy, or a combination of both. To date, chemotherapy for cancer of the head and neck has not yielded acceptable clinical results in sole-modality management of this disease. It has, however, shown some promise in combination therapy and is used for palliation (Gussack, Brantley, & Farmer, 1984). Current therapeutic methods may result in morbidity and have limitations. Surgery has the advantage of accurate determination of the extent of the lesion and its local spread, is usually well tolerated, and leaves normal local tissues relatively unaffected. Unfortunately, surgery potentially may be incomplete relative to the tumor excision. Surgery also often results in cosmetic deformity and functional deficits, such as loss of the larynx, loss of part of the jaw, or sensory and motor nerve deficits. Radiotherapy has the advantages of causing minimal cosmetic deformity and covering a wide therapeutic area, including potential micrometastasis that may be missed by surgery. Radiotherapy, however, results in wide-ranging side effects, including xerostomia, radiation caries, and the risk of osteoradionecrosis or perichondritis (Stecht, 2004). Radiation is less effective in dealing with the hypoxic centers of tumors, and these may give rise to recurrence. Combination therapy has the advantages of both surgery and radiotherapy in terms of cure, but unfortunately also carries the long-term functional and cosmetic disadvantages of both modalities (Jesse, 1978; Mady, Sader, Hoole, Zimmermann, & Horch, 2003; Theurer & Martin, 2003; Zelefsy et al., 1996; see also Chapters 7 and 10 in this text).

MANAGEMENT OF ORAL CANCER

Diagnosis, Prognosis, and Treatment Planning

Diagnosis

In general, the two main considerations in the management of oral cancer are elimination of disease and posttreatment rehabilitation. The key to elimination of disease is a comprehensive treatment plan based on a diagnosis that determines the name of the disease (e.g., squamous cell carcinoma, adenoid cystic carcinoma), its location (e.g., larynx, anterior two thirds of the tongue), and TNM clinical staging. Clinical outcome data, such as recurrence and disease-free survival rates, have been based on comparisons using TNM status as the independent variable. Therefore, the prospective choice of therapy and the retrospective response to therapy are based on this clinical staging system (Hermanek et al., 1997) (see Tables 13.1 and 13.2). In addition to clinical staging, a comprehensive approach to information gathering and decision making is a very important component of the overall management process (Singer, Phillips, Kramer, & Fu, 1998). A detailed management "care map" is included in Figure 13.1 for aid in the decision-making processes for all members of the team.

Tissue of Origin and Tumor Type

Although a variety of malignancies are possible in the head and neck (see Table 13.3), squamous cell carcinoma is the most common, comprising approximately 90% of all head and neck malignancies (Silverman, 1998). HNSCCa tends to invade locally and may spread to the regional lymph nodes of the neck. Therefore, local surgical excision of the tumor is often accompanied by radical neck dissection and/or radiotherapy of the neck. Recurrence of disease is often seen relatively early (within months) and is often identified at the surgical borders of the resection or in the neck. In contrast, adenoid cystic carcinoma has a tendency to be relatively slow growing and tends to track along nerve trunks and recur relatively late (up to 15 years after treatment), either at the local level or as metastasis to the lungs. Because of the tendency for spread along nerve trunks, local excision is often accompanied by wide beam radiotherapy (Shafer et al., 1983).

Location

Location of the lesion according to surface anatomy is extremely important in the management of head and neck cancer (see Figure 13.2). The decision as to whether or not the disease is treatable is often dictated by its location and continuity with vital structures. Intracranial spread or distant metastasis may prevent a curative approach. When resectable, disease location dictates the approach to be taken to eliminate disease and has significant implications with respect to posttreatment rehabilitation and quality of life (QOL) issues (Wolff, Leeper, Gratton,

(text continues on p. 272)

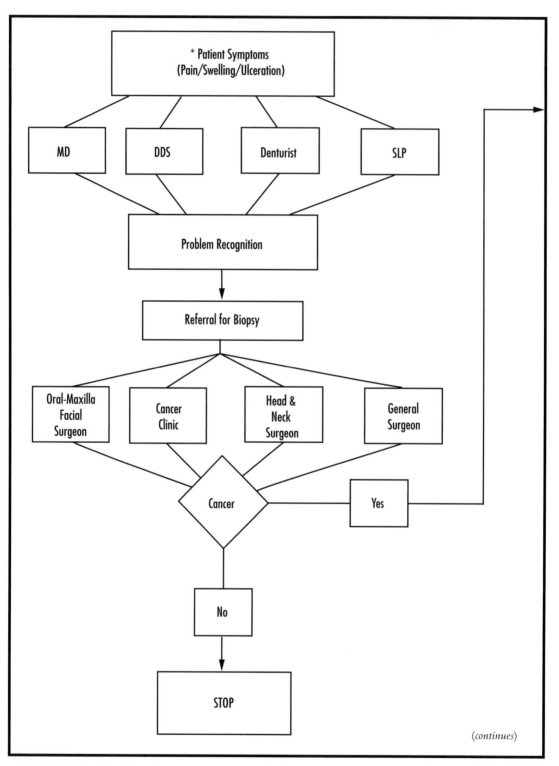

FIGURE 13.1. Multidisciplinary information gathering and synthesis care map. 1° = primary; 2° = secondary.

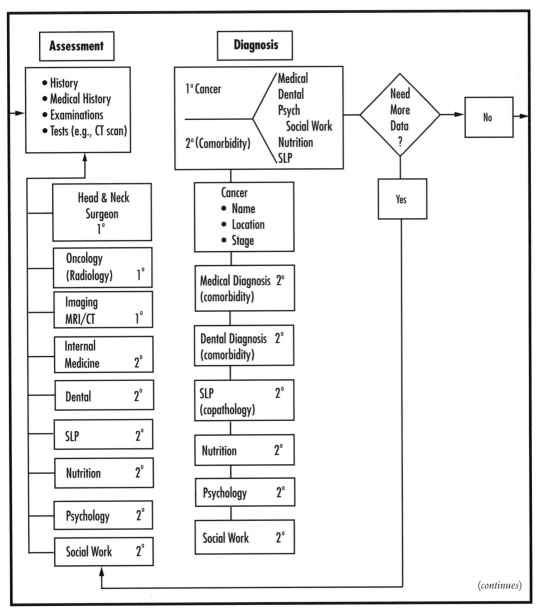

FIGURE 13.1. *Continued.*

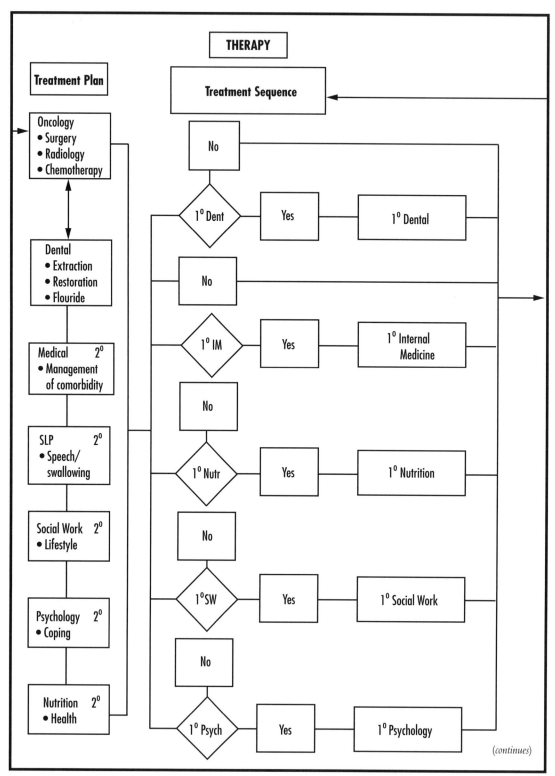

FIGURE 13.1. *Continued.*

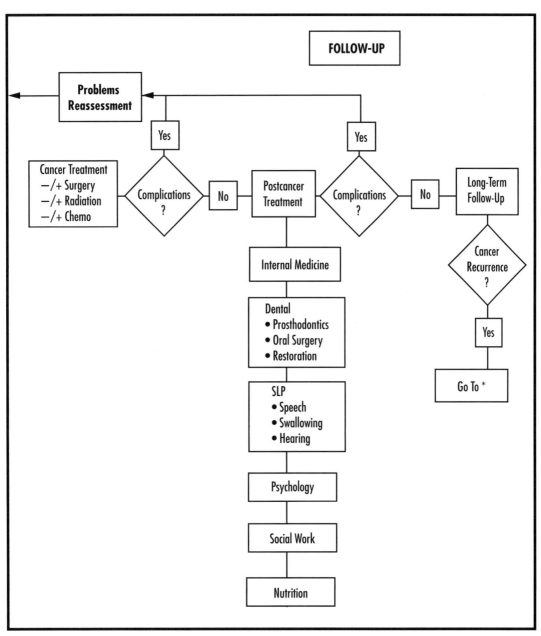

FIGURE 13.1. *Continued.*

TABLE 13.3

Examples of Malignancies of the Head and Neck

Skin Cancer

    Basal cell carcinoma

    Squamous cell carcinoma

    Malignant melanoma

Cancer of the Oral Epithelium

    Carcinoma in situ

    Verrucous carcinoma

    Squamous cell carcinoma

    Lymphoepithelial carcinoma

    Nasopharyngeal carcinoma

Malignant Salivary Gland Tumors

    Adenoid cystic carcinoma

    Polymorphous low-grade adenocarcinoma

    Mucoepidermoid carcinoma

    Acinic cell carcinoma

Sarcomas

    Osteosarcoma

    Chondrosarcoma

    Rhabdomyosarcoma

    Kaposi's sarcoma

Other Malignant Lesions

    Lymphomas

& Doyle, 2004; Wright, O'Brien, Lieberman, Bradfield, & Mennel, 1988). For example, wide beam radiotherapy for oral cancers often results in major damage to the salivary glands and subsequent xerostomia. Further, radiation damage to the bone and soft tissues of the mouth sets the stage for the potential development of osteoradionecrosis.

Imaging

The use of computer assisted tomography (CAT) or magnetic resonance imaging (MRI) helps the surgeon, radiation oncologist, and radiotherapist to determine the location and extent of cancer spread. These imaging techniques may reveal invasion of tumor into bone, extension to the base of skull, or major vascular involvement. These issues have significant implications with respect to modality of therapy (i.e., surgery, radiotherapy, or both).

Prognosis

The prognosis for a patient is multifactorial and includes the following considerations: overall health status, the type of tumor and location, the extent of spread and its resectability, TNM status, and the ability to rehabilitate the patient to an acceptable posttreatment QOL (Shafer et al., 1983).

Cure

On average, posttreatment survival for HNSCCa is in the range of 50% over 5 years. In general, the prognosis is poorer for larger or more posterior tumors, and poorer when there is regional nodal involvement or distant metastasis (Silverman, 1998).

Rehabilitation

Posttreatment rehabilitation has the goal of maintaining or replacing structures and function following either surgery, radiotherapy, or both. By its very nature, the treatment of cancer creates significant anatomical, functional, and cosmetic defects. In part, the choice of therapy depends on the team's ability to restore anatomy, function, or both to maintain an acceptable QOL for the patient (Leeper & Gratton, 1999).

Palliation

If the extent of disease is such that cure is unlikely and treatment would be debilitating, the offer of palliative care may be made. Palliative treatment may include noncurative radiation, surgery, or chemotherapy in an effort to control symptoms such as pain or difficulty with eating and breathing (Wright et al., 1988; see Chapter 28 in this text).

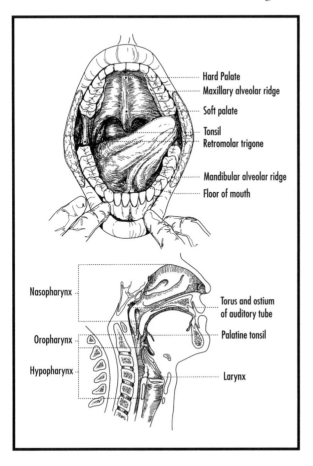

FIGURE 13.2. Surface anatomy of the head and neck.

Treatment Planning

Radiotherapy

Radiotherapy may be planned with or without surgery, depending on the type of tumor and its TNM status. It may precede or follow surgery on a planned basis or be required after failure to control disease following surgery (see Chapter 10 in this text). Typically, radiotherapy is delivered using an external beam approach to target the tumor from the outside with an attempt to spare contiguous normal structures as much as possible. In addition, external beam radiotherapy is often used to treat the regional lymph nodes of the neck (see Figure 13.3) on either a therapeutic or preventative basis. Brachytherapy, or the placement of radioactive grains or pellets near the site of the tumor to more directly deliver radiation to the tumor, is an alternative to external beam radiotherapy. Care must be taken with brachytherapy because of the danger of significantly higher radiation delivery to adjacent structures such as bone and the attendant risk of osteoradionecrosis (Wright et al., 1988).

Chemotherapy

Typically, chemotherapy is not the first-line therapy of choice for head and neck cancer. The use of chemotherapy is considered a palliative measure following the failure of surgery and radiation (Wright et al., 1988).

Surgery

The two major aims of surgery are tumor ablation and defect reconstruction. Tumor ablation requires the complete removal of the tumor at the local and regional levels. It is for this reason that (a) a margin of normal tissue must be removed at the local level and (b) radical neck surgery is often included in the surgical approach to eliminate nodal involvement (see Chapters 7 and 8 in this text).

Maxillary Surgery

The standard procedure for removal of cancer of the maxilla is partial maxillectomy (Spiro, Strong, & Shah, 1997) (see Figure 13.4). The surgical exposure of the site is achieved by either a transoral or transfacial approach. The expected defect may be relatively minor or quite extensive. The main components of the defect are the loss of the alveolus, the hard palate, and the soft palate (Kornblith, Zlotolow, & Gooen, 1996). The larger or more posterior the tumor in the oral cavity, the more the defect will involve all three structures. A significant posttreatment consequence of maxillary surgery is velopharyngeal incompetence. This occurs as a result of a defect between the mouth and the nasal cavity or as a result of loss of part (or all) of the soft palate. The anticipated margins of the surgical defect are determined, and the surgical cuts are accomplished using a combination of soft tissue dissection and bone cuts. The margins are then confirmed to be tumor free by either clinical or microscopic examination.

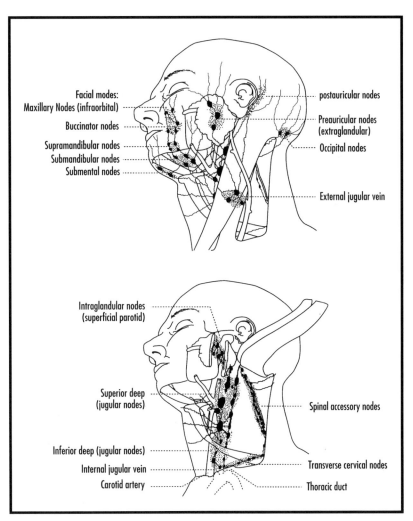

FIGURE 13.3. Lymph nodes of the head and neck.

Defect Obturation

Following tumor removal, the defect is packed with an antibacterial dressing and covered with a primary surgical splint or obturator. This surgical obturator is designed and fabricated on the basis of an understanding of the anticipated surgical margins using a preoperatively obtained model of the upper jaw. Ideally, this is done in consultation with the head and neck surgeon and the prosthodontist who will ultimately be providing the patient with the final prosthesis. The use of a surgical obturator permits very early rehabilitation and significantly reduces postsurgical morbidity by allowing for immediate oral function, including eating and speech. It also allows for guided healing of the initial defect along the contours of the immediate surgical obturator. At approximately 2 weeks postoperatively, the dressing is removed and an interim obturator is placed. This obturator provides ongoing restoration of velopharyngeal competence and maintenance of oral function while the defect heals. A more permanent obturator prosthesis is fabricated 2 to 4 months following surgery. Ideally, the prosthodontist works in conjunction with the speech pathologist in the design and evaluation of the obturator prosthesis to obtain optimal velopharyngeal function (Lapointe, Lampe, & Taylor, 1996).

Tongue, Floor of Mouth, and Mandibular Surgery

The range and scope of procedures employed for the removal of tumors of the lower jaw and tongue are much more extensive than those for the upper jaw. Complicating the situation further are the variable means of reconstructing these defects following ablative surgery.

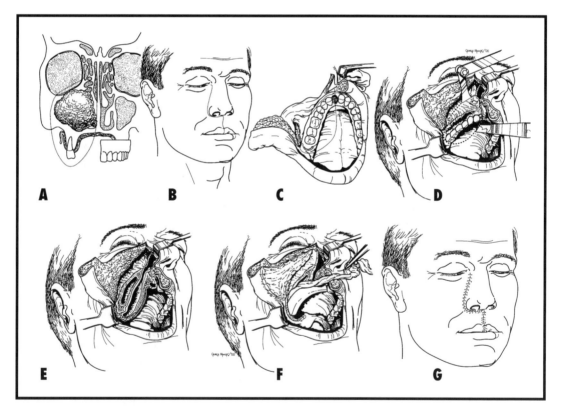

FIGURE 13.4. Maxillectomy surgery. (A) Location of tumor in the maxillary sinus with surgical margin indicated by the dotted line. (B) Facial incision for access to the underlying maxilla. (C) Intra-oral incision for tumor removal. (D) Bone cuts made with oscillating saw and osteotomes. (E) The final surgical defect. (F) The defect is lined on the inside of the cheek with skin graft, the defect is packed with medicated surgical dressing, and a surgical obturator prosthesis is used to create a floor for the defect and to restore the soft and hard palates. (G) Final closure of the facial incision.

Tongue and Floor of Mouth

For relatively small tumors of the tongue and floor of mouth, simple excision with primary closure is often employed. This results in a diminution of tongue volume and some tethering of the tongue (see Figure 13.5). As tumors become more extensive in size with posterior or deep spread, the volume of excision increases and the need for reconstruction beyond primary closure arises (see Figure 13.6). In these cases, larger surgical defects are reconstructed with flaps. These may be pedicled flaps, such as a pectoralis major (see Figure 13.7), or free microvascularized flaps, such as radial forearm (see Chapters 8 and 12 in this text). These flaps can result in relatively bulky, adynamic structures, with potential restrictions in tongue mobility and problems with deglutition, speech, and prosthetic rehabilitation (Silverman, 1998).

Mandibular Surgery

Cancer arising primarily from the jaw is relatively rare. Much more common is spread of cancer to the mandible from contiguous structures, such as the floor of mouth or the tongue. When this occurs, segmental or block resection of the lower jaw is required. Commonly, the overall resection is quite large, and reconstruction with pedicled or microvascularized free flaps is employed (see Figure 13.8). This surgery may be accompanied with bone or plate reconstruction of the continuity defect in the jaw (Wright et al., 1988).

THE ROLE OF THE DENTIST IN THE MANAGEMENT OF THE INDIVIDUAL WITH HEAD AND NECK CANCER

Screening

An important role for dentists is ongoing screening of their patients for diseases in the oral cavity, including cancer. Although oral cancer is relatively rare, dentists have an ideal opportunity to regularly and appropriately monitor patients for the development of disease. This screening includes clinical and radiographic examination and maintaining appropriate vigilance for new or undetected abnormalities.

System Entry

When a community dentist notes an abnormality in the tissues of the oral cavity and suspects malignancy, the patient is referred to either an oral and maxillofacial surgeon or a head and neck surgeon for biopsy, pathological evaluation, and diagnosis. If a lesion is confirmed to be malignant, the patient is entered into the system for comprehensive workup, detailed diagnosis, and treatment planning.

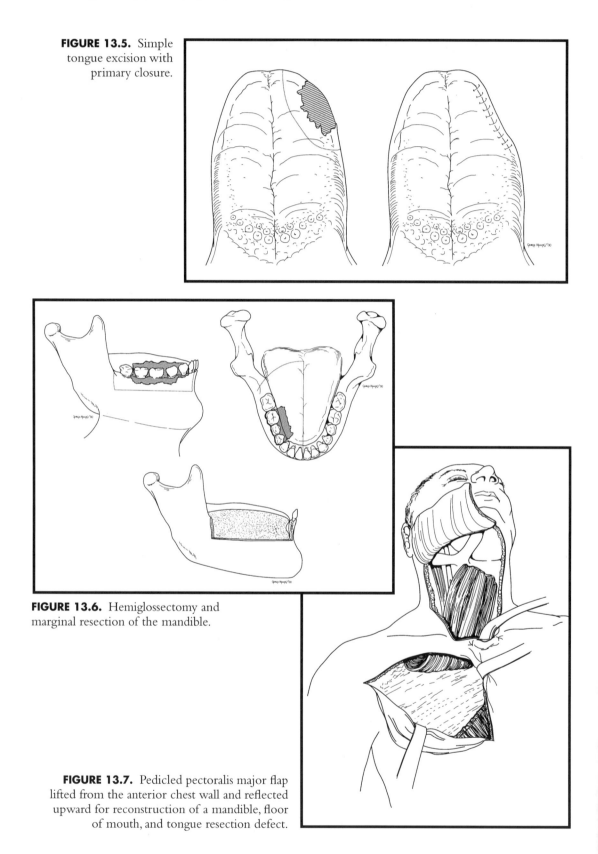

FIGURE 13.5. Simple tongue excision with primary closure.

FIGURE 13.6. Hemiglossectomy and marginal resection of the mandible.

FIGURE 13.7. Pedicled pectoralis major flap lifted from the anterior chest wall and reflected upward for reconstruction of a mandible, floor of mouth, and tongue resection defect.

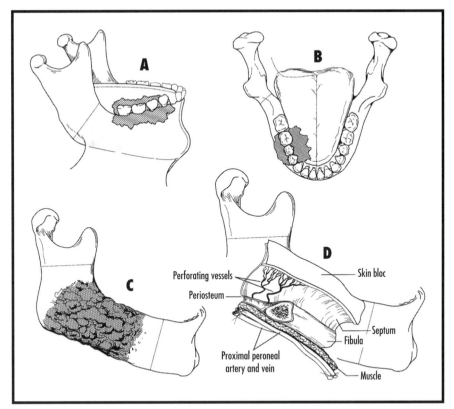

FIGURE 13.8. Extensive surgical defect (A and B) created by hemiglossectomy and segmental resection of the mandible (C). Defect reconstruction with microvascularized free fibula with soft tissue and skin (D).

Oncologic Diagnosis and Treatment Planning

On the basis of tumor type, location, TNM staging, and the patient's general health status and ability to undergo treatment, an oncologic treatment plan is developed (see Chapter 8 in this text). This plan can involve surgical removal of the lesion and regional nodal spread (neck dissection) and/or radiotherapy for local disease and regional nodal spread. In conjunction with the surgical treatment plan, a reconstruction treatment plan is usually devised. This plan may include primary closure, local or distant flap reconstruction, or the fabrication of a prosthesis (Beumer, DePaola, & Leupold, 1986).

Dentists as Members of the Head and Neck Cancer Team

Members of the head and neck cancer team typically include a general dentist with a particular interest in head and neck cancer, an oral and maxillofacial surgeon, and a prosthodontist. The general dentist assesses the patient's overall dental needs and provides and coordinates dental management. The oral and maxillofacial surgeon specializes in more complex surgery for the teeth and jaw and may be included in all phases of treatment, including pretreatment preparation of the jaw for radiation or surgery, the cancer surgery itself, and posttreatment reconstruction. The oral and maxillofacial surgeon often becomes involved when posttreatment extractions are required or when complications such as osteoradionecrosis become a factor. The prosthodontist offers expertise for the management of complex reconstructive needs, particulary in the area of maxillary reconstruction following maxillectomy surgery. As part of the head and neck cancer team, dentists are in a unique position to offer appropriate insight into the diagnosis and planning process for patients with oral cancer. Specifically, team dentists evaluate the individual's pretreatment dental status and offer input into the planning process.

Pretreatment Dental Evaluation and Recommendations

The most significant concerns for the head and neck team dentist are prevention of infection and osteoradionecrosis. From this perspective, the team dentist offers recommendations, taking into account the oncologic treatment plan. Careful preparation of the oral cavity for treatment must be carried out, particularly if radiotherapy is part of treatment. Potential interventions may include standard maintenance therapy (cleaning, restorations, etc.), topical fluoride applications, extractions of some or all of the teeth, prosthetics (dentures or primary, secondary, and tertiary obturators), dental implants, and ongoing reevaluation (before, during, and after treatment).

DIAGNOSIS, PREVENTION, AND TREATMENT OF OSTEORADIONECROSIS

In light of the potentially devastating effect of osteoradionecrosis (ORN), special consideration must be given to this problem. Radiotherapy is an effective modality for cancer treatment because of its ability to kill tumor cells. Unfortunately, radiation also has a deleterious effect on normal cells. The initial radiation damage is a result of direct cytotoxicity and causes acute mucositis and destroys salivary glands. Loss of salivary flow leads to a dry mouth or xerostomia, which in turn sets the stage for radiation caries. Radiation caries can result in extensive decay of the patient's dentition, particularly if oral hygiene and dental care are not ideal (Stokman et al., 2003). In general, in the longer term, damage to the small arterioles of the oral tissues results in a chronic state of hypoperfusion, hypoxia, and hypocellularity. For soft tissues, fibrosis and poor wound healing may follow even trivial damage. Radiated bone is also damaged and heals very poorly. If the bone is exposed by damage to the overlying soft tissue, either through trauma or further surgery (e.g., dental extractions), the healing potential is very poor and bone often dies (chronic ORN). Overt ORN is often precipitated by the rapid decay of teeth with infection and the need for extractions in the radiated field (Marx, 1983a).

Diagnosis of ORN

ORN can be very painful. On examination, ORN will be manifested as exposed bone plus or minus superficial infection. There may be bone exposure either orally or through the skin or both. Radiographically the bone appears moth eaten, and there may be a concomitant pathological fracture in the area. Osseous involvement may be very substantial, extending beyond the obvious clinical exposure or radiographic appearance. Physiological imaging, such as a technicium bone scan, is often used to help diagnose and delineate the extent of disease.

Prevention of ORN

Limiting radiation exposure to 60 CG or less has been noted to significantly reduce the incidence of ORN (Thorn, Hansen, Specht, & Bastholt, 2000). Careful assessment of and attention to the dentition prior to radiotherapy is required to eliminate active infection and to remove teeth that are likely to require extraction following radiotherapy. This includes teeth with significant periodontal disease, large caries, caries at the neck of the tooth, extensive restorations, root canal treatment, and teeth that are in the radiation field. For those teeth that are retained, scrupulous oral hygiene, fluoride treatment, and regular evaluation must be maintained. If teeth must be extracted following radiotherapy, prevention of ORN is a high priority. Individuals requiring extractions following radiotherapy are sent for hyperbaric oxygen (HBO) prophylactically (Marx, Johnson, & Kline, 1985). HBO therapy consists of having the patient undergo a series of "dives" inside a hyperbaric chamber. Typically, the patient is taken to two atmospheres of pressure and then given 100% oxygen to breathe. This results in increased concentrations of dissolved oxygen in blood and tissues. The course of up to 30 dives stimulates endothelial ingrowth into the hypoxic tissue. This neovascularization results in improved cellularity of the tissue and allows for more normal collagen formation and wound healing. HBO produces an improvement in the vascularity and oxygenation in the affected tissues, significantly reducing the risk of development of overt ORN following extractions (Marx, 1983b).

Treatment of ORN

The treatment of ORN is based on the extent of disease and is multimodal. Antibiotics are used to control superficial soft tissue infection. HBO therapy is used to improve the vascularity and oxygenation of both bone and the overlying soft tissue.

Surgery is used to eliminate the grossly affected parts of bone and then recon-struct with either plates or bone grafts (Balogh & Sutherland, 1983; Dempsey, Hines, Smith, & Sproat, 1997; Marx, 1983a) (see Figure 13.9 for an outline of the decision-making protocol and Figure 13.10 for a clinical example).

DENTAL IMPLANTS AND EXTRAORAL IMPLANTS FOR THE HEAD AND NECK CANCER PATIENT

The use of dental implants to support prostheses is a developing area for the head and neck cancer patient. Dental implants are metal (titanium) screws or cylinders that are placed into preplanned implant sites in the bone. The implants are al-lowed to heal and then, like tooth roots, can be used in a number of ways to sup-port either dental (see Figure 13.11) or facial prostheses (noses, ears, etc.). These can be particularly effective for patients who have surgical defects or recon-struction that renders the provision of standard dental prosthetics difficult, if not impossible.

Although versatile, implants have limitations. Sufficient, healthy bone must be present for implant placement with appropriate angulation and spacing to dis-tribute the forces placed on the prosthesis. Overloading of the appliance or indi-vidual implants will result in implant loosening and failure. The use of implants in radiated fields continues to be controversial, with a greater than normal risk of implant failure and the risk of inducing ORN (McGlumphy & Larsen, as cited in Peterson, Ellis, Hupp, & Tucker, 1998).

PROSTHETIC MANAGEMENT

Presurgical Dental Assessment and Management

Prosthodontic success in rehabilitation for the head and neck cancer patient is directly related to presurgical management. Communication and cooperation between the prosthodontist and the surgeon, radiation oncologist, chemothera-pist, oral surgeon, speech pathologist, and social worker will help to provide an effective and efficient plan of treatment (Leeper & Gratton, 1999). Once a diag-nosis is confirmed, the scheduling for definitive treatment generally is quite rapid. Within this limited time frame, dental status must be assessed and stabilized as required. The minimum dental management that must occur prior to surgery should include (a) oral prophylaxis, (b) management of acute infections of the oral cavity, (c) taking diagnostic impressions of existing oral structures and fab-rication of stone dental casts, (d) mounting of casts on an articulator to assess tooth–jaw relationship, (e) restoration of carious tooth structure and key teeth required to retain the forthcoming prostheses, and (f) extraction of teeth that cannot be restored or may compromise the surgical area.

(text continues on p. 286)

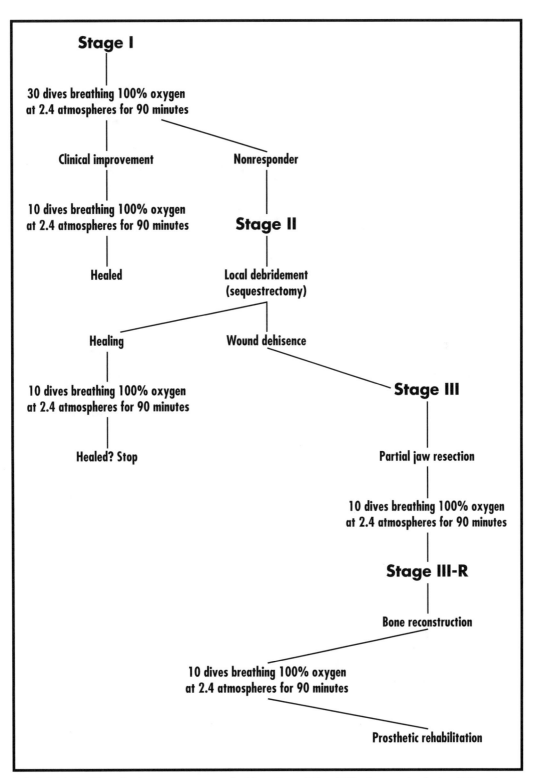

FIGURE 13.9. Hyperbaric oxygen protocols. *Note.* From "Cost Effectiveness Analysis of Hyperbaric Therapy in Osteoradionecrosis," by J. Dempsey, N. Hynes, T. Smith, and J. E. Sproat, 1997, *Canadian Journal of Plastic Surgery, 5,* p. 223. Copyright 1997 by Pulsus Group, Oakville, Ontario, Canada. Reprinted with permission.

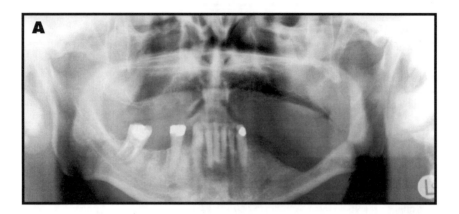

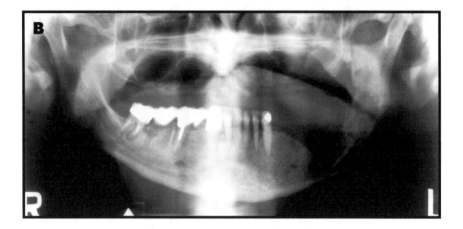

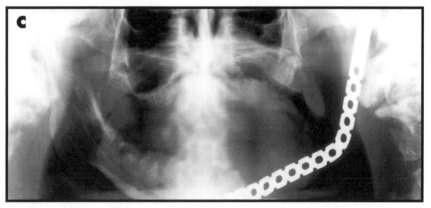

FIGURE 13.10. Osteoradionecrosis of the mandible. (A) Panoramic radiograph of a 56-year-old male immediately following surgery and radiotherapy. Resection of carcinoma of the left retromolar trigone included marginal resection of the mandible and radical neck dissection. (B) Panoramic radiograph of patient 2 years subsequent to surgery and radiation, presenting with a pathological fracture through osteoradionecrosis of the left mandible. (C) Panoramic radiograph of patient subsequent to hyperbaric oxygen and hemimandibulectomy with plate reconstruction.

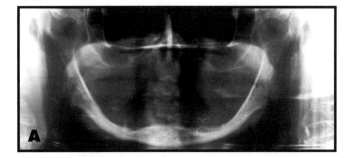

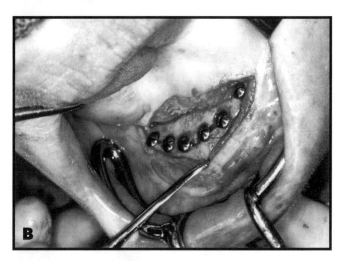

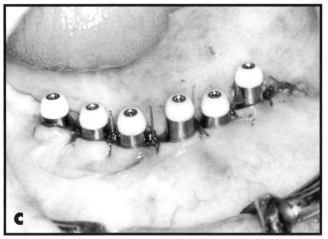

(continues)

FIGURE 13.11. Dental implant reconstruction following ablative surgery and free flap reconstruction. (A) Panoramic radiograph of 54-year-old male after resection of carcinoma of the floor of mouth indicating moderate to severe atrophy of the mandible. (B) Surgical insertion of implants into anterior mandible (note the skin of the microvascular reconstruction of the tongue and floor of mouth). (C) Surgical exposure of implants following 3-month period of osseointegration. (D) Panoramic radiograph indicating implants in position and underfunction with a fixed-detachable bridge. (E) Five-year postinsertion intraoral view of implant bridge in position (note shape and hypomobility of the tongue and floor of mouth). (F) Occlusion of implant-supported bridge in function with complete upper denture. (Prosthetics courtesy of Dr. David H. Charles.)

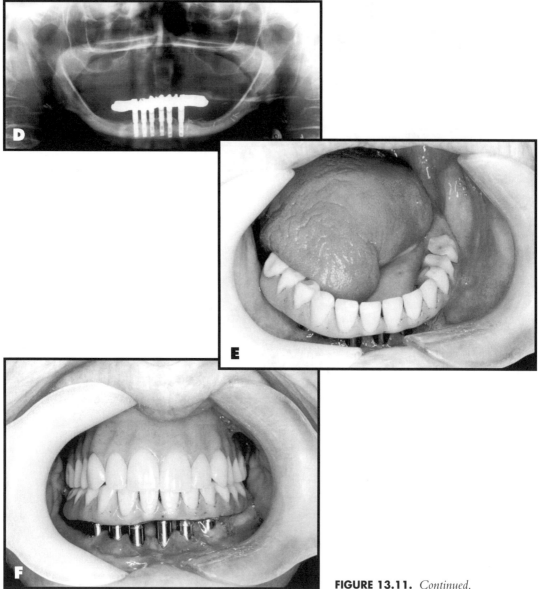

FIGURE 13.11. *Continued.*

Within this same time period, it is important for the maxillofacial team to meet with the patient and discuss the various stages of treatment and anticipated outcomes. Topics include the surgical site (location and extent), cosmesis, placement and timing of dental prostheses, alteration in mastication and swallowing behaviors, speech difficulties related to maxillary and mandibular deficiencies, and overall speech intelligibility. Reduction in the patient's anxiety about the forthcoming procedures and the effects on QOL may be dealt with by the team or by referral to a clinical psychologist or social worker. It is important to remind the patient of the time frame, from start to completion, of the surgical and rehabilitation processes and what might be expected at each stage of management.

Prosthetic Rehabilitation— Acquired Maxillary Defect

Residual defects resulting from surgical resection of a maxillary tumor from the maxilla compromise the function of the oral cavity. Resulting problems include leakage of food and fluid into the nasal cavity, impaired mastication, swallowing difficulties, hypernasality, nasal air emission, loss of articulatory precision, and reduced overall speech intelligibility. Obturation of the defect by a dental prosthesis is aimed at reducing or eliminating anatomical and functional deficiencies. Most patients treated surgically with partial or total resection of the maxilla (maxillectomy) have three different obturators at various stages of healing. At the time of surgery, a surgical obturator is placed and is retained from 7 to 10 days. An interim obturator is then fabricated shortly after initial wound healing has occurred, and the patient wears this until definitive healing of the defect has occurred (i.e., 3 to 6 months postsurgery). The fabrication and insertion of a definitive obturator occurs after wound healing is confirmed, generally 6 to 12 months postsurgery (Anderson, Awde, Leeper, & Sills, 1992; Beumer, Curtis, & Marunick, 1996; Desjardins, 1977, 1978).

The Surgical Obturator

The prosthodontist and surgeon consult on the site and extent of tissue to be removed during surgery. From the diagnostic cast provided by the prosthodontist, the surgeon outlines the anticipated hard and soft tissue areas to be resected. The diagnostic cast is then altered along the outlined surgical margins that estimate the topography of the anatomy postsurgery. The prosthodontist then authorizes the fabrication of the surgical obturator, covering as much of the defect as possible with the prosthesis. Typically, the splint (see Figure 13.12) is made

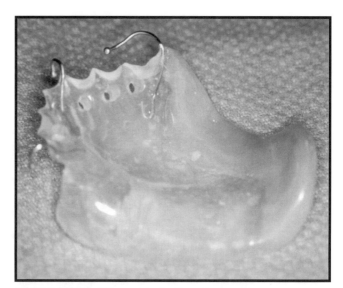

FIGURE 13.12. The surgical splint obturator.

of clear acrylic resin and is retained within the oral cavity with 18-gauge wire clasps embedded in the acrylic. Along the edges of the splint, small holes may be bored at interproximal areas to allow wire ligatures around the remaining teeth in the palatal arch. If the patient has few remaining teeth or if retention of the splint is in question, wires are passed over the zygomatic arch and then attached to the acrylic or screws are placed through the acrylic and into the residual osseous palate to secure the obturator in place. After a period of 7 to 10 days, the surgical splint is removed. Once the wire ligatures have been removed, the obturator will be modified by reduction or addition to accommodate for shrinkage of the wound site tissues and the potential loss of tissue bulk in the area. Reduction involves precise grinding and polishing of the acrylic. At this stage of healing, if additions to the obturator are required, it is accomplished using tissue-conditioning material applied to the obturator, aiding in prosthesis retention (Anderson et al., 1992; Desjardins, 1977).

In the case of the completely edentulous patient who has a clinically acceptable maxillary denture, the denture can be modified at the time of surgery within the surgical suite to act as the surgical obturator. When using the existing denture as the surgical obturator, the facial flange may have to be reduced to accommodate the surgical site. The posterior portion or soft palate region may have to be extended with tissue-conditioning material to obturate the surgical site, maximizing fit and thus optimizing function of the obturator (Beumer, Zlotolow, & Sharma, 1998). New complete dentures will be required in the definitive stage of obturation.

The surgical obturator allows for careful packing (dressing) of the wound site; keeps food and other debris from entering the wound; permits eating, drinking, and swallowing without a nasogastric tube; and allows immediate oral communication (Doyle, 1999; Leeper & Gratton, 1999). All of these functions enhance a patient's QOL.

The Interim Obturator

Depending on the progression of wound healing, the surgical obturator may be relined or modified to allow sufficient fit of the appliance for speech and deglutory function. As modifications are made, however, the prosthesis may become more bulky and less hygienic. When this occurs, it is desirable to replace the surgical obturator with an interim obturator (see Figure 13.13).

To make the interim obturator, the prosthodontist must take new impressions of the defect and entire maxillary region (both anterior and posterior). An acceptable impression will have an accurate representation of the features of the maxillary, palatal, and pharyngeal areas,

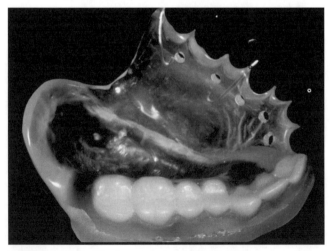

FIGURE 13.13. The interim obturator appliance.

capturing the detail and extent of the residual defect. On the new stone cast made from the impression, a simple design of the interim prosthesis is possible. The design typically follows the basic principles of removable prosthodontics and may include replacement of missing teeth in the visible areas of the anterior oral cavity. The prosthesis is developed in wax and trial fitted in the patient's mouth before being converted to processed acrylic resin. Because this version of the prosthesis will not be the final one, wrought wire clasps can be added to engage remaining teeth to aid in the retention of the interim obturator. At the time of initial insertion of the new interim obturator, areas of localized pressure on the oral mucosa must be identified with pressure indicator paste and then relieved. Reinstruction concerning insertion and removal of the new interim appliance should occur at this time. In addition, office visits are to be scheduled regularly to correct minor tissue irritations and to adjust clasp arms for comfortable fit and retention. Dental care of existing teeth must also continue during this interim period (Anderson et al., 1992; Desjardins, 1978; Leeper & Gratton, 1999).

The Definitive Obturator

Design of the definitive obturator prosthesis (see Figure 13.14) should begin after a majority of the wound healing has taken place, radiotherapy has been completed, adjustment to this course of treatment has been accepted, and the surgeon has determined that active pathology does not

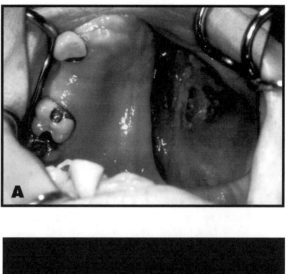

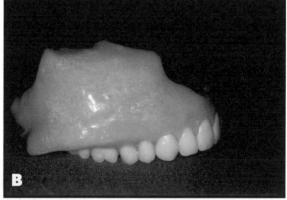

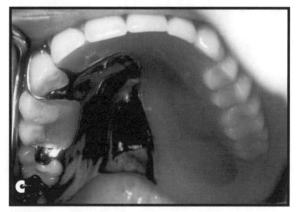

FIGURE 13.14. (A) The defect area for the definitive obturator appliance. (B) The definitive obturator appliance. (C) The definitive obturator appliance in position.

exist. The definitive obturator may be designed as a partial or complete denture. As with the interim obturator, impressions are again made, and stone casts are constructed and mounted on an articulator that simulates jaw movements. Acrylic bases support wax rims that are contoured for aesthetic and phonetic requirements. Artificial teeth are added to the wax bases. These wax prostheses are placed in the patient's mouth to check aesthetics, phonetics, occlusal relationships, and closure of the defect.

After the final contoured wax obturator is acceptable to both prosthodontist and patient, it is invested in a heavy metal flask, the wax is boiled away, and permanent acrylic resin is processed into the resulting void. In some clinical situations, a framework of chromium cobalt with clasps is adhered to the wax and then to the acrylic. These metal clasps engage remaining teeth to facilitate in the retention of the obturator. If the person is edentulous, complete upper and lower dentures may be fabricated. The approach for making this prosthesis is similar to that for normal dentures, except for those areas where a defect is present in the maxillary or near or in the soft palate area. Here, special techniques are used to decrease the weight of the obturator in the defect area by making the obturator "hollow." The "box-type" obturator fills the maxillary defect, but has a smooth "lid" attached to it on the oral side. The air-filled obturator segment fulfills the need for obturation while keeping weight on the defect at a minimum (Anderson et al., 1992; Desjardins, 1978; Leeper & Gratton, 1999).

Defect Management for the Partially Edentulous Individual

The typical protocol for treatment of partially edentulous individuals is developed following careful assessment of the remaining teeth and tissues in and around the surgical defect. Specific radiographs and a survey analysis from the diagnostic casts of the maxillary and mandibular arch segments are necessary to find optimum location for attachments of the denture components. Obviously, it is necessary to complete all restorative and periodontal procedures before proceeding. The person must have a good oral hygiene program under way and must understand the features of the prosthesis and his or her role in maintaining it for maximum usefulness. As with application of a partial denture for any person, the maxillofacial treatment must have a prosthesis with similar basic features, including support, bracing, and retentive components. The basic components of the prosthesis, namely the framework and the base area, are made in several steps. The framework is designed by the prosthodontist and fabricated in a chromium cobalt alloy and contains the supportive, bracing, and retentive elements of the design. The base area of the prosthesis is made with acrylic resin and covers the edentulous and defect area and provides a base for attachment of artificial teeth. With additional defects in the posterior area (soft palate), the partial denture may need a "tailpiece" or section to cover (obturate and/or lift) the defect in the soft tissue (see Figure 13.15). For either anterior (maxillary) or posterior (soft palate) defect areas, it is essential to achieve effective seals to eliminate leakage of food

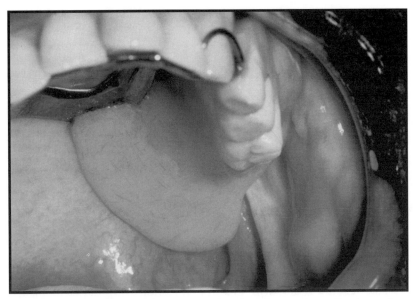

FIGURE 13.15. Obturator for the partially edentulous patient: Portions of hard and soft palate.

and fluid into the nasal passages and to normalize resonance balance during speech.

Again, internal bulky portions of the obturator may be made hollow to reduce weight. In addition, relining of the obturator–defect area with a soft malleable material will be necessary from time to time to maintain a viable seal. The same relining material may be used along the junction of the buccal and maxillary region where deep undercut areas (ablation of alveolar or palatal ridge) may cause the seal (retention) of the denture against the palatal area to become loosened (Anderson et al., 1992; Desjardins, 1978; Leeper & Gratton, 1999).

Defect Management for the Edentulous Individual

A major challenge for any prosthodontist is the fabrication of a prosthesis for the edentulous individual who has had a partial or total maxillectomy. The major problems are many, with size and shape of the defect primary, but with secondary features relating to the absence of supporting teeth and underlying bone, difficulty in achieving a sufficient seal (retention) to hold the denture in place, and potential movement of the obturator around the oral cavity during function. Ideally, the prosthodontist hopes to have the maxillary obturator contact the superior-lateral and posterior-lateral walls of the defect area, the medial area of the resected area, and the skin graft–mucosal scar band around the buccal or pharyngeal area of the defect. Developing a healthy understanding of the limitations of this appliance during swallowing and speech and the difficulties in developing a good path of insertion and removal are paramount, and appointments for adjustments and follow-up care are typically necessary to increase the chances for a successful outcome.

Prosthetic Rehabilitation of the Acquired Mandibular Defect

Not unlike persons requiring a complete lower denture, individuals who require oral surgery to remove portions of the mandible present a particular challenge for the prosthodontist. Typically, smaller cancerous lesions may be excised and will not affect the continuity of the mandible. Larger lesions may require surgery to the mandible, tongue, and floor of mouth, with osseous and soft tissue grafting a consideration. Anterior or lateral surgical excision of portions of the mandibular bone will necessitate stabilization of the remaining segments of the mandible with graft bone or surgical steel splints at the time of initial surgery or at the secondary surgical phase. Loss of the condylar portion of the mandible may necessitate reconstruction with costal cartilaginous rib graft or implantation of artificial condylar elements and body of the mandible to regain symmetry and function for mastication, swallowing, and speech (Adisman, 1990; Anderson et al., 1992; Leeper & Gratton, 1999).

Management for the Partially Edentulous Mandibulectomized Individual

Following surgery, some teams recommend fixation of the maxillary arch segments with ligature wires for 5 to 10 weeks to provide successful wound healing. Other approaches suggest no interarch fixation and beginning the individual on a program of physical therapy exercises shortly after primary wound healing. The purpose is to reduce tissue fixation and trismus in the temporomandibular joint region. Exercises involve progressively opening the mouth wider (passively and actively), closing with slight resistance, and moving the mandible away from the surgically resected side at about 3 weeks postsurgery.

As noted, a significant postsurgical complication for the mandilectomy patient is the severe deviation of the residual mandible to the surgical side. To counter this phenomenon, a removable partial denture can be fabricated with a "buccal flange." The purpose of this flange is to guide and train the muscles of mastication to allow for a more normal path of closure and maximum occlusal intercuspation with the opposing teeth in the maxillary arch. The prosthesis usually consists of a removable maxillary partial denture framework with a buccal guide bar and a lower removable partial denture with a buccal flange fabricated out of a chrome cobalt alloy. If the mandibular deviation is slight, a palatal occlusal ramp can be fabricated on the maxillary prosthesis, which functions the same as the buccal flange prosthesis by guiding the mandible to close laterally in a more acceptable occlusal relationship. Such prostheses are typically described as interim prostheses for classification and funding. In most cases, the developed occlusal contacts will occur when the mandible is in centric relation (with the condyle anteriorly and superiorly positioned in the glenoid fossa), hence eliminating extraneous tooth contacts on the nonresected side of the jaw. Obviously, the patient generally will gravitate to the nonresected side for mastication (Leeper & Gratton, 1999).

Defect Management for the Completely Edentulous and Mandibulectomized Individual

The anatomical and functional limitations of a complete lower denture are problematic in individuals who are edentulous. The loss of tissue in the floor of the mouth, including the tongue, buccal areas, and lip areas, further complicates the situation for placement of lower dentures (see Figure 13.16). The greater the loss of tissue in the mandible and surrounding areas, the more problematic become the support, retention, and stability of the mandibular denture. Also, the more the mandible and associated muscles of mastication have been surgically altered, the more the mandible will deviate to the surgical side, resulting in poor occlusal relationships bilaterally. Such occlusal relationships will impinge on mastication and tongue function for speech and swallowing. Other treatment modalities (e.g., radiotherapy, chemotherapy) can significantly affect the integrity of oral tissues and result in major tissue irritation dryness and possible ulceration, which contribute to the problematic use of a mandibular denture (Anderson et al., 1992; Leeper & Gratton, 1999).

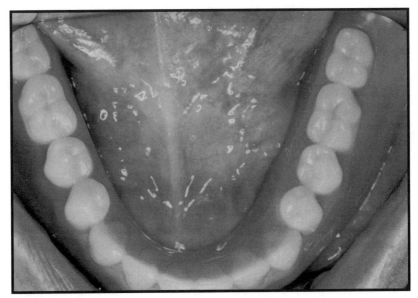

FIGURE 13.16. Appliance for completely edentulous mandibular defects.

Individuals with mandibular resections may be treated with rather simple, uncomplicated denture designs, with appropriate modifications of the mandibular area. Close adaptation of the denture base to the remnants of the mandibular ridge and extension of flanges to the limit of tissue tolerance (i.e., precise contouring of buccal flange to approximate but not interfere with the buccinator and masseter muscles) are necessary. In situations where the tongue is sutured to the resected side of the jaw, the depth of the residual sulcus will dictate whether it may be possible to engage the denture flange in that area to aid in prosthesis retention and stability.

Because the mandible cannot close in a consistently repeatable fashion, on the resected side, a flat occlusal scheme is used to counteract this motion. On the unresected side, a maxillary occlusal ramp made of acrylic resin may be placed lingually to the maxillary posterior teeth to guide jaw closure and tooth contact, improving stability of the prosthesis. Another option is to place a second row of maxillary teeth lingually to the conventionally placed maxillary teeth on the unresected side to allow for a broader occlusal table, providing stable occlusal contact with the mandible deviated to the surgical side, again minimizing denture dislodgment (Anderson et al., 1992; Leeper & Gratton, 1999).

PROSTHETIC REHABILITATION OF THE ACQUIRED SOFT PALATE DEFECT

The size, location, and condition of the tissues surrounding the soft palate defect govern the design of the appliance's velopharyngeal and pharyngeal sections. In addition, some patients may already have interim or definitive prostheses before the effects of radiation therapy lessen and the tissues in the velopharyngeal region heal. Obturators for defects of the entire soft palate take their shape from movements developed from the lateral and posterior pharyngeal walls. Impression techniques employing a variety of head and tongue movements help in producing the final obturator form. As with other ablated structures noted earlier, the posterior section is constructed of acrylic resin and relies on an internal framework for support and connection to the anterior base section. The internal framework provides a scaffolding on which impression materials (thermoplastic waxes, light curing resins) are layered to achieve the most physiologically acceptable form for breathing, swallowing, and speech. The obturator should be located at the level of the greatest pharyngeal wall movement and may not need to extend vertically more than 10 mm (Beumer, Curtis, & Firtell, 1979). Ideally, the obturator should be located in the region of the pharynx where normal palatal closure once occurred. Passive contact should exist between the acrylic of the obturator and the mucosa of the velopharynx and pharynx. During swallowing, coughing, and production of some posteriorly placed speech sounds (e.g., /k/, /g/), the nasopharyngeal section should not be displaced. Obturators in the soft palate area should incorporate a polished, convex superior surface and a concave palatal surface to minimize mucus accumulation and provide adequate tongue space for deglutition and speech.

PROSTHETIC RECONSTRUCTION OF THE ACQUIRED TONGUE DEFECT

Following medical treatment for head and neck cancer, the patient may be left with structural and functional deficits that adversely affect speech, mastication, or swallowing. These deficiencies may be the result of damaged sensory and motor control of the oropharyngeal structures, abnormal palatal configurations, or alterations in tissue size or dynamics of one of the major structures affecting speech and swallowing (e.g., the tongue). Many patients with partial glossectomy or poorly functioning tongue motion as a result of surgical excision or radionecrosis of lingual nerves may profit from alteration of the palatal region for better speech and swallowing. The principle put forward is that if the "floor" (tongue) of the mouth cannot be raised to the "roof" (alveolar area, hard palate), then the roof must be lowered to meet the floor. Using this lay principle, a number of clinical investigators (Aramany, Downs, Beery, & Aslan, 1982; Gillis & Leonard, 1983; Lauciello, Vergo, Schaaf, & Zimmerman, 1980; Leonard & Gillis, 1982; Logemann, Kahrilas, Hurst, Davis, & Krugler, 1989; Shimodaira, Yoshida, Yusa, & Kanazawa, 1998) have described and documented effective changes in speech and swallowing by employing both palatal drop and lingual augmentation prostheses for individuals with poor lingual motor form and control.

Following wound healing and revision of the surgical obturator for the maxillectomy or combined maxillary–mandibulectomy patient, the palatal drop prosthesis may be fabricated on the residual prosthesis or on the original preoperative complete or partial denture covering the maxillary region. A soft dental wax is adapted to the maxillary prosthesis and contoured in the palatal region to "drop" into the area of the mandibular region where there is no tongue (total ablation), a partial tongue, or limited motor control of the existing tongue. The shape of the wax modeling is related directly to the functional deficiencies of the tongue and is contoured so that the tongue can make contact with the maxillary region. This area is often irregular and must be "fitted" to the bottom (floor) structure of the mouth (mandible). A pressure-indicator paste is spread on the contoured wax in the palatal vault segment of the prosthesis, and the patient is asked to perform a series of phonetic and functional movements, with notation made of which segments of the residual tongue make contact with the soft wax (see Figure 13.17A). Modifications are made by heating the wax and recontouring the palatal configuration until the speech output reaches a more proficient level employing assessment tools (see later "Oral Articulatory Evaluation" section). Once the contour of the wax is deemed appropriate, the wax is replaced with autopolymerizing acrylic resin through a laboratory process performed by a maxillofacial dental technician. The processed palatal drop prosthesis is fit to the oral cavity, and the pressure-indicator paste is again applied to the palatal drop portion, with adjustments made to the acrylic to fine-tune speech and swallowing (see Figure 13.17B). A period of patient adaptation in which subtle modifications are made to the palatal drop prosthesis is normally required. These adjustments depend on a host of patient factors and cannot be predicted; however, they are

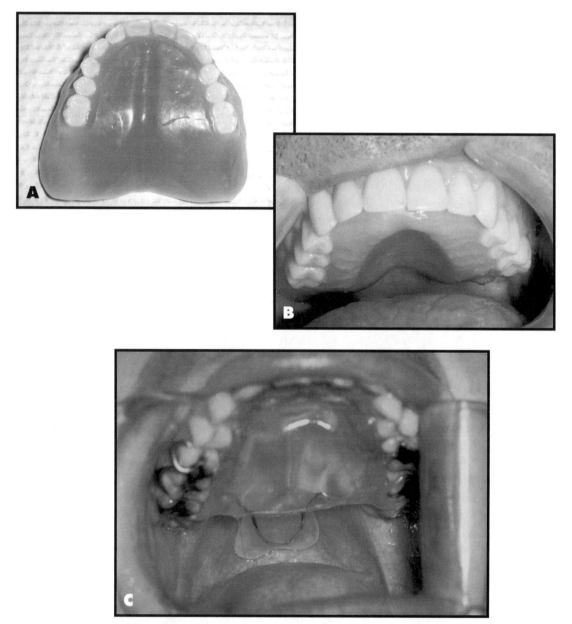

FIGURE 13.17. (A) Palatal drop appliance: Wax definition. (B) Palatal drop appliance in position. (C) Palatal drop appliance in conjunction with palatal lift appliance.

always anticipated. In addition, palatal drop prostheses may also be part of an obturator or soft palatal lift appliance (see Figure 13.17C). Obviously, attention to each component of these special appliances requires consistent recall and reevaluation for management of speech and swallowing difficulties (see Chapter 14 in this text).

DEFECT MANAGEMENT WITH IMPLANT-SUPPORTED PROSTHESES

Given the cautions noted earlier concerning instability of dental appliances for oral cancer defect management, it is important to note that osseointegrated dental implants have become a major technique for providing oral function in persons with appliance retention problems (Parel, Branemark, & Jansson, 1986a, 1986b). Osseointegrated dental implants (see Figure 13.18) are made of commercially pure titanium or a titanium alloy. The endosseous portion of the implant is cylindrical in shape, with screw threads or some other macroretentive feature, of various diameters and lengths. Classically, the implants are placed in the maxillary or mandibular bone in two surgical stages. The first stage is to raise a full thickness flap over the planned implant site. An osteotomy is prepared in the bone, sized for the particular implant to be used, through the use of three to four drills of incrementally larger diameter. Copious irrigation and light force are required to prevent overheating of the osseous tissue. The osteotomy is then tapped, creating threads that allow the implant to be threaded into place to achieve primary stability of the implant. A cover screw is placed on the exposed portion of the implant, and the flap is sutured in place. The implant is left to heal for 3 to 6 months to allow for proper integration. Osseointegration has occurred when there is "direct" bone contact with the implant, with the absence of any fibrous connective tissue. After the initial healing period, the second stage consists of uncovering the implant through the use of a flap or soft tissue punch and replacing the cover screw with an abutment that will penetrate through the overlying mucosa. After a brief period for soft tissue healing, fabrication of the prosthesis can be initiated utilizing the transmucosal abutments.

After preliminary impressions are made, a custom impression tray is constructed to carry the final impression material to the implant site. This final impression is made using special material to record the position of the abutments and surrounding tissue as accurately as possible. From the resulting master stone cast, a metal superstructure is made that will be used to retain the prosthesis. The final prosthesis will then be attached to the superstructure directly or designed as a removable or clip-on device. If rigidly attached, it will act as natural teeth and be cared for similar to normal dentition. If removable, it will have to be cared for like any other removable prosthesis (Anderson et al., 1992; Beumer et al., 1998; Leeper, Sills, & Charles, 1993).

Extraoral Implant Devices

Although a full discussion of extraoral implant devices is too extensive for the present context, it should be noted that osseointegrated implants are possible throughout the craniofacial area. Given the possibility that portions of the face, lip, nose, cheek, eye, and ear may be involved, and hence must be sacrificed surgically for treatment purposes, implants that aid in fixating prostheses to these

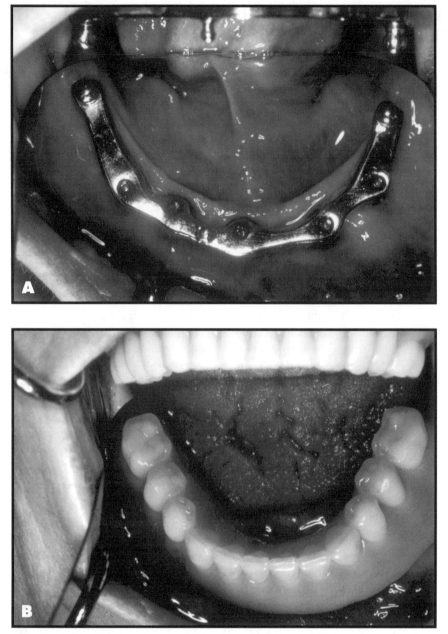

FIGURE 13.18. (A) Osseointegrated dental implants in mandible with bar attachment. (B) Implant with denture attached in place.

areas are important considerations (Anderson et al., 1992; Beumer et al., 1998). Planning for these extraoral devices commits the team of otolaryngology, maxillofacial, or plastic surgeons, as well as the prosthodontist and anaplastologist, to be involved in the plan of treatment. If the individual is to have a maxillary prosthesis in addition to a nose and eye prosthesis, it is important for each professional to know which component should be placed first, second, and third in the treatment plan. At each stage of treatment, the person and perhaps family members should be counseled by a psychologist or social worker concerning emotional issues. Speech pathology assessment and treatment should focus on eating, swallowing, and speech function at each stage of prosthodontic management.

COMMUNICATION REHABILITATION OF THE PROSTHETICALLY MANAGED INDIVIDUAL WITH ORAL CANCER

As another phase in the progression of treatment planning, a speech–language pathology consultation is an important part of the team approach because the maxillofacial patient is often left with serious communication and swallowing problems following surgery. Assessment of overall intelligibility and articulation, voice, and resonance abilities is necessary both before and after surgery.

Pre- and Postoperative Counseling for Communication Skills

Patients who undergo excision of a maxillary or mandibular oral tumor will profit from social and psychological counseling before, during, and after fitting of the oral dental obturator (Doyle, 1994; Kornblith et al., 1996). Kornblith et al. (1996) reported that the most significant predictor of the individual's adjustment and the perception of negative socioeconomic impact of cancer on his or her life was the "satisfactory functioning" (i.e., the "goodness of fit" for eating, swallowing, and speaking) of the obturator. Each session spent during the prosthodontic treatment phase is important in terms of dealing with the individual's feelings of satisfaction or lack thereof. It would seem that careful scrutiny of the patient's feelings, perhaps employing some standardized inventories or scales of social and psychological adjustment, would be beneficial (de Boer et al., 1995; Hassan & Weymuller, 1993; List et al., 1996; also see Chapter 28 in this text). In addition to counseling the patient, it is important to include the spouse, family, or caregivers in the various stages of prosthetic management (Doyle, 1994, 1999).

Oral Communication Assessment: Transdisciplinary Approaches

In addition to performing functional assessment of oral communication, speech–language pathologists, prosthodontists, and other members of the oral–maxillofacial health care team need to develop outcome measures. These measures are crucial because maxillofacial management requires several types of health care: surgery, radiotherapy, chemotherapy, dentistry, speech rehabilitation, and physical and occupational therapy. Furthermore, financial limitations imposed by the patient's personal finances or health insurance must be considered (Light, 1997).

Whereas surgery, radiation treatment, chemotherapy, and dental and prosthetic management are largely covered under many existing third-party payment systems, factors such as length of hospital stay, surgical and dental supplies, and loss of work for travel to receive treatment may not be covered. These issues need to be considered by the patient and other health care providers, who must rationalize costs and cost recovery for services provided. Thus, the restructuring of hospitals and "in-house" rehabilitation units, home care services, and other aspects of the health care system in North America (Moore, 1999) acknowledges that rehabilitation providers need to be "accountable" to the patient and to the various rehabilitative disciplines in order to justify reimbursement. Sharing reimbursement among health care providers (e.g., occupational therapy, physical therapy, neuropsychology) subsequently requires the speech–language pathologist, like the other health care providers, to justify his or her role in the rehabilitation of individuals receiving maxillofacial–prosthetic treatment.

The Speech–Language Pathologist's Role in Assessment

The role of the speech–language pathologist in the patient's evaluation process is focused on the estimation of speech disability accompanying maxillofacial defects. To provide the rehabilitation team with information concerning oral communication and related factors (e.g., swallowing, cosmesis, QOL issues), the speech–language assessment may employ perceptual, acoustical, and physiological measurement procedures related to overall communication skills. These evaluations include estimating the "normalcy" of articulation, voice quality, oral and nasopharyngeal resonance, articulation of specific speech sounds, and overall speech intelligibility (i.e., understandability).

Prior to assessment of speech production, the SLP needs to identify the individual's medical, psychological, social, and vocational–avocational characteristics. Case history information may lead to a more thorough understanding of the premorbid aspects of the patient's QOL (Doyle, 1994; see Chapter 28 in this text) and areas that may need special focus and attention postmanagement to achieve a more normal life. In addition, a detailed description of the anatomical site of the tumor should be noted and the defect classified for later comparative analysis purposes (Brown, Rogers, McNally, & Boyle, 2000; Spiro et al., 1997). One useful graphic descriptor of the oral–pharyngeal area has been developed by Jacobson, Franssen, Fliss, Birt, and Gilbert (1995). This "resection template" demarcates anatomic subsites for possible surgical excision in the oral and oropharyngeal cavities. Color coding and marking of 18 specific surgical areas allow for accurate detailing of site and extent of surgical excision for documentation and correlation with other physical and psychological factors that may influence functional outcomes.

Assessment of Oral-Motor and Communication Function

Systematic evaluation of the speech production mechanism involves assessment of each part of the vocal tract system (i.e., respiratory, laryngeal, velopharyngeal, and oral articulatory subsystems). Each may be evaluated individually with a variety of instrumental and perceptual techniques, but they are usually viewed in a holistic, interconnected, and coordinated fashion because speech is the result of movements and actions of a number of neuromuscular units. For example, information gained about articulatory precision in individuals with primary hard palate defects (e.g., oral–nasal fistulae resulting from partial surgical ablation) must be tempered with concerns about the effective airflow and acoustical tone through a potentially incompetent velopharyngeal mechanism (e.g., posterior defect of the soft tissue due to tissue shrinkage from radiation). Such considerations should be made before a decision is made about the primacy of articulation problems from anterior defects (the oral–nasal fistulae) on the distortion of overall speech performance (Leeper & Gratton, 1999; Leeper et al., 1993). One approach to speech management of oral–pharyngeal defects is based on a physiological model (Netsell & Daniel, 1979). As suggested by Netsell and Daniel, the goal of a physiological, acoustical, and perceptual evaluation of an individual's speech production mechanism is to determine the type and extent of disorder for each "valve" within the subsystem. This approach allows the speech–language pathologist to select and organize the management strategy based on knowledge of each component of the system. The functional components of the speech production system include the following: abdomen, diaphragm, rib cage (these components are considered the "chest wall" and provide the necessary aeromechanical driving force for speech and breathing), larynx, velopharyngeal port (velum, posterior pharyngeal wall, lateral pharyngeal walls), posterior aspects of tongue, anterior portions of tongue, mandible, and lips. Assessment of each of these components before and after prosthetic management is necessary to describe the efficiency of each component system and determine how each valve interacts with the others. A brief introduction to the assessment procedures employed by the speech–language pathologist when evaluating subsystems in patients with maxillofacial defects destined for prosthetic management is provided in the next subsections.

Respiratory Evaluation

Breath support is assessed to determine whether sufficient air is transported from the lungs through the larynx to the oral articulators to provide speech of reasonable loudness. Observation of chest wall activity during quiet breathing and during simple and complex speech acts allows for gross visual perception of the rate and excursion of respiratory activity. Some patients have respiratory irregularities or demonstrate reduced transglottal air pressure for phonation or impaired intraoral air pressure for certain consonant sounds (e.g., /p/). These respiratory issues may be due to advanced age, chronic pulmonary obstruction, or other breath support–limiting diseases (e.g., emphysema, asthma). Because those undergoing maxillofacial prosthetic treatment are at risk for loss of air pressure, they are usually referred to a pulmonary function laboratory in the hospital for standard spirometric evaluations (e.g., forced vital capacity [FVC], forced expiratory volume in 1 second [FEV1]). In addition, flow–volume loop characteristics are often collected (Leeper, Ahmad, Sills, & Gallie, 1989). Posttreatment, these measures are obtained with and without the prosthetic devices in place.

Another indirect method to assess respiratory support for phonation and speech is via measurement of subglottal air pressure (P_{sub}). Using electronic instrumentation, P_{sub} measures may be obtained (Holmes, Leeper, & Nicholson, 1994; Leeper & Graves, 1984; Warren, 1996; Wilson & Leeper, 1992) from the pressure and flow traces produced by measuring the peak intraoral air pressure output (as an estimate of alveolar air pressure) for repeated productions of a voiceless consonant (/p/) paired with a vowel. Patients with excessive air escape through oral or velopharyngeal defects that do not allow separation of the oral–nasal cavities will often overdrive the laryngeal system with higher than normal alveolar (lung) pressures. Hence, they show increased respiratory drive and rapidly deplete air volume. Differences in breath support with and without a temporary blockage of the oral–nasal defect may indicate potential for improvement in respiratory control for speech and breathing following prosthetic management.

It should be possible for the speech–language pathologist to indicate to the prosthodontist whether the individual obtaining treatment does or does not have the requisite breath support to produce words, short phrases, or sentences to communicate. If breath support is lacking, the speech–language pathologist should implement specific management procedures designed to increase depth of inhalation before speaking, sustain consistent breath output over the specific verbal duration, and develop strategies for the rapid and forceful inhalation of breath at certain word boundaries.

Intervention should be developed so that the individual using a dental obturator can obtain a minimum P_{sub} level of 3 cm H_2O for speech and sustain this level for at least 5 seconds. Specific techniques include (a) adjusting posture to enhance inhalatory and exhalatory strength, (b) binding the chest wall to maximize output levels, (c) learning the "feeling" of different levels of inhalation to support selected lengths of speech, (d) developing the proper chest wall shape (i.e., simultaneously adjusting rib cage and abdominal wall) for the most rapid adjustment of breath support for speech, and (e) improving the naturalness of speech phrasing using auditory or visual feedback about breathing pattern and speech quality (Leeper & Gratton, 1999; Yorkston, Beukelman, & Bell, 1988).

Phonatory Evaluation

As with the respiratory system, alterations in the oral–pharyngeal system can have "downstream" effects on how the vocal folds function as a voice source. Inability to rapidly adjust the muscles that attach to the larynx from above (e.g., stylohyoid, sternohyoid) may cause alterations in vocal frequency, intensity, and glottic closure and may further disrupt an already perturbed speech signal.

The phonatory system is initially evaluated at the perceptual level to determine whether pitch, loudness, vocal range, and quality are within normal limits for the individual's gender, age, and physical condition. Measurement of maximum phonation time for a vowel is used to relate respiratory capacity and glottal efficiency (Boone & McFarlane, 1988). Measures of laryngeal valving efficiency (laryngeal airway resistance) can also be assessed by recording intraoral air pressure as an estimate of P_{sub} (transglottal pressure) and transglottal airflow and considering the ratio of the two. Acoustical measures that correlate well with a listener's perception of vocal quality include average frequency, frequency range, and pitch variability (jitter), range of loudness (intensity measures) and loudness variability (shimmer), and signal-to-noise or harmonic-to-noise ratio (Leeper, Doyle, et al., 1993). These measures are noninvasive and may be obtained from acoustical recordings of sustained vowels or connected speech employing several types of commercial software packages during performance of gross maximal limits of voice production (Kent, Kent, & Rosenbek, 1987).

Assessment of the laryngeal subsystem should allow the speech–language pathologist to inform the prosthodontist about the efficiency of the respiratory and laryngeal subsystems for providing the necessary subglottal support for voicing of speech elements. The speaker must develop 3 cm H_2O of P_{sub} to generate voice, then have sufficient glottal closure to initiate and then sustain sound over 5 seconds. In addition, there should be enough flexibility to ensure pitch and loudness variability for expression of emphasis or meaning (e.g., contrastive stress).

A lack of any of these features means that the speech–language pathologist will need to use behavioral and prosthetic management methods to facilitate improved speech. Prosthetic management alone will be a primary factor by aiding in the development of sufficient upstream breath control (separation of nasal and oral cavities for added pneumatic strength). Pitch and loudness using biofeedback from instruments (e.g., computerized frequency–loudness systems) may improve phrasing and linguistic emphasis across various contexts (e.g., declarative, question statements). Voiced and voiceless distinctions may be improved by emphasizing increased intraoral breath pressure for voiceless elements, increasing duration of vowels before voiceless consonants, or using more forceful releases for voiceless consonants at the ends of words by employing biofeedback to improve overall intelligibility (Leeper & Gratton, 1999; Yorkston et al., 1988).

Resonatory Evaluation

Defects (both anterior and posterior) that affect velopharyngeal valving may cause intelligibility problems in the speech of individuals with orofacial deficits and may cause the listener to perceive deficits related to acoustical "damping" and a "muffled" voice (i.e., less intense oral output). Conversely, lack of normal nasal resonance on nasal sounds (/m/, /n/, /ng/) may cause the listener to perceive hyponasality (Sandor, Leeper, & Carmichael, 1997).

The least intrusive assessment approach is via listener judgments or psychophysical scaling of resonance balance. Such judgments serve as a pre–post clinical measure of speech change following prosthetic management and possibly the efficacy of intervention (Leeper, Sills, & Charles, 1993). Another less intrusive assessment tool, the Nasometer (by Kay Elemetrics, Lincoln Park, NJ), measures the ratio of acoustic nasal sound energy divided by the oral plus nasal sound energy (called "nasalance") during selected oral and nasal sound production. Nasalance values obtained from individuals undergoing prosthetic management may be compared to normative values (Seaver, Dalston, Leeper, & Adams, 1991).

Using commercially available pressure transducers, pneumotachographs, and computer acquisition hardware and software (Warren, 1979), measures of air pressure and airflow through the nose and mouth during speech production may be obtained (Leeper & Sills, 1986). The resultant pressure-flow signals can be applied for an estimation of opening (orifice area size) with and without the prosthesis (Warren & DuBois, 1964). Orifice area values above 20 mm^2 are generally considered problematic for velopharyngeal (VP) incompetence, whereas values less than approximately 20 mm^2 on nasal sounds (e.g., /m/) may relate to perception of speech as lacking appropriate nasal tone (i.e., hyponasal) (Warren, 1996). The same instrumentation may also be used to describe the nasal airway resistance during rest breathing. Measures of nasal airway resistance to the flow of air through that system are useful for describing alterations in the oropharyngeal airway before and following surgical or prosthetic management (Leeper & Gratton, 1999; Leeper, Janzen, Sills, Ahmad, & Seewald, 1994; Warren, Trier, & Bevin, 1974).

A more intrusive instrument for evaluation of the velopharyngeal port is a flexible fiberoptic nasendoscope (D'Antonio, Marsh, Province, Muntz, & Phillips, 1989) that allows direct optical viewing of the velopharyngeal mechanism and videorecording. Videonasendoscopy permits description of the movement of the velum and posterior pharyngeal wall and medialization of the lateral pharyngeal walls during speech and swallowing. The video may be synchronized with sound to document movement of the velopharyngeal mechanism during speech prior to and following prosthetic management, as well as for identifying the size, shape, and color of the tissues (Golding-Kushner, 1990).

The most invasive procedure available to describe the VP port mechanism is videofluoroscopy (Skolnick & Cohn, 1989). Videofluoroscopy of the velopharyngeal system is typically viewed separately by the dental oncology team (oral surgeon, prosthodontist, speech–language pathologist) for the same speech elements in a three-dimensional format (i.e., frontal, lateral, basal). The frontal view is useful for describing the height and movement of the lateral pharyngeal walls; the lateral view for detailing the lift, placement, and degree of closure of the velum (or its remnants) on the posterior pharyngeal wall; and the basal view for a three-dimensional image of the VP closure pattern during speech and swallowing, both prior to and following prosthetic management.

Pre- to postsurgery differences in resonance balance (normal, hypernasal, or hyponasal) that occur in relation to the management of the oropharyngeal defect should be assessed using a perceptual or instrumental approach. Information obtained from such assessment may provide valuable information to the speech–language pathologist, prosthodontist, and patient. With many assessment tools available, the speech–language pathologist will be able to indicate to the prosthodontist how much nasalization is present via perceptual, aerodynamic (VP orifice area), or acoustical (nasalance) measures; this information provides a measure of the separation between the oral and nasal passages and may be compared to nasendoscopy and videofluoroscopy evaluations. Such information may then be related to how nasalization affects overall speech intelligibility. Modifications of the interim and definitive prostheses by the prosthodontist should take into account the place and size of the defect that needs obturation or augmentation.

Treatment approaches by the speech–language pathologist following placement of a dental prosthesis may include (a) ensuring that both respiratory and laryngeal function are as efficient as possible, (b) increasing the precision of articulation (e.g., overarticulation of speech sounds), (c) increasing vocal intensity and effort to increase and direct vocal tone orally, (d) slowing the rate of articulation, and (e) increasing overall intelligibility by employing biofeedback of nasalization for selected high-frequency content words (Leeper & Gratton, 1999; Yorkston et al., 1988).

Oral Articulatory Evaluation

The effects on speech of the partial, subtotal, or total removal of the tongue or portions of the anterior maxilla or mandible may be devastating. With no or limited tongue mobility in the anterior oral cavity, eating, swallowing, and speech are often affected (Gillis & Leonard, 1983; Leonard & Gillis, 1982, 1990; Wheeler, Logemann, & Rosen, 1980).

The assessment of the articulatory aspects of speech is typically accomplished by employing perceptual and instrumental techniques. Articulation is rated either with formal inventories (e.g., *Templin–Darley Tests of Articulation*; Templin & Darley, 1969) or through informal assessments. Articulatory precision, speed and consistency of production, and stimulability are examined. As a more global description of articulation, a rating of proficiency using a 7-point equal-appearing interval scale or other types of scales (e.g., magnitude estimation, categorical) may be used to describe a combination of the parameters noted above. Finer details of consonant production may be conducted using one of several types of intelligibility tests initially designed for neurogenic dysarthrias of speech, but directly applicable to peripheral dysarthrias in persons having ablative surgery and subsequent prosthetic management (Kent, Weismer, Kent, & Rosenbek, 1989; Yorkston, & Beukelman, 1981; Yorkston, Beukelman, & Traynor, 1984). In addition, acoustic analyses (formant frequency, amplitude, and spectral moments) of certain vowels or consonants, either alone or in combination, have been used in relation to perceptual judgments of speech (Doyle, Leeper, Houghton-Jones, Heeneman, & Martin, 1996; Duncan, Leeper, & Gratton, 2000; Gillis & Leonard, 1983; Leonard & Gillis, 1982; Tobey & Lincks, 1989).

Another portion of the oral articulatory assessment involves the aeromechanical evaluation of oral port size (tongue–hard palate valving) (Warren & DuBois, 1964). The difference in technique from assessing the velopharyngeal port is that a mask covers the mouth rather than the nose. Differential pressure sensors are then placed in front of and behind the articulatory constriction (e.g., the tongue dorsum for /s/) for data collection prior to and following placement of an oral dental appliance.

The assessment component for oral articulation must be related to the prosthodontist and team members by the speech–language pathologist to answer these general queries: Is there an oral articulatory problem? How severe is the problem (to professional and patient)? How is severity of this subsystem compared to the others examined? Which, if any, subsystem has primacy over the other (in terms of severity) for management?

Management of oral articulatory problems should focus on therapy features. These include (a) improving place and manner of articulation through direct drills, (b) developing compensatory strategies for correct articulation when related structures have been ablated or modified, (c) increasing the opportunity for "contrastive" drills (e.g., *p*in vs. *b*in) to improve voicing contrasts or plosive requirements, (d) intelligibility drills to aid in compensatory articulation for the most "understandable" sound, (e) decreasing speech rate to aid in the compensatory aspects of articulation and improve intelligibility, and (f) assessing all articulatory features following any substantial modifications to the appliance or following subsequent surgeries (see Figure 13.1) (Leeper & Gratton, 1999; Yorkston et al., 1988).

Swallowing Evaluation

Many individuals with oral cancer demonstrate masticatory and swallowing difficulties, in addition to speech problems, following oral–maxillofacial surgery (DeNittis et al., 2001; Eisbruch et al., 2002; Haribhakti, Kavarana, & Tibrewala, 1993; Mady et al., 2003; Pauloski et al., 1993; Pauloski et al., 1994; Robbins, Bowman, & Jacob, 1987; Shimodaira et al., 1998; Wedel, Yontchev, Carlsson, & Ow, 1994; Wheeler et al., 1980). Physical and functional assessment and long-term follow-up with the obturator and subsequent modification of these dental appliances on swallowing should follow current standards of practice for management (Logemann, 1983, 1988). Further information concerning assessment and management of individuals with oral–maxillary prostheses is provided in Chapter 14 in this text.

POTENTIAL OUTCOME MEASURES OF COMMUNICATION SKILLS DURING REHABILITATION OF INDIVIDUALS WITH ORAL CANCER UNDERGOING PROSTHODONTIC MANAGEMENT

Measurement of outcomes following surgical resection, radiotherapy, and dental obturation of oral defects secondary to oral cancer is necessary for continuing management. It is also important that refinement of protocols and further research into the effectiveness of such protocols for certain clinical groups take place. As noted earlier, describing the effectiveness of certain management programs is essential in terms of the cost of treatment, the number of individuals needing management, and the effect on individuals' long-term lifestyle and everyday functioning. In additon, the overall effectiveness of each treatment plan can be evaluated. Pope and Tarlov (1991) described one model for evaluating outcomes in *Disability in America: Toward a National Agenda for Prevention*. In this document, four levels of assessment are recommended: (a) pathology—the cellular or tissue level of the disease; (b) impairment—the impact of the disease on each of several subsystems serving speech and swallowing; (c) function limitations—the individual's ability to perform certain daily tasks such as talking, eating, and swallowing; and (d) disability—the psychosocial level of the disease or disorder, including how the individual interacts with friends and family and is accepted or discriminated against at home, work, or leisure.

Mahanna, Beukelman, Marshall, Gaebler, and Sullivan (1998) reported their protocol for serving the four areas outlined above. To evaluate each area, the authors included in their assessment protocol the following items: (a) *pathology/ tissue level*—visual description and palpation of soft tissue irritation via prosthetics, and presence or absence of infection of the surgical site; (b) *impairment level*—evaluation of speech performance, including perceptual scaling of hyper-hyponasality, and aerodynamic studies of appropriate separation of the oral–nasal and pharyngeal components of speech; (c) *functional limitations*—computerized measures of speech intelligibility and rate of speech; and (d) *disability*—assessment via a Communication Effectiveness Index (Lomas et al., 1989), a self-administered visual analog scale to rate the patient's ability to communicate effectively before and following prosthodontic management of the oral defect. Mahanna et al. suggested that this approach to documenting outcomes at several physical, psychological, and social–societal levels is important for evaluating the effectiveness of obturator prosthetic treatments for individuals with oral cancers.

A similar approach was suggested by Light (1997), who surveyed speech–language pathologists and members of other rehabilitation disciplines who treat patients with oral cancers. Light suggested eight categories of functional assessment for evaluation of oral cancer patients needing maxillofacial prosthodontics. The categories included (a) total body function, including an oral–motor component; (b) oral–motor functional mechanisms; (c) speech intelligibility or articulation tests; (d) nasal emission tests; (e) swallowing assessment, including oral preparatory and transit phase times; (f) muscle movement, including nonspeech oral–motor maneuvers; (g) assessment of drooling; and (h) patient self-assessment of function status and improvement.

No matter which assessment tools are used pre- or postoperatively, it is important that some reliable and valid method of assessment be made across Pope and Tarlov's (1991) four levels of outcome assessment. Both perceptual and physical measures should be made at each time of obturator fitting (i.e., surgical splint, temporary, definitive), and changes in physical and psychosocial outcomes should be noted (Wolff et al., 2004). Modification of any protocol should occur when any one of the assessment tools fails to meet strict guidelines for validity and reliability of test instruments. Such modifications help the clinician meet the requirements of reduced cost to the health care system, improved strategies for training patients for prosthodontic care, and documenting the effectiveness of prosthodontic care (Leeper & Gratton, 1999).

SUMMARY

This chapter has addressed general dental issues, oral surgery, and prosthodontic and speech management of individuals with orofacial cancer who require maxillofacial rehabilitation. Current methods of assessment and management from a transdisciplinary approach have been described. Assessment of the respiratory, laryngeal, velopharyngeal, and oral articulatory systems prior to and following oral surgery, radiotherapy, or chemotherapy, and prosthodontics has been presented. Successful rehabilitation of patients with orofacial defects secondary to cancer demands a team of professionals, expert at each stage of surgical, dental, speech, and psychosocial care. In addition to the direct methods of dental, surgical, and prosthetic management described, techniques for documenting outcomes of management of oral cancer from prosthetic and communication viewpoints were addressed. These techniques will aid the rehabilitation team in documenting success for the rationalization of cost of care of their patients for their team approach to prosthetic management for oral cancer.

REFERENCES

Adisman, I. (1990). Prosthesis serviceability for acquired jaw defects. *Dental Clinics of North America, 34,* 265–284.

Anderson, J. D., Awde, J. D., Leeper, H. A., & Sills, P. S. (1992). Prosthetic management of the head and neck cancer patient. *The Canadian Journal of Oncology, 2*(3), 110–118.

Aramany, M. A., Downs, J. A., Beery, Q. C., & Aslan, F. (1982). Prosthodontic rehabilitation for glossectomy patients. *Journal of Prosthetic Dentistry, 48,* 78–81.

Balogh, J., & Sutherland, S. (1983). Osteoradionecrosis of the mandible: A review. *American Journal of Otolaryngology, 13,* 82.

Batsakis, J. G. (1979). Squamous cell carcinomas of the oral cavity and the oropharynx. In J. G. Batsakis (Ed.), *Tumors of the head and neck: Clinical and pathological considerations* (2nd ed.). Baltimore: Williams and Wilkins.

Beumer, J., Curtis, T. A., & Firtell, D. N. (1979). *Maxillofacial rehabilitation: Prosthodontic and surgical considerations.* St. Louis, MO: Mosby.

Beumer, J., Curtis, T., & Marunick, M. (1996). *Maxillofacial rehabilitation: Prosthodontic and surgical considerations.* St. Louis: Ishiyaki EuroAmerica.

Beumer, J., DePaola, L. G., & Leupold, R. J. (1986). Prosthetic management. In D. E. Peterson, E. G. Elias, & S. T. Sonis (Eds.), *Head and neck management of the cancer patient* (pp. 453–478). Boston: Martinus Nijhoff.

Beumer, J., Zlotolow, I., & Sharma, A. (1998). Restoration of palate, tongue–mandible, and facial defects. In S. Silverman (Ed.), *Oral cancer* (pp. 75–89). Hamilton: B.C. Decker.

Boone, D. R., & McFarlane, S. C. (1988). *The voice and voice disorders* (4th ed.). Englewood Cliffs: Prentice Hall.

Brown, J. S., Rogers, S. N., McNally, D. N., & Boyle, M. (2000). A modified classification for the maxillectomy defect. *Head & Neck, 22,* 17–26.

Cancer Care Ontario. (1999). *Ontario cancer registry.* Retrieved from www.cancercare.on.ca

Cann, C. I., Fried, M. P., & Rothman, K. J. (1985). Epidemiology of squamous cell cancer of the head and neck. *The Otolaryngologic Clinics of North America, 18,* 367–388.

D'Antonio, L. L., Marsh, J. L., Province, M. A., Muntz, H. R., & Phillips, C. J. (1989). Reliability of flexible nasopharyngoscopy for evaluation of velopharyngeal function in a clinical population. *Cleft Palate Journal, 26,* 217–224.

Davis, R. K. (1985). Prognostic variables in head and neck cancer. *The Otolaryngologic Clinics of North America, 18*(3), 411.

de Boer, M. F., Pruyn, J. F. A., van den Borne, B., Knegt, P. P., Ryckman, R. M., & Verwoerd, C. D. A. (1995). Rehabilitation outcomes of long-term survivors treated for head and neck cancer. *Head & Neck, 17,* 503–515.

Dempsey, J., Hynes, N., Smith, T., & Sproat, J. E. (1997). Cost effectiveness analysis of hyperbaric therapy in osteoradionecrosis. *Canadian Journal of Plastic Surgery, 5,* 221–229.

DeNittis, A. S., Machtay, M., Rosenthal, D. I., Sanfilippo, N. J., Lee, J. H., Goldfeder, S., Chalian, A. A., Weinstein, G. S., & Weber, R. S. (2001). Advanced oropharyngeal carcinoma treated with surgery and radiotherapy: Oncologic outcome and functional assessment. *American Journal of Otolaryngology, 22*(5), 329–335.

Desjardins, R. P. (1977). Early rehabilitative management of the maxillectomy patient. *Journal of Prosthetic Dentistry, 38,* 311–318.

Desjardins, R. P. (1978). Obturator design for acquired maxillary defects. *Journal of Prosthetic Dentistry, 39,* 424–435.

Doyle, P. C. (1994). *Foundations of voice and speech rehabilitation following laryngeal cancer* (pp. 97–122). San Diego: Singular.

Doyle, P. C. (1999). Postlaryngectomy speech rehabilitation: Contemporary concerns in clinical care. *Journal of Speech–Language Pathology and Audiology, 23,* 109–116.

Doyle, P. C. , Leeper, H. A., Houghton-Jones, C., Heeneman, H., & Martin, G. F. (1996). Perceptual characteristics of hemilaryngectomized and near-total laryngectomized male speakers. *Journal of Medical Speech–Language Pathology, 3,* 131–143.

Duncan, P., Leeper, H. A., & Gratton, D. (2000, November). *Fricative production in patients with oral cancer managed prosthetically.* Paper presented at the American Speech-Language-Hearing Association Annual Convention, Washington, DC.

Eisbruch, A., Lyden, T., Bradford, C. R., Dawson, L. A., Haxer, M. J., Miller, A. E., Teknos, T. N., Chepeha, D. B., Hogikyan, N. D., Terrell, J. E., & Wolf, G. T. (2002). Objective assessment of swallowing dysfunction and aspiration after radiation concurrent with chemotherapy for head–neck cancer. *International Journal of Radiation Oncology and Biological Physics, 53,* 23–28.

Elwood, J. M., & Gallagher, R. P. (1985). Factors influencing early diagnosis of cancer of the oral cavity. *Canadian Medical Association Journal, 33,* 651.

Franceschi, S., Bidoli, E., Herrero, R., & Munoz, N. (2000). Comparison of cancers of the oral cavity and pharynx worldwide: Etiological clues. *Oral Oncology, 36,* 106–115.

Gillis, R. E., & Leonard, R. J. (1983). Prosthetic treatment for speech and swallowing in patients with total glossectomy. *Journal of Prosthetic Dentistry, 50,* 808–814.

Golding-Kushner, K. J. (1990). Standardization for the reporting of nasopharyngoscopy and multiview videostroboscopy: A report from an international working group. *Cleft Palate Journal, 27,* 337–347.

Gussack, G. S., Brantley, B. A., & Farmer, J. C. (1984). Biology of tumors and head and cancer chemotherapy. *Laryngoscope, 94,* 1181–1187.

Hardie, J. (1987). Oral submucous fibrosis: A review with case reports. *Journal of the Canadian Dental Association, 5,* 391.

Haribhakti, V., Kavarana, N., & Tibrewala, A. (1993). Oral cavity reconstruction: An objective assessment of function. *Head & Neck, 15,* 119–124.

Hassan, S. J., & Weymuller, E. A. (1993). Assessment of quality of life in head and neck cancer patients. *Head & Neck, 15,* 485–496.

Hermanek, P., Hutter, R. V. P., Sobin, L. H., Wagner, G., & Wittekind, C. (1997). *TNM classification of malignant tumors* (4th ed.). Indianapolis, IN: Wiley.

Ho, T., Zahurak, M., & Koch, W. M. (2004). Prognostic significance of presentation-to-diagnosis interval in patients with oropharyngeal carcinoma. *Archives of Otolaryngology—Head and Neck Surgery, 130,* 45–51.

Holmes, L., Leeper, H. A., & Nicholson, I. (1994). Laryngeal airway resistance of older men and women as a function of vocal sound pressure level. *Journal of Speech and Hearing Research, 37,* 789–799.

Jacobson, M. C., Franssen, E., Fliss, D. M., Birt, B. D., & Gilbert, R. W. (1995). Free forearm flap in oral reconstruction: Functional outcome. *Archives of Otolaryngology—Head Neck Surgery, 121,* 959–964.

Jesse, R. H. (1978). Oral cancer. *American Cancer Society Monograph.* Reviewed in *Selected Readings in General Surgery, 10*(1), 3.

Kent, R. D., Kent, J. F., & Rosenbek, J. C. (1987). Maximum performance tests of speech production. *Journal of Speech and Hearing Disorders, 52,* 367–387.

Kent, R. D., Weismer, G., Kent, J. F., & Rosenbek, J. C. (1989). Toward phonetic intelligibility testing in dysarthria. *Journal of Speech and Hearing Disorders, 54,* 482–499.

Kornblith, A. B., Zlotolow, I. M., Gooen, J., Huryn, J. M., Lerner, T., Strong, E. W., Shah, J. P., Spiro, R. H., & Holland, J. C. (1996). Quality of life of maxillectomy patients using an obturator prosthesis. *Head & Neck, 18,* 323–334.

Lapointe, H. J., Lampe, H. B., & Taylor, S. M. (1996). Comparison of maxillectomy patients with immediate versus delayed obturator prosthesis placement. *Journal of Otolaryngology, 25*(5), 308–312.

Lauciello, F. R., Vergo, T., Schaaf, N. G., & Zimmerman, R. (1980). Prosthodontic and speech rehabilitation after partial and complete glossectomy. *Journal of Prosthetic Dentistry, 43,* 204–211.

Leeper, H. A., Ahmad, D., Sills, P. S., & Gallie, A. (1989). Pulmonary function characteristics of selected individuals with dysarthria: The effects of a palatal lift appliance. *Journal of Speech–Language Pathology and Audiology, 13,* 57–62.

Leeper, H. A., Doyle, P. C., Heeneman, H., Martin, G. F., Hoasjoe, D. K., & Wong, F. S. (1993). Acoustical characteristics of voice following hemilaryngectomy and near-total laryngectomy. *Journal of Medical Speech–Language Pathology, 1,* 89–94.

Leeper, H. A., & Gratton, D. G. (1999). Oral prosthetic rehabilitation of individuals with head and neck cancer: A review of current practice. *Journal of Speech–Language Pathology and Audiology, 23,* 117–133.

Leeper, H. A., & Graves, D. K. (1984). Consistency of laryngeal airway resistance in adult women. *Journal of Communication Disorders, 17,* 153–163.

Leeper, H. A., Janzen, V., Sills, P. S., Ahmad, D., & Seewald, C. (1994). Technique for assessing nasal airway resistance in patients treated prosthetically. *Journal of Prosthetic Dentistry, 72,* 210–216.

Leeper, H. A., & Sills, P. S. (1986). Prosthetic and speech management of patients with velopharyngeal incompetence. *Human Communication Canada, 10,* 5–20.

Leeper, H. A., Sills, P. S., & Charles, D. (1993). Prosthodontic management of maxillofacial and palatal defects. In K. T. Moller & C. D. Starr (Eds.), *Cleft palate: Interdisciplinary issues and treatment* (p. 145–188). Austin, TX: PRO-ED.

Leonard, R. J., & Gillis, R. E. (1982). Effects of a prosthetic tongue on vowel intelligibility and food management in a patient with total glossectomy. *Journal of Speech and Hearing Disorders, 47,* 25–29.

Leonard, R. J., & Gillis, R. E. (1990). Differential effects of speech prostheses in glossectomized patients. *Journal of Prosthetic Dentistry, 64,* 701–708.

Light, J. (1997). Functional assessment testing for maxillofacial prosthetics. *Journal of Prosthetic Dentistry, 77,* 388–393.

List, M. A., Ritter-Sterr, C. A, Baker, T. M., Colangelo, L. A., Matz, G., Pauloski, B. R., & Logemann, J. A. (1996). Longitudinal assessments of quality of life in laryngeal cancer patients. *Head & Neck, 18,* 1–10.

Logemann, J. A. (1983). *Evaluation and treatment of swallowing disorders.* San Diego: College-Hill Press.

Logemann, J. A. (1988). Swallowing physiology and pathophysiology. *Otolaryngology Clinics of North America, 21,* 613–623.

Logemann, J. A., Kahrilas, P. J., Hurst, P., Davis, J., & Krugler, C. (1989). Effects of intraoral prosthetics on swallowing in patients with oral cancer. *Dysphagia, 4,* 118–120.

Lomas, J., Pickard, L., Bester, S., Elbard, H., Finlayson, A., & Zoghaib, C. (1989). The Communication Effectiveness Index: Development and psychometric evaluation of functional communication measures for adult aphasia. *Journal of Speech and Hearing Research, 54,* 113–123.

Mady, K., Sader, R., Hoole, P. H., Zimmermann, A., & Horch, H. H. (2003). Speech evaluation and swallowing ability after intra-oral cancer. *Clinical Linguistics and Phonetics, 17,* 411–420.

Mahanna, G. K., Beukelman, D. R., Marshall, J. A., Gaebler, C. A., & Sullivan, M. (1998). Obturator prostheses after cancer surgery: An approach to speech outcome assessment. *Journal of Prosthetic Dentistry, 79,* 310–316.

Marx, R. E. (1983a). A new concept in the treatment of osteoradionecrosis. *Journal of Oral and Maxillofacial Surgery, 41,* 351–357.

Marx, R. E. (1983b). Osteoradionecrosis: A new concept of its pathophysiology. *Journal of Oral and Maxillofacial Surgery, 41,* 283–288.

Marx, R. E., Johnson, R. P., & Kline, S. N. (1985). Prevention of osteoradionecrosis: A randomized prospective clinical trial of hyperbaric oxygen vs. penicillin. *Journal of the American Dental Association, 111,* 49–54.

Moore, M. (1999). The human cost of Medicare reform. *ASHA Leader, 4*(14), 1–5.

Netsell, R., & Daniel, B. (1979). Dysarthria in adults: Physiologic approach to rehabilitation. *Archives of Physical Medicine and Rehabilitation, 60,* 502–508.

Parel, S. M., Branemark, P.-I., & Jansson, T. (1986a). Osseointegration in maxillofacial prosthetics: Part I. Intraoral applications. *Journal of Prosthetic Dentistry, 55,* 490–494.

Parel, S. M., Branemark, P.-I., & Jansson, T. (1986b). Osseointegration in maxillofacial prosthetics: Part II. Extraoral applications. *Journal of Prosthetic Dentistry, 55,* 600–606.

Parker, S., Tong, T., & Bolden, S. (1997). Cancer statistics, 1997. *California Cancer Journal Clinics, 47,* 3–26.

Pauloski, B., Logemann, J., Rademaker, A., McConnel, F., Heiser, M., Cardinale, S., Shedd, D., Lewin, J., Baker, S., Graner, D., Cook, B., Milianti, F., Collins, S., & Baker, T. (1993). Speech and swallowing function after anterior tongue and floor of mouth resection with distal flap reconstruction. *Journal of Speech and Hearing Research, 36,* 267–276.

Pauloski, B., Logemann, J., Rademaker, A., McConnel, F., Stein, D., Beery, Q., Johnson, J., Heiser, M., Collins, S., & Baker, T. (1994). Speech and swallowing function after oral and oropharyngeal resections: One-year follow-up. *Head & Neck, 16,* 313–322.

Peterson, L. J., Ellis, E., III, Hupp, J. R., & Tucker, M. R. (Eds.). (1998). *Contemporary oral and maxillofacial surgery.* St. Louis, MO: Mosby.

Pope, A., & Tarlov, A. (1991). *Disability in America: Toward a national agenda for prevention* (Executive Summary, pp. 1–31). Washington, DC: National Academy Press.

Robbins, K., Bowman, J., & Jacob, R. (1987). Postglossectomy deglutitory and articulatory rehabilitation with palatal augmentation prosthesis. *Archives of Otolaryngology—Head and Neck Surgery, 113,* 1214–1218.

Sandor, G. K. B., Leeper, H. A., & Carmichael, R. P. (1997). Speech and velopharyngeal function. *Oral and Maxillofacial Surgery Clinics of North America, 9,* 147–165.

Seaver, E. J., Dalston, R. M., Leeper, H. A., & Adams, L. E. (1991). A study of nasometric values for normal nasal resonance. *Journal of Speech and Hearing Research, 34,* 715–721.

Shafer, W. G., Hine, M. K., & Levy, B. M. (1983). *A textbook of oral pathology* (4th ed.). Philadelphia: Saunders.

Shimodaira, K., Yoshida, H., Yusa, H., & Kanazawa, T. (1998). Palatal augmentation prosthesis with alternative palatal vaults for speech and swallowing: A clinical report. *Journal of Prosthetic Dentistry, 80,* 1–3.

Silverman, S. (1998). *Oral cancer* (4th ed.). Hamilton, Ontario, Canada: Decker.

Singer, M., Phillips, T., Kramer, A., & Fu, K. (1998). Treatment. In S. Silverman (Ed.), *Oral cancer* (pp. 75–89). Hamilton, Ontario, Canada: Decker.

Skolnick, M. L., & Cohn, E. R. (1989). *Videofluoroscopic studies of speech in patients with cleft palate.* New York: Springer-Verlag.

Spiro, R. H., Strong, E. W., & Shah, J. P. (1997). Maxillectomy and its classification. *Head and Neck, 19,* 309–314.

Stecht, P. (2004). Oral complications in the head and neck radiation patient: Introduction and scope of the problem. *Supportive Care in Cancer, 10,* 36–39.

Stokman, M. A., Spijkervet, F. K., Burlage, F. R., Dijkstra, P. U., Manson, W. L., de Vries, E. G., & Roodenburg, J. L. (2003). Oral mucositis and selective elimination of oral flora in head and neck cancer patients receiving radiotherapy: A double-blind randomised clinical trial. *British Journal of Cancer, 88,* 1012–1016.

Templin, M., & Darley, F. (1969). *Templin–Darley Tests of Articulation.* Oakdale: University of Iowa.

Theurer, J. A., & Martin, R. E. (2003). Effects of oral cancer treatment: Speech, swallowing, and quality of life outcomes. *Journal of Speech–Language Pathology and Audiology, 27,* 190–201.

Thorn, J. J., Hansen, H. S., Specht, L., & Bastholt, L. (2000). Osteoradionecrosis of the jaws: Clinical characteristics and relation to the field of irradiation. *Journal of Oral and Maxillofacial Surgery, 58*(10), 1088–1093.

Tiecke, R. W. (1965). *Oral pathology.* New York: McGraw-Hill.

Tobey, E. A., & Lincks, J. (1989). Acoustic analyses of speech changes after maxillectomy and prosthodontic management. *Journal of Prosthetic Dentistry, 62,* 449–455.

Warren, D. W. (1979). PERCI: A method for rating palatal efficiency. *Cleft Palate Journal, 16,* 279–285.

Warren, D. W. (1996). Regulation of speech aerodynamics. In N.J. Lass (Ed.), *Principles of experimental phonetics* (p. 46–92). St. Louis, MO: Mosby-Year Book.

Warren, D. W., & DuBois, A. B. (1964). A pressure-flow technique for measuring velopharyngeal orifice area during spontaneous speech. *Cleft Palate Journal, 1,* 52–71.

Warren, D. W., Trier, W. C., & Bevin, A. G. (1974). Effect of restorative procedures on the nasopharyngeal airway in cleft palate. *Cleft Palate Journal, 11,* 367–373.

Wedel, A., Yontchev, E., Carlsson, G., & Ow, R. (1994). Masticatory function in patients with congenital and acquired maxillofacial defects. *Journal of Prosthetic Dentistry, 72,* 303–308.

Wheeler, R. L., Logemann, J. A., & Rosen, M. S. (1980). Maxillary reshaping prosthesis: Effectiveness in improving speech and swallowing of postsurgical oral cancer patients. *Journal of Prosthetic Dentistry, 43,* 313–319.

Wilson, J.V., & Leeper, H. A. (1992). Changes in laryngeal airway resistance in young adult men and women as a function of vocal sound pressure level and syllable context. *Journal of Voice, 6,* 235–245.

Wolff, T. J., Leeper, H. A., Gratton, D. G., & Doyle, P. C. (2004). The Psychosocial Aspects of Prosthetic Use Scale (PAPUS): Preliminary data. *Journal of Speech–Language Pathology and Audiology, 28,* 34–42.

Wright, J. M., O'Brien, J. C., Lieberman, Z. H., Bradfield, J. S., & Mennel, R. G. (1988). Treatment of oral cancer. In B. A. Wright, J. M. Wright, & W. H. Binnie (Eds.), *Oral cancer: Clinical and pathological considerations.* Boca Raton, FL: CRC Press.

Yorkston, K. M., & Beukelman, D. R. (1981). *Manual of the assessment of intelligibility of dysarthric speech.* Austin, TX: PRO-ED.

Yorkston, K. M., Beukelman, D. R., & Bell, K. R. (1988). *Clinical management of dysarthric speakers* (pp. 208–325). Boston: College-Hill.

Yorkston, K. M., Beukelman, D. R., & Traynor, C. D. (1984). *Computerized assessment of intelligibility of dysarthric speech.* Tigard, OR: C. C. Publications.

Zelefsky, M. J., Gaynor, J., Kraus, D., Strong, E. W., Shah, J. P., & Harrison, L. B. (1996). Long-term subjective functional outcome of surgery plus postoperative radiotherapy for advanced stage oral cavity and oropharyngeal carcinoma. *American Journal of Surgery, 171,* 258–262.

Chapter 14

Management of Swallowing Disorders in Individuals with Head and Neck Cancer

Cathy L. Lazarus

The treatment of head and neck cancer can result in a variety of changes, including those affecting voice, speech, swallowing, respiration, and appearance (Conley, 1962; Dejonckere & Hordijk, 1998; Lazarus, 1998; Logemann, 1985; McConnel, 1988; Sessions, Stallings, Brownson, & Ogura, 1973; Staple & Ogura, 1966). Management of these problems requires a team effort by professionals who typically include the surgeon, radiation oncologist, medical oncologist, speech–language pathologist, radiologist, maxillofacial prosthodontist, gastroenterologist, social worker (or psychiatrist), physical therapist, and oncology nurse. The speech–language pathologist and maxillofacial prosthodontist work fairly closely to rehabilitate speech and swallowing in those individuals diagnosed with head and neck cancer. The purpose of this chapter is to review management of swallowing disorders in the patient with head and neck cancer. This includes the normal timing, sequence, and types of interventions to improve swallow functioning.

PRETREATMENT REHABILITATION CONSIDERATIONS

To effectively rehabilitate swallowing in individuals with head and neck cancer, the speech–language pathologist must be part of the team that makes decisions about treatment. These decisions include the type of treatment, the schedule of treatment, and the timing of intervention. When an individual is newly diagnosed with head and neck cancer, his or her case is typically brought to a team, whose members review information such as findings on clinical examination, tumor histopathology, and tumor description by computerized tomographic (CT) imaging or magnetic resonance imaging (MRI). Based on this information, the tumor is then staged based on tumor site, size, histology, and degree of invasion into adjacent structures. Staging ranges from I to IV, with Stage IV tumors being larger and more invasive than lower stage tumors (American Joint Committee on Cancer, 1997; see also Chapter 13 in this text). The team discusses the individual's medical condition, as well as psychosocial and communication needs. The team then makes recommendations regarding treatment, taking into consideration the various factors, particularly tumor location, staging, and extent of disease. For example, tumor size and depth of invasion into adjacent structures may preclude surgery as an option. However, surgery may be the treatment of choice for smaller or less invasive tumors.

When surgical treatment is an option, the team considers how a particular surgery might affect swallowing (as well as voice and speech), because the extent of surgical resection and the type of surgical reconstruction can have an impact on swallow functioning (Colangelo, Logemann, & Rademaker, 2000; Jenkins, Lazarus, & Logemann, 1981; Lazarus, Logemann, Jenkins, & Ossoff, 1981; Logemann, 1984; McConnel et al., 1998). If, for example, a patient has a supraglottic tumor that extends laterally to the pharyngeal wall, surgery would likely require a supraglottic laryngectomy and partial lateral pharyngeal wall resection (see Chapter 11 in this text). The surgical inclusion of the lateral pharyngeal wall might interfere with bolus (food or liquid) clearance through the pharynx, because pharyngeal contraction might be compromised. If a partial laryngectomy procedure will result in reduced laryngeal elevation, or compromised supraglottic and glottic closure (see Chapter 11), swallowing will likely be affected (Jenkins et al., 1981; Lazarus et al., 1981; Logemann, 1984; Robb & Lewin, 2003; Samlan & Webster, 2002). For individuals with oral and oropharyngeal cancer, the surgeon must consider the amount of lingual tissue likely to remain after surgery; the amount of lingual tissue and lingual range of motion will have an effect on the individual's ability to chew and form a bolus, hold the bolus of food or liquid in the mouth, propel this bolus into the pharynx, and ultimately clear the bolus through the upper pharynx (Eisbruch et al., 2002; Graner et al., 2003; McConnel et al., 1994; McConnel et al., 1998; see also Chapters 8 and 13 in this text).

When surgery is not an option and organ preservation protocols of radiotherapy with or without chemotherapy are indicated, an individual's medical condition must be considered, because toxicity and side effects from chemotherapy such as immunosuppression can be severe and life threatening (Pfister et al., 1994; Vokes et al., 1995; see also Chapter 10 in this text). In addition, radiotherapy can result in mucositis and xerostomia (Peters et al., 1988), both of which can have a negative impact on swallowing.

Individuals about to undergo radiotherapy (either as primary cancer treatment or following surgery) are typically seen pretreatment (or presurgery) for a dental evaluation by the maxillofacial prosthodontist. Pretreatment dental extractions may be needed to lower the risk of postradiation damage to the teeth and bone and may also prevent osteoradionecrosis. Individuals about to undergo oral cancer resections are also typically seen pretreatment by the maxillofacial prosthodontist (see Chapter 13 in this text). The prosthodontist assesses the individual's dental condition, particularly if that individual is to undergo postoperative radiotherapy, to determine if any teeth require extraction. The prosthodontist also assesses dentition to determine whether some teeth can be salvaged to act as an anchor for a palatal lowering (augmentation) prosthesis, which can improve swallowing (and speech) following partial tongue resection (Cantor, Curtis, Shipp, Beumer, & Vogel, 1969; J. W. Davis, Lazarus, Logemann, & Hurst, 1987; Leonard & Gillis, 1990; K. T. Robbins, Bowman, & Jacob, 1987; Skoner et al., 2003; Wheeler, Logemann, & Rosen, 1980). Construction of this prosthesis requires collaboration between the prosthodontist and speech–language pathologist (see Chapter 13 in this text).

PRETREATMENT COUNSELING

Once the treatment type and schedule have been decided, individuals with head and neck cancer and significant others are seen by the speech–language pathologist for pretreatment counseling (see Chapter 15 in this text). Counseling is designed to (a) inform the individual about the types of swallowing problems he or she may experience during or after treatment; (b) discuss the role of the team members, particularly that of the speech–language pathologist, in the individual's swallowing rehabilitation; and (c) discuss the role of the individual and family members in the rehabilitation process. Counseling is designed to let the individual know that he or she will be followed during and after treatment, as needed, for rehabilitation of swallowing. This knowledge typically reduces the person's anxiety level, resulting in improved compliance with posttreatment swallow therapy. Pretreatment counseling also communicates that the individual will play a role in his or her own rehabilitation. The individual's attention to his or her self-care and follow-through with practice of swallow exercises will permit optimal rehabilitation (see Chapter 15 in this text).

POSTTREATMENT INTERVENTION

In the first few days posttreatment, the speech–language pathologist sees the individual to provide counseling and to answer any new questions (see Chapter 15). At this time, the speech–language pathologist reassures the individual that he or she will receive a clinical and, if needed, an instrumental swallow assessment. The individual is also informed that he or she will likely be given swallow exercises to practice on a brief but frequent and daily basis. Prior to this first posttreatment visit, the speech–language pathologist obtains information about the exact treatment the individual received and any complications that occurred during the course of treatment. For example, if the individual underwent surgery, information about the precise location and extent of surgical resection and type of reconstruction should be obtained (see Chapter 12 in this text), because the nature of the surgery can have an impact on swallow functioning and the final outcome of swallowing intervention. Final tumor pathology and pathology of the resected margins around the tumor (i.e., whether margins are free of disease or residual tumor is in surrounding tissue) can provide some indication of the individual's prognosis in terms of cancer survival. The location and extent of surgical resection and the nature of reconstruction must always be considered.

Once healing is complete in individuals having undergone surgery, the speech–language pathologist conducts an assessment of the postsurgical anatomy and the physiology of the oral, pharyngeal, and laryngeal structures (see Chapter 13). Labial, lingual and mandibular range of motion is assessed, as is oral sensation. This evaluation also includes a voice evaluation, articulation assessment, and clinical examination of swallowing.

The results of this assessment may indicate the need for an instrumental assessment to examine swallow physiology. Types of instrumental assessment include (a) videofluoroscopy, the modified barium swallow, which can be conducted alone or paired with manometry, the latter to assess pressures generated on the bolus within the oral cavity, oropharynx, or hypopharynx; (b) scintigraphy; (c) videoendoscopy; and (d) ultrasound (Hamlet, Muz, Farris, Kumpuris, & Jones, 1992; Langmore, Schatz, & Olsen, 1988; Logemann, 1983, 1993; McConnel, 1988; Muz, Mathog, Miller, Rosen, & Borrero, 1987; Shawker, Sonies, Hall, & Baum, 1984). *Videofluoroscopy* allows for visualization of the entire upper aerodigestive tract (i.e., the oral cavity, nasopharynx, oropharynx, hypopharynx, larynx, upper airway, and cervical esophagus), any structural abnormalities, disorders of movement in these structures, and bolus flow in relation to the structural and movement abnormalities during the entire oropharyngeal swallow. In addition, the presence, etiology, timing, and approximate percentage of aspiration can be determined (Logemann, 1993). *Scintigraphy* captures a view of the bolus flow through the upper aerodigestive tract and can quantify the percentage of aspiration (Hamlet et al., 1992; Muz et al., 1987); however, the upper aerodigestive tract structures are not visualized and, therefore, the nature of the physiological swallow abnormality causing aspiration cannot be definitively determined. *Videoendoscopy* does not visualize the swallow event, but it does provide information about bolus flow and laryngeal structural movement prior to and after the swallow (Langmore et al., 1988; Logemann, Rademaker, Pauloski, Ohmae, & Kahrilas, 1998). It also can be used as a biofeedback tool for various breath-hold maneuvers used in swallow rehabilitation (Martin, Logemann, Shaker, & Dodds, 1993; Mendelsohn & Martin, 1993). *Ultrasound* provides information about tongue, hyoid, and lateral pharyngeal wall motion during swallowing, but it does not visualize the entire pharynx, larynx, and cervical esophagus (Miller & Watkin, 1997; Shawker et al., 1984). Once the assessments of swallowing are completed, diet recommendations and a treatment plan can be determined.

NORMAL SWALLOWING

Normal swallowing involves movement and coordination of oral, pharyngeal, laryngeal, and esophageal structures to propel a bolus through the upper aerodigestive tract into the stomach. Swallowing is divided into four phases: oral preparatory, oral, pharyngeal, and esophageal (Logemann, 1993). During the oral preparatory phase, the bolus (i.e., ball of food or liquid) is prepared (e.g., chewed) to be swallowed. During the oral phase, the tongue propels the bolus into the pharynx. The pharyngeal phase consists of the pharyngeal swallow, during which the bolus travels through the pharynx into the esophagus. During the esophageal phase, the bolus travels from the region of the upper esophageal sphincter into that of the lower esophageal sphincter and through this lower sphincter into the stomach.

Oral Preparatory Phase

During the oral preparatory stage, liquid and food are tasted, sensed for texture, and masticated. During mastication and bolus formation, the lips are sealed to prevent spillage of material out of the mouth. Adequate buccal tone is needed to prevent spillage into the lateral oral sulci. Adequate range of motion for the tongue, particularly in the lateral plane, is required to move the food onto the lateral teeth for mashing and also to retrieve the masticated food from the lateral teeth, lateral sulci, and hard palate (Abd-El-Malek, 1939). A rotary jaw movement, which is rapid and highly regular (Palmer, Rudin, Lara, & Crompton, 1992), occurs during chewing. In addition, the palate is lowered against the posterior tongue, thereby creating a glossopalatal seal or sphincter (Dantas, Dodds, Massey, Shaker, & Cook, 1990) and preventing premature spillage of oral contents into the pharynx. Palatal lowering also creates a wider nasal passageway for breathing during chewing (Logemann, 1983). Saliva mixes with the food or liquid, and a cohesive bolus results (Abd-El-Malek, 1939). Once the bolus is well chewed or of a liquid or paste consistency, it is cupped on the tongue and is ready to be swallowed (Whillis, 1946). The tongue then elevates and seals the bolus against the palate (Kahrilas, Lin, Logemann, Ergun, & Facchini, 1993; Shawker, Sonies, Stone, & Baum, 1983). The tongue seal is maintained with the lateral and anterior margins of the tongue against the upper alveolar ridge. Cranial nerves V (trigeminal), VII (facial), X (vagus), and XII (hypoglossal) are involved in the motor activity executed during this phase of swallowing.

Oral Phase

The oral phase of the swallow begins when the tongue initiates bolus propulsion posteriorly through the oral cavity (Logemann, 1983). To propel the bolus posteriorly, the mid-tongue progressively elevates from front to back, applying pressure on the bolus tail (i.e., the trailing edge of the bolus) (Kahrilas et al., 1993). As the oral portion of the tongue propels the bolus posteriorly in the mouth, the tongue base moves anteriorly in a ramplike, grooved position to allow the leading edge of the bolus (the bolus head) to flow posteriorly into the pharynx (Hamlet, Stone, & Shawker, 1988; Kahrilas et al., 1993; Shedd, Scatliff, & Kirchner, 1960). Elevation of the velum eliminates the glossopalatal sphincter and allows bolus flow over the posterior tongue (Dodds et al., 1989). The velum then elevates against the posterior pharyngeal wall to seal the nasopharynx from the oropharynx and prevent nasal regurgitation (Bosma, 1957). In addition, the side walls of the nasopharynx, created by the superior pharyngeal constrictors, move medially to create a circular closure of the nasopharynx (Dodds, Stewart, & Logemann, 1990).

Triggering of the Pharyngeal Swallow

The oral and pharyngeal phases are tightly coupled in time. The pharyngeal phase typically begins when the bolus head reaches the posterior oral cavity, at the approximate location of the anterior faucial arches (i.e., palatoglossus muscle) (Logemann, 1983). The triggering mechanism for the pharyngeal swallow is complex and currently not well understood. Receptors involved in triggering of the pharyngeal swallow have been found on the anterior faucial arches, posterior faucial arches, posterior pharyngeal wall, tongue base, soft palate, uvula and tonsil, and epiglottis, the most sensitive of these areas being the anterior faucial arch region (Månsson & Sandberg, 1974, 1975; Pommerenke, 1928; Sinclair, 1970). These receptors are sensitive to light touch, stroking, deep pressure, and chemical and thermal input (Fujiu, Toleikis, Logemann, & Larson, 1994; Månsson &

Sandberg, 1974, 1975; Pommerenke, 1928; Pouderoux, Logemann, & Kahrilas, 1996; Sinclair, 1970). Cranial nerves V (trigeminal), IX (glossopharyngeal), and X (vagus) provide peripheral innervation for the sensory component involved in deglutition and provide sensory information from the oral cavity, oropharynx, and larynx.

Peripheral sensory and motor information converges upon cranial nerve nuclei within the central nervous system, specifically the brainstem. Afferent (sensory) information from cranial nerves VII (facial), IX (glossopharyngeal), and X (vagus) is received within the solitary nucleus (Carpenter, 1991). Afferent information from cranial nerves V, VII, IX, and X is also received within the spinal, mesencephalic, and principal sensory nucleus of cranial nerve V (Carpenter, 1991). Brainstem motor nuclei include the trigeminal motor nucleus, which provides input to the trigeminal nerve; the nucleus ambiguus (NA) and retrofacial nucleus, which provide input to the motor components of cranial nerves IX and X; the dorsal motor nucleus, which provides input to cranial nerve X; the accessory nucleus, which provides input to cranial nerve XI; and the hypoglossal nucleus, which provides input to the hypoglossal nerve (Carpenter, 1991; Ezure, Oku, & Tanaka, 1993).

Two regions in the brainstem are involved in the central pattern generator (CPG) for swallowing. These include a dorsal swallowing center, located in the region of the nucleus tractus solitarius (NTS) and the adjacent reticular formation, and a ventral swallowing center, located in the region of the NA and adjacent reticular formation (Amri, Car, & Jean, 1984; Kessler & Jean, 1985). The dorsal center is thought to program and initiate the motor sequence for swallowing that is to be relayed to the ventral swallowing center. The ventral center is believed to be the "switching" center, serving to trigger and modulate motoneuron activity (inhibition and excitation) involved in swallowing (Amri et al., 1984; Jean, 1984). Both centers are believed to contain swallowing interneurons, the dorsal center relaying to the ventral center and the ventral center relaying to motoneurons (Kessler & Jean, 1985). Continuous sensory feedback influences the neurons of the CPG in order to modulate the central program, with the swallowing neurons receiving sensory information from the region of the neural tract that is under their control (Jean, 1990). Sensory fibers conveying tactile, proprioceptive, and gustatory information converge within the NTS and likely convey information via interneurons to the dorsal pattern generator for the programming of swallowing. In addition to brainstem input, cortical input modulates swallowing (Amri et al., 1984; Car, Jean, & Roman, 1975).

Pharyngeal Phase

Several pharyngeal muscular events occur during the pharyngeal phase of swallowing, including (a) closure of the nasopharynx to prevent nasal reflux; (b) rapid, posterior motion of the tongue base to propel the tail of the bolus through the oropharynx; (c) sequential contraction of the pharyngeal constrictors to propel

the bolus through the pharynx; (d) airway closure; (e) hyoid and laryngeal elevation and anterior movement; and (f) upper esophageal sphincter (UES) relaxation and opening.

As the bolus tail passes over the tongue base during the pharyngeal phase of
the swallow, the tongue base moves in a rapid manner posteriorly to meet the anteriorly bulging posterior pharyngeal wall, thus driving the bolus through the
pharynx (Cerenko, McConnel, & Jackson, 1989; Kahrilas et al., 1993; Kahrilas,
Logemann, Lin, & Ergun, 1992). During bolus transport through the pharynx,
there is an aborally propagated contraction of the pharyngeal constrictors in the
horizontal plane simultaneous with pharyngeal shortening in the vertical plane
(Atkinson, Kramer, Wyman, & Ingelfinger, 1957; Kahrilas et al., 1992; Palmer,
Tanaka, & Siebens, 1988). The hyoid and larynx elevate and move anteriorly
(Ramsey, Watson, Gramiak, & Weinberg, 1955). This anterior–superior laryngeal
and hyoid motion places the larynx in a protected position to prevent aspiration
of the bolus into the airway (Ramsey et al., 1955). In addition, the anterior traction force of the larynx opens the cricopharyngeal region or UES (Asoh &
Goyal, 1978; Kahrilas, Logemann, Krugler, & Flanagan, 1991).

Airway protection during the pharyngeal phase of swallowing involves closure of the supraglottic larynx, or laryngeal vestibule, and closure of the true
vocal folds (Adran & Kemp, 1952, 1956, 1967; Ekberg, 1982; Logemann et al.,
1992). Closure of the laryngeal vestibule during swallowing involves two mechanisms: (a) inversion or lowering of the epiglottis, with downward tilting past
horizontal to maximally protect the larynx, and (b) contact of the epiglottic base
with the arytenoids (Adran & Kemp, 1952, 1956, 1967; Ekberg, 1982; Logemann
et al., 1992). Supraglottic laryngeal closure also involves apposition of the ventricular bands (i.e., false vocal folds) (Adran & Kemp, 1956). The downward tilting of the epiglottis is believed to result primarily from the biomechanical effects
of posterior motion of the tongue base, forces from the bolus, and laryngeal and
hyoid elevation and associated anterior motion (Adran & Kemp, 1967; Logemann
et al., 1992; Vandaele, Perlman, & Cassell, 1995). The aryepiglottic muscles assist in
epiglottic inversion, but only to a small degree (Donner, Bosma, & Robertson,
1985). The supraglottic closure involves apposition of the epiglottic base to the
arytenoid cartilages as a result of active muscular movement involving anterior
tilting of the arytenoid cartilages to meet a bulging epiglottic base (Adran &
Kemp, 1967; Ekberg, 1982; Logemann et al., 1992). Closure of the larynx also
occurs at the level of the glottis, with approximation of the true vocal folds
(Adran & Kemp, 1956; Ohmae, Logemann, Kaiser, Hanson, & Kahrilas, 1995).
Vocal fold closure occurs as the larynx elevates approximately 50% of its maximum during the pharyngeal swallow (Flaherty, Seltzer, Campbell, Weisskoff, &
Gilbert, 1995).

The cricopharyngeal muscle is attached anteriorly to the lamina of the
cricoid cartilage (Pick & Howden, 1974). Thus, there is a musculoskeletal (i.e.,
muscular cartilaginous) component to the UES. During the pharyngeal swallow,
the initial component of UES opening involves the cessation of resting muscular
activity (i.e., relaxation) in the UES region. The now relaxed, compliant UES

muscular region opens due to the forward traction on this region by the anterior displacement of the larynx. The UES region is further distended by intrabolus pressure (Asoh & Goyal, 1978; Cook et al., 1989; Kahrilas, Dodds, Dent, Logemann, & Shaker, 1989).

Bolus Effects on Swallowing

Bolus volume and viscosity can alter the timing and extent of structural movement, as well as the degree of muscle activity for normal swallowing. Several aspects of the oral and pharyngeal phases of swallowing are altered with bolus volume. Duration of laryngeal vestibule closure, anterior and superior hyolaryngeal movement, and UES opening during swallowing increase with bolus volume (Dantas, Kern, et al., 1990; Jacob, Kahrilas, Logemann, Shah, & Ha, 1989; Logemann et al., 1992). A shorter duration of tongue base contact to the posterior pharyngeal wall has been observed with an increase in bolus volume (Bisch, Logemann, Rademaker, Kahrilas, & Lazarus, 1994; Lazarus, Logemann, Rademaker et al., 1993). Laryngeal vestibule closure has been found to occur earlier in relation to UES opening with increasing bolus volume, providing additional airway protection (Bisch et al., 1994). The extent of pharyngeal structural movement has been found to increase with bolus volume, including increased extent of vertical and anterior hyoid and laryngeal movement, superior upper esophageal sphincter movement, and width of UES opening (Adran & Kemp, 1952; Dodds et al., 1988; Jacob et al., 1989; Kahrilas et al., 1989). Increases in lingual, submental, and laryngeal muscle activity also have been found with increasing bolus volume (Cook et al., 1989; Jacob et al., 1988; Miller & Watkin, 1996; Palmer, Perlman, McCulloch, Vandaele, & Luschei, 1994; Shaker, Cook, Dodds, & Hogan, 1988). Finally, intrabolus pressure and bolus velocity through the UES have been found to increase with bolus volume (Ergun, Kahrilas, Lin, Logemann, & Harig, 1993; Kahrilas et al., 1991).

Bolus viscosity also alters various aspects of both the oral and pharyngeal phases of swallowing, including systematic increases in lingual, submental, and hyolaryngeal muscle activity with increases in viscosity during oral phase swallowing (Dantas & Dodds, 1990; Jacob et al., 1988; Miller & Watkin, 1996; Palmer et al., 1994; Palmer et al., 1992; Pouderoux & Kahrilas, 1995; Reimers-Neils, Logemann, & Larson, 1994; Shaker et al., 1988; Takahashi & Nakazawa, 1991). Systematic increases in extent of vertical and anterior hyoid and laryngeal motion and width of UES opening during swallowing with increasing bolus viscosity have also been found (Dantas, Kern, et al., 1990; Ekberg, Liedberg, & Owall, 1986). The timing of the swallow varies with bolus viscosity, including oral containment time, total swallow duration, oral transit time, and pharyngeal transit time, all of which increase with bolus viscosity (Dantas & Dodds, 1990; Palmer et al., 1992; Reimers-Neils et al., 1994). Other temporal changes in oropharyngeal structural movement include increased oral transit and pharyngeal transit duration, duration of laryngeal vestibule closure, and increased duration of UES opening during swallowing with increased bolus viscosity (Bisch et al., 1994;

Dantas & Dodds, 1990; Dantas, Kern, et al., 1990; J. Robbins, Hamilton, Lof, & Kempster, 1992).

RADIOGRAPHIC EVALUATION OF SWALLOWING

Radiographic examination via the modified barium swallow (MBS) is commonly used to evaluate swallowing in those treated for head and neck cancer (Logemann, 1983, 1993). The MBS utilizes fluoroscopy and is typically videotaped. The individual is typically seated upright, with the oral cavity, pharynx, larynx, and cervical esophagus visualized. Calibrated bolus volumes of liquids, pastes, and masticated consistencies are typically presented. The individual's oropharyngeal swallow physiology is identified, as are any anatomic or physiologic swallowing disturbances. Once the physiologic swallowing disorders have been defined, the cause, timing, and approximate percentage of aspiration is determined, as is the approximate percentage of oral and pharyngeal residue. Based on the nature of the swallowing disorder(s), appropriate postures or maneuvers are introduced to determine whether bolus flow or oral and pharyngeal structural movement can be altered for a safer swallow. Postures are designed to compensate for a swallowing problem, altering the bolus flow within the oral cavity and pharynx (Kahrilas et al., 1991; Logemann, 1993; Logemann, Kahrilas, Kobara, & Vakil, 1989; Logemann, Rademaker, Pauloski, & Kahrilas, 1994; Rasley et al., 1993; Shanahan, Logemann, Rademaker, Pauloski, & Kahrilas, 1993; Welch, Logemann, Rademaker, Pauloski, & Kahrilas, 1993). Table 14.1 presents the rationales for using the various postures, based on the type of disorder identified radiographically. Maneuvers are designed to alter the timing, extent, or duration of oral and pharyngeal structural movement during the swallow (Kahrilas et al., 1991; Lazarus, 1993; Lazarus, Logemann, & Gibbons, 1993; Logemann, 1993). Table 14.2 provides information on the indications for the various swallow maneuvers, based on the type of swallowing disorder.

Once the anatomic and physiologic disorders of swallowing have been identified and the appropriate postures, maneuvers, or some combination determined, the speech–language pathologist then ascertains the optimal bolus type and volume that can be swallowed safely (see Table 14.3). If no volume or viscosity can safely or efficiently be taken by mouth, even with use of specific postures or maneuvers (or a combination of the two), nonoral diet recommendations are provided. Even if the individual does not aspirate, the efficiency of the swallow must be considered when making oral or nonoral diet recommendations. Individuals are supposed to avoid a specific food or liquid if it takes them longer than 10 seconds to propel the bolus into the pharynx or if they aspirate greater than 10% of the bolus (Logemann & Bytell, 1979). If postures or maneuvers allow for safe oral intake, the speech–language pathologist recommends the safest bolus volumes and viscosities, as well as the postures or maneuvers that the individual must use when taking nutrition by mouth. When making diet recommendations, the speech–language pathologist must be aware of the individual's level of fatigue while performing swallow maneuvers in the X-ray suite. If a

TABLE 14.1

Rationales for Postures That Assist Swallowing Disorders

Disorder Observed on VFG	Posture Applied	Rationale
Inefficient oral transit (reduced bolus propulsion by oral tongue)	Head back	Uses gravity to clear oral cavity
Delay in triggering pharyngeal swallow	Chin tuck	Widens valleculae to prevent bolus entering airway; pushes epiglottis posteriorly, increasing airway protection
Reduced posterior motion of tongue base (residue in valleculae)	Chin tuck	Pushes tongue base backward toward pharyngeal wall
Unilateral laryngeal dysfunction (aspiration during swallow)	Head rotated to damaged side	Places extrinsic pressure on thyroid cartilage, increasing adduction
Reduced laryngeal closure (aspiration during swallow)	Chin tuck, head rotated to damaged side	Puts epiglottis in more protective position, narrows laryngeal entrance, increases glottic closure by applying extrinsic pressure
Reduced pharyngeal contraction (residue spread throughout pharynx)	Lying down on one side	Eliminates gravitational effect on pharyngeal residue
Unilateral pharyngeal paresis (residue on one side of pharynx)	Head rotated to damaged side	Eliminates damaged side from bolus path
Unilateral oral and pharyngeal weakness on same side (residue in mouth and pharynx on same side)	Head tilt to stronger side	Directs bolus down stronger side
Cricopharyngeal dysfunction (residue in pyriform sinuses)	Head rotated	Pulls cricoid cartilage away from posterior pharyngeal wall, reducing resting pressure in cricopharyngeal sphincter

Note. VFG = videofluorographic examination.
From "Role of the Modified Barium Swallow in Management of Patients with Dysphagia," by J. Logemann, 1997, *Otolaryngology—Head and Neck Surgery, 116,* p. 336. Copyright 1997 by Harcourthealth. Reprinted with permission.

person exhibits fatigue when employing a maneuver during swallowing, it is unlikely that this person will be able to maintain adequate oral nutrition using the maneuver during meals. In this case, the individual should be instructed to practice to build up tolerance for and improve performance with the maneuver.

Upon completion of the videofluorographic evaluation of swallowing, individuals are followed for intensive daily swallow therapy while in the hospital and, as needed, are seen for outpatient swallow therapy following discharge. If individuals undergo postoperative radiotherapy, they should be followed during their treatment. Individuals tend to become fatigued during the radiotherapy and

TABLE 14.2
Rationales for Maneuvers that Can Alter Swallow Physiology
and Improve Swallowing Functioning

Swallow Maneuver	Disorder Observed on VFG	Rationale
Supraglottic swallow	Reduced or late vocal cord closure; delayed pharyngeal swallow	Voluntary breath hold usually closes vocal folds before and during swallow
Super supraglottic swallow	Reduced closure of airway entrance	Effortful breath hold tilts arytenoid forward, closing airway entrance before and during swallow
Effortful swallow	Reduced posterior movement of tongue base	Effort increases posterior tongue base movement
Mendelsohn maneuver	Reduced laryngeal movement	Laryngeal movement opens UES, prolonging laryngeal elevation prolongs UES opening
	Discoordinated swallow	Normalizes timing of pharyngeal swallow events

Note. VFG = videofluorographic examination; UES = upper esophageal sphincter.
From "Role of the Modified Barium Swallow in Management of Patients with Dysphagia," by J. Logemann, 1997, *Otolaryngology—Head and Neck Surgery, 116,* p. 337. Copyright 1997 by Harcourthealth and Jeri Logemann. Reprinted with permission.

TABLE 14.3
Rationales for Appropriate Bolus Types by Swallowing Disorder

Swallowing Disorder	Easiest Food Consistencies	Consistencies To Avoid
Reduced range of tongue motion	Thick liquid initially, then thin liquid	Thick foods
Reduced tongue coordination	Liquid	Thick foods
Reduced tongue strength	Thin liquid	Thick, heavy foods
Delayed pharyngeal swallow	Thick liquids and thicker foods	Thin liquids
Reduced airway closure	Pudding and thick foods	Thin liquids
Reduced laryngeal movement/ cricopharyngeal dysfunction	Thin liquid	Thicker, higher viscosity foods
Reduced pharyngeal wall contraction	Thin liquid	Thick, higher viscosity foods
Reduced tongue base posterior movement	Thin liquid	Higher viscosity foods

Note. From "Therapy for Oropharyngeal Swallowing Disorders," by J. A. Logemann, 1996, in *Deglutition and Its Disorders: Anatomy, Physiology, Clinical Diagnosis, and Management* (p. 452), by A. Perlman and K. Schulze-Delrieu (Eds.), San Diego: Singular. Copyright 1996 by Singular Publishing Group and Jeri Logemann. Reprinted with permission.

will likely practice their swallow exercises less frequently; however, they should still be monitored during this period for any new complaints or swallowing problems related to the radiotherapy (i.e., pain on swallowing, reduced ability to trigger a swallow, or reduced salivary flow, all of which might result in reduced ability to manipulate a bolus within the mouth or propel a bolus into the pharynx).

SWALLOWING REHABILITATION AFTER PARTIAL LARYNGECTOMY

As noted previously, swallowing difficulties are not uncommon in those diagnosed with head and neck cancer. Such swallowing abnormalities must always be considered in those individuals who undergo conservative, partial laryngectomy procedures for treatment of laryngeal tumors. Given that a variety of partial laryngectomy procedures may be employed dependent upon the size and location of a laryngeal tumor, swallowing concerns specific to particular surgical procedures must be addressed. The extent of swallowing dysfunction and the length of rehabilitation after partial laryngectomy procedures will depend on the extent of surgical resection and whether the individual will be treated with postoperative radiotherapy (Jenkins et al., 1981; Lazarus et al., 1981; Logemann, 1984; Sessions & Zill (1979); Smith, Kotz, Beitler, & Wadler, 2000; see also Chapter 11 in this text). Within the following sections, postsurgical swallowing concerns for two types of partial laryngectomy procedures are addressed, those pertaining to hemilaryngectomy and those particular to supraglottic laryngectomy. Information presented relates to the postsurgical changes that will be observed, the influence of anatomical changes on swallowing function, and therapeutic considerations.

Hemilaryngectomy

Those individuals treated with hemilaryngectomy typically resume swallow function within 7 to 10 days of surgery, with no swallowing abnormalities (Logemann, 1984). If surgery, however, involves resection of other structures (i.e., extended hemilaryngectomy), such as a portion or all of the arytenoid cartilage or extension into the anterior commissure with a portion of the opposite vocal fold, swallowing problems can occur (Pressman & Bailey, 1978). Duration of rehabilitation will depend on the extent of tissue resected. Following extended hemilaryngectomy procedures, individuals are typically given airway closure exercises, such as the supraglottic or super-supraglottic swallow, to improve supraglottic and glottic closure for swallowing (Logemann, 1993; Martin et al., 1993). Vocal fold adduction exercises also are introduced to improve glottic closure for swallowing and voice (Logemann, 1983).

Postures may be helpful to eliminate aspiration, which typically occurs during the swallow because of reduced airway closure. Head rotation to the surgical side helps close the glottis because of extrinsic pressure on the thyroid cartilage (Logemann, Kahrilas, Kobara, & Vakil, 1989; Logemann, Rademaker, et al.,

1994). If aspiration cannot be eliminated, head rotation can be combined with chin-tuck posture, the latter of which places the airway in a more protected position, with the tongue base situated closer to the pharyngeal wall (Logemann, 1993; Shanahan et al., 1993; Welch et al., 1993). Individuals usually only need to use these postures for a short time and can regain swallow function within a month or so.

Supraglottic Laryngectomy

After supraglottic laryngectomy, individuals typically experience swallowing difficulty because the supraglottic structures, including the false vocal folds and epiglottis, are resected (Ogura & Biller, 1969). Supraglottic airway closure must be accomplished by tongue base–arytenoid contact, with anterior tilting of the arytenoids to the epiglottic base (Logemann, Gibbons, et al., 1994). If the supraglottic region, or laryngeal vestibule, does not close completely, material can enter the vestibule before or during the swallow. Some or all of this penetrated material can enter the airway after the swallow. Therefore, postsurgically, these individuals are typically instructed in (a) the super–supraglottic swallow, to improve laryngeal vestibule and glottic closure for swallowing (Logemann, Pauloski, Rademaker, & Colangelo, 1997b), and (b) exercises designed to improve tongue-base posterior motion, including tongue-base retraction exercises, the effortful swallow, and the tongue-hold maneuver (Fujiu & Logemann, 1996; Logemann, 1993; Veis, Logemann, & Colangelo, 2000). These tongue-base exercises are designed specifically to improve posterior motion of the tongue-base. The tongue-hold maneuver is also designed to increase anterior motion of the posterior pharyngeal wall for improved tongue base–pharyngeal wall contact and improved bolus clearance past the tongue base (Fujiu & Logemann, 1996). If aspiration cannot be eliminated with the super–supraglottic swallow maneuver (Logemann et al., 1992; Logemann, et al., 1997b), the chin-tuck posture can be combined with this maneuver to help deflect material away from the airway. If this combination of posture and maneuver does not eliminate aspiration, an individual can be placed in the side-lying position. In this position, residual material will remain on the lateral pharyngeal wall, rather than dumping into the airway by gravity after the swallow (Logemann, 1993).

    If the use of postures, maneuvers, or a combination of the two eliminates aspiration on thin liquids, some individuals can safely swallow thicker consistencies, such as thick liquids. They might, however, need to use these postures or maneuvers during meals to prevent aspiration. Some individuals learn to use the supraglottic swallow automatically over the course of a few months. Others, however, need to consciously focus on using this maneuver during meals, particularly with liquids. Following standard supraglottic laryngectomy, the time to achieve normal swallowing typically takes 28 days (Logemann, 1984); however, if the individual is to undergo postoperative radiotherapy, resumption of normal swallowing can take several months. Even if a person resumes normal swallowing after surgery, once radiotherapy begins, swallowing may deteriorate. Therefore, it is very important to follow individuals during radiotherapy so that swallow therapy can be introduced, if needed.

Some individuals may require an extended supraglottic laryngectomy, a procedure that includes structures other than those typically resected in the standard supraglottic laryngectomy (Ogura, Sessions, & Ciralsky, 1975). Depending on the location of the tumor, surgery may require extension into the tongue base or may involve resection of a portion or all of one arytenoid cartilage. Resection of these structures will likely compromise airway protection for swallowing. With a fair amount of tongue base resected, material tends to fall over the remaining tongue base directly into the airway. With resection involving the arytenoid cartilage, glottic closure is typically compromised, resulting in aspiration during the swallow (Lazarus et al., 1981; Logemann, 1984). After extended supraglottic laryngectomy, individuals are often seen for a lengthy period of swallow rehabilitation. They often take primary nutrition by gastrostomy tube while practicing their swallow exercises. Unfortunately, despite intensive swallow rehabilitation, some individuals are unable to safely or efficiently take any nutrition by mouth and require permanent gastrostomy; similar difficulties may be observed in those treated with organ preservation methods (Carrara-de-Angelis, Feher, Barros, Nishimoto, & Kowalski, 2003).

SWALLOWING REHABILITATION AFTER TOTAL LARYNGECTOMY

Individuals having undergone total laryngectomy are not typically referred for assessment of swallowing. Following total laryngectomy, individuals can no longer aspirate because the airway and esophagus have been separated. Mild swallowing problems can occur, however, due to the structural changes resulting from total laryngectomy (McConnel, 1988). These can include mildly impaired tongue function for manipulation of foods or liquids after the hyoid bone has been resected. In addition, patients may find it difficult to swallow particular types of foods because pharyngeal swallowing pressures required to propel a bolus through the pharynx are higher after total laryngectomy than in healthy individuals (McConnel, 1988). Although there are no data that demonstrate the efficacy of swallowing exercises following total laryngectomy, it makes sense to provide exercises designed to improve pressures on the bolus and bolus clearance through the pharynx for individuals with pharyngeal pressure problems. These would include tongue-base range-of-motion and strengthening exercises, such as the tongue-hold maneuver, effortful swallow, and tongue-base retraction exercise (Fujiu & Logemann, 1996; Logemann, 1993).

Hypopharyngeal or esophageal stenoses can interfere with bolus passage through the pharynx and esophagus (R. K. Davis, Vincent, Shapshay, & Strong, 1982). Surgeons typically dilate the pharynx or esophagus to improve bolus flow for swallowing. Scar tissue (otherwise known as a pseudoepiglottis) can develop at the base of the tongue and can impede the flow of material through the upper pharynx (Muller-Miny, Eisele, & Jones, 1993). This problem requires surgical resection of the scar tissue. Individuals having undergone total laryngectomy may find mealtime less enjoyable due to reduced or altered taste sensation that may occur with postoperative radiotherapy (Schwartz, Weiffenbach, Valdez, & Fox, 1993). Less enjoyment of meals can also be attributed to the impairment of olfaction that many individuals who undergo total laryngectomy experience (van Dam, et al., 1999). The speech–language pathologist should work closely with the social worker and may also work with the dietician, psychologist, or psychiatrist to support the individual treated for head and neck cancer and ensure optimal recovery of swallow (and communication) functioning.

SWALLOWING REHABILITATION OF INDIVIDUALS WITH PHARYNGEAL WALL RESECTION

Tumors of the pharyngeal wall are typically resected and reconstructed using some type of muscle flap or skin graft. This surgery typically results in swallowing problems, because resecting part of the pharyngeal wall can interfere with the sequential contraction of the pharyngeal constrictors that occurs during the pharyngeal swallow. This interference typically results in reduced bolus clearance through the pharynx and pharyngeal residue after the swallow. The speech–language pathologist can ask the patient to rotate the head to the side of the surgery to improve pressure generation and bolus clearance through the pharynx (Logemann, 1993; Ohmae, Ogura, Kitahara, Karaho, & Inouye, 1998). If pharyngeal residue cannot be eliminated and the individual is aspirating this residue after the swallow, a side-lying position can be used, with the patient lying on the unoperated side. This posture allows the residue to remain on the pharyngeal wall rather than entering the airway after the swallow (Logemann, 1993). The patient can then safely reswallow this residue while lying down. If the size or location of the resection is such that bolus clearance through the pharynx is severely affected, a thin liquid diet may be indicated, because thicker viscosity materials would be propelled and cleared through the pharynx less efficiently and would result in a greater amount of pharyngeal residue (Logemann, 1993).

SWALLOWING REHABILITATION OF INDIVIDUALS UNDERGOING SURGICAL ORAL CANCER TREATMENT

Swallowing rehabilitation begins soon after surgery, once suture lines have healed sufficiently to allow active range-of-motion and resistance exercises. At the initial postoperative clinical evaluation, the speech–language pathologist should inspect the patient's oral cavity to determine the location and amount of tissue resected and the size and location of flaps. An oral-motor assessment should be performed, including assessment of labial, lingual, and velar range of motion for isolated and rapidly repeated nonspeech and speech movements. Labial and lingual sensation and strength should also be assessed. A bedside swallow examination should be performed. Assessment of lingual ability to seal a bolus against the palate and lateralize a bolus to the teeth for chewing can be accomplished using a rolled up piece of gauze (Logemann, 1983). Once material (usually liquids) is given to the individual, the clinician should make a judgment about oropharyngeal transit times and degree of laryngeal elevation during the swallow (Logemann, 1983). The clinician should inspect the oral cavity after each swallow to determine the presence, amount, and location of any oral residue. The clinician should also note any symptoms of aspiration, including gurgly, wet-sounding voice quality, coughing, or throat clearing (Linden, Kuhlemeier, & Patterson, 1993; Logemann, Veis, & Colangelo, 1999; see also Chapter 13 in this text).

If the individual has a tracheostomy tube that is not capped, the patient should be instructed to occlude the end of the tube with a finger during the swallow (Logemann, Pauloski, & Colangelo, 1998; Muz, Hamlet, Mathog, & Farris, 1994). If further assessment of swallowing is needed, the patient should undergo videofluorographic (VFG) examination of swallowing. VFG assessment of swallowing is often warranted in this population to further define any abnormal oropharyngeal swallow physiology. Furthermore, VFG assessment will also identify whether swallowing disorders result in aspiration, which may be silent (i.e., a cough is not immediately produced in response to material entering the airway) on clinical examination (Garon, Engle, & Ormiston, 1996; Kidd, Lawson, Nesbitt, & MacMahon, 1993; Logemann, 1983; Lundy et al., 1999; Pauloski et al., 2002; Pauloski et al., 2004; C. H. Smith, Logemann, Colangelo, Rademaker, & Pauloski, 1999; Sorin, Somers, Austin, & Bester, 1988; Splaingard, Hutchins, Sulton, & Chaudhuri, 1988).

Tracheostomy tubes should be maintained during the initial week(s) following surgery. Both clinical and X-ray examinations of swallowing can be completed with the tracheostomy tube in place. Unless the tracheostomy tube has an overinflated cuff that is impinging on the esophagus and perhaps interfering with bolus clearance through the upper pharynx (Pinkus, 1973), the tracheostomy tube will likely not interfere with swallowing. Furthermore, it is helpful for the patient to have the tracheostomy tube, which allows for easier expectoration of secretions and can provide the clinician with useful information about aspiration of foods or liquids (for those who are able to expectorate aspirated material through the tracheostomy tube).

For individuals with nasogastric tubes, it is best to maintain the tube during the early postoperative days, because it is prudent to maintain nutrition while the individual is learning swallow maneuvers and practicing swallowing exercises (see Al-Othman, Amdur, Morris, Hinerman, & Mendenhall, 2003). Removal of a nasogastric tube does not motivate an individual to eat but rather can increase anxiety about whether adequate oral nutrition will be maintained. At the early stages of swallow rehabilitation, an individual's swallow may be very inefficient and the individual may need time and practice before being able to use swallow maneuvers during meals well enough to meet his or her nutritional needs. Thus, having the nasogastric tube in place will reduce the individual's anxiety about trying to meet these nutritional needs. Reducing the person's anxiety level may also provide greater motivation and energy to practice the prescribed swallow exercises.

The nature of swallowing problems exhibited by patients surgically treated for oral cancer will depend on the amount of tissue resected and the type of reconstruction (Fujiu, Logemann, & Pauloski, 1995; Hirano et al., 1992; McConnel et al., 1994; McConnel et al., 1998; Pauloski et al., 1994; Teichgraeber, Bowman, & Goepfert, 1986; see also Chapter 13 in this text). Individuals frequently have impairments affecting lip closure, bolus formation, sealing against the hard palate, vertical tongue motion, anteroposterior tongue motion, and triggering of the pharyngeal swallow. In addition, oral residue in the surgical defect, in the floor of mouth, and on the tongue and palate is also common (Conley, 1962; Logemann & Bytell, 1979; Shedd et al., 1960). Individuals who undergo anterior tongue resections may experience difficulty maintaining an anterior lingual–palatal seal, with hard palate residue and residue in the anterior sulcus that the tongue is unable to clear. They may also experience problems with bolus control for chewing. A palatal augmentation prosthesis may eliminate these problems, or at least reduce the amount of anterior oral cavity residue (J. W. Davis et al., 1987; Wheeler et al., 1980).

Patients with lateral–posterior composite resections may have a similar difficulty maintaining a lingual–palatal seal, but on the side of and along the anteroposterior length of the resection. This can result in residue that is typically found in the lower sulcus on the operated side, particularly in that the floor of the mouth and the mandible are often resected in a lateral–posterior composite resection. Again, a palatal augmentation prosthesis should improve lingual–palatal contacts along the length of the resected tongue for improved bolus control and propulsion through the pharynx, as well as reduce residue from the lower sulcus. If greater than 50% of the tongue is resected, a palatal augmentation prosthesis should be constructed soon after surgery. The prosthesis should be constructed so that the palatal vault (i.e., augmentation to the prosthesis) is lowered to meet the residual tongue or floor of mouth (the latter in the case of a total glossectomy). Following total or subtotal glossectomy, patients are typically unable to chew effectively.

Pharyngeal disorders frequently seen following anterior and posterior tongue resections include reduced pharyngeal contraction, reduced tongue-base posterior motion, reduced hyoid motion, and reduced laryngeal elevation and laryngeal vestibule closure for swallowing (Pauloski, Logemann, Fox, & Colangelo, 1995; Pauloski et al., 1994). In addition, oropharyngeal swallow efficiency, a summary measure of swallowing function, is often reduced and has been correlated with extent of lingual tissue resected (Fujiu et al., 1995; Rademaker, Pauloski, Logemann, & Shanahan, 1994).

The type of surgical reconstruction can have an impact on swallow function. Patients tend to have better swallow function and earlier return to oral nutrition when the surgical defect is closed primarily (i.e., the surgeon does not use a flap reconstruction, but rather sutures remaining tissues together) (Hirano et al., 1992; McConnel et al., 1994; McConnel et al., 1998; Pauloski, Logemann, Colangelo, Rademaker, & McConnel, 1995; Teichgraeber et al., 1986). If flaps are used, free flap reconstruction, such as the radial free forearm flap, can result in less tethering of the tongue and less interference with bolus flow than bulkier flaps, such as the pectoralis major myocutaneous flap. In addition, with reanastomosis of nerves during reconstruction of some free flaps, such as the radial forearm flap, sensation can be maintained (hence the term "sensate flap") (Urken, Moscoso, Lawson, & Biller, 1994). To what extent this sensate flap improves swallow function, however, is not as yet known. Tumor stage has been correlated with swallow function (Hirano et al., 1992). Typically poorer swallow function occurs as tumor stage increases because larger tumors require larger surgical resections and large, bulky flaps for reconstruction, which can interfere with bolus control, flow, and clearance through the oral cavity and oropharynx (DeNittis et al., 2001; see also Chapter 8 in this text).

Patients should be given swallow exercises as soon as healing is complete. Range-of-motion exercises for the jaw should be given, particularly if the person has undergone hemimandibulectomy and if postoperative radiotherapy is planned. These exercises should work on increasing jaw opening, lateral movement of the jaw, and circular jaw movement for chewing (Logemann, 1983). Clinicians should instruct individuals to practice these exercises during the course of postoperative radiotherapy in an effort to reduce the risk of developing trismus (reduced jaw opening). Individuals who undergo procedures requiring splitting and resuturing of the lips (i.e., mandibulotomy or hemimandibulectomy) also may need lip range-of-motion and strengthening exercises to improve closure for swallowing, as well as for speech. Tongue range-of-motion exercises also are given as soon as healing is complete, to increase range of motion in the vertical, anterior–posterior, and lateral planes (Logemann, Pauloski, Rademaker, & Colangelo, 1997a).

Speech exercises also are typically provided at this time, to improve lingual range of motion and precision of lingual–palatal contacts for both speech and swallowing. Individuals may be given tongue strengthening exercises, with active resistance against a tongue depressor along the lateral tongue margins and on elevation with the tongue to improve lingual strength. If a sufficient amount of tongue remains after the resection to allow for lingual–palatal contact, exercises may be provided to improve the lingual–palatal seal (to maintain a bolus against the palate) and to work on the sequential front-to-back elevation of the mid-tongue while maintaining the palatal seal along the anterior and lateral tongue margins for the oral phase of the swallow. This tongue strengthening can be accomplished using a rolled up gauze (4 × 4 inch) squeezed against the palate with the tongue. The gauze is also effective to work on lateral lingual motion for chewing, with the person attempting to maneuver the gauze with the tongue to the lateral molars or gums and to retrieve it from these lateral margins. Once the individual exhibits good ability to perform this exercise, food boluses can be introduced, typically beginning with pureed or very soft foods. For those unable to maintain a lingual–palatal seal or lateralize gauze to the teeth, however, food should not be introduced until after construction of a palatal augmentation-lowering prosthesis. Individuals should be instructed to practice swallow exercises for 2 to 3 minutes, 5 to 8 times per day, and should be seen daily while in the hospital. Upon discharge, follow-up should be scheduled weekly for at least 4 to 6 weeks. Individuals should also be instructed to continue daily practice of exercises during radiotherapy and for approximately 4 to 6 weeks after completion of radiotherapy. Reevaluation of swallowing during or after radiotherapy may be needed because swallow functioning may deteriorate.

Individuals treated for oral cancer may need to use compensatory postures to improve swallow efficiency. These postures can include a head tilt toward the nonsurgical side, which will allow material to flow along the unoperated side of the oral cavity and can improve bolus control (Logemann, 1983, 1993). If anterior–posterior tongue motion is reduced, the head-back posture can be used to facilitate and speed oral transit and bolus clearance through the oral cavity (Logemann, 1983). When using the head-back posture, the person should be instructed to use a voluntary airway closure maneuver when swallowing, such as the super-supraglottic swallow, to eliminate the risk of aspiration before the swallow (Kahrilas et al., 1991). The head-tilt posture can be combined with the head-back posture to improve bolus clearance through the oral cavity. Patients who undergo composite resection (anterior or lateral–posterior) may demonstrate delayed triggering of the pharyngeal swallow and may benefit from thermal or tactile stimulation of the swallow to improve the speed of swallow triggering (Lazzara, Lazarus, & Logemann, 1986; Rosenbek, Roecker, Wood, & Robbins, 1996).

Delayed triggering of the pharyngeal swallow may be due to reduced oropharyngeal sensation that can occur after oral cancer surgery (Aviv, Hecht, Weinberg, Dalton, & Urken, 1992). If a portion of the tongue base is included in the resection, bolus clearance past the tongue base can be affected, as can supraglottic airway protection. In this case, tongue-base range-of-motion exercises should be provided. These exercises are designed to improve tongue-base range of motion in the posterior direction (i.e., toward the posterior pharyngeal wall) (Logemann, 1993; Veis et al., 2000). The individual may benefit from eating or drinking using the effortful swallow, perhaps combined with the chin-tuck posture to improve bolus clearance past the tongue base (Logemann, 1993). The chin-tuck posture combined with the super-supraglottic swallow can improve airway protection both before and during the swallow (Logemann, 1985). Following total or subtotal glossectomy, individuals frequently swallow effectively and efficiently using a "dump-and-swallow" method. This technique involves taking a large sip of liquid from a cup, filling the pharynx, and repeatedly swallowing while maintaining airway closure during and between each swallow (Logemann, 1983).

INTRAORAL PROSTHETICS: PALATAL LOWERING OR AUGMENTATION PROSTHESIS

In addition to using postures or maneuvers to improve swallowing, intraoral prosthetics can be constructed to further improve swallow (and speech) functioning. Individuals with any degree of tongue resection are good candidates for a palatal augmentation prosthesis. The maxillofacial prosthodontist typically sees the individual after healing, usually within 4 to 6 weeks postsurgery (or 4 to 6 weeks postradiotherapy) to take a dental impression for construction of the prosthesis base plate. Once the plate has been constructed, the speech–language pathologist and maxillofacial prosthodontist work collaboratively to construct the augmentation portion of the prosthesis (Davis et al., 1987; Wheeler et al., 1980; see also Chapter 13 in this text). The prosthodontist provides expertise in design and construction of the prosthesis, while the speech–language pathologist provides expertise in the anatomy and physiology of speech and swallowing so as to ensure that the prosthesis will effectively maximize the patient's speech and swallowing function. Individuals typically require 5 or 6 weekly visits for construction and modification of the prosthesis. Individuals need to demonstrate good dental hygiene; adequate care and maintenance of dentures, if worn; good manual dexterity because the prosthesis is removed at night; and motivation to wear the prosthesis for communication and swallowing.

During construction of the prosthesis, wax is added to the base plate so that the residual tongue can contact the wax. The speech–language pathologist determines where wax should be added so that the tongue can contact the augmented palate for speech, as well as for swallowing. The speech–language pathologist examines the intraoral anatomy (i.e., the amount and location of remaining lingual tissue, and the size and location of flaps) and range of tongue motion to determine how much wax is needed to lower the palatal vault to the residual tongue. The individual is instructed to elevate the tongue to the augmented palate and to run the tongue along the palate to determine whether enough wax has been added to ensure lingual–palatal contact. Bolus control maneuvers, such as sealing a piece of gauze against the palate with the tongue, are also used during construction of the augmentation to ensure that enough wax has been added to assist in the oral phase of swallowing. Wax is added to areas of the prosthesis where the tongue is not making adequate contact and is removed from locations where it interferes with tongue motion.

The speech–language pathologist instructs the individual to repeat words with stop and affricate consonants including /t/, /d/, /k/, /g/, /ʧ/, and /ʤ/ to determine whether enough wax has been added for precise contact with the tongue. The clinician also instructs the individual to repeat words with initial tip–alveolar |s| and blade–palatal (|ʃ|) fricative phonemes to determine the location and amount of wax needed to maintain a medial airstream. The clinician can insert a gloved finger into the oral cavity to feel for lateral air emission during production of initial fricatives, and additional wax can be added until the lateral airstream can no longer be felt or heard. For persons treated with total glossectomy, the palatal augmentation prosthesis is typically fairly large, because the augmentation portion needs to be near the remaining muscles composing the floor of mouth in order to assist with bolus control and bolus clearance through the oral cavity. Once the optimum amount and location of wax has been added to the plate, the wax is replaced by hardened plastic. Additional swallow and speech exercises are given to the individual to perform with the prosthesis in place to maximize use of the prosthesis for swallowing and speech.

Once the prosthesis has been constructed and the individual has had a few weeks to wear the prosthesis during meals and while practicing speech and swallow exercises, a VFG examination of swallowing may be indicated to determine whether the prosthesis is assisting in swallow function. The VFG study also allows the clinician to determine whether additional modification to the prosthesis is needed. VFG examination will reveal how well the prosthesis assists in bolus control and movement through the oral cavity, including the speed and efficiency of bolus propulsion during the oral phase. In addition, the speed and efficiency of bolus movement and clearance through the pharynx during the swallow can also be visualized (J. W. Davis et al., 1987; Logemann, Kahrilas, Hurst, Davis, & Krugler, 1989).

REHABILITATION OF INDIVIDUALS WITH CANCER OF THE PALATE

Individuals treated surgically for cancer of the hard palate are typically seen preoperatively by the maxillofacial prosthodontist. A temporary maxillary obdurator is constructed and placed in the surgical defect at the time of surgery. It is then replaced by a permanent removable obdurator. If the soft palate is included in the resection, a palatal bulb obdurator is added to the back portion of the prosthesis once healing is complete to improve velopharyngeal closure for swallowing and speech. If lateral and posterior pharyngeal walls are preserved during surgery, resonance can be fairly normal and nasal reflux might not occur, because the lateral and posterior pharyngeal walls contract medialward to contact the palatal bulb and assist in the circular closure of the velopharyngeal mechanism. If, however, a portion of the lateral or posterior pharyngeal walls is resected or pharyngeal wall tissue becomes fibrotic after radiotherapy, the pharyngeal walls may not move enough to contact the bulb, resulting in hypernasality and nasal reflux of food or liquids during swallowing.

SWALLOWING REHABILITATION OF INDIVIDUALS TREATED WITH RADIOTHERAPY

Radiation Effects

Irradiation to the head and neck can result in changes to the tissues, muscles, dentition, and bone that can have an impact on swallowing. Changes to the tissues of the oral cavity and oropharynx include mucositis and erythema (Arcuri & Schneider, 1992; see also Chapter 10 in this text). In addition, changes to the pharyngeal structures can occur postradiotherapy, with skin thickening, increased density of subcutaneous fat, and thickening of the epiglottis (Redvanly, Hudgins, Gussack, Lewis, & Crocker, 1992). In addition to tissue effects, other physiologic effects of radiotherapy, particularly to the oral and oropharyngeal regions, can include pain, burning sensation, altered tactile sensation, altered or reduced taste sensation, reduced dental sensation, bone changes (including osteoradionecrosis), trismus (restriction in mouth opening), and changes in the oral flora (Abu Shara et al., 1993; Arcuri & Schneider, 1992; Aviv et al., 1992; Ichimura & Tanaka, 1993; Knowles, Chalian, & Shidnia, 1986; Schwartz et al., 1993; see also Chapters 7, 10, and 13 in this text).

Later physiologic changes following radiotherapy (at least 6 months after treatment) involve vascular damage, which can result in reduction of blood supply to the muscles and replacement with collagen and eventual tissue fibrosis (Bentzen, Thames, & Overgaard, 1989; Ben-Yosef & Kapp, 1992; Brown, Fixsen, & Plowman, 1987; Law, 1981). These changes can occur up to 15 years postradiotherapy (Bentzen, Turesson, & Thames, 1990) and can affect swallowing long after radiation treatment (Lazarus, 1993). Both acute and late effects of radiotherapy to the head and neck appear to be dose dependent, including total dose, dose per fraction, and total treatment time (Bentzen et al., 1990; Karasek, Constine, & Rosier, 1991; Maciejewski, Withers, Taylor, & Hliniak, 1990).

Xerostomia (i.e., reduced salivary flow) can be a very troublesome side effect of radiotherapy. Persons treated with radiotherapy to the head and neck demonstrate significantly lower salivary flow rates than healthy individuals (Kuo et al., 1993; Schwartz et al., 1993; Stokman et al., 2003). Lowest salivary flow rates have been found when individuals receive bilateral radiation treatment to the neck (Law, 1981). There is often no recovery of salivary function over time (Kuo et al., 1993; Liu, Fleming, Toth, & Keene, 1990). Individuals are typically given artificial saliva products to add some moisture to the oral cavity; however, some people find these products to be greasy or the effects short lasting, and they prefer to carry water bottles. Drugs (e.g., Pylocarpine) are available to stimulate and increase saliva production (Cooper, Fu, Marks, & Silverman, 1995), but individual reports of increased salivary flow have been variable. Xerostomia can result in difficulty swallowing, with the reduced ability to manipulate a bolus within the mouth, which can result in delayed triggering of the pharyngeal swallow (Hamlet et al., 1997; Hughes et al., 1987; Månsson & Sandberg, 1975).

Radiotherapy can also reduce muscle strength, an effect that can persist over time (Jentzsch et al., 1981; Lazarus, 1996; Stinson et al., 1991). Muscle wasting and loss of movement have also been observed as early and late complications following radiotherapy to skeletal muscle (Brown et al., 1987). Radiotherapy is known to affect swallowing, primarily due to tissue fibrosis, and can affect tongue strength, triggering of the pharyngeal swallow, and pharyngeal phase structural movement (Lazarus, 1996, 1997; Lazarus et al., 1996). The pharyngeal phase muscular activity can be reduced in rate, range, timing, and coordination, with a reduction in pharyngeal contraction, tongue-base posterior motion, hyoid motion, laryngeal elevation, and closure of the laryngeal vestibule and glottis for swallowing (Lazarus et al., 1996). Movement of the pharyngeal structures has been found to be sluggish and reduced in maximum extent, particularly tongue base–to–pharyngeal wall motion and contact, hyolaryngeal elevation, and laryngeal vestibule closure during the swallow (Eisele, Koch, Tarazi, & Jones, 1991; Ekberg & Nylander, 1983; Kendall, McKenzie, Leonard, & Jones, 1998; Kotz, Abraham, Beitler, Wadler, & Smith, 1999; Lazarus, 1997; Lazarus et al., 1996). These motility disorders can result in reduced ability to clear a bolus from the pharynx and aspiration of food or liquid after the swallow (Lazarus, 1997; Lazarus et al., 1996). Aspiration can also occur during the swallow because of reduced laryngeal vestibule and glottic closure (Lazarus, 1997; Lazarus et al., 1996). Oropharyngeal swallow efficiency has also been found to be reduced in patients treated with primary radiotherapy, as well as in individuals treated surgically with postoperative radiotherapy (Lazarus, 1996, 1997; Lazarus et al., 1996; McConnel et al., 1994; Pauloski, Rademaker, Logemann, & Colangelo, 1998).

Swallow Management

Individuals who have undergone surgery and who receive postoperative radiotherapy should be followed during the course of their treatment to monitor changes. Radiotherapy is typically given once daily for approximately 35 treatments; however, other treatment regimens are often used (e.g., twice-daily treatments in conjunction with chemotherapy, with schedules of 1 week of treatment, 1 week without, for 10 weeks). Practice of swallow exercises should be encouraged, but the speech–language pathologist must consider how much the patient can tolerate. Those individuals complaining of fatigue or oral and pharyngeal soreness due to mucositis may not feel up to practicing exercises. Swallowing should be monitored, and complaints should be addressed promptly. If swallowing complaints relate to pain and soreness, diet should be appropriately modified, typically by a downgrade to a softer or liquid diet. If an individual appears to demonstrate a physiologic swallowing problem, a clinical and perhaps radiographic assessment of swallowing is warranted, and the clinician might recommend diet changes, swallow therapy, or both. Patients should be encouraged to continue practice of swallow exercises postradiotherapy, because radiotherapy can result in late tissue changes and deterioration of swallowing over time (Lazarus, 1993).

Swallowing Rehabilitation of Individuals Treated with Primary Radiotherapy (Organ Preservation Treatment)

Organ-sparing (nonsurgical) radiotherapy protocols have become increasingly common as an option for patients with larger, typically unresectable tumors of the head and neck (see Chapters 10 and 11 in this text). Cure rates following organ-preservation treatments are comparable to those after surgical treatment (Hirsch et al., 1991; Taylor et al., 1989; Taylor et al., 1997; Vokes, Moran, Mick, Weichselbaum, & Panje, 1989; see also Chapter 10 in this text). Although the organ is preserved anatomically, function may not be spared, particularly for swallowing (Kendall et al., 1998; Kotz et al., 1999; Lazarus, 1997; Lazarus et al., 1996; Murry, Madasu, Martin, & Robbins, 1998; Rademaker et al., 2003). Often the side effects of radiotherapy are heightened with concomitant chemotherapy, resulting in a greater degree of mucositis, pain, and soreness (Peters et al., 1988; see also Chapter 10 in this text). Swallowing problems are similar to those seen after postsurgical radiotherapy (Lazarus, 1997; Lazarus et al., 1996); however, dysphagic individuals may require longer periods of time for swallowing rehabilitation because the side effects (i.e., mucositis, tissue changes, and edema) of the combined radiotherapy and chemotherapy can take months to subside.

Individuals about to undergo organ-preservation treatments are not typically referred to speech–language pathologists. Therefore, it is imperative for a speech–language pathologist to become a team member and educate other members of the team about possible swallowing problems posttreatment. Persons about to undergo organ-preservation protocols for head and neck cancer treatment should be counseled pretreatment, with discussion about swallowing problems that might occur during or after treatment (see also Chapters 11 and 15 in this text). In addition, although no data are available at this time, it seems prudent that the patient be given prophylactic swallow exercises in an effort to prevent swallowing problems and to maintain swallow function during and after treatment. Tongue strengthening, tongue-base range-of-motion, laryngeal elevation, and closure exercises are all important. Individuals may not feel well enough to practice during their treatment; however, they should be encouraged to practice after completion of treatment when they begin to feel better.

SUMMARY

This chapter has presented information on the types of treatments for head and neck cancer and the effects of these treatments on swallow function. By understanding these effects, a more comprehensive program of management can be pursued. Additionally, when swallowing problems occur, they can be identified and addressed promptly. Furthermore, the role of the speech–language pathologist in management of swallowing disorders has been described, including pretreatment counseling, clinical and instrumental swallow assessment, therapeutic intervention, and collaborative construction and management of intraoral prosthetics.

REFERENCES

Abd-El-Malek, S. (1939). Observations on the morphology of the human tongue. *Journal of Anatomy, 73,* 201–210.

Abu Shara, K. A., Ghareeb, M. A., Zaher, S., Mobacher, A., Khalifa, M. C., & Saleh, S. Z. (1993). Radiotherapeutic effect on oropharyngeal flora in patients with head and neck cancer. *Journal of Laryngology and Otology, 107,* 222–227.

Adran, G. M., & Kemp, F. H. (1952). The protection of the laryngeal airway during swallowing. *British Journal of Radiology, 25,* 406–416.

Adran, G. M., & Kemp, F. H. (1956). Closure and opening of the larynx during swallowing. *British Journal of Radiology, 29,* 205–208.

Adran, G. M., & Kemp, F. H. (1967). The mechanism of the larynx: II. The epiglottis and closure of the larynx. *British Journal of Radiology, 29,* 205–208.

Al-Othman, M. O., Amdur, R. J., Morris, C. G., Hinerman, R. W., & Mendenhall, W. M. (2003). Does feeding tube placement predict for long-term swallowing disability after radiotherapy for head and neck cancer? *Head & Neck, 25,* 741–747.

American Joint Committee on Cancer. (1997) *Manual for the staging of cancer* (5th ed.). Philadelphia: Lippincott.

Amri, M., Car, A., & Jean, A. (1984). Medullary control of the pontine swallowing neurons in sheep. *Experimental Brain Research, 55,* 105–110.

Arcuri, M. R., & Schneider, R. L. (1992). The physiological effects of radiotherapy on oral tissue. *Journal of Prosthodontics, 1,* 37–41.

Asoh, R., & Goyal, R. K. (1978). Manometry and electromyography of the upper esophageal sphincter in the opossum. *Gastroenterology, 74,* 514–520.

Atkinson, M., Kramer, P., Wyman, S. M., & Ingelfinger, F. J. (1957). The dynamics of swallowing: I. Normal pharyngeal mechanisms. *Journal of Clinical Investigation, 36,* 581–598.

Aviv, J. E., Hecht, C., Weinberg, H., Dalton, J. F., & Urken, M. L. (1992). Surface sensibility of the floor of the mouth and tongue in healthy controls and in radiated patients. *Otolaryngology— Head and Neck Surgery, 107,* 418–423.

Bentzen, S. M., Thames, H. D., & Overgaard, M. (1989). Latent-time estimation for late cutaneous and subcutaneous radiation reactions in a single-follow-up clinical study. *Radiotherapy and Oncology, 15,* 267–274.

Bentzen, S. M., Turesson, I., & Thames, H. D. (1990). Fractionation sensitivity and latency of telangiectasia after postmastectomy radiotherapy: A graded-response analysis. *Radiotherapy and Oncology, 18,* 95–106.

Ben-Yosef, R., & Kapp, D. S. (1992). Persistent and/or late complications of combined radiation therapy and hyperthermia. *International Journal of Hyperthermia, 8,* 733–745.

Bisch, E. M., Logemann, J. A., Rademaker, A. W., Kahrilas, P. J., & Lazarus, C. L. (1994). Pharyngeal effects of bolus volume, viscosity, and temperature in patients with dysphagia resulting from neurologic impairment and normal subjects. *Journal of Speech and Hearing Research, 37,* 1041–1049.

Bosma, J. F. (1957). Deglutition: Pharyngeal stage. *Physiological Reviews, 37,* 275–300.

Brown, A. P., Fixsen, J. A., & Plowman, P. N. (1987). Local control of Ewing's sarcoma: An analysis of 67 patients. *The British Journal of Radiology, 60,* 261–268.

Cantor, R., Curtis, T. A., Shipp, T., Beumer, J., & Vogel, B. S. (1969). Maxillary speech prostheses for mandibular surgical defects. *Journal of Prosthetic Dentistry, 22,* 253–260.

Car, A., Jean, A., & Roman, C. (1975). A pontine primary relay for ascending projections of the superior laryngeal nerve. *Experimental Brain Research, 22,* 197–210.

Carpenter, M. B. (1991). *Core text of neuroanatomy* (4th ed., pp. 134–181). Baltimore: Williams & Wilkins.

Carrara-de-Angelis, E., Feher, O., Barros, A. P., Nishimoto, I. N., & Kowalski, L. P. (2003). Voice and swallowing in patients enrolled in a larynx preservation trial. *Archives of Otolaryngology— Head and Neck Surgery, 129,* 733–738.

Cerenko, D., McConnel, F. M. S., & Jackson, R. T. (1989). Quantitative assessment of pharyngeal bolus driving forces. *Otolaryngology—Head and Neck Surgery, 100,* 57–63.

Colangelo, L., Logemann, J., & Rademaker, A. (2000). Tumor size and pre-treatment speech and swallowing in patients with resectable tumors. *Otolaryngology—Head and Neck Surgery, 122,* 653–662.

Conley, J. J. (1962). The crippled oral cavity. *Plastic and Reconstructive Surgery, 30,* 469–478.

Cook, I. J., Dodds, W. J., Dantas, R. O., Massey, B., Kern, M. K., Lang, I. M., Brasseur, J. G., & Hogan, W. J. (1989). Opening mechanism of the human upper esophageal sphincter. *American Journal of Physiology: Gastrointestinal Liver Physiology, 20,* G748–G759.

Cooper, J. S., Fu, K., Marks, J., & Silverman, S. (1995). Late effects of radiation therapy in the head and neck region. *International Journal of Radiation Oncology, Biology, Physics, 31,* 1141–1164.

Dantas, R. O., & Dodds, W. J. (1990). Effect of bolus volume and consistency on swallow-induced submental and infrahyoid electromyographic activity. *Brazilian Journal of Medical Biologic Research, 23,* 37–44.

Dantas, R. O., Dodds, W. J., Massey, B. T., Shaker, R., & Cook, I. J. (1990). Manometric characteristics of glossopalatal sphincter. *Digestive Diseases and Sciences, 35,* 161–166.

Dantas, R. O., Kern, M. K., Massey, B. T., Dodds, W. J., Kahrilas, P. J., Brasseur, J. G., et al. (1990). Effect of swallowed bolus variables on oral and pharyngeal phases of swallowing. *American Journal of Physiology: Gastrointestinal Liver Physiology, 21,* G675–G681.

Davis, J. W., Lazarus, C., Logemann, J. A., & Hurst, P. S. (1987). Effect of a maxillary glossectomy prosthesis on articulation and swallowing. *Journal of Prosthetic Dentistry, 57,* 715–720.

Davis, R. K., Vincent, M. E., Shapshay, S. M., & Strong, M. S. (1982). The anatomy and complications of "T" versus vertical closure of the hypopharynx after laryngectomy. *Laryngoscope, 92,* 16–20.

Dejonckere, P., & Hordijk, G. (1998). Prognostic factors for swallowing after treatment of head and neck cancer. *Clinical Otolaryngology, 23,* 218–223.

DeNittis, A. S., Machtay, M., Rosenthal, D. I., Sanfilippo, N. J., Lee, J. H., Goldfeder, S., Chalian, A. A., Weinstein, G. S., & Weber, R. S. (2001). Advanced oropharyngeal carcinoma treated with surgery and radiotherapy: Oncologic outcome and functional assessment. *American Journal of Otolaryngology, 22,* 329–335.

Dodds, W. J., Man, K. M., Cook, I. J., Kahrilas, P. J., Stewart, E. T., & Kern, M. K. (1988). Influence of bolus volume on swallow-induced hyoid movement in normal subjects. *American Journal of Roentgenology, 150,* 1307–1309.

Dodds, W. J., Stewart, E. T., & Logemann, J. A. (1990). Physiology and radiology of normal oral and pharyngeal phases of swallowing. *American Journal of Radiology, 154,* 953–963.

Dodds, W. J., Taylor, A. J., Stewart, E. T., Kern, M. K., Logemann, J. A., & Cook, I. J. (1989). Tipper and dipper types of oral swallows. *American Journal of Radiology, 153,* 1197–1199.

Donner, M. W., Bosma, J. F., & Robertson, D. L. (1985). Anatomy and physiology of the pharynx. *Gastrointestinal Radiology, 10,* 196–212.

Eisbruch, A., Lyden, T., Bradford, C. R., Dawson, L. A., Haxer, M. J., Miller, A. E., Teknos, T. N., Chepeha, D. B., Hogikyan, N. D., Terrell, J. E., & Wolf, G. T. (2002). Objective assessment of swallowing dysfunction and aspiration after radiation concurrent with chemotherapy for head–neck cancer. *International Journal of Radiation Oncology, Biology, Physics, 53,* 23–28.

Eisele, D. W., Koch, D. G., Tarazi, A. E., & Jones, B. (1991). Aspiration from delayed radiation fibrosis of the neck. *Dysphagia, 6,* 120–122.

Ekberg, O. (1982). Closure of the laryngeal vestibule during deglutition. *Acta Otolaryngologie, 93,* 123–129.

Ekberg, O., Liedberg, B., & Owall, B. (1986). Barium and meat: A comparison between pharyngeal swallow of fluid and solid boluses. *Acta Radiologica Diagnosis, 27,* 701–704.

Ekberg, O., & Nylander, G. (1983). Pharyngeal dysfunction after treatment for pharyngeal cancer with surgery and radiotherapy. *Gastrointestinal Radiology, 8,* 97–104.

Ergun, G. A., Kahrilas, P. J., Lin, S., Logemann, J. A., & Harig, J. M. (1993). Shape, volume, and content of the deglutitive pharyngeal chamber imaged by ultrafast computerized tomography. *Gastroenterology, 105,* 1396–1403.

Ezure, K., Oku, Y., & Tanaka, I. (1993). Location and axonal projection of one type of swallowing interneurons in cat medulla. *Brain Research, 632,* 216–224.

Flaherty, R. F., Seltzer, S., Campbell, T., Weisskoff, R. M., & Gilbert, R. J. (1995). Dynamic magnetic imaging of vocal cord closure during deglutition using echoplanar magnetic resonance imaging techniques. *Gastroenterology, 109,* 843–849.

Fujiu, M., & Logemann, J. A. (1996). Effect of a tongue-holding maneuver on posterior pharyngeal wall movement during deglutition. *American Journal of Speech–Language Pathology, 5*, 23–30.

Fujiu, M., Logemann, J. A., & Pauloski, B. R. (1995). Increased postoperative posterior pharyngeal wall movement in patients with anterior oral cancer: Preliminary findings and possible implications for treatment. *American Journal of Speech–Language Pathology, 4*, 24–30.

Fujiu, M., Toleikis, J. R., Logemann, J. A., & Larson, C. R. (1994). Glossopharyngeal evoked potentials in normal subjects following mechanical stimulation of the anterior faucial pillar. *Electroencephalography and Clinical Neurophysiology, 92*, 183–195.

Garon, R. B., Engle, M., & Ormiston, C. (1996). Silent aspiration: Results of 1,000 videofluoroscopic swallow evaluations. *Journal of Neurologic Rehabilitation, 10*, 121–126.

Graner, D. E., Foote, R. L., Kasperbauer, J. L., Stoeckel, M. A., Okuno, S. H., Olsen, K. D., Sabri, A. N., Maragos, N. E., Cha, S. S., Sargent, D. J., & Strome, S. E. (2003). Swallow function in patients before and after intra-arterial chemoradiation. *Laryngoscope, 113*, 573–579.

Hamlet, S., Faull, J., Klein, B., Aref, A., Fontanesi, J., Stachler, R., Shamsa, F., Jones, L., & Simpson, M. (1997). Mastication and swallowing in patients with postirradiation xerostomia. *International Journal of Radiation Oncology, Biology and Physics, 37*, 789–796.

Hamlet, S., Muz, J., Farris, R., Kumpuris, T., & Jones, L. (1992). Scintigraphic quantification of pharyngeal retention following deglutition. *Dysphagia, 7*, 12–16.

Hamlet, S. L., Stone, M., & Shawker, T. H. (1988). Posterior tongue grooving in deglutition and speech: Preliminary observations. *Dysphagia, 3*, 65–68.

Hirano, M., Kuroiwa, Y., Tanaka, S., Matsuoka, H., Sato, K., & Yoshida, T. (1992). Dysphagia following various degrees of surgical resection for oral cancer. *Annals of Otology, Rhinology and Laryngology, 101*, 138–141.

Hirsch, S. M., Caldarelli, D. D., Hutchinson, J. C., Holinger, L. D., Murthy, A. K., Showel, J. L., & Taylor, S. G. (1991). Concomitant chemotherapy and split-course radiation for cure and preservation of speech and swallowing in head and neck cancer. *Laryngoscope, 101*, 583–586.

Hughes, C. V., Baum, B. J., Fox, P. C., Marmary, Y., Yeh, C., & Sonies, B. C. (1987). Oral-pharyngeal dysphagia: A common sequela of salivary gland dysfunction. *Dysphagia, 1*, 173–177.

Ichimura, K., & Tanaka, T. (1993). Trismus in patients with malignant tumours in the head and neck. *The Journal of Laryngology and Otology, 107*, 1017–1020.

Jacob, P., Kahrilas, P. J., Logemann, J. A., Shah, V., & Ha, T. (1989). Upper esophageal sphincter opening and modulation during swallowing. *Gastroenterology, 97*, 469–478.

Jacob, P., Kahrilas, P. J., Logemann, J. A., Tracy, J., Lazarus, C., & McLaughlin, B. (1988). Bolus viscosity and volume affect strap muscle EMG activity during swallowing. *Gastroenterology, 95*, 873.

Jean, A. (1984). Brainstem organization of the swallowing network. *Brain, Behavior and Evolution, 25*, 109–116.

Jean, A. (1990). Brainstem control of swallowing: Localization and organization of the central pattern generator for swallowing. In A. Taylor (Ed.), *Neurophysiology of the jaws and teeth* (pp. 294–321). London: Macmillan.

Jenkins, P., Lazarus, C., & Logemann, J. (1981, November). *Functional changes after hemilaryngectomy.* Paper presented at the annual convention of the American Speech-Language-Hearing Association, Boston.

Jentzsch, K., Binder, H., Cramer, H., Glaubiger, D. L., Kessler, R. M., Bull, C., Pomeroy, T. C., & Gerber, N. L. (1981). Leg function after radiotherapy for Ewing's sarcoma. *Cancer, 47*, 1267–1278.

Kahrilas, P. J., Dodds, W. J., Dent, J., Logemann, J. A., & Shaker, R. (1989). Upper esophageal sphincter function during swallowing. *Gastroenterology, 95*, 52–62.

Kahrilas, P. J., Lin, S., Logemann, J. A., Ergun, G. A., & Facchini, F. (1993). Deglutitive tongue action: Volume accommodation and bolus propulsion. *Gastroenterology, 104*, 152–162.

Kahrilas, P. J., Logemann, J. A., Krugler, C., & Flanagan, E. (1991). Volitional augmentation of upper esophageal sphincter opening during swallowing. *American Journal of Physiology: Gastrointestinal Liver Physiology, 23,* G450–G456.

Kahrilas, P. J., Logemann, J. A., Lin, S., & Ergun, G. A. (1992). Pharyngeal clearance during swallowing: A combined manometric and videofluoroscopic study. *Gastroenterology, 103,* 128–136.

Karasek, K., Constine, L. S., & Rosier, R. (1991). Sarcoma therapy: Functional outcome and relationship to treatment parameters. *International Journal of Radiation Oncology, Biology, Physics, 21*(Suppl. 1), 167–168.

Kendall, K. A., McKenzie, S. W., Leonard, R. J., & Jones, C. (1998). Structuralmobility in deglutition after single modality treatment of head and neck carcinomas with radiotherapy. *Head & Neck, 20,* 720–725.

Kessler, J. P., & Jean, A. (1985). Identification of the medullary swallowing regions in the rat. *Experimental Brain Research, 57,* 256–263.

Kidd, D., Lawson, J., Nesbitt, R., & MacMahon, J. (1993). Aspiration in acute stroke: A clinical study with videofluoroscopy. *Quarterly Journal of Medicine, 86,* 825–829.

Knowles, J. C., Chalian, V. A., & Shidnia, H. (1986). Pulp innervation after radiation therapy. *The Journal of Prosthetic Dentistry, 56,* 708–711.

Kotz, T., Abraham, S., Beitler, J., Wadler, S., & Smith, R. V. (1999). Pharyngeal transport dysfunction consequent to an organ-sparing protocol. *Archives of Otolaryngology—Head and Neck Surgery, 125,* 410–413.

Kuo, W., Wu, C. C., Lian, S. L., Ching, F. Y., Lee, K. W., & Juan, K. H. (1993). The effects of radiation therapy on salivary function in patients with head and neck cancer. *Kaohsiung Journal of Medical Science, 9,* 401–409.

Langmore, S. E., Schatz, K., & Olsen, N. (1988). Fiberoptic endoscopic examination of swallowing safety: A new procedure. *Dysphagia, 2,* 216–219.

Law, M. P. (1981). Radiation-induced vascular injury and its relation to late effects in normal tissues. In *Advances in radiation biology* (Vol. 9, pp. 37–73). New York: Academic Press.

Lazarus, C. L. (1993). Effects of radiation therapy and voluntary maneuvers on swallow function in head and neck cancer patients. *Clinics in Communicative Disorders, 3,* 11–20.

Lazarus, C. L. (1996). Effects of radiotherapy on tongue strength and swallowing. *Dysphagia, 11,* 161.

Lazarus, C. L. (1997). *The effects of radiotherapy on tongue strength and swallowing in oral and oropharyngeal cancer patients.* Unpublished doctoral dissertation, Northwestern University, Evanston, IL.

Lazarus, C. (1998). Communication problems in individuals with head and neck cancer. *Topics in Geriatric Rehabilitation, 14,* 44–55.

Lazarus, C., Logemann, J. A., & Gibbons, P. (1993). Effects of maneuvers on swallowing function in a dysphagic oral cancer patient. *Head & Neck, 15,* 419–424.

Lazarus, C., Logemann, J., Jenkins, P., & Ossoff, R. (1981, November). *Extent of supraglottic laryngectomy and functional status.* Paper presented at the annual convention of the American Speech-Language-Hearing Association, Boston.

Lazarus, C., Logemann, J. A., Pauloski, B. R., Colangelo, L. A., Kahrilas, P. J., Mittal, B. B., & Pierce, M. (1996). Swallowing disorders in head and neck cancer patients treated with radiotherapy and adjuvant chemotherapy. *Laryngoscope, 106,* 1157–1166.

Lazarus, C. L., Logemann, J. A., Rademaker, A. W., Kahrilas, P. J., Pajak, T., Lazar, R., & Halper, A. (1993). Effects of bolus volume, viscosity, and repeated swallows in nonstroke subjects and stroke patients. *Archives of Physical Medicine and Rehabilitation, 74,* 1066–1070.

Lazzara, G., Lazarus, C., & Logemann, J. A. (1986). Impact of thermal stimulation on the triggering of swallowing reflex. *Dysphagia, 1,* 73–77.

Leonard, R. J., & Gillis, R. (1990). Differential effects of speech prosthesis in glossectomized patients. *Journal of Prosthetic Dentistry, 64,* 701–708.

Linden, P., Kuhlemeier, K. V., & Patterson, C. (1993). The probability of correctly predicting sub-glottic penetration from clinical observations. *Dysphagia, 8,* 170–179.

Liu, R. P., Fleming, T. J., Toth, B. B., & Keene H. J. (1990). Salivary flow rates in patients with head and neck cancer 0.5 to 25 years after radiotherapy. *Oral Surgery, Oral Medicine and Oral Pathology, 70,* 724–729.

Logemann, J. A. (1983). *Evaluation and treatment of swallowing disorders.* San Diego, CA: College-Hill.

Logemann, J. (1984, November). *Recovery of vocal tract control after partial laryngectomy.* Paper presented at the annual convention of the Speech-Language-Hearing Association, San Francisco.

Logemann, J. (1985). Aspiration in head and neck surgical patients. *Annals of Otology, Rhinology and Laryngology, 94,* 373–376.

Logemann, J. A. (1993). *Manual for the videofluorographic study of swallowing* (2nd ed.). Austin, TX: PRO-ED.

Logemann, J. (1996). Therapy for oropharyngeal swallowing disorders. In A. Perlman & K. Schulze-Delrieu (Eds.), *Deglutition and its disorders: Anatomy, physiology, clinical diagnosis, and management.* (pp. 449–461). San Diego, CA: Singular.

Logemann, J. (1997). Role of the modified barium swallow in management of patients with dysphagia. *Otolaryngology—Head and Neck Surgery, 116,* 335–338.

Logemann, J., & Bytell, D. (1979). Swallowing disorders in three types of head and neck surgical patients. *Cancer, 81,* 469–478.

Logemann, J. A., Gibbons, P., Rademaker, A. W., Pauloski, B. R., Kahrilas, P. J., Bacon, M., Bowman, J., & McCracken, E. (1994). Mechanisms of recovery of swallow after supraglottic laryngectomy. *Journal of Speech and Hearing Research, 37,* 965–974.

Logemann, J. A., Kahrilas, P. J., Cheng, J., Pauloski, B. R., Gibbons, P. J., Rademaker, A. W., & Lin, S. (1992). Closure mechanisms of laryngeal vestibule during swallowing. *American Journal of Physiology: Gastrointestinal Liver and Physiology, 25,* G338–G344.

Logemann, J. A., Kahrilas, P. J., Hurst, P., Davis, J., & Krugler, C. (1989). Effects of intraoral prosthetics on swallowing in patients with oral cancer. *Dysphagia, 4,* 118–120.

Logemann, J., Kahrilas, P., Kobara, M., & Vakil, N. (1989). The benefit of head rotation on pharyngoesophageal dysphagia. *Archives of Physical Medicine and Rehabilitation, 70,* 767–771.

Logemann, J. A., Pauloski, B. R., & Colangelo, L. (1998). Light digital occlusion of the tracheostomy tube: A pilot study of effects on aspiration and biomechanics of the swallow. *Head & Neck, 20,* 52–57.

Logemann, J. A., Pauloski, B. R., Rademaker, A. W., & Colangelo, L. A. (1997a). Speech and swallowing rehabilitation for head and neck cancer patients. *Oncology, 5,* 651–659.

Logemann, J. A., Pauloski, B. R., Rademaker, A. W., & Colangelo, L. (1997b). Super-supraglottic swallow in irradiated head and neck cancer patients. *Head & Neck, 19,* 535–540.

Logemann, J. A., Rademaker, A. W., Pauloski, B. R., & Kahrilas, P. J. (1994). Effects of postural change on aspiration in head and neck surgical patients. *Otolaryngology—Head and Neck Surgery, 4,* 222–227.

Logemann, J. A., Rademaker, A. W., Pauloski, B. R., Ohmae, Y., & Kahrilas, P. J. (1998). Normal swallowing physiology as viewed by videofluoroscopy and videoendoscopy. *Folia Phoniatrica et Logopaedica, 50,* 311–319.

Logemann, J. A., Veis, S., & Colangelo, L. (1999). A screening procedure for oropharyngeal dysphagia. *Dysphagia, 14,* 44–51.

Lundy, D. S., Smith, C., Colangelo, L., Sullivan, P., Logemann, J. A., Lazarus, C. L., Newman, L. A., & Murry, T. (1999). Aspiration: Etiology and implications. *Otolaryngology—Head and Neck Surgery, 120,* 474–478.

Maciejewski, B., Withers, R., Taylor, J., & Hliniak, A. (1990). Dose fractionation and regeneration in radiotherapy for cancer of the oral cavity and oropharynx. Part 2. Normal tissue responses: Acute and late effects. *International Journal of Radiation Oncology, Biology, Physics, 18,* 101–111.

Månsson, I., & Sandberg, N. (1974). Effects of surface anesthesia on deglutition in man. *Laryngoscope, 27,* 427–437.

Månsson, I., & Sandberg, N. (1975). Oro-pharyngeal sensitivity and elicitation of swallowing in man. *Acta Otolaryngologica, 79,* 140–145.

Martin, B. J. W., Logemann, J. A., Shaker, R., & Dodds, W. J. (1993). Normal laryngeal valving patterns during three breath-hold maneuvers: A pilot investigation. *Dysphagia, 8,* 11–20.

McConnel, F. M. S. (1988). Analysis of pressure generation and bolus transit during pharyngeal swallowing. *Laryngoscope, 98,* 71–78.

McConnel, F. M. S., Logemann J. A., Rademaker, A. W., Pauloski, B. R., Baker, S. R., Lewin, J., Shedd, D., Heiser, M. A., Cardinale, S., Collins, S., Graner, D., Cook, B. S., Milianti, F., & Baker, T. (1994). Surgical variables affecting postoperative swallowing efficiency in oral cancer patients: A pilot study. *Laryngoscope, 104,* 87–90.

McConnel, F. M. S., Pauloski, B. R., Logemann, J. A., Rademaker, A. W., Colangelo, L., Shedd, D., Carroll, W., Lewin, J., & Johnson, J. (1998). Functional results of primary closure vs. flaps in oropharyngeal reconstruction. *Archives of Otolaryngology—Head and Neck Surgery, 124,* 625–630.

Mendelsohn, M. S., & Martin, R. S. (1993). Airway protection during breath-holding. *Annals of Otology, Rhinology and Laryngology, 102,* 941–944.

Miller, J. L., & Watkin, K. L. (1996). The influence of bolus volume and viscosity on anterior lingual force during the oral stage of swallowing. *Dysphagia, 11,* 117–124.

Miller, J. L., & Watkin, K. L. (1997). Lateral pharyngeal wall motion during swallowing using real time ultrasound. *Dysphagia, 12,* 125–132.

Muller-Miny, H., Eisele, D. W., & Jones, B. (1993). Dynamic radiographic imaging following total laryngectomy. *Head & Neck, 15,* 342–347.

Murry, T., Madasu, R., Martin, A., & Robbins, K. T. (1998). Acute and chronic changes in swallowing and quality of life following intraarterial chemoradiation for organ preservation in patients with advanced head and neck cancer. *Head & Neck, 20,* 31–37.

Muz, J., Hamlet, S., Mathog, R., & Farris, R. (1994). Scintigraphic assessment of aspiration in head and neck cancer patients with tracheostomy. *Head & Neck, 16,* 17–20.

Muz, J., Mathog, R. H., Miller, P. R., Rosen, R., & Borrero, G. (1987). Detection and quantification of laryngotracheopulmonary aspiration with scintigraphy. *Laryngoscope, 97,* 1180–1185.

Ogura, J. H., & Biller, H. F. (1969). Conservation surgery in cancer of head and neck. *Otolaryngologic Clinics of North America, 2,* 641–655.

Ogura, J. H., Sessions, D. G., & Ciralsky, R. H. (1975). Supraglottic carcinoma with extension to the arytenoid. *Laryngoscope, 85,* 1327–1331.

Ohmae, Y., Logemann, J. A., Kaiser, P., Hanson, D. G., & Kahrilas, P. J. (1995). Timing of glottic closure during normal swallowing. *Head & Neck, 17,* 394–402.

Ohmae, Y., Ogura, M., Kitahara, S., Karaho, T., & Inouye, T. (1998). Effects of head rotation on pharyngeal function during normal swallow. *Annals of Otolaryngology, Rhinology and Laryngology, 107,* 344–348.

Palmer, P. M., Perlman, A. L., McCulloch, T. M., Vandaele, D. J., & Luschei, E. S. (1994, November). *The effect of bolus volume on electromyography of select oral, laryngeal and pharyngeal muscles.* Paper presented at the annual meeting of the Dysphagia Research Society, McClean, VA.

Palmer, J. B., Rudin, N. J., Lara, G., & Crompton, A. W. (1992). Coordination of mastication and swallowing. *Dysphagia, 7,* 187–200.

Palmer, J. B., Tanaka, E., & Siebens, A. A. (1988). Motions of the posterior pharyngeal wall in swallowing. *Laryngoscope, 98,* 414–417.

Pauloski, B. R., Logemann, J. A., Colangelo, L. A., Rademaker, A. W., & McConnel, F. M. S. (1995, November). *Speech and swallow characteristics of surgically treated oral cancer patients.* Paper presented at the annual meeting of the American Speech-Language Hearing Association, Orlando, FL.

Pauloski, B. R., Logemann, J. A., Fox, J. C., & Colangelo, L. A. (1995). Biomechanical analysis of the pharyngeal swallow in postsurgical patients with anterior tongue and floor of mouth resection and distal flap reconstruction. *Journal of Speech and Hearing Research, 39,* 110–123.

Pauloski, B. R., Logemann, J. A., Rademaker, A. W., McConnel, F. M. S., Stein, D., Beery, Q., Johnson, J., Heiser, M. A., Cardinale, S., Shedd, D., Graner, D., Cook, B., Milianti, F., Collins, S., & Baker, T. (1994). Speech and swallowing function after oral and oropharyngeal resections: One-year follow-up. *Head & Neck, 16,* 313–322.

Pauloski, B. R., Rademaker, A. W., Logemann, J. A., & Colangelo, L. (1998). Speech and swallowing in irradiated and nonirradiated postsurgical oral cancer patients. *Otolaryngology—Head and Neck Surgery, 118,* 616–624.

Pauloski, B. R., Rademaker, A. W., Logemann, J. A., Lazarus, C. L., Newman, L., Hammer, A., MacCracken, E., Gaziano, J., & Stachowiak, L. (2002). Swallow function and perception of dysphagia in patients with head and neck cancer. *Head & Neck, 24,* 555–565.

Pauloski, B. R., Rademaker, A. W., Logemann, J. A., McConnel, F. M. S., Heiser, M. A., Cardinale, S., Lazarus, C. L., Pelzer, H., Stein, D., & Beery, Q. (2004). Surgical variables affecting swallowing in patients treated for oral/oropharyngeal cancer. *Head & Neck, 26,* 625–636.

Peters, L. J., Harrison, M. L., Dimery, I. W., Fields, R., Goepfert, H., & Oswald, M. J. (1988). Acute and late toxicity associated with sequential bleomycin-containing chemotherapy regimens and radiation therapy in the treatment of carcinoma of the nasopharynx. *International Journal of Radiation Oncology, Biology, Physics, 14,* 623–633.

Pfister, D. G., Bajorin, D., Motzer, R., Scher, H., Luoison, C., Harrison, L., et al. (1994). Cisplatin, fluorouracil, and leucovorin: Increased toxicity without improved response in squamous cell head and neck cancer. *Archives of Otolaryngology—Head and Neck Surgery, 120,* 89–95.

Pick, T. P., & Howden, R. (Eds.). (1974). *Gray's anatomy.* London: Running Press.

Pinkus, N. B. (1973). The dangers of oral feeding in the presence of cuffed tracheostomy tubes. *The Medical Journal of Australia, 1,* 1238–1240.

Pommerenke, W. T. (1928). A study of the sensory areas eliciting the swallowing reflex. *The American Journal of Physiology, 84,* 36–41.

Pouderoux, P., & Kahrilas, P. J. (1995). Deglutitive tongue force modulation by volition, volume and viscosity in humans. *Gastroenterology, 108,* 1418–1426.

Pouderoux, P., Logemann, J. A., & Kahrilas, P. J. (1996). Pharyngeal swallowing elicited by fluid infusion: Role of volition and vallecular containment. *American Journal of Physiology: Gastrointestinal Liver Physiology, 33,* G347–G354.

Pressman, J. J., & Bailey, B. J. (1978). The surgery of cancer of the larynx with special reference to subtotal laryngectomy. In J. C. Snidecor (Ed.), *Speech rehabilitation of the laryngectomized* (2nd ed., pp. 16–49). Springfield, IL: Thomas.

Rademaker, A. W., Pauloski, B. R., Logemann, J. A., & & Shanahan, T. K. (1994). Oropharyngeal swallow efficiency as a representative measure of swallowing function. *Journal of Speech and Hearing Research, 37,* 314–325.

Rademaker, A. W., Vonesh, E. F., Logemann, J. A., Pauloski, B. R., Liu, D., Lazarus, C. L., Newman, L. A., May, A. H., MacCracken, E., Gaziano, J., & Stachowiak, L. (2003). Eating ability in head and neck cancer patients after treatment with chemoradiation: A 12-month follow-up study accounting for dropout. *Head & Neck, 25,* 1034–1041.

Ramsey, G. H., Watson, J. S., Gramiak, R., & Weinberg, S. A. (1955). Cinefluorographic analysis of the mechanism of swallowing. *Radiology, 64,* 498–518.

Rasley, A., Logemann, J. A., Kahrilas, P. J., Rademaker, A. W., Pauloski, B. R., & Dodds, W. J. (1993). Prevention of barium aspiration during videofluoroscopic swallowing studies: Value of change in posture. *American Journal of Roentgenology, 160,* 1005–1009.

Redvanly, R. D., Hudgins, P. A., Gussack, G. S., Lewis, M., & Crocker, I. R. (1992). CT of muscle necrosis following radiation therapy in a patient with head and neck malignancy. *American Journal of Neuroradiology, 13,* 220–222.

Reimers-Neils, L., Logemann, J. A., & Larson, C. (1994). Viscosity effects on EMG activity in normal swallow. *Dysphagia, 9,* 101–106.

Robb, G. L., & Lewin, J. S. (2003). Speech and swallow outcomes in reconstructions of the pharynx and cervical esophagus. *Head & Neck, 25,* 232–244.

Robbins, K. T., Bowman, J. B., & Jacob, R. F. (1987). Postglossectomy deglutitory and articulatory rehabilitation with palatal augmentation prostheses. *Archives of Otolaryngology—Head and Neck Surgery, 113,* 1214–1218.

Robbins, J., Hamilton, J. W., Lof, G. L., & Kempster, G. B. (1992). Oropharyngeal swallowing in normal adults of different ages. *Gastroenterology, 103,* 823–829.

Rosenbek, J. C., Roecker, E. B., Wood, J. L., & Robbins, J. (1996). Thermal application reduces the duration of stage transition in dysphagia after stroke. *Dysphagia, 11,* 225–233.

Samlan, R. A., & Webster, K. T. (2002). Swallowing and speech therapy after definitive treatment for laryngeal cancer. *Otolaryngology Clinics of North America, 35,* 1115–1133.

Schwartz, L. K., Weiffenbach, J. M., Valdez, I. H., & Fox, P. (1993). Taste intensity performance in patients irradiated to the head and neck. *Physiology & Behavior, 53,* 671–677.

Sessions, D. G., Stallings, J. O., Brownson, R. J., & Ogura, J. H. (1973). Total glossectomy for advanced carcinoma of the base of the tongue. *Laryngoscope, 83,* 39–50.

Sessions, D. G., & Zill, R. (1979). Deglutition after conservation surgery for cancer of the larynx and hypopharynx. *Otolaryngology—Head and Neck Surgery, 87,* 779–796.

Shaker, R., Cook, I. J. S., Dodds, W. J., & Hogan, W. J. (1988). Pressure-flow dynamics of the oral phase of swallowing. *Dysphagia, 3,* 79–84.

Shanahan, T. K., Logemann, J. A., Rademaker, A. W., Pauloski, B. R., & Kahrilas, P. J. (1993) Chin-down posture effect on aspiration in dysphagic patients. *Archives of Physical Medicine and Rehabilitation, 74,* 736–739.

Shawker, T. H., Sonies, B., Hall, T. E., & Baum, B. F. (1984). Ultrasound analysis of tongue, hyoid, and larynx activity during swallowing. *Investigative Radiology, 19,* 82–86.

Shawker, T. H., Sonies, B., Stone, M., & Baum, B. J. (1983). Real-time ultrasound visualization of tongue movement during swallowing. *Journal of Clinical Ultrasound, 11,* 485–490.

Shedd, D. P., Scatliff, J. H., & Kirchner, J. A. (1960). The buccopharyngeal propulsive mechanism in human deglutition. *Surgery, 48,* 846–853.

Sinclair, W. J. (1970). Initiation of reflex swallowing from the naso- and oropharynx. *American Journal of Physiology, 218,* 956–960.

Skoner, J. M., Andersen, P. E., Cohen, J. I., Holland, J. J., Nansen, E., & Wax, M. K. (2003). Swallowing function and tracheotomy dependence after combined modality treatment including free tissue transfer for advanced-stage oropharyngeal cancer. *Laryngoscope, 113,* 1294–1298.

Smith, C. H., Logemann, J. A., Colangelo, L. A., Rademaker, A. W., & Pauloski, B. R. (1999). Incidence and patient characteristics associated with silent aspiration in the acute care setting. *Dysphagia, 14,* 1–7.

Smith, R. V., Kotz, T., Beitler, J. J., & Wadler, S. (2000). Long-term swallowing problems after organ preservation therapy with concomitant radiation therapy and intravenous hydroxyurea: Initial results. *Archives of Otolaryngology—Head and Neck Surgery, 126,* 384–389.

Sorin, R., Somers, S., Austin, W., & Bester, S. (1988). The influence of videofluoroscopy on the management of the dysphagic patient. *Dysphagia, 2,* 127–135.

Splaingard, M. L., Hutchins, B., Sulton, L. D., & Chaudhuri, G. (1988). Aspiration in rehabilitation patients: Videofluoroscopy vs. bedside clinical assessment. *Archives of Physical Medicine and Rehabilitation, 69,* 637–640.

Staple, T. W., & Ogura, J. H. (1966). Cineradiography of the swallowing mechanism following supraglottic subtotal laryngectomy. *Journal of Radiology, 87,* 226–230.

Stinson, S. F., DeLaney, T. F., Greenberg, J., Yang, J. C., Lampert, M. H., Hicks, J. E., Venzon, D., White, D. E., Rosenberg, S. A., & Glatstein, E. J. (1991). Acute and long-term effects on limb function of combined modality limb sparing therapy for extremity soft tissue sarcoma. *International Journal of Radiation Oncology, Biology, Physics, 21,* 1493–1499.

Stokman, M. A., Spijkervet, F. K., Burlage, F. R., Dijkstra, P. U., Manson, W. L., de Vries, E. G., & Roodenburg, J. L. (2003). Oral mucositis and selective elimination of oral flora in head and neck cancer patients receiving radiotherapy: A double-blind randomised clinical trial. *British Journal of Cancer, 88,* 1012–1016.

Takahashi, J., & Nakazawa, F. (1991). Effects of viscosity of liquid foods on palatal pressure. *Journal of Texture Studies, 22,* 13–24.

Taylor, S. G., Murthy, A. K., Caldarelli, D. D., Showel, J. L., Kiel, K., Griem, K. L., Mittal, B. B., Kies, M., Hutchinson, J. C., Holinger, L. D., Campanella, R., Witt, T. R., & Hoover, S. (1989). Combined simultaneous cisplatin/fluorouracil chemotherapy and split course radiation in head and neck cancer. *Journal of Clinical Oncology, 7,* 846–856.

Taylor, S. G., Murthy, A. K., Griem, K. L., Recine, D. C., Kiel, K., Blendowski, C., Bull Hurst, P., Showel, J. T., Hutchinson, J. C., Campanella, R. S., Chen, S., & Caldarelli, D. D. (1997). Concomitant cisplatin/5-FU infusion and radiotherapy in advanced head and neck cancer: 8-year analysis of results. *Head & Neck, 19,* 684–691.

Teichgraeber, J., Bowman, J., & Goepfert, H. (1986). Functional analysis of treatment of oral cavity cancer. *Archives of Otolaryngology—Head and Neck Surgery, 112,* 959–965.

Urken, M. L., Moscoso, J. F., Lawson, W., & Biller, H. F. (1994). A systematic approach to functional reconstruction of the oral cavity following partial and total glossectomy. *Archives of Otolaryngology—Head and Neck Surgery, 120,* 589–601.

Vandaele, D. J., Perlman, A. L., & Cassell, M. D. (1995). Intrinsic fibre architecture and attachments of the human epiglottis and their contributions to the mechanism of deglutition. *Journal of Anatomy, 186,* 1–15.

van Dam, F. S. A. M., Hilgers, F. J. M., Emsbroek, G., Touw, F. I., van As, C. J., & de Jong, N. (1999). Deterioration of olfaction and gustation as a consequence of total laryngectomy. *Larynogoscope, 109,* 1150–1155.

Veis, S., Logemann, J. A., & Colangelo, L. (2000). Effects of three techniques on maximum posterior movement of the tongue base. *Dysphagia, 15,* 142–145.

Vokes, E. E., Kies, M., Haraf, D. J, Mick, R., Moran, W. J., Kozloff, M., Mittal, B., Pelzer, H., Wenig, B., Panje, W., & Weichselbaum, R. R. (1995). Induction chemotherapy followed by concomitant chemoradiotherapy for advanced head and neck cancer: Impact on the natural history of the disease. *Journal of Clinical Oncology, 13,* 876–883.

Vokes, E. E., Moran, W. J., Mick, R., Weichselbaum, R. R., & Panje, W. R. (1989). Neoadjuvant and adjuvant methotrexate, cisplatin, and fluorouracil in multimodal therapy of head and neck cancer. *Journal of Clinical Oncology, 7,* 838–845.

Welch, M., Logemann, J. A., Rademaker, A. W., Pauloski, B. R., & Kahrilas, P. J. (1993). Changes in pharyngeal dimensions affected by chin tuck. *Archives of Physical Medicine and Rehabilitation, 74,* 178–181.

Wheeler, R. L., Logemann, J. A., & Rosen, M. S. (1980). Maxillary reshaping prostheses: Effectiveness in improving speech and swallowing in postsurgical oral cancer patients. *Journal of Prosthetic Dentistry, 43,* 313–319.

Whillis, J. (1946). Movements of the tongue in swallowing. *Journal of Anatomy, 80,* 115–116.

PART III

Chapter 15

Counseling the Laryngectomized Patient and Family

Considerations Before, During, and After Treatment

Leslie E. Glaze

A laryngectomy patient and his or her family will face enormous emotional challenges based on the loss of normal communication and the potentially life-threatening diagnosis of cancer. Communication is the very essence of the human connection, and at the time of the diagnosis, patients facing laryngectomy cannot fully comprehend the impact of permanent loss of normal voice. Therefore, they will need abundant and competent support from the moment of diagnosis and throughout the recovery period to achieve the ultimate desired goal: transition to a well-rehabilitated individual with effective alaryngeal speech. This chapter provides supportive information for speech–language pathologists who work with laryngectomized individuals and their families. This chapter focuses especially on the critical counseling role that a speech–language pathologist must fill pre- and postoperatively to create a clinical relationship with the patient and family that fosters open communication, trust, and a basis for effective clinical treatment.

Counseling, in the broadest sense, includes a range of interpersonal activities—including teaching, listening, empathizing, advocating, and affirming—that contribute to the emotional well-being of another individual. Traditionally, a counselor serves a role of giving information and advice. Luterman (1996), however, broadened this traditional definition of counselor as an "informer" and thoroughly cast aside the notion of counselor as "persuader." Rather, he redefined the role of a counselor as a professional who *listens to* and *values* the needs of the client, in a mutually trusted exchange that allows the client to become "better able to contend successfully with the specific problem at hand" (p. 5). Information provided must be clear, reliable, and accurate (Anderson & Doyle, 2000).

Indeed, evidence in the literature strongly supports the need for professionals to foster open discussion with patients and families about their feelings related to cancer recovery. Mesters et al. (1997) studied 133 head and neck cancer patients at four points in time: just before treatment, and at 6 weeks, 13 weeks, and 1 year following treatment. Patients self-rated their tendencies to discuss cancer openly. Those with increased tendencies toward open discussion generally showed more positive rehabilitation outcomes, including higher self-esteem, fewer negative feelings, more sense of control, and fewer psychological and physical complaints. To achieve clinical competence and comfort in this area, a speech–language pathologist must be prepared to learn effective communication counseling skills (Gilmore, 1997). Apart from directing the actual speech treatment program, speech–language pathologists have several counseling responsibilities to the laryngectomy patient and family:

- to provide information about alaryngeal speech rehabilitation
- to determine the patient's functional communication needs through careful interviews with the patient, spouse, family, or friends
- to build an effective professional relationship based on trust
- to monitor and empathize with the patient's emotional transitions
- to monitor and facilitate the patient's overall rehabilitation toward full recovery and renewed quality of life

355

Certainly, the speech–language pathologist is not the only team member who will counsel the patient and family through this process. Many professionals assist in the diagnosis, treatment, and rehabilitation of a laryngectomized individual, including the medical physician, head and neck surgeon, oncology nurse, radiologist, hospital nursing staff, physical therapist, dietician, respiratory therapist, dentist, prosthedontist, and speech–language pathologist. A multidisciplinary team with good intercommunication is essential to positive outcomes for patients with head and neck cancer, especially in advanced carcinomas (Blair & Callender, 1994).

In most practices, however, the head and neck surgeon, the oncology nurse, and the speech–language pathologist are the individuals who have the long-term responsibility for coordinating the patient's care and monitoring the patient's progress from diagnosis to full rehabilitation. The head and neck surgeon has primary responsibility for the surgery and the medical recovery. The oncology nurse will teach the patient new self-care routines to manage the stoma and ease adjustments to changes in eating, breathing, and other body functions. The speech–language pathologist's role begins preoperatively but extends well into the postoperative period, as long as alaryngeal speech treatment is needed. As one of these key professional caregivers, the speech–language pathologist must be prepared to consult with laryngectomy patients and their families before and after surgery, to meet their critical needs for emotional support, trust, and content information. Consequently, there are two parallel purposes of this chapter: (a) to highlight appropriate interpersonal communication techniques and (b) to provide a comprehensive summary of the relevant content information for pre- and postoperative consultation with patients and families. This chapter begins with suggestions for general counseling interactions for use with patients, spouses, families, and friends. The last portion provides specific guidelines for useful content information in the pre- and postoperative and rehabilitation periods.

EFFECTIVE COMMUNICATING AND COUNSELING FOR THE PATIENT AND FAMILY

Providing Emotional Support

As soon as the patient receives the cancer diagnosis, a new and unfamiliar wave of information, emotion, and activity is set in motion. Often, patients report that they feel an overriding sense of loss of control. Not only are they powerless to control the cancer growth, but they must suddenly have trust in many other individuals who will decide what treatment options are available, when these medical processes should occur, and what outcomes are expected. For the patient, this need to rely on so many unfamiliar professionals and their respective disciplines can be overwhelming (Doyle, 1994; Levine, 1996–1997; Salmon, 1986, 1991; see also Chapter 26 in this text). Preoperatively, the first task of the speech–language pathologist must be to meet the patient and family and establish whatever tentative rapport can be achieved (often in only one brief consultation). Even if time constraints prevent sufficient opportunity for informative discussion, the speech–language pathologist can provide assurance to the patient and family that he or she will be there to help postoperatively.

Most head and neck cancer patients have never required the services of a speech–language pathologist previously, and they do not relish the thought of needing to learn a new form of speech production. Thus, this news of the cancer diagnosis and the prospect of a laryngectomy surgery are overwhelmingly negative. The speech–language pathologist must recognize and accept the potential (and justifiable) frustration, anger, sadness, and even disbelief that patients and families may express pre- and postoperatively. Luterman (1996) and Salmon (1991; see also Chapter 3 in this text) both liken this emotional process to the well-known grief cycle stages associated with death described by Elizabeth Kubler-Ross (1974). This series of transitions for the patient and family may not occur in any predictable form or order, but they most definitely constitute an evolving process of realizing, grappling with, accepting, and ultimately adapting to change. For some patients, the negative overtones of this cycle may be pervasive. Chaturvedi, Shenoy, Prasad, Senthilnathan, and Premlatha (1996) determined that some ineffective coping techniques, including a sense of hopelessness and fatalism, were common in a series of 50 patients diagnosed with head and neck cancer. Henderson and Ord (1997) reported a suicide incidence of 1.2% (3 out of 241) in patients diagnosed with head and neck cancer and noted that some other patients in the same series refused treatment and counseling altogether. Terrell, Nanavati, Esclamado, Bradford, and Wolf (1999) administered a multidimensional quality-of-life rating instrument to 397 head and neck cancer patients. Of four factors (emotional well-being, pain, eating, and communication), low emotional well-being scores correlated most directly with the patients' perceived effects of head and neck cancer as an "overall bother." All of these findings suggest that while patients are adapting to changes in physical structure, communication, and eating, most do struggle with their emotional adjustments to life after surgery (see Terrell et al., 2004).

Hammerlid, Persson, Sullivan, and Westin (1999) reported an important positive benefit of psychosocial counseling in head and neck cancer patients. A yearlong psychoeducational group therapy program resulted in significantly improved ratings for social and emotional functions and overall quality of life as compared to a no-treatment control group. Thus, this information underscores the need to establish a basis for discussing and reconciling emotional adjustments to head and neck cancer. Speech–language pathologists can assist the patient and family, by listening actively and sensitively, to support them through the early emotional adjustments to the cancer diagnosis, the pending surgery, and later, the learning curve toward effective alaryngeal speech (American Cancer Society, 1995; Casper & Colton, 1998; Doyle, 1994; Keith & Thomas, 1996; Salmon, 1986; see also Chapters 3 and 5 in this text).

Based on clinical experience, several counseling techniques may enhance communications between clinicians and patients at all phases of the patient–clinician relationship.

1. Listen actively and without judgment; accept the patient's and family's emotions and do not try to modify their feelings. Intense sadness, confusion, anger, worry, fear, and frustration are likely to be honest reactions. When clinicians demonstrate tolerance for these feelings, even if they are negative, patients may be encouraged to maintain open communication that is essential for effective rehabilitation.

2. If a patient or spouse appears desperate or inconsolable, enlist the assistance of the referring physician, a professional counselor, and with the family's permission, a member of the clergy, to offer stronger support for the patient to guide him or her toward hope and reconciliation.

3. Do not intervene or take sides if patients or family members appear to disagree or argue. Understand that in all periods of stress, old anxieties or struggles may resurface. In both pre- and postoperative periods, the patient and family may feel helpless and experience a sense of emotional crisis, especially if they have not yet perceived the inevitable "peaks and valleys" of the rehabilitation process. The observations and impressions a clinician may form from any single session may not be representative of the long-term prognosis for rehabilitation.

4. Empathize and encourage, but do not attempt to minimize or "cheerlead" the situation. Encourage the patient's feelings of hopefulness and draw from other positive experiences with patient outcomes and typical recovery patterns to bolster the patient's understanding that good times and satisfaction still lie ahead. Consider the following set of verbal messages that could be provided to a patient facing postoperative blues and the relative effects of each:

   ◪ Well-intended but potentially alienating approach:
     "I'd like you to try to look on the bright side. You recovered from the surgery so quickly! I understand what this must feel like, but please don't worry. Although it's difficult not to be able to speak as you have for so many years, there are many alaryngeal speech alternatives, and I know that we will be able to find one that works well for you. Many others have done it. I am certain that you will, too!"

While seemingly positive and upbeat, this statement devalues the patient's sad feelings and suggests that he or she should feel better based on the speech–language pathologist's convictions.

   ◪ Better approach:
     "I can tell that you are sad. I can't begin to know what you are really feeling right now, but I can share with you my experience from many other patients. They tell me consistently that it is entirely normal to feel isolated and depressed at times, and that there will continue to be some ups and downs throughout this rehabilitation. But frankly, I would worry about a patient who doesn't express any sadness or depression during this process. I'm glad that you feel that you can share your thoughts with me.

Is there any information or assistance I can provide to help you through this transition today?"

This alternative statement affirms the patient's ability to "be true" to his or her own emotions. The speech–language pathologist provides support to all patients without presuming to know personally what each patient is feeling. Finally, this statement does not insist, coerce, or persuade the patient to "give up" the real emotion he or she is experiencing.

5. Despite the speech–language pathologist's best efforts to communicate clearly and sensitively, some patients will not agree with a well-intended approach. The source of disagreement is important. Sometimes, patients may be simply unhappy with the unwelcome, if justifiable call for lifestyle changes (e.g., need to end smoking following the surgery or to abandon fishing from a canoe in favor of a more stable boat). At other times, the source of the patient's disagreement may be completely unrelated to the clinical process per se. Nonetheless, professionals have the responsibility to maintain a universal positive regard for individuals and to take the emotional "high road" when patients disregard a recommendation or choose alternative paths than the ones that have been planned. The following anecdote illustrates the need for clinicians to be unwavering in their consistent positive support of patients, even if the pleasantries do not appear to be reciprocal:

> One former patient described himself as a "loner" and indeed, he spoke little, avoided eye contact, and responded to questions with terse, sarcastic remarks. Nonetheless, he came consistently to therapy, achieving and maintaining consistent progress during each session. I provided functional home exercises for him to practice speech with others, such as conversations with neighbors, getting directions from a store clerk, and asking for the correct time from strangers. To my knowledge, he had not conducted any of these speech tasks. Nonetheless, after about a month, he had developed very functional artificial larynx speech and I anticipated that he might wish to end treatment because he did not seem to enjoy it. One day, he arrived looking and appearing different—hint of a smile, with a bit more eye contact. As we began the usual greetings, he said, "Sorry I'm not much of a talker. I'm better now. Thanks for waiting for me." When I asked him what he meant by "waiting for him," he said, "It was just nice that you never gave up on me."

6. Share control of the clinician–patient relationship in counseling and rehabilitation by offering patients options for what information and how much they wish to hear in a given session. This is especially helpful when time is limited. Luterman (1996) recommended that the clinician announce how many minutes are left in the session and ask the client what questions are highest on his or her priority list for discussion. This tactic ensures that the session includes essential components of the planned session, while meeting the particular interests of the patient on that day.

7. Elicit the patient's suggestions for what goals he or she may have for treatment. This is the clinician's opportunity to encourage both basic functional needs, such as being able to communicate on the telephone, and advanced communication skills, such as

carrying on a conversation in a busy social environment. By requesting some goal directions from the patient, the clinician can devise functional outcome measures that embed practical motivations for each individual.

Establishing Trust

Before, during, and after treatment, skillful clinicians strive to achieve a level of trust with the patient and family. Obviously, this trust must be developed and granted over time and is earned based on the clinician's ability to consistently provide accurate and competent information, while maintaining sensitive yet direct honesty with the patient. Interacting with laryngectomized individuals has some distinct characteristics that are nearly unique among the broad range of communication disorders. First, laryngectomized patients are usually cognitively intact and entirely capable of equal partnership with clinicians in describing their needs and interests in the rehabilitation process. Second, these individuals have just faced and will hopefully overcome a life-threatening disease. Their emotional adjustments to a potentially deadly encounter with cancer may have long-standing repercussions in their own ability to become fully rehabilitated socially as well as physically. Third, these patients have been permanently deprived of their ability to communicate normally (Eadie & Doyle, 2004). In the process of speech rehabilitation, patients will undoubtedly have frustrating, humiliating, and sometimes embarrassing moments when messages cannot be delivered with the accustomed rate, style, independence, and intelligibility that they enjoyed preoperatively. The following anecdote demonstrates such a moment:

> One patient came to a session, grinning from ear to ear, prepared to tell a joke using his artificial larynx speech. To my dismay, I tracked only part of the anecdote and missed the entire punch line! To understand the quip, I was forced to question him and guess repeatedly at the phrase. He restated the punch line using other words, and finally resorted to writing the original words on paper. I finally got the message and laughed at the joke, but the cadence and "snap" of the humor was long gone for both of us. He understood my need to insist that I "get" the message rather than just smile and pretend, but it was a frustrating moment for both of us.

Clinicians must advocate strongly for patients to experience successful independent communication. To achieve that goal, however, the learning curve will usually require direct (though diplomatic) feedback regarding alaryngeal speech intelligibility.

    Some clinicians may feel that it is kinder to protect patients from repeated failure by pretending to understand, thinking that they deserve this (false) encouragement after surviving the significant ordeal of a cancer diagnosis and surgery. Most patients, however, report that they can tell very quickly when listeners are "pretending." Instead, the clinician must always be true to his or her patient by maintaining a commitment to honest feedback about speech intelligibility.

This honesty is the foundation of the trust that clinicians hope to develop with patients. This same honesty can also serve as a model for patients, to give them the courage to enable other listeners to be candid as well. A well-rehabilitated laryngectomized speaker will be able to say with pride, "If you can't understand me, just say so! I'll be happy to repeat it."

Because voice and personality are so closely related, loss of voice is also a loss of identity (Casper & Colton, 1998), and patients may find that they are unable to recover the same communication style as they experienced preoperatively. Indeed, Karnell, Funk, and Hoffman (2000) determined that social/role functioning correlated significantly with quality-of-life ratings in head and neck cancer patients. A person with a loud, boisterous, or life-of-the-party personality will not enjoy the same volume, speech rate, or spontaneity following surgery. Nonetheless, this outgoing personality trait may be the very asset that contributes to a positive course of speech rehabilitation. One former patient who was a traveling salesman continued to enjoy his "gift of gab" on the road using an artificial larynx, which he had deliberately selected based on his ability to speak faster and louder, as he had before. Another laryngectomized speaker who was employed in a retail setting opted for a tracheostoma valve so that she could be "hands free" to talk on the telephone and write at the same time.

Laryngectomy patients will also be forced to adjust to physical disfigurement due to the presence of a stoma, tissue scarring, and change in neck size. These visible changes may challenge the patients' self-esteem even beyond the need to develop alaryngeal speech communication (Doyle, 1999; Ramirez et al., 2003). In one study, quality-of-life measures were obtained in a self-report comparison between advanced head and neck cancer patients treated with conventional surgery and those treated with a nonsurgical organ-preservation protocol. Findings revealed that the category of "physical disfigurement associated with surgery" resulted in lower quality-of-life ratings and lower overall mental health indicators for the postsurgical patients (McDonough et al., 1996; Terrell, Fisher, & Wolf, 1998; Terrell et al., 2004). Similar findings were revealed in a comparison of patients with T1 glottic carcinoma with patient groups that received total laryngectomy or commando procedures (de Boer et al., 1995). Greater levels of psychosocial distress were reported for patients who underwent more significant physical disfigurement, but positive outcomes were most closely associated with open discussion of the illness and perceptions of adequate information from professionals (de Boer et al., 1995). In a separate study, Glicklich, Goldsmith, and Funk (1997) determined that a specific quality-of-life measure designed for head and neck cancer patients was more sensitive to patient perceptions than a general quality-of-life probe. Specifically, ratings of appearance (due to physical disfigurement) were captured strongly by the head and neck survey but not by the general probe.

Evidence is clear, therefore, that physical disfigurement is a profound underlying concern that does affect postsurgical quality of life in head and neck cancer patients. The speech–language pathologist can support patients' adjustment by being willing to foster their sense of comfort with the physical changes following surgery, and by counseling them to achieve the most natural social adaptations to changes in neck covering and management of sneezing, coughing, and secretions. Shirley Salmon (personal communication, 1984) used to liken the stoma to "a new nose," which accurately describes the function of the stoma while softening the anxiety and strangeness that patients may feel in having a new opening in the body. Beyond the associated health benefits of stoma covers, patients are obviously well aware of the need to keep the stoma covered for their own privacy and for public comfort. The following anecdote illustrates this issue well:

> One day a patient came into the clinic, red in the face and visibly upset. He had just entered the building from outside, where the wind was blowing so hard that it had actually blown his stoma bib out of his collar and up over his shoulder. When he had reached the elevator, he was still readjusting the cover, to the stares of others waiting in the elevator. His question for me was insightful: "Should I have been embarrassed?"

The role of counselor should include helping patients come to terms with their new physical structures, including comfort in protecting the stoma, without shame or embarrassment. In a successful rapport between patient and clinician, neither party should be embarrassed to discuss these issues.

Educating Patients and Families

Delivering information to patients and families can occur in many modalities: informal conversation, supportive written handouts or booklets, videotape demonstration, and "on-call" phone contacts. Many supplemental videotapes, Web sites, visual diagrams, and written summaries are available for the patient and family to review at home (Gress, 2004; Keith, 1991; Keith & Thomas, 1996; Salmon, 1986, 1991; see also Chapter 25 in this text). The American Cancer Society, the International Association of Laryngectomees, and other publishers have worthy reading materials and visual aids to underscore the information provided in a preoperative consultation. Often, patients will later concede that "information overload" at an early consultation prevents them from understanding new descriptions and explanations until they have had a chance to review materials a second time at home. After reading these materials at leisure and in relaxed surroundings, patients and families appear to know more about the condition and the expectations. They also report feeling more prepared to consider new information, and more confident in their ability to ask questions, to advocate for individual needs, and to fulfill a role as an equal partner in postoperative care.

The old adage that "there's no such thing as a stupid question" can be a point of encouragement for patients and their families, who are often worried about appearing unwise or incompetent to professionals. Thus, many feel embarrassed, unprepared, or poorly qualified to seek answers to their questions. Some patients are intimidated by the medical setting under any circumstances, which creates an underlying power imbalance between patient and caregiver. Facing a diagnosis of head and neck cancer is frightening, bewildering, and unfamiliar. This combination of events would cause many patients and families to lose confidence in their own abilities to manage a large set of new information. Some patients will relegate the question-asking duties to another family member, a trusted friend, or even a clergyman or community elder.

The role of the speech–language pathologist is twofold, then. First, the clinician must create an environment in which patients and families feel that they can ask all questions (even more than once) safely, comfortably, and confidently. Second, the clinician must be prepared to treat each question respectfully and confidentially, and make certain that responses are honest, accurate, tactful, and timely. Skilled clinicians will ensure that information is described clearly, using short, simple, and direct language without jargon. Patients and families are usually unfamiliar with most of the new terms related to alaryngeal physical care and speech rehabilitation. Consider, for example, the following message delivered by a speech–language pathology student to a patient at bedside:

◲ Well-intended but potentially alienating approach:
"Mr. Jones, just as soon as you are out of the ICU and the NG tube is removed, we'll be able to get you started talking with a Servox."

◲ Better approach:
"Mr. Jones, that feeding tube through your nose will come out as soon as the physician has determined that all of the wounds in your neck have healed and you are discharged from the intensive care unit. At that time, we'll let you begin using an artificial larynx device to talk."

Although the first message was accurate and well meant, the clinician may have confused the patient by assuming that he understood the meaning of "ICU," "NG," and "Servox." Beyond that, she did not tell him why the information is relevant. Instead, a short description of the place (intensive care unit), the function of the NG (nasogastric) tube (feeding tube though your nose), and the Servox device (the artificial larynx) would have reinforced the information for the patient.

Counseling a Spouse, Children, and Friends

The powerlessness expressed by many patients when they first receive a diagnosis of cancer is compounded for a spouse or significant other. These partners not only share in the shock and fear of the initial news, but must also stand aside while loved ones undergo the surgery and rehabilitation. Although spouses can be the best advocates for patients, they do experience their own set of emotional roller coasters. They may feel fear over the diagnosis, resentment at the need to take on a new and unfamiliar role, confusion in response to the patient's needs (how much help to provide), and a difficult adjustment to the loss of familiar communication patterns. All of these responses are entirely normal, especially in the early weeks. As with patients, spouses who appear indifferent and unconcerned may not be accepting the information completely or may be showing signs of latent anger or fear (see Chapter 3 in this text). Spouses often express anger at the situation, but most feel that they are not entitled to complain when it is the patient and not they who must face the cancer. There are also more significant worries, sometimes over loss of family income, the change in dominant roles (even temporarily), and the nagging fear of recurrence and survival (Levine, 1996–1997; Salmon, 1986; see also Chapters 28 and 29 in this text).

The speech–language pathologist may provide the following recommendations to spouses for support.

1. Allow the patient to do as much as he or she is able to do, once recovery from surgery is complete. One spouse expressed fear preoperatively that she would have to pay all the bills and do all the driving, two roles her husband had always taken before. When I asked her why she felt she had to take on these tasks, she responded, "Shouldn't I?" Do not allow subtle guilt or fear over the patient's diagnosis to eradicate the time-honored and traditional roles that have been comfortable in the past.

2. Seek out the mutual support of other spouses, through the International Association of Laryngectomees and American Cancer Society laryngectomy clubs. Often these groups provide a range of activities, including formal group discussions facilitated by a leader, informal coffee chats during meeting times, and periodic service projects. This spouse-to-spouse exchange can be invaluable, as they share both challenges and triumphs from experience.

3. Avoid speaking for the patient and encourage independent communication to the maximum extent possible. If other friends, family members, or strangers cannot understand a patient, it is fine to provide tactful "interpretation," but advise the speech–language pathologist, who will address these functional deficits directly in the speech therapy plan.

4. Retain time and comfort for oneself, recognizing that spouses also need emotional reserve to support others. Share any new concerns about adjustments and changes with the patient, to emphasize and maintain the partnership that has formed the basis for the relationship.

When the patient and spouse appear to work together easily and share a sense of optimism, the clinician can feel more assured that they will be able to communicate well through the process. Usually, as the rehabilitation process unfolds, adjustments move slowly into place and aggravations, although real, become anecdotal and hopefully laughable, especially between spouses whose love sustains them through this difficult transition. One spouse bemoaned the fact that they had worn a path in their carpeting from the kitchen to the TV room, because her husband's esophageal voice was too soft to allow him to "holler" from room to room to speak with her anymore (see Chapter 3 in this text). A favorite anecdote came from a female laryngectomy patient who captured the essence of spousal love and support in her description of her first night home after her surgery:

> Their bedtime routine had always been to whisper "I love you" to each other in the dark before drifting off to sleep. As she lay in the dark, without a voice, she felt heartbroken at the realization that she could no longer do this. After a few moments, she rolled over, put on her light, and wrote a brief note to her husband: "I love you." Then, she handed the note to him. He took it, stared at it a moment, rolled over, turned on his light, put on his glasses, and read it. "I love you, too," he said. Then, they went to sleep.

Children are surprisingly resilient, and most of their fears are confined to concerns about the loved one's prognosis and mortality. Once these issues are resolved, children seem to adapt easily to changes in speech and voice after listening to an alaryngeal speaker. In fact, the alaryngeal speech component is often a source of interest and novelty to children. Many become rapidly adept at understanding alaryngeal speech, and are interested in knowing more about the mechanics of producing esophageal speech or using an artificial larynx. Their interest and their tolerance for differences in speech production can be very encouraging for patients. One former patient reported that his granddaughter took him (and his artificial larynx device) to her kindergarten class for show and tell. Others have reported humorous escapades with children who are intrigued by the artificial larynx speech quality. On a more serious note, many patients have given extensively of their time and their wisdom by visiting elementary, middle, and high schools to warn of the dangers of smoking and to provide cancer awareness. These patient–heroes have spoken to literally thousands of groups, and the impact can be profound. The following is a poignant example of that very same impact:

> A patient was walking down a hospital corridor. A young child was ahead of him, walking with his mother. When he heard the patient speaking, using his artificial larynx, he whirled around, eyes widened. The patient took the time to explain that he was using an artificial larynx because his voice box had been removed after he got cancer from smoking cigarettes. The child nodded silently, then turned to his mother and said, "Please stop smoking."

Support from friends and acquaintances outside the family circle is another critical asset to the rehabilitation process. Because friends in social settings, the neighborhood, and the workplace are less directly affected by the emotional intensity of the surgery, they may supply a needed diversion for the patient and family. Patients who have friends that they can trust will also rely on their advice about the realities of speech intelligibility, appearance, and other physical changes following surgery. Friends can provide the essential motivation for the patient to move beyond the dependence on immediate family members to reestablish communicative independence in a larger arena of social contacts. When peers accompany patients to the clinic, they are often able to assess and report very accurately and candidly about the patient's observable progress.

> One former patient was quite timid about her appearance and about her use of the artificial larynx. Although she left therapy each week with some functional speech tasks to conduct with others, she was reluctant to try them. Fortunately, a close friend picked her up every day, made her walk around the local mall, and insisted that the patient order her own lunch. Gradually, the patient widened her scope of "comfortable" communication surroundings.

Nonetheless, some patients have disappointing experiences with friends who seem to withdraw from the patient following surgery, especially if they fear that any diagnosis of cancer is terminal (Casper & Colton, 1998; Doyle, 1994; see also Chapter 28 in this text). When this happens, the speech–language pathologist needs to remind patients and families of the potential for individuals to feel conflicted about their own fears of the cancer diagnosis or discomfort with alaryngeal speech intelligibility. The greater the self-esteem garnered by the patient, the more he or she is able to confront good friends and invite them to rekindle the relationship, albeit under slightly different speech circumstances.

THE TIME COURSE OF INFORMATION, REACTION, AND RECONCILIATION

Information Patients Need Preoperatively

The most critical speech–related information the patient needs to know boils down to this: "You will lose your larynx" and "There is oral speech after laryngectomy." The speech–language pathologist, however, needs to impart other important information. Appendix 15.A provides an example of a list that the clinician can use to make sure that he or she covers all topics at the preoperative consultation.

Doyle (1994) and Salmon (1991) asserted that there are four essential content areas that must be communicated to a patient preoperatively:

1. The patient will have postsurgical changes in anatomy and physiology.
2. The patient will have no voice in the early postoperative period, and immediately after surgery, the patient will need to write, use a communication board, or use gestures.
3. Several alaryngeal speech alternatives are available, and nearly every patient is able to achieve functional alaryngeal oral communication.
4. The speech–language pathologist will be available to assist the patient throughout the entire course of speech rehabilitation.

Patients must understand the changes in anatomy and physiology that will occur following surgery. At the minimum, it is essential that the clinician take time to review the differences in breathing, sneezing, coughing, and eating. By using clear and well-drawn visual aids of the anatomy before and after surgery, the speech–language pathologist can verify that the patient understands the following:

- The larynx will be removed, and the patient will not be able to speak immediately.
- With the loss of the larynx, both vocal communicative and nonspeech sounds will be lost, including audible laughing, crying, humming, snoring, throat clearing, coughing, whispering, and grunting.
- The trachea will be cut and diverted forward to the neck to create a stoma for breathing.
- There will be many early adjustments to stoma care, including managing secretions, crusting, suctioning, and use of saline.
- The patients will experience changes in tasting and smelling.

Moss (1988) and others (e.g., Gargan, 1969) who have described the experience from a patient's perspective assert that it is often true that patients listen to but do not "hear" some of the vital messages that surgeons and clinicians provide in the hectic preoperative period. Luterman (1996) also emphasized the difficulty patients may experience in hearing and absorbing information in the early period following the shock of a new diagnosis. Extreme examples are reported of patients who deny any recall of early critical messages, such as the diagnosis of cancer, the need to remove the whole larynx, the need for a stoma, or the fact that voice will be lost. For this reason, it may be useful for the speech–language pathologist to confirm the patient's understanding of the impending surgery by asking, "Tell me in your own words what the doctor has told you." This approach also ensures that the surgeon, not the speech–language pathologist, has provided the patient with the medical diagnosis and surgical plan.

After describing basic changes in anatomy and physiology, the speech–language pathologist can ask the patient, for example, "Now that you've heard this information, can you take a look at this postsurgical drawing and tell me, if you need to sneeze, where do you put the handkerchief?" It is also important for the clinician to reiterate what functions will remain intact (or nearly so, barring extensive supraglottic surgery or other compromise) once the healing is complete, including speech articulation skills, swallowing, visual and gestural expressions, and humor.

In the next segment of preoperative consultation, patients need to be given realistic information about the options for optimal alaryngeal rehabilitation. Patients have a right to know that there is oral speech after surgery, and they may wish to be informed briefly of the various options, including esophageal voice, tracheoesophageal puncture, artificial larynx devices, or a combination (Eksteen, Rieger, Nesbitt, & Seikaly, 2003). At all times, it is important for the clinician to present a fair and unbiased view of the options available, balanced with respect for the patient's tentative preferences, if any.

Some surgeons express definite preferences for one or another form of alaryngeal speech. The clinician, however, has a responsibility to apprise the patient and family of all viable forms of alaryngeal speech that may be appropriate for an individual, including the relative merits, detractors, costs, time demands, learning curves, and other factors (Doyle, 1994). The amount of information and detail presented in the preoperative discussion need not be exhaustive, and should be gauged to the extent of the patient's and family's interests (Gress, 2004). Any explanation of the alaryngeal speech alternatives should be unbiased, so that patients understand that there are many choices for consideration after surgery.

Although the preoperative counseling session is an ideal opportunity for the speech–language pathologist to form a preliminary opinion of the patient's potential to successfully acquire various alaryngeal speech methods, it is not possible to predict with certainty. For example, a patient who presents with severe hearing loss preoperatively may well have difficulty self-monitoring new artificial larynx speech intelligibility. Although some patients may appear to have a poor likelihood to achieve a specific alaryngeal speech type, surprises certainly can and do occur. One former patient displayed a significant hand tremor preoperatively, leading me to presume that he would have difficulty with artificial larynx sound control. Although the tremor required him to grip the device more forcefully, he did achieve very satisfactory sound timing with his device and developed good artificial larynx speech intelligibility. Casper and Colton (1998) reported on the advantages of listening to preoperative speech patterns to enhance the transition to alaryngeal speech. Presurgical speech characteristics, such as stuttering, foreign accent dialects, articulatory weakness, and rapid speech rate, may all influence the clinician's ability to target approaches to optimal speech intelligibility. Speech–language pathologists can also assess other information, such as writing skills and legibility, sociocommunicative needs, and plans for return to work, if applicable.

An important high point of preoperative interviews is a chance to discuss patients' hobbies, so that they can feel encouraged to plan on a realistic return to life and its pleasures following laryngectomy. Most hobbies, such as fishing, hunting, sports, cooking, gardening, and crafts, are completely attainable postsurgery. This topic also provides a useful opportunity for the clinician to learn about any avocations at home, work, or elsewhere that would require special accommodations following surgery. One former patient had no extraordinary communication demands, but had a passion for his hobby, refinishing antique furniture. With this information, we were able to order a specialized stoma vent for him to use when around the various chemicals and paints needed for that activity.

Information Patients Need Postoperatively as Inpatients

Patients report that after arriving in the postsurgical intensive care unit, their first hours awake are often filled with initial relief at having survived the surgery, followed by fear of seeing the stoma. For most, there is less pain and discomfort associated with the recovery than they had anticipated. The oncology or ward nurse has an immense responsibility in these early days, helping the patient to view and care for the stoma for the first time, and teaching him or her about feedings, wound healing, and other physical changes following surgery. Although the patient has received many explanations about the removal of the larynx, the initial sight of the predetermined communication system (writing or picture board) brings about fresh realization. In his 1969 autobiography titled *Why Me?* William Gargan, a former actor who underwent a laryngectomy, wrote about his experience:

> A nurse indicated a pad at my side … I wrote on the pad, "Pretty flowers." … Now, it registered. No sound came out. I couldn't speak because my voice box was gone. All the words of the past weeks about the operation and the loss of my speech had not really meant anything. I had lost the power of speech, that marvelous gift that separates men from animals. Gone. Totally gone. It was a feeling I would experience on and off for days … (p. 33)

In the immediate period postlaryngectomy, there will be many silent hours, and the potential for feelings of social isolation and desperation are obviously increased (Stemple, Glaze, & Gerdeman Klaben, 2000). Ironically, this feeling of communication deprivation may be increased even when there are many supportive family members around at bedside, for this is also the patient's time to realize that he or she cannot participate in the conversation normally. Often, a visit from the speech–language pathologist or a qualified laryngectomy visitor will be of more interest to the patient than it was preoperatively, because the motivation for addressing speech rehabilitation options is now acutely evident. Appendix 15.B provides an example of a list of issues that the speech–language pathologist should cover during this early postoperative consultation period.

Once the patient has been moved from the intensive care unit to a regular hospital floor, the speech–language pathologist may make regular bedside visits to introduce the artificial larynx and begin formal therapy, if possible. Ideally, the patient will be able to participate in initial sessions of alaryngeal speech therapy as an inpatient. Being able to use an artificial larynx and communicate orally, even minimally, is an enormous boon for most patients and families. Patients may also experience spontaneous esophageal speech sounds this early, which can be a helpful sign, especially for future esophageal or tracheoesophageal speech users. Regardless of the method of alaryngeal speech, the inpatient period is a useful time to establish a working relationship, begin direct alaryngeal speech therapy, secure an artificial larynx device for the patient, and specify plans for outpatient therapy, as needed.

Preparing Patients and Families for Homecoming

Leaving the hospital for home is an important milestone for the patient and family, because it signals that the patient is now firmly on the road to recovery. The initial euphoria at being released from the hospital and returned to one's own surroundings is sometimes met with ambiguous or wary feelings of malaise. Patients are now able to envision firsthand the multitude of small differences that will require accommodation once they are discharged (see Appendix 15.C). Many circumstances will remind the patient and family members again and again of the permanent changes that have occurred following surgery. These include answering the telephone, calling from room to room, maintaining a foothold in an active conversation, and speaking over the noise of a television or radio. Other physical changes affect showering, elimination, dressing comfortably and fashionably with stoma protection in mind, food tastes, and smell. Many laryngectomy patients recall those first few days at home with conflicting emotions, including joy at being home again and frustration at the larger understanding of what is lost and different following surgery, but most feel some tentative hope at the prospect of the rehabilitation path ahead.

Information Patients and Families Need in the Early Months Postsurgery

In the early months after surgery, a patient and family finally receive the full view of how life is to be following the laryngectomy. Most of the important information about the immediate prognosis for recovery or recurrence is known at this time. Whether a patient heals quickly, receives radiation treatment, achieves intelligible speech rapidly, returns to work, and other important factors will determine how quickly the patient and family will reconcile the diagnosis of cancer and the rehabilitative aftermath. The acute levels of attention and crisis that surrounded the period before, during, and immediately after surgery have subsided. Most patients report that the familiar dips into sadness and isolation lessen, although they do continue as new situations arise (Bjordal & Kaasa, 1995). One patient reported sudden dismay during hunting season, a full 6 months postsurgery, when he realized that he was not going to be able to lift his rifle due to loss of shoulder strength following a radical neck dissection. Another was surprised to realize that he could not "call" out his ball during a picnic volleyball game. These small recognitions continue to unfold as seasons and activities change across time, usually bringing with them creative accommodations, rather than the emotional challenge of earlier weeks.

This early period following surgery is an optimal time to seek group support in local alaryngeal speech clubs or chapters of the International Association of Laryngectomees. For patients, spouses, and other family members, the group exchange is informative and relaxing, and it provides a necessary outlet for new families to share questions and concerns with those who have longer postlaryngectomy experiences. Appendix 15.D lists several questions that may encourage an open dialogue between the clinician and the patient.

Toward Total Rehabilitation

How do clinicians and patients assess when to end treatment? Ultimately, the decision to separate from the therapeutic relationship is left to the patient and family. Three characteristics, however, seem to signal the appropriate time to end a successful course of treatment. First, patients have achieved superior alaryngeal speech skills, so that their ability to monitor and modify their own speech is as good as the clinician's external feedback, which has now become superfluous. Second, patients have returned to their lives and reentered all of the desired social and work-related activities and settings. The third indicator is perhaps more subtle, but equally vital: Patients appear to truly emerge from a long period of self-absorption and focus, and show interest in offering support to other new laryngectomy patients and families. This providing of service to the head and neck cancer community may take several forms. Some individuals participate strongly in alaryngeal groups or clubs, taking roles as club officers, for example. Others seek specialized training to become qualified alaryngeal visitors for new patients. Some create or join campaigns to speak to children about the risks and outcomes of tobacco and alcohol use. Some advocate in local and state government arenas for antitobacco legislation. The essence of this final transition is that the laryngectomized speaker has achieved the admirable goal of becoming a well-rehabilitated laryngectomee. This demonstrated commitment to provide service back to the community is a clear and final indicator that this individual is no longer a cancer "victim."

SUMMARY

For the speech–language pathologist to provide effective pre- and postoperative counseling for laryngectomy patients and families requires many qualifications, some of which are based on years of experience and lessons learned from many patients. Clinicians must be prepared to provide a comprehensive core of essential information to patients and families. They must also demonstrate specialized counseling skills to communicate with this special population. Overall, a speech–language pathologist must be prepared to listen actively to what the patient, spouse, and other caregivers or family members are saying about individual or collective concerns. Professionals must avoid the tendency to presume or guess needs and, instead, remain flexible and tolerant to accommodate the infinite variability in patient comfort, recovery patterns, and paths toward recovery and reconciliation.

Appendix 15.A

Information To Impart at Preoperative Consultation

- Introduce yourself and provide a written card with your name, professional title, telephone number, and address.
- Review the patient's medical information and check that the patient understands the physician's surgical plan. If these plans do not correspond to information you have received in the referral, clarify the mismatch and verify that the surgeon is apprised of any misunderstanding.
- Discuss the physical changes that the patient will expect postoperatively, including creation of a stoma for breathing, coughing, and sneezing, and the need for stoma care (with nurse's help). Describe the need to be fed through an intravenous tube, followed by the nasogastric tube, in the early days postsurgery. Emphasize that a return to oral eating will occur after the physician has determined that tissue healing is complete.
- Describe the communication alternatives immediately postsurgery, including writing or using a communication board. Estimate the timing of initial alaryngeal speech trials.
- Present a brief but comprehensive description of the plan for alaryngeal speech therapy. Unless a primary tracheoesophageal puncture is planned, describe all three formats: artificial larynx, esophageal speech, and tracheoesophageal puncture.
- Confirm your commitment to maintain consistent contact with the patient and manage the alaryngeal speech rehabilitation program. Estimate when speech therapy will begin and how long it will last.
- If time permits, arrange for a hearing test for the patient and spouse.
- Offer to arrange for a meeting with a qualified laryngectomy visitor, if the physician permits and the patient or family wish to have this contact.
- Offer to make other referrals, as desired, to counseling professionals, a member of the clergy, or others.

Appendix 15.B

Information To Impart at Postoperative Inpatient Consultation

- Discuss progress in general health recovery, including breathing, eating, sleeping, stoma care, and general comfort.
- Verify that the patient is using some form of written or picture communication to express needs.
- Review what is known about the remaining medical treatment plan (e.g., progress with nasogastric tube feedings, waiting for fistula to heal, other issues).
- Present the artificial larynx, usually with an oral adapter, and begin speech practice at bedside. Arrange for the patient to order a device or to receive a loaner to take home.
- Arrange a schedule for outpatient speech therapy sessions, as needed.
- Provide the patient and family with supportive written materials made available from the American Cancer Society or the International Association of Laryngectomees. Offer to secure more references, if desired.
- If not arranged preoperatively, offer to arrange a meeting with a qualified laryngectomy visitor, if the physician permits and the patient or family wish to have this contact.
- If not arranged preoperatively, offer to make other referrals, as desired, to counseling professionals, a member of the clergy, or others.
- Confirm the local emergency response. The 911 dispatcher and paramedics should be notified about the patient's status as a "neck breather" for resuscitation purposes. Provide the dispatcher with the patient's name, address, telephone number, and emergency contacts. Confirm that the dispatcher understands that the patient may not be able to speak on the telephone in the early weeks after returning home. This is especially critical for patients who live alone.
- Encourage the patient to order a Medic-Alert bracelet that says "neck breather," and place a "neck breather" resuscitation card in his or her wallet and car.

Appendix 15.C

Information To Impart at Postoperative Outpatient Consultation

- Consider the patient's socioemotional adjustments to communication with spouse, family, friends, and coworkers. Invite the patient to self-assess his or her progress in these areas.
- Determine whether there are any unforeseen barriers to artificial speech communication discovered in various speaking environments (e.g., ambient noise, listener's hearing loss). Continue to probe for insights on the patient's individual functional communication needs at home, at work, and in social settings.
- If not already done, arrange for a hearing test for the patient and spouse.
- Begin formal alaryngeal speech therapy, as planned.

Appendix 15.D

Conversation Starters
Questions To Encourage Open Discussion

1. Changes associated with treatment of head and neck cancer are significant and can be a source of enormous stress for patients, for families, and for other loved ones. Clinicians should seek further information by asking, "Right now, are there other forms of stress, usual or unusual, that are troubling you as you go through this process?"

    Comment: Speech–language pathologists enter the lives of laryngectomy patients with a singular focus on the professional role in rehabilitating head and neck cancer and alaryngeal speech. It is unfair, however, for the clinician to presume that this is the sole experience a patient has that is causing unusual stress. Rather, it is useful to know whether other *concurrent stresses are influencing the patient's ability to comply with recommendations or focus attention on speech rehabilitation.*

2. You have taken enormous responsibility and shown great courage throughout this transition. Who supports you when you need help or need someone to back you up?

    Comment: It is also useful to know what coping strategies and support individuals are available to patients and spouses or other loved ones *who must shoulder the primary burdens of rehabilitation. The response to this question will also provide the clinician with information about other trusted caregivers in the family's circle of support.*

3. You have already been through the diagnosis, the surgery, and the early adjustments to a new breathing pattern and a new voice. What do you miss most from your old voice, and what are the hardest parts of this transition to a new voice?

    Comment: This query can be a useful probe for understanding what functional limits are still troublesome to the patient who is in the process of achieving functional alaryngeal speech. Responses to this question can also provide a benchmark for setting longer term goals for treatment outcome and patient satisfaction. At some point in the weeks past surgery, some patients begin to express reluctance at complaining or calling attention to their disability. Although this may be an important positive step toward reconciliation to the surgery, it is also a critical time to ensure that patients are not "burying" specific goals that might be achieved, with help from the clinician.

---

4. How do you express yourself when you are angry or sad? How do you let others know when you are upset?

Comment: Following laryngectomy surgery, patients often express pain at the loss of the ability to express negative emotions, because crying, shouting, and screaming are lost abilities. Even rapid and loud speech rate (associated with anger) is significantly attenuated in all alaryngeal speech forms. Clinicians must ensure that patients have identified functional alternatives for these emotional outbursts and that they are not allowing negative emotions to go unsaid.

---

5. How confident are you in your ability to communicate independently? For example, how comfortable would you feel

- approaching an unfamiliar store clerk with a special request?
- managing a complex phone conversation with an unfamiliar listener?
- giving detailed directions to a stranger?

Comment: Progress in functional speech therapy may be evident in the treatment environment, but realistic goals extend far beyond the therapy room. It is the clinician's responsibility to verify that patients achieve sufficient self-confidence with their new speech mode that they can take initiatives to address unfamiliar listeners spontaneously. Because alaryngeal speech is an "invisible" disability, unfamiliar listeners are not expecting the perceptual difference in alaryngeal speech. Many patients report that they have learned to anticipate (albeit uncomfortably) the "surprise in the eyes" when they first speak to a stranger. Nonetheless, this achievement is a hallmark of total rehabilitation for laryngectomy speakers.

---

6. Restoring satisfactory quality of life is essential for laryngectomized individuals to achieve complete rehabilitation. Would you find it helpful to speak with a counselor about the special challenges and difficulties you have faced in this transition?

Comment: Many patients may have lingering doubts and dissatisfaction weeks, months, and even years after surgery. By offering patients the potential for more extensive counseling from a professional, speech–language pathologists acknowledge to them that this is a justifiable option and that additional help is available to them, whether or not they choose to participate. Clinicians fully expect that patients will achieve a renewed sense of optimism and purpose as they recover physical health; if, however, the corresponding mental health recovery does not occur, patients will never achieve the comfortable satisfaction of a complete rehabilitation.

REFERENCES

American Cancer Society. (1995). *First steps: Helping words for the laryngectomee.* Atlanta: Author.

Anderson, C., & Doyle, P. C. (2000, July). *A retrospective examination of information provision following total laryngectomy.* Paper presented at the 5th International Conference on Head and Neck Cancer, San Francisco.

Bjordal, K., & Kaasa, S. (1995). Psychological distress in head and neck cancer patients 7–11 years after curative treatment. *The British Journal of Cancer, 71,* 592–597.

Blair, E. A., & Callender, D. L. (1994). Head and neck cancer: The problem. *Clinics in Plastic Surgery, 21*(1), 1–7.

Casper, J. K., & Colton, R. H. (1998). Clinical manual for laryngectomy and head/neck cancer rehabilitation (2nd ed.). In R. T. Wertz (Series Ed.), *Clinical competence series.* San Diego, CA: Singular.

Chaturvedi, S. K., Shenoy, A., Prasad, K. M., Senthilnathan, S. M., & Premlatha, B. S. (1996). Concerns, coping and quality of life in head and neck cancer patients. *Support Care Cancer, 4,* 186–190.

de Boer, M. F., Pruyn, J. F., van den Borne, B., Knegt, P. P., Ryckman, R. M., & Verwoerd, C. D. (1995). Rehabilitation outcomes of long-term survivors treated for head and neck cancer. *Head & Neck, 17,* 503–515.

Doyle, P. C. (1994). *Foundations of voice and speech rehabilitation following laryngeal cancer.* San Diego, CA: Singular.

Doyle, P. C. (1999). Postlaryngectomy speech rehabilitation: Contemporary considerations in clinical care. *Journal of Speech–Language Pathology and Audiology, 23,* 109–116.

Eadie, T. L., & Doyle, P. C. (2004). Auditory–perceptual scaling and quality of life in tracheoesophageal speakers. *Laryngoscope, 114,* 753–759.

Eksteen, E. C., Rieger, J., Nesbitt, M., & Seikaly, H. (2003). Comparison of voice characteristics following three different methods of treatment for laryngeal cancer. *Journal of Otolaryngology, 32,* 250–253.

Gargan, W. (1969). *Why me? An autobiography by William Gargan.* Garden City, NY: Doubleday.

Gilmore, S. I. (1997). Laryngectomy. In T. A. Crowe (Ed.), *Applications of counseling in speech–language pathology and audiology* (pp. 189–202). Baltimore: Williams & Wilkins.

Gliklich, R. E., Goldsmith, T. A., & Funk, G. F. (1997). Are head and neck specific quality of life measures necessary? *Head & Neck, 19,* 474–480.

Gress, C. D. (2004). Preoperative evaluation for tracheoesophageal voice restoration. *Otolaryngology Clinics of North America, 37*(3), 519–530.

Hammerlid, E., Persson, L.-O., Sullivan, M., & Westin, T. (1999). Quality-of-life effects of psychosocial intervention in patients with head and neck cancer. *Otolaryngology—Head and Neck Surgery, 120,* 507–516.

Henderson, J. M., & Ord, R. A. (1997). Suicide in head and neck cancer patients. *Journal of Oral and Maxillofacial Surgery, 55,* 1217–1221.

Karnell, L. H., Funk, G. F., & Hoffman, H. T. (2000). Assessing head and neck cancer patient outcome domains. *Head & Neck, 22,* 6–11.

Keith, R. L. (1991). *Looking forward: A guidebook for the laryngectomee* (2nd ed.). New York: Thieme Medical.

Keith, R. L., & Thomas, J. E. (1996). *A handbook for the laryngectomee* (4th ed.). Austin, TX: PRO-ED.

Kubler-Ross, E. (1974). *On death and dying.* New York: Macmillan.

Levine, S. K. (1996–1997). Emotional aspects of laryngectomees. In J. Lauder (Ed.), *Self help for the laryngectomee* (pp. 77–81). San Antonio, TX: Lauder Enterprises.

Luterman, D. M. (1996). *Counseling persons with communication disorders and their families* (3rd ed.). Austin, TX: PRO-ED.

McDonough, E. M., Varvares, M. A., Dunphy, F. R., Dunleavy, T., Dunphy, C. H., & Boyd, J. H. (1996). Changes in quality-of-life scores in a population of patients treated for squamous cell carcinoma of the head and neck. *Head & Neck, 18,* 487–493.

Mesters, I., van den Borne, H., McCormick, L., Pruyn, J., de Boer, M., & Imbos, T. (1997). Openness to discuss cancer in the nuclear family: Scale, development, and validation. *Psychosomatic Medicine, 59,* 269–279.

Moss, D. G. (1988). *Why didn't they tell me? Questions and answers for the laryngectomee.* Seattle, WA: Laryngectomee Supply.

Ramirez, M. J., Ferriol, E. E., Domenech, F. G., Llatas, M. C., Suarez-Varela, M. M., & Martinez, R. L. (2003). Psychosocial adjustment in patients surgically treated for laryngeal cancer. *Otolaryngology—Head and Neck Surgery, 129,* 92–97.

Salmon, S. J. (1986). Adjusting to laryngectomy. In W. H. Perkins & J. L. Northern (Series Eds.) & J. C. Shanks (Vol. Ed.), *Seminars in speech and language: Vol. 7. Current strategies of rehabilitation in the laryngectomized patient* (No. 1, pp. 67–94). New York: Thieme Medical.

Salmon, S. J. (Ed.). (1991). Some thoughts about counseling: A speech pathologist's perspective. In S. J. Salmon & K. H. Mount (Eds.), *Alaryngeal speech rehabilitation: For clinicians by clinicians* (pp. 29–53). Austin, TX: PRO-ED.

Stemple, J. C., Glaze, L. E., & Gerdeman Klaben, B. (2000). *Clinical voice pathology: Theory and management* (3rd ed.). San Diego, CA: Singular.

Terrell, J. E., Fisher, S. G., & Wolf, G. T. (1998). Long-term quality of life after treatment of laryngeal cancer. *Archives of Otolaryngology—Head and Neck Surgery, 124,* 964–971.

Terrell, J. E., Nanavati, K., Esclamado, R. M., Bradford, C. R., & Wolf, G. T. (1999). Health impact of head and neck cancer. *Otolaryngology—Head and Neck Surgery, 120,* 852–859.

Terrell, J. E., Ronis, D. L., Fowler, K. E., Bradford, C. R., Chepeha, D. B., Prince, M. E., Teknos, T. N., Wolf, G. T., & Duffy, S. A. (2004). Clinical predictors of quality of life in patients with head and neck cancer. *Archives of Otolaryngology—Head and Neck Surgery, 130,* 401–408.

Chapter 16

Taking It to the Limits
Achieving Proficient Esophageal Speech

Minnie S. Graham

Because no two clients are exactly alike, no two therapies are ever exactly alike. In the process of meeting the challenges of alaryngeal speech, both the clinician and the laryngectomee must give their best performance. (Graham, 1997, p. 182)

Since 1980, thanks to developments in space-age technology and incredible advances in medical science, the array of communication options available to the alaryngeal speaker has increased and improved considerably. The three most frequently used means of communication are artificial larynx speech, esophageal speech, and tracheoesophageal (TE) speech (Eksteen, Rieger, Nesbitt, & Seikaly, 2003). In a survey of over 200 individuals who underwent laryngectomy in the United States (Palmer & Graham, 2004), 55% reported use of the artificial larynx (see Chapter 22 in this text), 20% esophageal speech, and 17% TE speech as their primary method of communication. Both the TE voice prosthesis and the artificial larynx offer immediate and functional communication for most individuals who try them (Singer, 2004). Esophageal speech has not benefited directly from technology, nor is it considered part of the fast track to regaining communication after laryngectomy. Why, then, does esophageal speech remain such a strong contender among the alaryngeal speech methods?

The purpose of this chapter is to advocate for and provide detailed information about esophageal speech and esophageal speech instruction. Herein is a discussion of the advantages and disadvantages of esophageal speech, candidate selection, and prognosis for acquisition of esophageal speech. A review of the literature is used to support a hierarchical approach to esophageal speech training. Three specific techniques are described for insufflating the esophagus: the injection method for obstruents, the injection method for sonorants and vowels, and the inhalation method. Goals and therapeutic activities that support a systematic approach to esophageal speech training are identified and accompanied by discussions of potential problems and their resolution. The chapter concludes with information relevant to the advanced esophageal speaker who frequently uses combined methods of air intake to achieve proficient esophageal speech.

ADVANTAGES OF ESOPHAGEAL SPEECH

Esophageal speech has several important advantages over other alaryngeal speech methods. First, there is no equipment to purchase, maintain, repair, or replace. Second, as Bennett and Weinberg (1973) reported, listeners prefer esophageal speech over the mechanical sound produced by the artificial larynx. Third, esophageal speech has been rated superior to artificial laryngeal speech by listeners using a number of variables, including vocal quality, pitch, speech rate, articulatory precision, intensity, naturalness, and intelligibility (Doyle, Danhauer, &

Reed, 1988; Kalb & Carpenter, 1981; Shames, Font, & Matthews, 1963; Williams & Watson, 1985). Fourth, without an external device to manipulate, both of the person's hands are free to drive, write, fish, cook, and take pictures (Casper & Colton, 1998; Doyle, 1994). Finally, as opposed to TE speech, no additional primary or secondary surgical procedure is required (Singer, 2004). Therefore, esophageal speech offers certain advantages to the individual that other types of alaryngeal speech do not.

DISADVANTAGES OF ESOPHAGEAL SPEECH

Esophageal speech cannot match the pitch variations, loudness level, rate, and intelligibility of laryngeal speech (Carpenter, 1991; DiCarlo, Amster, & Herer, 1955; Doyle, 1994; Hyman, 1955; Robbins, 1984; Robbins, Fisher, Blom, & Singer, 1984; Snidecor & Curry, 1959, 1960; Tikofsky, 1965; Weinberg, Horii, & Smith, 1980). The fundamental frequency for esophageal speech, both in males and females, is approximately 65 Hertz (Hz), or half that of the average adult male laryngeal speaker (Doyle, 1994; D. E. Martin, 1994a; Robbins et al., 1984). A fundamental frequency of 65 Hz in a female alaryngeal speaker means her voice is approximately two octaves lower than the mean fundamental frequency of the female laryngeal speaker. Thus, the potential exists for the gender of the female esophageal speaker to be misidentified in the absence of visual or other identifying characteristics (Shanks, 1994b; Weinberg & Bennett, 1972a, 1972b).

Esophageal speech has been reported to be 6 to 10 decibels (dB) lower in intensity than laryngeal speech (Baken, 1987; Berry, 1978; Robbins et al., 1984; Snidecor & Isshiki, 1965; Weinberg et al., 1980). In conditions of competing noise, intelligible esophageal speech may be difficult (Horii & Weinberg, 1975; Shanks, 1994a). Casper and Colton (1998) and Hoops and Noll (1969) observed that the speaking rate of the alaryngeal speaker tends to be slower than that of the laryngeal speaker. Snidecor and Curry (1959) reported a mean rate of 113 words per minute in their "superior" esophageal subjects, a rate that is approximately two thirds the average rate of 150 to 165 words per minute for laryngeal speakers (Shanks, 1994a). Naive listeners rate esophageal speech intelligibility from 54.9% (Shames et al., 1963) to 78.5% (Kalb & Carpenter, 1981) at the word level, and from 54% (Clayton, 1976) to 75.1% (Hoops & Curtis, 1971) at the sentence level. Following a survey of 10 studies involving listener comprehension of esophageal speech, Casper and Colton (1998) reported an overall 71.3% intelligibility rating. Thus, even the most proficient esophageal speaker may experience difficulty with pitch variation, volume, rate, and intelligibility when compared to the laryngeal speaker.

FACTORS TO CONSIDER IN CANDIDATE SELECTION

A variety of factors influence the determination of whether to initiate esophageal speech training with certain individuals. Casper and Colton (1998) provided examples of individuals who might not be appropriate esophageal speech candidates: patients who had undergone extensive surgery involving the pharynx, esophagus, tongue, or mandible; patients with coexisting multiple and serious medical conditions; patients with significant hearing loss; patients using a TE prosthesis (see Chapters 12 and 17 in this text); and patients disinterested in learning esophageal speech. Gilmore (1999) identified six categories of variables influential to esophageal speech acquisition—physical, social, occupational, psychological, training, and idiopathic. For example, hearing loss, motor speech disorders, surgical complications, and concurrent medical conditions are all considered negative physical factors. Coughing, modifications in breathing, increased mucus, cosmetic alterations, and noises or mannerisms associated with air intake must be dealt with on a daily basis (see Chapter 28 in this text). Gilmore observed that, following laryngectomy, some individuals experience a reduction in income, recognition, and social status, as well as loss of normal interactions with family, friends, and society. Occupational factors such as change of employment, forced retirement, unemployment, demotion, or transfer also may occur. Certain emotions, attitudes, and behaviors may influence the individual's attempts to deal with loss and grief related to these changed circumstances. Furthermore, Gilmore asserted that the competence and effectiveness of the alaryngeal rehabilitation team have a direct effect on the individual's acquisition of esophageal speech. Finally, there may be idiopathic, or unexplainable, factors that prevent an individual from acquiring esophageal speech (Duguay, 1999; Gilmore, 1999). Thus, there appear to be myriad reasons why an individual may not be an appropriate candidate for esophageal speech training. The success of the speech rehabilitation effort is dependent on the identification of these factors and the determination of whether or not these variables can be reduced or eliminated (see Chapter 5 in this text). Gilmore (1999) suggested a preventive therapeutic approach to anticipate and manage problems "before patterns of speech failure become firmly entrenched" (p. 261).

PROGNOSIS FOR ACQUIRING ESOPHAGEAL SPEECH

With the knowledge that so many factors have the potential to interfere with the rehabilitation process, one can appreciate how the decision to pursue esophageal speech training does not guarantee acquisition of functional esophageal speech. "Functionality" has been described as the individual's ability to produce "esophageal speech that is sufficiently intelligible, fluent, and comfortable to support resumption of the communication functions assumed prior to laryngectomy" (Gilmore, 1999, p. 222). The failure to acquire functional esophageal speech ranges from 40% (Gardner & Harris, 1961; H. Martin, 1963; Putney, 1958) to 74% (Gates et al., 1982). King, Fowlks, and Pierson (1968) and Salmon (1983) estimated the failure rate at close to 60%. Gilmore (1999) cited improper training factors (related to the alaryngeal rehabilitation team) as one of the reasons the individual may not attain functional esophageal speech. Casper and Colton (1998) and Doyle (1994) reported that many potential esophageal speakers must devote a substantial amount of time (as well as financial commitment) to speech therapy instruction and practice. The number of tasks facing the esophageal speaker-in-training is daunting. The client is challenged to (a) produce esophageal voicing using the various methods of air intake, (b) refine articulatory precision, (c) increase the number of syllables spoken per air charge, (d) manipulate pitch using intonation and stress, and (e) maintain appropriate rate and phrasing (Doyle, 1994; Hyman, 1994a; Shanks, 1994a; see also Chapter 6 in this text). For these reasons, esophageal speech training must be approached in an organized and sequential manner with goals clearly delineated (Snidecor, 1974). The progression through a hierarchy of easy to more difficult tasks is well documented in the literature and supports the probability of successful acquisition of esophageal speech (see Chapter 3 in this text).

THE ESOPHAGEAL SPEECH TRAINING HIERARCHY: A REVIEW OF THE LITERATURE

There have been substantial contributions to the literature regarding esophageal speech training. The common thread connecting the therapeutic approaches and techniques is the support for a hierarchy, an organized sequence of tasks leading to proficiency of esophageal speech. The various perspectives differ in terms of which method of air intake to introduce first, the order of therapeutic goals, and the phonetic context of stimuli.

In the description of his nine-stage sequence for acquiring esophageal speech, Snidecor (1974) stated that the client must first learn to move the air in and out of the esophagus using "easy" vowels such as /ɑ/, /i/, and /o/. One-syllable stimuli composed of plosives plus vowels (e.g., "pie") are followed by functional, single-syllable words (e.g., "stop" and "thanks").[1] By the fourth step, the client is expected to produce two-syllable words. In the process, the client strives to produce both syllables on one injection. During production of simple three- to four-syllable phrases (e.g., "open the door"), therapy emphasis is on phrasing and articulatory precision. Snidecor proposed a hierarchy for articulation practice beginning with unvoiced consonants and advancing to contrastive drill practice (e.g., "fit" vs. "feet"). The goal of effecting changes in pitch and loudness to code stress is deferred to the final stages of treatment. The esophageal speaker initially reads aloud and then later engages in active conversation, striving to increase the rate of speaking while maintaining intelligibility. Because esophageal speech is limited in pitch and loudness variations when compared to laryngeal speech, Snidecor (1974) offered the esophageal speaker several compensatory strategies to improve intelligibility: (a) stand closer to and face the listener during conditions of competing noise; (b) encourage a hearing impaired spouse or

---

[1]A variety of speech practice materials for the alaryngeal speaker are found in the following publications: Emerson and Witteman (1995), Graham (1997), Keith and Thomas (1989, 1996), and Lauder (1999).

friend to use a hearing aid; (c) on the telephone, position the mouthpiece against the lips while speaking; and (d) identify oneself as female (as appropriate) at the beginning of the telephone conversation.

Diedrich and Youngstrom (1966) advocated the use of three methods of air intake for esophageal speech production. Esophageal speech training begins with the consonant method of injection: unvoiced plosives /p/, /t/, and /k/; fricatives /s/ and /ʃ/; and affricate /ʧ/ are produced in consonant–vowel (CV) arrangements. Second, the inhalation method is taught for phonation of the low back vowel /ɑ/. Instructions for the injection method using tongue pumping appear in the next paragraph. Once the concept of three methods of air intake has been mastered, the client is ready to begin practice and to "develop efficient and intelligible speech" (p. 118). The second stage consists of stimuli arranged at succeeding levels of difficulty. Diedrich and Youngstrom advised against moving too quickly through the lower levels to reach multisyllabic words and phrases. At each level of the hierarchy, control and stabilization are emphasized. The first stimuli in the second stage are one-syllable words beginning with obstruents. The clinician alerts the client to any secondary characteristics exhibited (e.g., stoma noise, extraneous facial movements, klunking, and bodily tension). Single-syllable words beginning with sonorants, vowels, and voiced obstruents are practiced at the next level. In time, two-syllable words and phrases utilizing obstruents to facilitate air intake are introduced. Improved control of the air returning from the esophagus increases the individual's ability to prolong vowels (duration of phonation), an important milestone for progressing further up the hierarchy (Berlin, 1963). By the three- to five-syllable level, the esophageal speaker is reading aloud, focusing on articulation, phrasing, sound blending, rate, inflection, and stress. Premature emphasis on loudness, when esophageal speech has not been firmly established, may result in secondary behaviors (e.g., stoma noise, increased bodily tension, overarticulation). Not until the client is engaging in spontaneous phrases and sentences in conversation is loudness addressed. To increase loudness, Diedrich and Youngstrom (1966) suggested increased oral openness, digital pressure against the neck (site of the neoglottis), and contraction of the abdominal muscles. These techniques, when accompanied by pitch variation and inflection, serve to improve loudness, as well as the intelligibility and naturalness of the communication.

Gardner (1971) was another supporter of teaching esophageal speech in hierarchical phases beginning with consonant–vowel–consonant (CVC) words using unvoiced plosives and the fricative /s/ in the initial position (consonant method of injection). Next, instruction for the tongue pump method is given, followed by introduction of the inhalation method. Regardless of the method of air intake, Gardner encouraged the use of plosives to facilitate speech production. For example, at the two-syllable word level, an unvoiced obstruent initiates the second syllable (e.g., "thirsty," "fireside," "ketchup"). To produce syllables that begin with a vowel, the injection method using tongue pumping and the inhalation method is taught. The vowel /ɑ/ is then introduced, and stimulus items are expanded to include all vowels, including diphthongs. Control of the air charge is encouraged by having the individual alternate syllable combinations ("pot–pie") and prolong the vowels. At the two-syllable word level, all voiced plosives, fricatives, and the affricate /ʤ/ are practiced. Finally, the nasals /m/, /n/, and /ŋ/; the lateral /l/; and the glides /r/, /j/, and /w/ are added. At the phrase level, the esophageal speaker strives for greater fluency and control of expelled air by practicing multisyllabic words without plosives. In longer phrases and sentences, goals relating to rate, prosody, pitch range, inflection, and loudness are included. Precise articulation is the key to overall intelligibility. The client improves articulation accuracy (and thus intelligibility) by practicing vowel and consonant contrasts (e.g., "sit" vs. "seat," "my" vs. "by") and by focusing on word final consonants (e.g., "dig," not /dɪg-ʌ/ or /dɪ/).

Hyman (1994b) agreed with Gardner's (1971) recommended use of plosives and sibilants in CVC arrangements to facilitate movement of air into the esophagus during the early stages of esophageal speech training. Practice begins with single syllables, leading up to multiple repetitions of the syllable. In addition to improving articulatory precision, Hyman expected the client to vary the duration, intonation, and loudness of the stimuli. His suggestions for improving loudness were similar to those offered by Diedrich and Youngstrom (1966). Pitch fluctuations are encouraged by using a continuous glide of the vowel /ɑ/ and by practicing questions (e.g., "How are you?"). To progress up the hierarchy, the variety of plosive and sibilant sounds within the CVC context is increased. Eventually, multisyllabic words and phrases that contain plosives, sibilants, nasals, consonant clusters, the glottal /h/, and vowels are added to the repertoire.

Thus, esophageal speech training is firmly grounded in the philosophy that there is a sequence of activities that must be presented and accomplished for the client to progress toward the goal of functionality. Regardless of their differences in instruction, all of these clinicians (Diedrich & Youngstrom, 1966; Gardner, 1971; Hyman, 1994b; Snidecor, 1974) recognized the facilitative power of the unvoiced (and voiced) obstruents for producing esophageal speech, especially in the early stages of therapy.

HOW UNVOICED AND VOICED OBSTRUENTS FACILITATE AIR INTAKE

Compression of the intraoral and pharyngeal air occurs naturally as the tongue (and sometimes the lips) forms the obstruents in speech production (Diedrich & Youngstrom, 1966). Due to their high intraoral pressures, the unvoiced obstruents (/p/, /t/, /k/, /s/, /ʃ/, and /ʧ/) and /s/ blends (/sp/, /st/, /sk/) are particularly effective for injecting air into the esophagus to achieve voicing for the succeeding vowel (Diedrich, 1999; Diedrich & Youngstrom, 1966; Duguay, 1999; Salmon, 1994). For this air injection to occur at the single-word level, the obstruent must be in the initial, or releasing, position of the syllable (e.g., /p/ in "pie"). In two or more syllables, the presence of obstruents and the coarticulation effect (where one sound influences the adjacent sound) assist in the production of sonorants and vowels. Duration of speaking time may be increased by using the available obstruents to "inject" air (Diedrich, 1999; Edels, 1983; Gardner, 1971; Weiss, Gordon, & Lillywhite, 1987). For example, in the phrase "stack it up," air injection occurs during the obstruents /st/, /k/, and /t/, resulting in voicing of the vowels /æ/, /ɪ/, and /ʌ/, respectively.

In laryngeal speech, the vocal folds are adducted and vibrating during voiced consonant production and are abducted during unvoiced consonant production. In esophageal (and TE) speech, the pharyngoesophageal (PE) segment is the source of vibration. Unlike the vocal folds, the PE musculature is not designed to make voiced–voiceless consonant distinctions. Christensen, Weinberg, and Alfonso (1978) found voice onset time (VOT) for voiceless consonants produced by esophageal speakers to be significantly shorter than that of laryngeal speakers. The end result in the esophageal speaker is that the consonant is likely to be voiced as air returning from the esophagus vibrates the PE segment, regardless of the speaker's intent (e.g., "tie" is perceived by the listener as "die"). Doyle et al. (1988) and Sacco, Mann, and Schulz (1967) confirmed this observation by studying listener ratings of intelligibility of voiced and unvoiced obstruents in esophageal speech. In the Sacco et al. study, listeners perceived voiced consonants correctly 76% of the time; however, unvoiced consonants were interpreted accurately only 60% of the time. Horii and Weinberg (1975) showed that intelligibility ratings for unvoiced consonants decreased even further when produced during competing white noise. Sacco et al. suggested that the esophageal speaker should compensate for decreased listener comprehension of the voiced–voiceless distinction by shortening the vowel adjacent to the voiceless consonant and lengthening the vowel for the voiced counterpart.

Based on the information from the literature, there are at least two reasons to introduce unvoiced obstruents first in esophageal speech training. First, unvoiced obstruents create greater intraoral air pressure, enhancing the opportunity for air to move past the PE segment and into the upper esophagus. This increases the chance that the beginning esophageal speaker will achieve voicing during early practice sessions. Second, the vowel following the voiceless obstruent should be voiced briefly, a feat within reach of the new esophageal speaker who does not yet have sufficient control of the returning air to prolong vowels (duration of phonation). This strategy also promotes successful productions at the early stages of the hierarchy. Thus, in early esophageal speech training, the literature supports the selection of certain obstruents based on their ability to increase intraoral air pressure and to move air into the upper esophagus. In addition, researchers and clinicians have provided information about which vowels are more facilitative.

THE VOWEL HIERARCHY

All vowels require voicing; however, vowel production does not increase intraoral air pressure that is sufficient to move air into the upper esophageal segment. To facilitate esophageal voicing, an action that does increase intraoral pressure (i.e., inhalation, obstruent production, or tongue pumping) must precede the vowel. The selection of a vowel hierarchy is based not on the ability to build intraoral air pressure, but rather on the position of the tongue. Not infrequently, the client experiences reduction in tongue mobility following laryngectomy due to the dissection of lingual muscles and their attachments to the hyoid bone. Lingual exercises may assist the client in regaining movement. In the early stages of esophageal speech training, however, vowels that are made with the tongue low in the mouth are considered more facilitative. Among others, Diedrich and Youngstrom (1966), Duguay (1999), and Hyman (1994b) have established a sequence of vowels to facilitate esophageal speech acquisition. The low back vowel /ɑ/ is considered an "easy vowel" because the tongue is positioned low and posteriorly in the mouth in a "resting" position. Duguay (1999) suggested that the vowels /e/, /ɛ/, /ʌ/, /ɑ/, /ɔ/, /aɪ/, and /ɪ/ are appropriate for use in early esophageal speech instruction. For all these vowels, with the exception of /aɪ/ and /ɪ/, the height of the tongue is at mid or low positions in the mouth during production (Nicolosi, Harryman, & Kresheck, 1983). Use of vowels that require less complex lingual positioning may increase the level of success in early esophageal speech tasks.

The critical elements for the construction of an activity hierarchy may be found in the writings and research of such successful clinicians as Diedrich and Youngstrom (1966), Duguay (1999), Gardner (1971), Hyman (1994b), Salmon (1994), and Snidecor (1974). Their findings are summarized as follows:

- Unvoiced obstruents—plosives /p/, /t/, and /k/; fricatives /s/ and /ʃ/; and affricate /tʃ/—are easier to produce than voiced obstruents. The production of unvoiced obstruents facilitates air injection by creating greater intraoral air pressure than voiced cognates. Instruction for words beginning with sonorants and vowels is usually delayed until after unvoiced obstruents have been introduced.
- Mid, low, central, and back vowels (/o/, /ɔ/, /ʌ/, /ə/, /æ/, /e/, /ɛ/, /ɑ/) require minimal tongue movement. These vowels are given preference over high and front vowels in the early stages of esophageal speech training.
- The length of productions in early esophageal speech training is limited to single syllables. Following successful productions at the single-syllable level, the sequence of productions increases to two-syllable words, three- to four-syllable phrases, sentences, oral reading, structured conversation, and finally, spontaneous conversation.[2]

FURTHER CONSIDERATIONS FOR SUCCESSFUL ESOPHAGEAL SPEECH TRAINING

As mentioned earlier in this chapter, the literature reports a failure rate for learning esophageal speech that ranges from 40% to 74%, with an average rate close to 60%. The alaryngeal speech rehabilitation team needs to be aware of factors that

---

[2]In Graham's (1997) appendixes, more than 10,700 stimuli are arranged by level of difficulty for the various methods of alaryngeal speech.

are important to the success of esophageal speech training and acquisition. First, the speech clinician must possess a certain level of competency and effectiveness in alaryngeal speech rehabilitation. Second, the client must be committed to regular attendance for therapy sessions and follow through with home practice. Third, the client must have the cognitive capacity, anatomical structures, and physiological capabilities to learn and effectively use various methods of air intake for esophageal speech.

To initiate the rehabilitative process, the physician determines when the patient has healed sufficiently to begin esophageal speech training. Typically, instruction may begin as soon as the nasogastric (NG) tube has been removed, provided there is no fistula or any other condition with the potential to interfere with air intake (Duguay, 1999).

Doyle (1994), Duguay (1999), and Gardner (1971) advocated providing all patients with an artificial larynx either during the preoperative counseling session or within a few days after surgery. Even if the artificial larynx will not be the long-term primary method of communication, the individual will have an immediate and viable means of communicating with his or her family, hospital personnel, and the community. In particular, reliance on the artificial larynx may reduce the client's anxiety to communicate while attempting to learn esophageal speech.

As a primary player on the alaryngeal speech rehabilitation team, the client must have a basic understanding of the role of the oral–pharyngeal–esophageal structures in esophageal speech. Simplistic diagrams of the pre- and postoperative anatomy of these structures are used to identify the lips, tongue, hard and soft palates, pharynx, PE segment, and esophagus. The client learns that, although deflated at rest, the esophagus is expanded to accommodate the injected air during esophageal speech. Patient education is a powerful component of the therapeutic relationship in terms of improving motivation and promoting self-instruction. Additional considerations for patient instruction include the following:

1. There must be congruence between (a) the selection of vocabulary, the complexity of instructions, and the redundancy of information in therapy and (b) the client's cognitive and educational levels. Visual aids or models are used to explain new terms (e.g., Postlaryngectomy Training Aid Set published by InHealth Technologies, Carpinteria, California). Instructions should be simple, direct, and given in a step-by-step manner. If misunderstood, directions should be repeated or presented in a different way.

2. Visual, auditory, and tactile feedback assists the client in learning target behaviors and in reducing or eliminating undesired behaviors. Written instructions and word lists are provided for home practice. The clinician may demonstrate for the client his or her clinical observation of certain behaviors, such as devoicing of the final consonant in words (e.g., "I heard you say /pɪk/ not /pɪg/"). Both the clinician and client can perform audio- and videotape analysis of the individual's productions. In the presence of hearing loss, the client may not hear excessive stoma noise, so tactile instruction is helpful (Graham, 1997). Placement of the client's fingers in front of the stoma allows him or her to feel the expulsion of air (Casper & Colton, 1998; Diedrich & Youngstrom, 1966; Doyle, 1994; Weinberg, 1983). To promote sensory awareness while the client is learning to inject and return the air in a timely manner, the clinician can ask the client to focus on

the sensation of fullness in the neck at the level of the PE segment (Casper & Colton, 1998).

3. Following the earliest successful productions of esophageal speech, the client should be encouraged to describe the behavior in his or her own words. The clinician can use such descriptors as "I rolled the air back with my tongue," "I squeezed the air back up into my mouth," and "I said the word with more energy" to prompt the client to perform and describe the behavior in future productions.

4. The client should practice the injection and inhalation methods of air intake using the motto "Easy in, easy out." To facilitate the return of air from the esophagus to the oral cavity, the thoracic and abdominal muscles are contracted; however, the alaryngeal speaker should not take deep breaths or push. Forceful exhalations coupled with muscle contraction result in stoma noise (i.e., an audible blast of air from the stoma). Stoma noise is distracting to the listener and impedes intelligibility. In addition, such effortful speech is fatiguing (Snidecor, 1974).

5. The beginning esophageal speaker often has not learned sufficient control of the air charge to prevent movement of the air downward into the stomach. Bloating, belching, and gas are frequent consequences of prolonged practice sessions. At least in the early stages of esophageal speech training, the clinician should hold shortened practice sessions (Doyle, 1994; Graham, 1997) and suggest that the client avoid eating immediately prior to speech practice.

6. Articulatory precision and appropriate rate and phrasing are critical components of intelligibility, and their importance in esophageal speech therapy should not be minimized.

7. Emphases on pitch and loudness variations are considered advanced level skills. Premature attention to pitch variations and loudness may result in undesired secondary behaviors (e.g., stoma noise and increased muscular tension).

8. Excessive stoma noise, facial grimacing, klunking, and bodily tension are extraneous nonverbal behaviors that can distract from and impair communicative effectiveness. The clinician and client should be on guard as to the prevention, reduction, or elimination of these behaviors throughout therapy.

9. The simplicity and naturalness of the injection method for obstruents make this method a good starting point in therapy. Either the injection method for sonorants and vowels or the inhalation method are introduced next. Based on the individual's performance, one or both methods are developed.

10. In the early stages of esophageal speech, the client receives instruction in all three methods of air intake and learns to differentiate these methods. In the intermediate and advanced stages of esophageal speech, the client integrates and applies this knowledge to select the appropriate method(s) of air intake based on the phonetic context of the utterance.

THE ANATOMY AND PHYSIOLOGY OF ESOPHAGEAL SPEECH METHODS

The basis for all the methods of esophageal speech lies in the understanding of the reconstructed anatomy and its function following laryngectomy. During a total laryngectomy, the larynx is removed and the upper portion of the trachea is pulled forward and attached superiorly to the sternum. The reconstructed pharynx is joined directly to the esophageal opening. The junction at which the hypopharynx joins the esophagus is called the pharyngoesophageal (PE) segment (Diedrich, 1999; Edels, 1983). Located anterior to cervical vertebrae 4 through 7, the PE segment is composed of striated muscle: the cricopharyngeus muscle, the lower strands of the inferior pharyngeal constrictor, and the superior esophageal sphincter (Diedrich, 1999; Diedrich & Youngstrom, 1966; Zemlin, 1998). The PE segment, also called the neoglottis, is the source of vibration during esophageal speech (Diedrich & Youngstrom, 1966; Edels, 1983; D. E. Martin, 1994b). Inferior to the PE segment, the upper esophagus serves as the reservoir of air for alaryngeal speech production (Diedrich, 1999; Edels, 1983; D. E. Martin, 1994b).

Even at rest, the air pressure within the nasal, oral, and pharyngeal cavities is positive in contrast to the negative air pressure in the esophagus (Edels, 1983). The air pressure in the esophagus has been measured at between -4 mm and -7 mm Hg (millimeters of mercury) below atmospheric pressure during nonspeaking conditions (Dey & Kirchner, 1961; Duguay, 1999; Edels, 1983). According to the laws of physics, air from an area of higher pressure will tend to move into an area of lower pressure until the two pressures are equalized. The differential between air pressure in the nasal and oropharyngeal cavities and air pressure in the esophagus supports the use of the injection and inhalation methods of esophageal speech.

Two methods for moving air from the oral cavity into the esophagus are possible: injection and inhalation (Diedrich, 1999; Duguay, 1999; Edels, 1983; Salmon, 1994). During the *injection method*, lip and tongue movements increase the already positive air pressure in the oral cavity, forcing air through the closed PE segment and into the upper portion of the esophagus (Duguay, 1999). Thoracic and abdominal muscles then tighten, preventing the air from moving further down the esophagus. The trapped air courses upward through the PE segment, setting the surrounding pharyngeal–esophageal musculature into vibration, and creating sound. As the individual articulates the desired syllable(s), the vibrations are given resonance within the oropharyngeal and nasal cavities (Edels, 1983). In contrast to the injection methods of esophageal insufflation, the inhalation method requires a pressure differential to be created passively. Both approaches to esophageal air insufflation are addressed in subsequent sections of this chapter.

Two subtypes of the injection process can be identified based on the manner of articulation: the *injection method for obstruents* and the *injection method for sonorants and vowels*. Plosives, fricatives, and affricates are obstruents—that is, during their production, the breath stream is partially or totally obstructed and intraoral air pressure is high. In contrast, vowels and sonorants (nasals, glides, and laterals) are made with a relatively unobstructed flow of air, and their production alone does not increase intraoral air pressure.

The Injection Method for Obstruents

The injection method for obstruents is achieved by producing a syllable that begins with a plosive, fricative, or affricate (e.g., "patch," "soup," or "church"), thus increasing the positive air pressure within the oral cavity (Edels, 1983; Shanks, 1986). Strength of articulatory contact (e.g., of the lip and tongue musculature) builds and compresses intraoral air pressure sufficient to overcome the resistance of the closed PE segment (Doyle, 1994; Edels, 1983). Air is then forced past the PE segment into the esophagus (Diedrich, 1999). Voicing occurs as the air is redirected into the oral cavity, thereby vibrating the PE segment. The functionality of the method is boosted by the estimated frequency of occurrence of 36% for obstruents in English (Weiss et al., 1987). Particularly during connected speech, the esophageal speaker will benefit from the natural occurrence of obstruents among the phrases or sentences. The injection method for obstruents is referred to using various terms: consonant press, consonant injection, "Dutch method" of air injection, or plosive injection (Duguay, 1999; Edels, 1983; Salmon, 1994).

The Injection Method for Sonorants and Vowels

The esophageal speaker cannot rely solely on the injection method for obstruents to move air into the esophagus. All syllables do not begin with a plosive, fricative, or affricate; in fact, sonorants and vowels account for approximately 62% of English productions (Weiss et al., 1987). To become a proficient esophageal speaker, the individual must also learn the injection method for sonorants and vowels (or the inhalation method, to be discussed subsequently). Because the production of a sonorant or vowel does not increase intraoral air pressure, a lip or tongue seal is used to trap the air and the tongue moves the air toward the PE segment. In the literature, this method has many names, including tongue pump, glossopharyngeal press, and glossopharyngeal closure (Diedrich, 1999; Duguay, 1999; Edels, 1983; Salmon, 1994; Weinberg & Bosma, 1970). Pumping action of the tongue reduces the size of the oral cavity, compressing the air (and increasing intraoral air pressure). According to Edels (1983), the compressed air forces the PE segment open (and, in some individuals, the musculature of the PE segment relaxes as well), allowing the air to slip into the esophagus. As in the injection method for obstruents, velopharyngeal closure prevents air escape into the nasal cavity (Diedrich, 1999; Doyle, 1994; Duguay, 1999; Edels, 1983).

The Inhalation Method

Both subtypes of the injection method rely on an increase in intraoral pressure, which in turn overcomes the muscular resistance of the PE segment, forcing air from the oral and pharyngeal cavities downward into the esophagus. The inhalation method is based on the concept of increasing the negative pressure below the level of the PE segment so that air is sucked, rather than forced, into the upper esophageal reservoir (Edels, 1983). In the inhalation method, neither the lips nor the tongue is actively involved; the velopharyngeal port may be open or closed (Diedrich, 1999; Diedrich & Youngstrom, 1966; Duguay, 1999; Salmon, 1994). A quick short breath is taken in through the stoma. As the diaphragm moves downward, there is a sharp increase in the negative pressure of the thoracic cavity where the esophagus is located (Edels, 1983). A vacuum effect is created in the esophagus as the negative air pressure increases to approximately -15 mm Hg (from -4 to -7 mm Hg at rest) (Edels, 1983; Salmon, 1994). Now there is an even greater discrepancy between the relative positive air pressure in the oropharyngeal cavity (above the PE segment) and the negative air pressure in the esophagus (below the PE segment). Air flows from the oropharynx past the PE segment and into the upper esophagus in an attempt to equalize the air pressures. Several clinicians believe the PE segment must be relaxed voluntarily during the inward airflow (Diedrich, 1999; Duguay, 1999; Edels, 1983; see also Chapter 21 in this text). Once air has entered the upper esophagus, the PE sphincter closes, trapping the air in the esophagus. The procedure for return of the air to the oropharynx parallels that of the injection method for obstruents. As is true for the other methods of esophageal speech, air return for voicing is facilitated by the recoiling and elastic properties of the esophageal walls, increased air pressure in the esophagus, diaphragmatic tension, and abdominal muscle contractions (not pushing) (Diedrich, 1999; Duguay, 1999). The vibrated air is articulated into speech by movements of the lips and tongue (Diedrich & Youngstrom, 1966; Duguay, 1999). Resonance occurs as the sound passes through the pharynx into the oral or nasal cavities.

INTRODUCING ESOPHAGEAL SPEECH METHODS

The esophageal speaker is introduced to and encouraged to learn all three methods of air intake: the injection method for obstruents, the injection method for sonorants and vowels, and the inhalation method (Diedrich & Youngstrom, 1966; Duguay, 1999; Edels, 1983; Gardner, 1971; Salmon, 1994; Snidecor, 1974). The injection method for obstruents employs "natural" speaking movements; that is, all the client needs to do is produce the plosive, fricative, or affricate. Because the injection method for obstruents so closely resembles the oral movements of laryngeal speech, it is usually taught first and is a required method for all esophageal speakers. Use of the injection method for obstruents, however, is appropriate only in instances where the word begins with an obstruent.

The client has a choice of air intake methods for words that begin with sonorants and vowels: the injection method for sonorants and vowels or the inhalation method. Neither method is superior to the other (Diedrich & Youngstrom, 1966); in fact, some therapists encourage the esophageal speaker to try both (Keith, 1977; Snidecor, 1978). Therefore, both methods should be discussed and demonstrated. The client's success with one or the other method is the determining factor for final selection (Salmon, 1994). If the individual is experiencing difficulty with one method, Gardner (1971) suggests trying the other. For the person who can belch voluntarily, the inhalation method may be the method of choice because the two physical acts are similar; however, the inhalation method involves controlled air release for speech production (Keith, 1977; Lauder, 1999).

During the beginning and intermediate stages of esophageal speech training, each method of air intake is practiced in separate activities. The client needs to understand which method of air intake to use to produce the target phoneme. Proficiency at the advanced levels of esophageal speech, however, means the speaker must learn to apply two or more of the air intake methods to accommodate the variety of phonemic arrangements that occur in regular speech. Snidecor (1974, 1978) concluded that superior esophageal speakers used a combination of all three methods of air intake during connected speech, and that the preferred method of air intake varied among the individual speakers. Thus, although one method may be primary, proficient esophageal speakers will use a combination of methods to insufflate the esophageal reservoir.

Teaching the Injection Method for Obstruents

For the injection method for obstruents (IMO), plosives, fricatives, and affricates are used to facilitate the movement of air from the oropharyngeal cavity into the esophagus. Initially, the client is instructed to produce an energized /p/, adding the back vowel /ɑ/. Tight lip contact for the /p/ builds positive air pressure behind the point of articulatory contact in the oral cavity. The compressed air is forced through the PE segment into the upper esophagus. Return of the air to the oral cavity is enhanced by tightening of the thoracic and abdominal muscles; the PE segment is vibrated and the vowel /ɑ/ is given voicing.

The Hierarchy: Restricted Phonetic Context and Controlled Length of Production

Not all obstruents are equal in their ability to inject air into the esophagus, nor are all of them produced with the same ease. Consequently, a hierarchy of the most to the least facilitative consonants has been established (see Table 16.1). As reported in the literature (Diedrich, 1999; Diedrich & Youngstrom, 1966; Duguay, 1999; Moolenaar-Bijl, 1953; Salmon, 1994), due to their high intraoral pressures, the unvoiced obstruents (/p/, /t/, /k/, /s/, /ʃ/, and /tʃ/) and /s/ blends (/sp/, /st/, /sk/) are the most effective for injecting air into the esophagus to achieve voicing for the succeeding vowel. Thus, the unvoiced plosives, fricatives, and affricates appear at Levels I and II of the IMO hierarchy.

A hierarchy has also been established regarding tongue position and ease of vowel production. Vowels made with the tongue in the mid or low position in the mouth use less muscular effort than vowels produced with higher and more frontal tongue positions (Diedrich & Youngstrom, 1966; Duguay, 1999; Hyman, 1994b). The mid and low vowels /ɑ/, /oʊ/, /ɔ/, /ʌ/, /ə/, /æ/, /eɪ/, and /ɛ/ are

(text continues on p. 399)

TABLE 16.1

Hierarchy for Teaching the Injection Method for Obstruents

Level	No. of Syllables	Phonetic Context: Obstruents	Phonetic Context: Vowels		Examples of Stimuli
I	1	Unvoiced: /p/, /t/, /k/, /f/, /s/, /ʃ/, /θ/, /ʧ/, /sp/, /st/, /sk/, and /h/ as a "modified" /k/	Mid and low: /ɑ/, /oʊ/, /ɔ/, /ʌ/, /ə/, /æ/, /eɪ/, and /ɛ/	/p/	pop, poach, paw, putt, pack, pace, pet
				/t/	toss, tote, talk, tuck, task, teach, tech
				/k/	cop, coat, caught, cut, cat, cape, keg
				/f/	fog, foam, fought, fuss, fact, face, fetch
				/s/	sock, soap, saw, some, sat, safe, self
				/ʃ/	shot, show, shawl, shut, shack, shade, shed
				/θ/	thought, thorn, thaw, thumb, thatch, thank, theft
				/ʧ/	chop, chose, chaw, chunk, champ, chase, check
				/sp/	spa, sport, spawn, spud, span, space, spend
				/st/	start, stove, stalk, stuff, staff, state, step
				/sk/	scar, scope, scald, scum, scab, skate, sketch
				/h/	hot, hope, hawk, hunt, had, haste, help
II	1	Same as Level I	Other: /u/, /ʊ/, /ɝ/, /i/, /ɪ/, /aɪ/, /aʊ/, and /ɔɪ/	/p/	pool, put, purse, pea, pig, pipe, pout, poi
				/t/	two, took, turn, tea, tip, tight, town, toy
				/k/	cool, cook, curve, key, kiss, kite, couch, coy
				/f/	food, foot, first, fee, fit, five, foul, foil
				/s/	soup, soot, sir, seat, sick, sight, sour, soy
				/ʃ/	shoo, should, sure, she, ship, shy, shout
				/θ/	third, think, thin, thigh
				/ʧ/	chew, church, cheese, chin, chime, chow, choy
				/sp/	spoon, spur, speak, spill, spy, spout, spoil
				/st/	stoop, stood, stir, steel, stick, style, stout, stoic
				/sk/	school, skirt, ski, skip, sky, scout
				/h/	who, hood, her, he, hit, hide, how, hoist
III	1	Voiced: /b/, /d/, /g/, /v/, /z/, /ð/, and /ʤ/	Mid and low: /ɑ/, /oʊ/, /ɔ/, /ʌ/, /ə/, /æ/, /eɪ/, and /ɛ/	/b/	ball, bowl, bought, bug, bath, bake, bed
				/d/	dot, dough, dawn, dust, dad, date, debt
				/g/	gone, go, gawk, gum, gap, gate, guest

(continues)

TABLE 16.1 *Continued.*
Hierarchy for Teaching the Injection Method for Obstruents

Level	No. of Syllables	Phonetic Context: Obstruents	Phonetic Context: Vowels	Examples of Stimuli	
III (continued)				/v/	vote, vault, van, vase, vet
				/z/	zap, zone, Zack, zest
				/ð/	though, the, that, they, them
				/dʒ/	job, joke, jaw, just, jab, jail, gem
IV	1	Same as Level III	Other: /u/, /ʊ/, /ɜ/, /i/, /ɪ/, /aɪ/, /aʊ/, and /ɔɪ/	/b/	boot, bush, bird, beat, big, by, bow, boy
				/d/	due, dirt, deed, dig, dime, doubt
				/g/	goof, good, girl, geese, give, guy, gown
				/v/	verse, vim, vice, vow, voice
				/z/	zoo, zinc, zip, zounds
				/ð/	these, this, thy, thou
				/dʒ/	juice, germ, jeep, gym, gibe, joy
V	1	Unvoiced blends: /pl/, /pr/, /tr/, /tw/, /kl/, /kr/, /fl/, /fr/, /sl/, /sm/, /sn/, /sw/, /ʃr/, /θr/, /spl/, /spr/, /str/, and /skr/	All	/pl/	plot, plus, plan, plume, plain, please, plow, ploy
				/pr/	prod, probe, praise, press, prune, preach, proud
				/tr/	trot, troll, truck, trap, trade, true, treat, trim, try
				/tw/	twirl, tweak, twist, twice
				/kl/	clock, close, claw, class, clay, clue, clear, clown
				/kr/	crow, crawl, crunch, crack, crate, crude, cry
				/fl/	flop, flow, flat, flame, flesh, flute, flea, flight
				/fr/	frog, frame, fresh, fruit, free, frisk, fright
				/sl/	slot, slow, slaw, slam, slate, slurp, slick, slouch
				/sm/	small, smoke, smack, smell, smooth, smith
				/sn/	snow, snap, snail, sneeze, snip, snide, snout
				/sw/	swap, sway, sweat, swoop, swirl, sweet, switch
				/ʃr/	shrub, shred, shrewd, shriek, shrimp, shroud
				/θr/	throat, thrust, thrash, thread, threw, three, thrill
				/spl/	splash, splurge, spleen, split, splice
				/spr/	sprung, sprang, spread, spruce, spring, sprite
				/str/	stroke, straw, strut, stray, street, strip, stripe
				/skr/	scratch, scrape, screw, scream, script, scribe

(continues)

TABLE 16.1 *Continued.*
Hierarchy for Teaching the Injection Method for Obstruents

Level	No. of Syllables	Phonetic Context: Obstruents	Phonetic Context: Vowels	Examples of Stimuli		
V *(continued)*		Voiced blends: /bl/, /br/, /dr/, /gl/, and /gr/		/bl/ block, blow, bluff, black, bless, blue, blur /br/ broke, brush, brag, brake, bread, breathe, broil /dr/ drop, drove, draw, drag, drape, dream, drip, dry /gl/ gloss, glow, glad, glue, gleam, glitch, glide /gr/ grow, grudge, grass, grade, grew, green		
VI	2	Unvoiced occurring in the releasing position for both syllables	All	pop top pig pen teacher toy car ketchup coupon faucet fountain	soak socks suit coat shopper sure thing thirsty thankful chicken choice cut	speed trap spot check stone cold stove top sketch pad scared stiff
VII	2	Unvoiced occurring in the releasing position of first word or syllable	All	pitch dark push back tomboy towel dry	same day season shadow sugar	sports dial speed bump stood there store bought
	2	Voiced occurring in the re-leasing position of second word or syllable		cough drop cougar feel good phone bill	Thursday thunder chew gum chalkboard	schedule scolded
VIII	2	Voiced: /b/, /d/, /g/, /v/, /z/, /ð/, and /ʤ/	All	birthday back door done that double good-bye grapevine	veggie vision zigzag zebra these girls those jewels	jet black jazz band

(continues)

TABLE 16.1 *Continued.*
Hierarchy for Teaching the Injection Method for Obstruents

Level	No. of Syllables	Phonetic Context: Obstruents	Phonetic Context: Vowels	Examples of Stimuli
IX	3–4	Voiced and unvoiced in the releasing positions of both syllables	All	pickup truck salt and pepper baked potato downtown shopping Don't count on Ted thumbs up sign keep a secret decaf coffee vintage cars frozen pot pies just between them stabbing back pain
X	5–6	Same as Level IX	All	take a bus or taxi skipped to the back page cowboy's silver buckle Barbara called the doctor. credit card debit sunset at six-thirty snapshots from vacation pecan pie for dessert found a parking space days in December the best I can do vacation schedule

paired with the unvoiced obstruents in Level I (see Table 16.1). The remaining vowels, /u/, /ʊ/, /ɝ/, /i/, /ɪ/, /aɪ/, /aʊ/, and /ɔɪ/, are introduced in Level II.

In addition to restricting the phonetic context of practice stimuli, the length of productions must also be controlled. During the first five levels of IMO, the length of utterance remains at one-syllable productions. The beginning esophageal speaker spends much time practicing control of the air returning from the esophagus. Increased skill will allow the client to extend voicing to two or more syllables on one air charge. For this reason, the hierarchy for length of utterance begins with single-syllable words and advances to two-syllable, three- to four-syllable, and finally five- to six-syllable words and phrases (see Table 16.1).

The hierarchy for teaching the IMO is divided into 10 levels of stimuli based on the arrangement of phonetic context (obstruent and vowel combinations) and the number of syllables (length of utterance). Each level is described herein, and examples of stimuli are given in Table 16.1.

◢ Level I: Single-Syllable Words Beginning with Unvoiced Obstruents Plus Mid and Low Vowels

The phonetic context for Level I is limited to the unvoiced obstruents: plosives /p/, /t/, and /k/; fricatives /f/, /s/, /ʃ/, and /θ/; the affricate /ʧ/; and the /s/ blends /sp/, /st/, and /sk/. The glottal glide /h/, although technically not an obstruent, is included if the esophageal speaker produces it as a modified /k/ (very light velar contact to simulate hissing). The clinician is reminded of Diedrich and Youngstrom's (1966) observation that, to inject air using IMO, the obstruent must occur in the initial, or releasing, position of the syllable. For example, in the word /tæp/, the /t/ is in the releasing position of the syllable and the /p/ is in the arresting position. Air has the potential to be injected on the /t/ but not on the /p/ in this arrangement.

The selected consonants release the consonant–vowel (CV) or consonant–vowel–consonant (CVC) syllable and are combined with vowels that are made with mid or low tongue positions in the mouth. Phonetic context includes the low back vowel /ɑ/, the mid back vowels /oʊ/ and /ɔ/, the mid central vowels /ʌ/ and /ə/, the low front vowel /æ/, and the mid front vowels /e/ and /ɛ/. Examples of single-syllable words that begin with one of the unvoiced obstruents plus a mid or low back vowel appear in Table 16.1, Level I.

◢ Level II: Single-Syllable Words Beginning with Unvoiced Obstruents Plus Other Vowels

To ensure successful progression in the hierarchy and to easily identify specific problem areas that may arise, only one phonetic element is changed per level. At Level II, only the phonetic context for the vowels is changed. The unvoiced obstruents introduced at Level I are retained and combined with vowels that have higher and more frontal tongue positions. The vowels used are the high back vowels /u/ and /ʊ/; the mid central semi-vowel /ɝ/; the high front vowels /i/ and /ɪ/; and the diphthongs /aɪ/, /aʊ/, and /ɪ/.

⏺ Level III: Single-Syllable Words Beginning with Voiced Obstruents Plus Mid and Low Vowels

At Level III, the client practices stimulus words beginning with the voiced plosives /b/, /d/, and /g/; the voiced fricatives /v/, /z/, and /ð/; and the voiced affricate /dʒ/. To facilitate production of the newly introduced voiced obstruents, the phonetic context for vowels is limited to mid and low vowels.

⏺ Level IV: Single-Syllable Words Beginning with Voiced Obstruents Plus Other Vowels

Now that the client can successfully combine voiced obstruents with mid and low vowels at the single-syllable level, he or she is ready to add the more difficult vowels—those made with high or frontal tongue positions—into the training hierarchy. The length of the stimulus remains at one syllable.

⏺ Level V: Single-Syllable Words Beginning with Unvoiced and Voiced Obstruent Blends

The phonetic context for Level V is based on the individual's proven ability to produce one-syllable words initiated with any obstruent in combination with any vowel. At this level, all the obstruent blends (/pl/, /pr/, /bl/, /br/, /tr/, /tw/, /dr/, /kl/, /kr/, /gl/, /gr/, /fl/, /fr/, /sl/, /sm/, /sn/, /sw/, /ʃr/, /θr/, /spl/, /spr/, /str/, /skr/) are introduced in combination with all the vowels. The client must increase duration of phonation to include the blend and the vowel (e.g., /b/, /r/, and /ə/ in the stimulus word /brəʃ/).

⏺ Level VI: Two-Syllable Words and Phrases: Unvoiced Obstruents

At Level VI, the length of utterance is increased to two syllables. In connected speech, air may be injected on the obstruents that occur throughout the utterance. When two or more syllables are placed together in an utterance, their production resembles one long continuous word and an obstruent in the arresting position of one syllable has the potential to release the following syllable. For example, in the phrase "stick it up,", /k/ both arrests the first syllable and releases the second; also, /t/ both arrests the second syllable and releases the third. In this application, /k/ and /t/ are referred to as double consonants; that is, they serve two functions by arresting one syllable and releasing the following syllable.

    Unvoiced obstruents are used to release both syllables. This choice is based on the decision to change only one factor of the production hierarchy at a time. The client is encouraged to blend the two syllables together. For example, the phrase "keep out" should be said like one word /kipaʊt/ instead of two separate words /kip/ and /aʊt/ so that the air injection on /p/ will give voicing to the diphthong /aʊ/.

⏻ Level VII: Two-Syllable Words and Phrases: Unvoiced and Voiced Obstruents

At this level, the length of utterance is held at two syllables and an unvoiced obstruent remains in the releasing position of the first syllable. To increase the level of difficulty, a voiced obstruent releases the second syllable. As shown in Table 16.1, the stimuli include short phrases such as "stood there" and "cough drop."

⏻ Level VIII: Two-Syllable Words and Phrases: Voiced Obstruents

The last phonetic context to be practiced at the two-syllable level is voiced obstruents in the releasing position of both syllables. At this level of the hierarchy, the presence of voiced obstruents in both syllables exercises and expands the client's control of the returning air from the esophagus.

⏻ Level IX: Three- to Four-Syllable Phrases and Sentences with Unvoiced and Voiced Obstruents in the Releasing Positions

Entry into Level IX means the esophageal speaker has a strong foundation in the practice of voiced and unvoiced obstruents combined with any vowel in one- to two-syllable words and phrases. At this level, it is no longer necessary to separate out the unvoiced–voiced components. The client is ready to expand his or her repertoire to include three- and four-syllable phrases and sentences. The stimuli should be spoken with as natural a rhythm as possible to emphasize the coarticulatory effects of connected speech. For example, the phrase "take it easy" must be said as if it were one long word, /tɛkɪtizi/, so that the /t/ in "take" releases the first syllable, the /k/ in "take" releases the second syllable, the /t/ in "it" releases the third syllable, and the /z/ releases the fourth syllable.

⏻ Level X: Five- to Six-Syllable Phrases and Sentences with Unvoiced and Voiced Obstruents in the Releasing Positions

Using word lists of five- to six-syllable phrases and sentences, the client continues at Level X to practice injecting air on obstruents while increasing the duration of the utterance. Restricted phonetic context dictates that obstruents be located strategically throughout the utterance to release every syllable. For the utterance "snack on cheese and crackers," the client must blend the words to take advantage of the coarticulatory effect (e.g., he or she must say /snækɑntʃizænkrækɚz/).

Learning the Injection Method for Obstruents Is Not Enough
While learning the IMO, the client does not practice syllables that are released by sonorants or vowels (e.g., "No one knew our name"). For the client who is

proficient only for the IMO, an air charge for this utterance would not be possible. During the production of sonorants and vowels, intraoral air pressure is not increased and air is not forced down through the PE segment. The reality is that the esophageal speaker must have another way of getting air into the upper esophagus for words that begin with sonorants and vowels. In addition to the IMO, the esophageal speaker must also learn either the injection method for sonorants and vowels or the inhalation method.

Teaching the Injection Method for Sonorants and Vowels

Unlike the IMO, the injection method for sonorants and vowels (IMSV) cannot rely on the production of specific consonants to transfer air from the oral cavity into the esophagus. Instead, actions of the lips and tongue compress the intraoral air and inject the air into the esophagus *prior* to sonorant or vowel production. The IMSV is also known as the glossopharyngeal press, tongue pump, and glossal press (Diedrich & Youngstrom, 1966; Doyle, 1994; Edels, 1983; Salmon, 1994).

Accompanied by velopharyngeal closure (to prevent nasal air escape), the lips or tongue forms a seal so that the air in the oral cavity is pressed against the posterior wall of the pharynx, down through the PE segment, and into the upper esophagus. Some individuals describe flattening the tongue against the hard and soft palates to move the trapped air posteriorly with even greater force. Other users of the IMSV use an anterior-to-posterior rocking motion of the tongue to "sweep the air back." Although the manner for moving air into the esophagus using the IMSV is different from using the IMO, the process of returning air to the oral cavity is the same. The elasticity of the esophageal walls, positive air pressure in the thoracic cavity, diaphragmatic tension, air pressures in the stomach, and abdominal muscle contractions all contribute to increased air pressure within the esophagus. The returning air overcomes the resistance of the PE segment, setting the PE segment into vibration (Edels, 1983).

Whereas the IMO is a natural behavior, the IMSV requires the client to master sequencing and timing of the labial and lingual movements. Air must be moved posteriorly prior to speaking. There are a variety of approaches to compressing the air within the oral cavity for posterior movement. Therapy time must be dedicated to finding the combination that is most successful for the individual client. Four options for labial and lingual posturing are described.

Option 1: Lip Seal, Tongue Pump
1. Use the tongue to capture the ball of air that is present in the middle of the mouth. Position the ball of air between the hard palate and the tongue. Another idea: Place the tongue tip in the position to make a /t/. Hold the tip and sides of the tongue—not the middle of the tongue—firmly against the hard palate.
2. Close the lips tightly.

3. Press the tongue against the hard palate, pumping the ball of air backwards into the throat.

4. As the ball of air goes down into the neck, quickly but gently squeeze the air back up.

5. Open the mouth and say /ɑ/.

Option 2: No Lip Seal, Tongue Pump
Same as Option 1, except leave the lips slightly parted.

Option 3: Lip Seal, Tongue Sweep

1. Use the tongue to capture the ball of air that is present in the middle of the mouth. Position the ball of air between the hard palate and the tongue. Another idea: Place the tongue tip in the position to make a /t/. Hold the tip and sides of the tongue—not the middle of the tongue—firmly against the hard palate.

2. Close the lips tightly.

3. Use an anterior to posterior rocking or rolling motion of the tongue to sweep the ball of air down into the throat (without swallowing).

4. As the ball of air goes down into the neck, quickly but gently squeeze the air back up.

5. Open the mouth and say /ɑ/.

Option 4: No Lip Seal, Tongue Sweep
Same as Option 3, except leave the lips slightly parted.

The Hierarchy: Restricted Phonetic Context and Controlled Length of Production

To ensure that the client is learning to inject air via the tongue pump or sweep method and not relying on the presence of an obstruent to move the air back, none of the stimulus words should contain obstruents. The stimuli used for the IMSV are restricted to a sonorant or a vowel in the releasing position of syllables. Diedrich (1999) and Moolenaar-Bijl (1953) suggested that mid and low vowels be selected for the introductory level of the activity hierarchy because of the facilitative position of the tongue during production. Stimulus length begins with one-syllable and advances to two-, three- to four-, and finally five- to six-syllable words and phrases. Based on this hierarchy of restricted phonetic context and the length of utterance, there are seven levels of stimuli (see Table 16.2).

⌐ Level I: Single-Syllable Words Beginning with Mid and Low Vowels

At the first level, the single-syllable stimulus words begin with a vowel selected from a restricted phonetic context of mid and low vowels: the low back vowel

(text continues on p. 406)

TABLE 16.2

Hierarchy for Teaching the Injection Method for Sonorants and Vowels or the Inhalation Method

Level	No. of Syllables	Phonetic Context: Sonorants	Phonetic Context: Vowels	Examples of Stimuli	
I	1	None	Mid and low: /ɑ/, /oʊ/, /ɔ/, /ʌ/, /æ/, /eɪ/, and /ɛ/	/ɑ/	a, arch, are
				/oʊ/	own, oak, oar
				/ɔ/	all, ought, awe
				/ʌ/	of, ugh, up
				/æ/	at, act, add
				/eɪ/	ate, aim, ace
				/ɛ/	edge, air, ebb
II	1	None	Other: /u/, /ʊ/, /ɝ/, /i/, /ɪ/, /aɪ/, /aʊ/, and /ɔɪ/	/u/	ooze, ooh'd
				/ʊ/	oops
				/ɝ/	urge, earl, irk
				/i/	eat, eel, ease
				/ɪ/	it, is, in, if
				/aɪ/	I, ice, eyes
				/aʊ/	out, ouch, owl
				/ɔɪ/	oil, oink
III	1	/w/, /l/, /r/, /j/, /m/, and /n/	Mid and low: /ɑ/, /oʊ/, /ɔ/, /ʌ/, /æ/, /eɪ/, and /ɛ/	/w/	walk, won't, want, once, wag, wait, west
				/l/	lock, load, law, luck, last, lace, let
				/r/	rock, roast, raw, rut, ran, rate, red
				/j/	yacht, yoke, yaw, yam, yank, yet
				/m/	mom, more, maw, must, main, met
				/n/	not, no, gnaw, nut, nap, name, nest
IV	1	Same as Level III	Other: /u/, /ʊ/, /ɝ/, /i/, /ɪ/, /aɪ/, /aʊ/, and /ɔɪ/	/w/	wound, wood, were, wee, wit, why, wow
				/l/	look, loon, learn, leak, lit, lie, loud, loin
				/r/	roost, rook, reed, rip, right, round, Roy
				/j/	you, yearn, you're, yeast, year, yipes, yowl
				/m/	move, merge, meet, miss, my, mouth, moist
				/n/	new, nook, nurse, neat, knit, nice, now, noise

(continues)

TABLE 16.2 *Continued.*
Hierarchy for Teaching the Injection Method for Sonorants and Vowels or the Inhalation Method

Level	No. of Syllables	Phonetic Context: Sonorants	Phonetic Context: Vowels	Examples of Stimuli	
V	2	Occurring in the releasing position for one or both syllables	Occurring in the releasing position for one or both syllables	winner eyewash airless room rates lemon	our lunch enough orange none are almost	arrow an egg ill will young men railroad
VI	3–4	Same as Level V	Same as Level V	lawn mower Where are you? I'm all out. ran a mile only one way mirror image annual rains		You'll learn more. near our woods lone man running memory loss minimum wage weenie roast online remark
VII	5–6	Same as Level VI	Same as Level VI	I owe you a meal. numerous remarks early one morning e-mail anywhere way in or way out Loan me your remote. No way are you early!		a well-known airline really low on money only nine more minutes Leonard married Molly. No one knew our name. really in a rush a lean, mean Marine

/ɑ/, the mid back vowels /oʊ/ and /ɔ/, the mid central vowels /ʌ/ and /ə/, the low front vowel /æ/, and the mid front vowels /e/ and /ɛ/.

❏ Level II: Single-Syllable Words Beginning with Other Vowels

Following successful productions of words beginning with mid and low vowels, single syllables beginning with all other vowels are introduced. At Level II, the restricted phonetic context consists of the high back vowels /u/ and /ʊ/, the mid central semi-vowel /ɝ/, the high front vowels /i/ and /ɪ/, and the diphthongs /aɪ/, /aʊ/, and /ɔɪ/.

❏ Level III: Single-Syllable Words Beginning with Sonorants plus Mid and Low Vowels

Next, the client is ready to try production of single syllables beginning with the sonorants /w/, /l/, /r/, /j/, /m/, and /n/ coupled with mid and low vowels.

❏ Level IV: Single-Syllable Words Beginning with Sonorants plus Other Vowels

As shown in Table 16.2, at Level IV, high front, mid central, and high back vowels and diphthongs follow sonorants within the CV or CVC arrangement. This is the last level of the IMSV hierarchy to use single-syllable stimuli.

❏ Level V: Two-Syllable Words Beginning with Sonorants and Vowels

Entry to Level V means the client can produce single-syllable words beginning with any sonorant or vowel using the IMSV (see later section titled "Phases for Teaching All Methods of Esophageal Speech" for discussion regarding production accuracy). Length—the production of two-syllable words—is the addition to Level V. Both syllables must contain either a sonorant or vowel in the releasing position. During Levels V, VI, and VII, the client demonstrates control of the returned air by increasing the number of syllables per air charge.

❏ Levels VI and VII: Multisyllabic Phrases and Sentences with Sonorants and Vowels

The length of stimuli increases at Level VI to three to four syllables and increases at Level VII to five to six syllables. The stimuli remain free of any obstruents that might assist the client in loading air into the upper esophagus. The goal is to increase the efficiency of each injection by increasing the number of syllables said on one exiting air charge. In addition to the individual's level of muscular control of the returning air, the capacity of the esophageal reservoir governs the number of syllables that can be produced on one air charge.

Teaching the Inhalation Method

The esophageal speaker has two options for moving air from the oral cavity into the upper esophagus to produce syllables that begin with a sonorant or vowel. In the previously described IMSV method, lip and tongue movements inject or *force* air from the oral cavity through the PE segment and into the upper esophagus. An alternative method, the inhalation method, increases the negative pressure within the esophagus so that oral air is literally *sucked* (as opposed to forced) through the PE segment and into the upper esophagus.

Belching, a behavior normally associated with the digestive act, is a classic example of how the inhalation method works. Unfortunately, naturally occurring eructation is usually abrupt, uncontrolled, and short in duration. Nonetheless, the client's ability to belch at will is a favorable prognostic sign for learning the inhalation method (Doyle, 1994). Speech instruction should focus on teaching the client to control and prolong the expelled air for the purpose of esophageal speech. Because the terms *belch* or *burp* are regarded as socially unacceptable behaviors, the term *inhalation method* is used exclusively throughout therapy.

An understanding of how the technique works may be useful to the individual who is learning the inhalation method. By taking a short, swift air intake through the stoma (Salmon, 1994), the diaphragm contracts, pushing the stomach downward toward the intestines. The esophagus, which is attached to the stomach superiorly, is lengthened slightly and its volume increased. Momentarily, the negative air pressure within the esophagus almost doubles (Atkinson, Kramer, Wyman, & Inglefinger, 1957; Duguay, 1999). The air pressure in the oral and oropharyngeal areas is closer to the atmospheric air pressure and is positive in relation to the negative air pressure in the esophagus (Diedrich, 1999). Air under positive pressure will move toward an area of negative air pressure to equalize the pressure in both areas (Duguay, 1999). Thus, quick inhalation of air through the stoma creates enough of a vacuum within the upper esophagus to pull or suck the air in the oral and oropharyngeal cavities into the esophagus (Diedrich, 1999; Duguay, 1999). *Note:* The inhalation must occur quickly; if air is inhaled slowly, the two air pressures equalize slowly and the vacuum effect is not as dramatic.

To facilitate movement of air from the oral cavity into the upper esophagus, the client is instructed to "breathe in quickly" (as if gasping in surprise), "sniff," "suck air," or "yawn" (Diedrich & Youngstrom, 1966). The tongue is not active in the process and should lie in the floor of the mouth. Some clients report that parting their lips and jutting the chin slightly forward during inhalation is helpful. The sound of the air being sucked through the PE segment may be heard as a "click" in a quiet environment. The client tightens the abdominal muscles and the muscles surrounding the esophagus to squeeze the air back up toward the oral cavity for the production of a syllable beginning with either a vowel (e.g., /ɑ/) or a sonorant (e.g., /m/). Forceful exhalation of lung air through the stoma is discouraged; such effort typically results in stoma noise, and does not facilitate speech production.

The Hierarchy: Restricted Phonetic Context and Controlled Length of Production

Like the IMSV, the purpose of the inhalation method is to move air into the upper esophagus prior to speech production. Unlike the IMO, neither the IMSV nor the inhalation method is dependent on the productions of specific consonants to facilitate air intake.

The practice stimuli for the inhalation method are identical to the practice stimuli for the IMSV (see Table 16.2). Only sonorants and vowels appear in the releasing position of syllables. The hierarchy of stimuli are the same as for the IMSV. Length of stimuli range from one syllable (Level I) and advance to five- to six-syllable phrases and sentences (Level VII).

GOAL SETTING AND PROBLEM SOLVING FOR ALL METHODS OF ESOPHAGEAL SPEECH

Regardless of the method of air intake for esophageal speech—the IMO, the IMSV, or the inhalation method—the speech production goals and the design of the practice stimuli parallel one another. There are two categories of goals in esophageal speech training: voicing and intelligibility. The *voicing* goals are consistency of voicing, quality of voicing, and latency (Berlin, 1963; Snidecor, 1978; Weinberg et al., 1980). Voicing goals focus on the client's ability to move air into the esophagus, return the air to the oral cavity, and produce esophageal quality of voicing, all in a reliable and timely manner. As esophageal speech emerges, the goals for *intelligibility*—articulatory precision, appropriate rate of speech, and attention to nonverbal behaviors associated with speaking—are addressed. All of these goals are discussed in the following subsections.

Goal 1: Consistency of Voicing

The first step in esophageal speech training involves learning how to transfer air from the oral cavity into the upper esophagus and return it on demand. The ability to consistently move the air from the oral cavity into the upper esophagus and return the air to the oral cavity, vibrating the PE segment in the process, is the foundation for successful esophageal speech.

Problem Solving: Inconsistent or No Voicing

Progress at the lower levels of the hierarchy may be slow as the individual develops control over the air in–air out process. Visual, auditory, and tactile stimulation are used to review and reinforce the instructions for the specific method of air intake with the client. Performance anxiety may be lessened by the presence of a relaxed, optimistic, and supportive learning environment, and this may facilitate voice acquisition.

Injection Method for Obstruents. Initially, the client may be able to achieve voicing with certain obstruents only (e.g., the plosives /p/ or /t/). To accommodate the key sound(s), specific phoneme practice lists are created by the clinician for use in therapy. For example, if /p/ is the key sound, then the practice list at Level I might have these words: *pot, poke, pest, pause, pump, pad, pie, pain, pop,* and *peg.*

Consistency of voicing and articulatory precision are interrelated goals (see Goal 4). The IMO requires vigorous movements of the articulators to build the intraoral air pressure. For various reasons, the client may have poor lingual or labial strength. Oral–facial exercises are used to strengthen the musculature and assist in imploding the air for speech. Firm approximation of the lips for /pɑ/ can be monitored by placing a piece of paper or the client's fingertips in front of the lips for visual and tactile feedback. Mirror practice is most effective for monitoring the visual obstruents /p/, /t/, /f/, /s/, /ʃ/, /ʧ/, and /sp/; however, tactile sensation provides more appropriate feedback for the other obstruents. The production of /t/ can be described as follows: "Press the tongue tip firmly against the alveolar ridge; now bounce the tongue away and say /tɑ/." To facilitate /f/, the client presses the upper teeth firmly against the lower lip, "exploding the /fɑ/." The obstruents /s/, /ʃ/ and /ʧ/ can be practiced first in isolation—the goal is to create an audible hissing sound—and then paired with a low or mid vowel for voicing (see Table 16.1, Level I).

Injection Method for Sonorants and Vowels. The client should try all four methods of pumping or sweeping the air with the tongue into the oropharynx. A diagram of the lateral view of the head and neck can be used to show the direction of air movement. Using both hands (one to represent the tongue and the other to represent the hard and soft palates), the clinician illustrates the positioning and movements of the tongue against the hard and soft palates. Visualization of sucking through a straw may assist the client in finding proper tongue tip placement and producing an anterior to posterior wavelike action of the tongue.

Problem Solving: The Hypertonic or Spasmodic Pharynx

A hypertonic, or overly tense, PE segment is limited in its ability to vibrate for speech production. Therefore, failure to achieve consistency of voicing may be due to increased tonicity of the pharyngeal constrictor following total laryngectomy (Blom, Singer, & Hamaker, 1985; Singer & Blom, 1981). Elevated tension in the pharyngeal walls can trap the air intake, thus preventing the return of air to the oral cavity and forcing the air into the stomach (Casper & Colton, 1998; Singer, Blom, & Hamaker, 1986). Other causes, such as stenosis, postradiation edema, or tumor recurrence, also may narrow the oropharynx and PE segment (Casper & Colton, 1998). Alternative explanations may also exist based on careful review of the literature (see Chapter 6 in this text).

Blom et al. (1985) reported an incidence of PE spasm in 40% of a group of individuals who had failed to acquire esophageal speech. In a radiologic study of 134 poor and failed esophageal speakers, McIvor, Evans, Perry, and Cheesman (1990) identified varying degrees of narrowing of the pharynx (hypertonic pharynx, spastic pharynx, or stricture of the pharynx) in 85% of these individuals. Singer and Blom (1981) found that dilations, muscle relaxants, anticholinergic drugs, and tranquilizers were ineffective in relieving the tightened PE segment.

Procedures that have been successful in relaxing the hypertonic or spasmodic pharyngeal constrictor include pharyngeal constrictor myotomy (Singer & Blom, 1981), pharyngeal plexus neurectomy (Singer et al., 1986), and botulinum toxin injections (Blitzer, Komisar, Baredes, Brin, & Stewart, 1995). Surgical myotomy, the dissection of select fibers on one side of the pharyngeal constrictor, is the treatment of choice for individuals with increased PE segment tone (McIvor et al., 1990; Singer, 1988; Singer & Blom, 1981; Singer et al., 1986). Singer et al. (1986) suggested that a pharyngeal plexus neurectomy be performed during primary laryngectomy for all patients. They proposed that the procedure might accelerate the rate of acquisition for esophageal speech and effect a more natural vibratory quality due to the lowered airflow resistance at the PE segment.

Relatively new in its use with alaryngeal patients is Botox, a potent neurotoxin that inhibits the release of acetylcholine within 24 to 78 hours of administration into the cricopharyngeus muscle and adjacent area. Blitzer et al. (1995) reported a 20% to 60% improvement in their laryngectomized subjects' TE speech after Botox injection. The beneficial effects last approximately 3 to 4 months (Blitzer et al., 1995; Terrell, Lewin, & Esclamado, 1995). Although the use of Botox to improve TE speech has been widely reported, discussion of its application to relax the pharyngeal constrictor for improvement of esophageal speech is more recent (Lewin, 1998, 1999).

Blom et al. (1985) and Gilmore (1999) recommended a proactive approach to identifying those individuals who may be at risk for failure at learning esophageal speech. They suggested routine administration of the esophageal insufflation test at the initiation of esophageal speech training. By not delaying the evaluation, the clinician will not subject the individual to "sufficient failure to undermine self-confidence or motivation to continue pursuing esophageal speech" (Gilmore, 1999, p. 250).

Problem Solving: The Hypotonic Pharynx or PE Segment

Approximately 15% of the individuals who can inject air into the esophagus (using either the IMO or IMSV) but who cannot return it for speech production are found to have a hypotonic pharynx; that is, the pharyngeal walls and the fibers that compose the PE segment have very low muscular tension. Although air may have been injected into the upper esophagus, the low resistance of the pharyngeal musculature results in weak or no vibration of the PE segment (McIvor et al., 1990). For some individuals with a hypotonic pharynx, external digital pressure applied to the anterior or lateral portion of the neck at the level of the PE segment during air return mechanically narrows pharyngeal walls; the PE segment then vibrates, and voicing occurs (McIvor et al., 1990; Singer et al., 1986).

Goal 2: Esophageal Quality of Voicing

The alaryngeal speaker's voicing can be defined as either pharyngeal or esophageal in quality. Esophageal quality of voicing occurs when air has been successfully injected or inhaled into the upper esophagus and returned to the oral cavity, vibrating the PE segment so that the tone created is consistent, sufficient in duration, relatively free of strain, and capable of pitch variation (Gilmore, 1999; D. E. Martin, 1994a). The assumptions are that the esophageal speaker has moved the air from the oral–nasal cavities into the upper esophageal reservoir and that the PE segment and surrounding musculature have offered sufficient resistance to the returning air so that vibration occurs (Gilmore, 1999; D. E. Martin, 1994b).

Problem Solving: Pharyngeal Quality Using Injection Method

To achieve esophageal quality of voicing, the client must make lip and/or tongue movements that create sufficient air pressure to overcome the resistance of the PE segment. If the injection is weak or improper movements are used, the air fails to reach the level of the PE segment and upper esophagus and may be trapped in the hypopharynx. If the air turbulence is sufficient to vibrate the pharyngeal walls, pharyngeal quality of voicing is the consequence (Damsté, 1994). Common among new esophageal speakers, pharyngeal voicing is somewhat higher in pitch, shorter in duration, and lower in volume than esophageal quality speech (Weinberg & Westerhouse, 1973).

Cut-away illustrations of the head and neck are used to show the client where the injected air is supposed to go. Placement of the hand against the side of the neck at the site of the PE segment may help the client understand how far down the air has to be moved. Relaxation exercises to reduce tension in the shoulders, neck, and jaw may be paired with visualization of openness in the throat (e.g., during chewing or yawning). For the IMO, CV stimuli that use vowels that encourage openness of the throat (e.g., /ɑ/, /aʊ/, or /ɔ/) are selected. Throughout esophageal speech practice, the pharyngeal area should remain open and relaxed. Lowering of the chin and "thinking low pitch" may facilitate relaxation of the client's oropharyngeal area.

Problem Solving: Pharyngeal Quality Using Inhalation Method

Because oropharyngeal openness is an integral step in the inhalation method, pharyngeal quality of voicing generally does not occur. If there is tension in the muscles adjacent to the PE segment, the client is encouraged to breathe or sniff in quickly through the stoma and to imitate the openness of a yawn.

Goal 3: Latency

There are two interpretations of *latency* in the alaryngeal speech rehabilitation literature: production latency and duration of phonation latency. *Production latency* is a measure of the amount of time that elapses between the injection of air and the return of air for voicing. Ideally, there should be no more than 1 second between the command to speak and the production of the target utterance. The second type of latency, *duration of phonation,* is defined as the length of time that voicing can be sustained on one air charge. In the beginning stages of therapy, when control of the air is minimal, the anticipated length of phonation is one syllable per air charge. Practice will permit the esophageal speaker to increase the duration of single vowels to 2 seconds or more, or to say 2 or more syllables on one injection or inhalation. "A duration of 2 seconds or better is pretty good and may be adequate for producing connected speech, especially if the speaker uses multiple methods of air charging" (D. E. Martin, 1994a, p. 333).

Berlin (1963) proposed that production latency is a better indicator of proficient esophageal speech than the number of syllables that can be produced on one air charge (duration of phonation). He observed that esophageal speakers who are rated as good speakers have production latencies of .5 second or less. Therapy time may be better spent learning to frequently and efficiently reinflate the esophagus (while maintaining smoothness and continuity of connected speech) than striving endlessly to increase the number of syllables said on one injection.

Problem Solving: Delayed Latency Related to Searching Behaviors

Injection Methods. Inappropriate extraneous behaviors, such as lip pursing, multiple injections, groping for lip or tongue placement, and facial grimacing, may increase the latency of production and are distracting to the listener. Visual and tactile feedback may assist the client in eliminating these undesired "preparatory" behaviors. Anatomical illustrations (e.g., for IMSV, "Place your tongue tip here and flatten the blade of your tongue against the roof of your mouth") or a mirror (e.g., for IMO, "Look at your mouth as you make the /t/; your lips are slightly apart and your tongue tip is up") may serve as useful instructional tools. In their earliest speech attempts, some clients may be able to produce voicing consistently only on certain consonants or vowels (e.g., /pɑp/ but not /tɑp/, or /æt/ but not /ɪt/). To simplify the therapy task, a word list composed of stimuli beginning with these specific consonants or vowels (termed "key sounds") is used. Smooth, continuous production is encouraged, and the client is told to "make the contact, do the contact, and say the word."

Inhalation Method. Physical behaviors are often used to teach the inhalation method (e.g., yawning, sucking, or covering the stoma momentarily during inhalation attempts). These facilitating techniques should be discarded as soon as the client has the idea of inhalation. Otherwise, these behaviors may become habituated, resulting in a prolonged preparatory phase with exaggerated oral opening, chin jutting, shoulder raising, or gasping. The concept of "easy in, easy out" should be reinforced.

Problem Solving: Short Duration of Phonation for Vowels

Due to poor control of the air charge, early esophageal speech productions tend to be abrupt and brief. Specific therapy practice, focusing on prolonging the vowels in the utterance, will improve control of the returning air charge. A series of short words (e.g., *pot, tap, cot* for IMO, or *up, on, lake* for IMSV or inhalation method) are used as warm-ups at the beginning of each session, with the reminder to the client to "stretch out the vowel as long as you can." The goal is to achieve a minimum of 2 seconds' duration of the vowel, signifying increased control of the air charge.

Goal 4: Articulatory Precision

Voicing in esophageal speech is the result of vibration of the PE segment; however, the articulators are responsible for shaping the sound into meaningful speech. Articulatory precision is fundamental to the intelligibility of esophageal speech. The client must be vigilant regarding the accuracy of the consonant and vowel productions. As discussed earlier in this chapter, listener distinctions between voiced–voiceless consonants are made difficult due to the absence of the vocal folds (Christensen et al., 1978; Doyle et al., 1988; Horii & Weinberg, 1975; Sacco et al., 1967). The production of the nasals /m/, /n/, and /ŋ/ requires an open velopharyngeal port. The glottal /h/, made by exhaling air through partially adducted vocal folds by the laryngeal speaker, requires compensatory articulatory movements by the esophageal speaker to achieve a similar effect.

Problem Solving: Imprecise Articulation

Using the IMO, energetic articulatory contacts during the production of plosives, fricatives, and affricates are necessary to build enough intraoral pressure to overcome the resistance of the PE segment so that the air is forced into the esophagus.

Preoperative speech patterns related to foreign accent, regional dialect, dysarthria, or an articulation disorder will have an influence on the intelligibility of esophageal speech. As a consequence of the laryngectomy procedure, in which mandibular and lingual muscle attachments to the hyoid bone are severed, the individual almost always experiences a dysarthric component of speech postoperatively. To improve articulatory strength, range of motion, and control, oral–facial exercises are recommended. Laying a strong foundation of articulatory precision at the single-syllable level is an excellent investment for more advanced esophageal speech activities that follow.

Problem Solving: Ill-Fitting Dentures

Radiation treatments may result in atrophy of gum tissue. Dentures or other dental appliances may slip during esophageal speech, interfering with the injection methods and with articulatory precision. Denture adhesive is a quick fix; however, a referral to the dentist or prosthodontist for long-term adjustment of the appliance is recommended.

Problem Solving: Hearing Loss

In their study of 90 male esophageal speakers, Kahane and Irwin (1975) found high-frequency hearing losses among the majority of esophageal speakers 60 years of age or older. These older speakers also demonstrated higher stoma noise ratings than younger esophageal speakers. A high-frequency hearing loss can impair the individual's ability to receive auditory feedback during speech production (i.e., fricative production). Thus, self-monitoring for stoma noise is significantly impaired. Till, England, and Law-Till (1987) reported a reduction in stoma noise in their patients who used a microphone placed at the stoma and received feedback via headphones. In the absence of critical auditory information, clients may be taught to rely on visual cues such as mirror feedback (Weinberg, 1983) and tactile cues such as location of the tongue tip against the alveolar ridge for the production of /s/ or placement of the fingertips in front of the stoma to monitor for escaping air (Diedrich & Youngstrom, 1966; Weinberg, 1983).

Problem Solving: Voiced Versus Unvoiced Obstruents Using IMO

As discussed earlier in this chapter, listeners of esophageal speech more often perceive obstruents as voiced, regardless of the speaker's intent. For example, "tie" is heard as "die." Sacco et al. (1967) proposed that the length of voicing for the accompanying vowel is the source of confusion between voiced and unvoiced consonant productions. Voiced consonants are usually accompanied by longer vowel production (and voice onset time) than are unvoiced consonants. As a compensatory strategy, Sacco et al. recommended that the esophageal speaker use shorter vowel duration when the adjacent consonant is unvoiced. Consonant contrast drills using voiced and unvoiced cognates in the initial position (e.g., *pan* vs. *ban, tall* vs. *doll,* and *sue* vs. *zoo* [Hyman, 1994a; Nichols, 1976]) or in the final position (e.g., *lit* vs. *lid, slap* vs. *slab,* and *buck* vs. *bug* [Hyman, 1994a; Nichols, 1977]) are helpful in teaching the client this technique.

Problem Solving: Lack of Nasal Resonance for Nasal Sounds

Injection Methods. During air intake for the IMO and IMSV, there must be velopharyngeal closure to prevent air escape through the nasal cavity. As a result of frequent air intake for esophageal speech, the client tends to maintain velopharyngeal closure, a behavior that is nonproblematic unless nasals are present. If the nasals /m/, /n/, and /ŋ/ are produced with a closed velopharyngeal port, they are perceived by the listener as the plosives /b/, /d/, and /g/, respectively (Diedrich & Youngstrom, 1966; Duguay, 1999). Contrastive drills using plosives and nasals are helpful in restoring appropriate nasal resonance (e.g., *my* vs. *by, name* vs. *dame,* and *wing* vs. *wig;* [Graham, 1997]).

Inhalation Method. Denasalization of /m/, /n/, and /ŋ/ is less likely to occur using the inhalation method because the velopharyngeal port is kept open while air is sucked from the nasal and oral cavities into the esophagus. If the esophageal speaker has difficulty achieving appropriate nasality, contrastive drills with consonants can be practiced.

Problem Solving: The Glottal Fricative /h/

Many esophageal speakers accept their inability to produce the glottal fricative /h/ and simply rely on being understood within the context of the utterance (e.g., "Two 'eads are better than one"). Because it takes the laryngeal speaker slightly longer to say "hand" than to say "and," Duguay (1999) suggested that the esophageal speaker slightly prolong the vowel following the /h/ (e.g., "a-a-and" vs. "and"). The purpose is to allow the listener to mentally fill in the missing /h/. In another approach, Shanks (1994a) and Hyman (1994b) described how to make a brief linguavelar contact (a softened /k/) with air turbulence that closely resembles the /h/. The substituted sound approximates the frication produced in the German word /"ich"/. Contrast drills can be used to practice distinguishing between word pairs such as *air–hair, and–hand, eat–heat, Ike–hike, owe–hoe,* and so forth (Duguay, 1999).

Goal 5: Appropriate Rate of Speech

Rate can be defined as the number of syllables or words spoken within a certain time period. The mean speaking rate for superior esophageal speakers is 113 words per minute (Snidecor & Curry, 1959), approximately two thirds the average speaking rate for a laryngeal speaker (Shanks, 1994a). The slower rate for esophageal speakers is explained by the necessity for frequent air intake to charge the esophagus with air. Speaking rates differ among esophageal speakers; superior esophageal speakers have a faster speaking rate than do poor esophageal speakers, indicating that the superior speakers have mastered the air intake procedures (Hoops & Noll, 1969; Shipp, 1967).

Rate, however, is only one factor in the complex mix that determines intelligibility of speech. Articulatory precision has an even greater influence on intelligibility than does rate (Hyman, 1994a). The third factor, meaningful phrasing, adds a naturalness of communication component to the equation. Defining what is an appropriate rate from an evaluation and teaching perspective is an elusive task. Choosing to increase or decrease rate without considering the esophageal speaker's skills in articulation or phrasing almost always has a negative effect on intelligibility (Hoops & Noll, 1969; D. E. Martin, 1994a; Shipp, 1967).

Problem Solving: Rate of Speech Too Fast

If the rate of production exceeds the limits of the client's articulatory control or bypasses the prosodic elements of phrasing, intelligibility suffers. Articulatory precision and meaningful phrasing are prerequisites to increasing the rate of speech. Specific attention to oral–facial exercises (see "Goal 4: Articulatory Precision") and contrastive consonant drills will improve articulatory control. Inserting brief pauses in longer utterances (four- to five-syllable sentences or longer) will enhance the naturalness of communication and contribute to the listener's comprehension. The speaker can learn to slow a fast rate of speech by imagining one's listener "having to take notes of the conversation."

Problem Solving: Rate of Speech Too Slow

Listeners may perceive esophageal speakers with too slow a speech rate as below average in their speaking ability. In the early stages of esophageal speech training, the emphasis is on consistency of voicing, articulatory precision, and short latency of production. The length of stimuli is limited to one and two syllables. With advancement to longer phrases and sentences, the client is expected to blend the syllables into connected speech in a timely manner. The perception of a slow speech rate may be attributed to vowels that are drawn out excessively, a syllable-by-syllable rhythm, and long pauses for air charging. To improve the listener's perception of a more natural rate and prosody, therapy activities can alternately address shortening the vowel length, blending syllables, pausing for emphasis, and improving the timeliness and efficiency of the injection or inhalation methods.

Goal 6: Attention to Nonverbal Behaviors Associated with Speaking

Observation of a good communicator reveals a number of desirable nonverbal behaviors—frequent eye contact with the listener, hand gestures and facial expressions that are congruent with the verbal message, variations in pitch and loudness, pauses for emphasis, and interjections (e.g., "um," "er," "oh!" and light laughter). The goal for the esophageal speaker is to adopt, as much as possible, the speech mannerisms that signal relaxed and natural communication. Some alaryngeal speakers were good communicators preoperatively and resume their good speech habits spontaneously; other individuals may benefit from instruction and practice in becoming better communicators.

In the process of learning esophageal speech, the individual may acquire certain behaviors that detract from or interfere with effective communication. Multiple injections or inhalations, excessive stoma noise, facial grimaces, extraneous head movements, and loss of eye contact are among the undesirable behaviors. Without exception, these mannerisms are caused by excessive tension associated with the process of air intake and return for esophageal speech. Excessive muscle tension sabotages the goal of fluent, easily produced esophageal speech. Unless identified and remediated early in therapy, these behaviors have the potential to become habituated and highly resistant to rehabilitation efforts.

Problem Solving: Multiple Injections or Inhalations

The proficient esophageal speaker is able to move air into the upper esophagus on the first attempt—one consonant production for the IMO, one tongue or lip press for the IMSV, or one quick inhalation for the inhalation method. During the learning process, however, the client may, in an effort to achieve voicing, make multiple attempts to get the air down. The resulting behaviors—double injections using repetitions of a single consonant (e.g., /p-p-pɑ/), two or more lip or tongue presses, or repeated gulping of air—are inefficient. Multiple injections or inhalations fatigue the alaryngeal speaker, distract the listener, interfere with the naturalness of communication, and overfill the esophagus so that air accumulates in the stomach (as gas). To avoid such unpleasant side effects and the possible formation of a bad habit, the client should be instructed to inject (or inhale) once per trial. A second chance is readily given, but each attempt at air intake is considered a separate trial.

Problem Solving: Excessive Stoma Noise

The laryngeal speaker relies on the controlled and prolonged exhalation of lung air to vibrate the vocal folds and produce voicing. Although the esophageal speaker no longer has access to lung air for speech production, the natural impulse is to exhale while speaking (Snidecor & Isshiki, 1965). Forceful exhalation through the trachea results in audible air turbulence or stoma noise. Stoma noise, another behavior that is distracting to the listener, as well as fatiguing for the alaryngeal speaker, tends to appear early in therapy. There must be a determined effort to suppress the stoma noise from the onset. The client must take responsibility for decreasing if not eliminating the stoma noise using self-monitoring skills. Individuals with high-frequency hearing loss are significantly impaired in their ability to monitor for stoma noise (Kahane & Irwin, 1975). In the absence of auditory feedback, tactile sensation (fingertips in front of the stoma) may be the primary means for detecting escaping air. Contrastive practice—discerning between forceful and gentle exhalations—may also be of benefit to the client.

Problem Solving: Facial Grimacing, Extraneous Head Movements, and Loss of Eye Contact

All of these behaviors—facial grimacing, extraneous head movements, and loss of eye contact—are the consequence of excessive tension. Relaxation exercises are used to decrease tension in the oral, facial, and shoulder muscles. Visual feedback (i.e., via a mirror) during speech practice helps the client identify and lessen extraneous head, neck, and shoulder movements. Eye contact can be improved through mirror practice and reminders from the clinician or other listeners.

PHASES FOR TEACHING ALL METHODS OF ESOPHAGEAL SPEECH

All methods of air intake for esophageal speech share the same six goals: appropriate esophageal quality, consistency of voicing, latency, articulation, rate, and nonverbal behaviors. At each level of the hierarchy for a specific method of air intake, all six goals are addressed. From a hierarchical perspective, asking the client to attend to all six goals within a single activity is an unreasonable expectation (at least at the onset of each level). Because the client is vulnerable to information overload, practice activities for the six goals are divided into initial, intermediate, and advanced phases at each level of the hierarchy.

The Initial Phase

In the initial phase, one goal is selected per therapy activity. Within the overall therapy session, there may be several activities that use a particular method of air intake; however, only one goal is addressed in each activity. For example, the first activity may focus only on consistency of voicing using the IMO. When the client is working on consistency of voicing, feedback is given regarding consistency of voicing only, and errors related to the other five goals are not mentioned. If articulation precision is the goal of the second activity, feedback is limited to information about articulatory movements and precision. When the client demonstrates the ability to focus on individual goals at a specific level of production with 90% accuracy over three consecutive sessions, the intermediate phase is begun (remaining at the same level of the hierarchy).

Intermediate Phase

In the intermediate phase, two goals are targeted per activity. For example, one activity may focus on consistency of voicing *and* esophageal quality of production while using the IMSV method. Another activity may pair articulatory precision *and* phrasing as goals. Activities using various two-goal combinations are presented until the client achieves at least 90% overall accuracy for the paired goals.

Advanced Phase

The advanced phase targets all six goals—consistency of voicing, esophageal quality, latency, articulation, phrasing, and nonverbal behaviors—within the same activity. Before progressing to the next level of the hierarchy for a specific method of air intake, the client must achieve 90% performance for all six goals at the current level. The same pattern of cycling through the three phases occurs at the next level of production.

CLINICIAN- AND CLIENT-GENERATED FEEDBACK: DEVELOPING SELF-MONITORING SKILLS

Throughout esophageal speech training, clinician feedback that is information specific and supportive is critical to the client's understanding and mastery of the air intake and speech production process. Visual, auditory, and tactile demonstrations and feedback are valuable learning tools for the client. The client benefits from identification of error behavior, followed by the clinician's suggestions for improvement; however, feedback regarding how or why a particular production was successful may be equally beneficial. Without the ability to judge his or her own productions, the client is dependent on external feedback.

The development of self-monitoring skills by the client is an important factor in learning esophageal speech, and thus is included in the planning of every therapy session. The individual who possesses successful self-monitoring and self-correction skills has the advantage of being able to maintain and improve his or her speech productions in all environments. Transference from clinician- to client-generated feedback occurs gradually. When a new level, phase, or goal for the method of air intake is introduced, feedback is given solely by the clinician. After a period of time, the client is encouraged to make decisions about the accuracy of his or her productions. The clinician either concurs or disagrees with the client's evaluation. The long-term goal is for the individual to independently and correctly self-monitor for all six goals at all levels of esophageal production. The client's progression toward such independent behavior is recorded on activity score sheets and later transferred to his or her daily log.

The Activity Score Sheet

An activity score sheet (see example in Figure 16.1) is used to organize the esophageal speech training session. For *each* activity, the clinician selects the following:

- the method of air intake (IMO, IMSV, or inhalation)
- the phase (number of goals for the activity)
- goal(s) for the activity

ACTIVITY SCORE SHEET
FOR TEACHING ESOPHAGEAL SPEECH

Name _____ Date _____

Method of
Air Intake:
  ❑ Injection of obstruents
  ❑ Injection of sonorants and vowels
  ❑ Inhalation

Phase:
  ❑ Initial (one goal)
  ❑ Intermediate (two goals)
  ❑ Advanced (multiple goals)

Goal(s):
  ❑ Consistency of voicing   ❑ Articulation
  ❑ Esophageal quality   ❑ Rate
  ❑ Latency   ❑ Nonverbal behaviors

Level of
Production:
  ❑ Single-syllable words   ❑ Three- to four-syllable words/phrases
  ❑ Two-syllable words/phrases   ❑ Five- to six-syllable words/phrases

Target
Sounds:
  ❑ Unvoiced obstruents   ❑ Mid and low vowels
  ❑ Voiced obstruents   ❑ Other vowels
  ❑ Obstruent blends   ❑ Sonorants
  ❑ Specific consonant _____

Monitoring:
  ❑ Clinician
  ❑ Client/clinician
  ❑ Client

	Stimuli	Accuracy	Comments
1			
2			
3			
4			
5			
6			
7			
8			
9			
10			
	Total Correct		
	Percent Correct		

FIGURE 16.1. Example of an activity score sheet for teaching esophageal speech. *Note.* Adapted from *The Clinician's Guide to Alaryngeal Speech Therapy* (p. 124), by M. S. Graham, 1997, Boston: Butterworth-Heinemann. Copyright 1997 by Butterworth-Heinemann. Adapted with permission.

- level of production (length of stimuli)
- target sounds (based on the method of air intake and phonetic context)
- monitoring (clinician only, client–clinician, or client only)

After determining the goal(s) for the activity, the clinician selects 10 stimuli for the level of production in which the client has demonstrated 70% to 80% success. Practice at this level of accuracy is motivating because the client is able to experience success while still challenging his or her learning. Advancement to the next phase or to the next level of the hierarchy is based on 90% accuracy on three consecutive sets of stimuli at the current phase or level of production. Scores for the client's productions are entered as correct (+) or incorrect (−) in the Accuracy column. Some clinicians prefer to use a more sophisticated level of scoring by further describing correct responses as immediate, delayed, assisted, or self-corrected.

COMBINING THE METHODS OF ESOPHAGEAL SPEECH

According to the literature (Moolenaar-Bijl, 1953; Nicolosi, Harryman, & Kresheck, 1983; Salmon, 1994; Shanks, 1996), many, if not most, proficient esophageal speakers use more than one method of air intake. Salmon (1994) and Shanks (1996) encourage experimentation among the methods; Moolenaar-Bijl (1953) asserts that no one method of air intake is superior to the other. In beginning esophageal speech training, the selection of which method to present first is based on ease of production by the individual client (Shanks, 1996).

To facilitate understanding and mastery of the various methods of air intake—IMO, IMSV, and the inhalation method—therapy activity hierarchies are separated up to and including the five- to six-syllable phrase and sentence levels of production. Stimuli that highlight the appropriate phonetic context for the specific method of air intake are used. The client may experience differing levels of success among the esophageal speech methods. The terminal goal for the esophageal speaker is to be able to produce any utterance, regardless of phonetic context or syllable length, with minimal effort and with maximal intelligibility.

The decision to combine several methods of esophageal speech into one therapy activity is based on the client's ability to perform at 90% or higher accuracy for all six goals at the five- to six-syllable phrases and sentences level of production using (a) the injection method for obstruents and (b) the injection method for sonorants and vowels *or* the inhalation method. The mixed methods of air intake are begun when the client demonstrates quality esophageal speech with short latency, precise articulation, appropriate rate, and few, if any, undesired nonverbal behaviors.

Goal Setting for the Combined Methods of Esophageal Speech

The advanced goals emphasize the intelligibility and communicative effectiveness of esophageal speech: articulatory precision, appropriate rate and phrasing, pitch control via intonation and stress, increased loudness, and attention to nonverbal behaviors associated with speaking. There are no restrictions on phonetic context; all consonants and vowels are included at all levels of production. Length of utterance follows a hierarchy from two- to four-syllable phrases and sentences (Level I) to spontaneous conversation (Level VI).

Goal 1: Articulatory Precision

Although articulatory precision is considered a basic skill for learning esophageal speech, its importance to intelligibility continues through the advanced level. Specific practice may highlight fricative production (e.g., /s/, /f/); nasal resonance for /m/, /n/, and /ŋ/; compensatory movements for /h/; voiced–unvoiced consonant contrasts (e.g., /p/ vs. /b/); and other consonant contrasts (e.g., "I can say *may*, I can say *bay*, and I can say *pay*").

Goal 2: Appropriate Rate and Phrasing

Appropriate rate and phrasing are dependent on the individual's articulatory control and latency of production. Attempting an increase in speech rate without consideration of the client's level of articulatory precision and ability to move air in and out of the upper esophagus in a timely manner may result in decreased intelligibility (Hoops & Noll, 1969; D. E. Martin, 1994a; Shipp, 1967). Superior esophageal speakers are described by their listeners as having good articulation, effective phrasing and pause time, and a faster speaking rate than poor esophageal speakers (Hoops & Noll, 1969; D. E. Martin, 1994a; Shipp, 1967). In addition, listeners in Berlin's (1963) study observed that good esophageal speakers have production latencies of .5 second or less.

The stimuli in advanced esophageal speech practice are composed using unrestricted phonetic context. The client is instructed to examine the stimulus phrase, sentence, or reading passage and to predict where air intake should occur using the IMO and the IMSV or the inhalation method. Obstruents in the releasing position of syllables are circled in red to emphasize that their production naturally facilitates air intake. In the absence of a preceding obstruent, the IMSV or inhalation method must be used to produce sound for syllables that begin with a sonorant or vowel. The places where air intake is needed are marked with a red slash, indicating the client needs to inject or inhale *prior* to speech production.

Most new esophageal speakers benefit from practicing frequent and efficient reinsufflation of the esophagus while maintaining the flow of connected speech. Attention is given to the grouping of syllables and words to form meaningful phrases (e.g., "I went / to the store / to buy milk / bread and eggs"). The suggestion to pause or perform air intake where a comma or period occurs in the written text may promote more natural phrasing.

Goal 3: Pitch Control Using Intonation and Stress

Through selectively tightening or expanding the vibrating pharyngeal walls, the client can exert some control over pitch variation during esophageal speech. According to Hyman (1994b), the esophageal speaker has the potential to alter pitch by as much as two octaves. Activities include intoning /ɑ/ beginning at the lowest note and moving up the scale to the highest note and then gliding back down the scale. Hyman recommends that the client ask questions ending with an upward inflection (e.g., "Hello?"). Reciting poems, rhymes, and limericks also may improve pitch flexibility due to the prosodic nature of verse. Contrastive stress drills are used to reinforce intonation and inflection. For example, the client may be asked several questions to which the designated response is "Today is Tuesday." When asked "Is today Wednesday?" the emphasis will be on the word "Tuesday." In response to "Was yesterday Tuesday?" the stress will be on the word "today."

Another type of intonational practice activity involves selecting a neutral utterance and producing it with various emotional overlays (e.g., "The door is open" is repeated several times to convey alternately happiness, sadness, anger, and surprise). In group situations, listeners are asked to identify the emotion the client is attempting to convey (via intonation and stress).

Goal 4: Increased Loudness

The esophageal speaker enjoys neither the intensity nor the range of loudness that the laryngeal speaker possesses. Esophageal speech is approximately 6 to 10 dB lower in intensity than is laryngeal speech (Robbins et al., 1984). The esophageal speaker's range of loudness is 20 dB, whereas the laryngeal speaker's range is 45 dB (D. E. Martin, 1994a).

The laryngeal speaker increases loudness by increasing the flow of lung air through the vocal folds. The esophageal speaker who tries this technique will experience a blast of air from the stoma and no significant increase in loudness. The size and flexibility of the pharyngeal cavity are primary determinants of the potential intensity available to the esophageal speaker. Loudness is not encouraged during early esophageal speech training when the individual is still learning how to move air in and out of the esophagus without forceful exhalation; rather, the emphasis is placed on reducing or eliminating stoma noise.

In advanced training—because the client has learned to produce esophageal speech without pushing—increased loudness becomes a goal. Contraction of the abdominal muscles (without forceful exhalation), finger pressure against the neck (at the level of the PE segment), sitting or standing upright, and increased oral opening may enhance loudness. Contrastive practice may assist the client in distinguishing between the feel of a loud versus a confidential voice.

Most of the suggestions to increase loudness are compensatory in nature. The client may choose to implement environmental controls to heighten intelligibility. Compensatory strategies include facing the listener, relying on the listener's speech-reading abilities, turning down or off competing noise (TV, radio), announcing the topic of the conversation, and using gestures and writing as supplements to speech. For the listener with hearing impairment, the client may need to use the artificial larynx or writing. A personal amplifier with microphone will boost loudness for the person who plans to lecture to a group or speak in a noisy environment.

Goal 5: Attention to Nonverbal Behaviors Associated with Speaking

By the advanced stage of esophageal speech training, negative behaviors—stoma noise, klunking, double injections, facial grimacing, and muscular tension—should have been reduced, if not eliminated. Attention is then directed toward promoting positive nonverbal behaviors associated with speaking, and thus enhancing the communicative effectiveness of the esophageal speaker. Contributors to the natural appearance of communication include eye contact and accompanying facial and hand gestures that are congruent with the verbal message.

Some individuals may devote so much time to the process of esophageal speech that they neglect the characteristics of being a good communicator. Group therapy is an opportune time to discuss being sensitive to the listener's needs, observing the rules of turn-taking, adhering to the time limits of specific conversations, and checking with the listener to be sure the message has been understood.

Levels of Production

To reach the advanced stage, the esophageal speaker must have demonstrated that he or she can produce five- to six-syllable utterances using a specific method of air intake within a restricted phonetic context. In this last sequence of the hierarchy, the client is expected to use a combination of air intake methods to produce stimuli created from an unrestricted phonetic context of consonants and vowels. To facilitate success in combining the esophageal speech methods, Level I of the advanced production begins with two- to four-syllable phrases and sentences. The hierarchy for teaching the combined methods of esophageal speech is divided into six levels of stimuli based on the length of utterance.

> ❏ Level I: Two- to Four-Syllable Phrases and Sentences
> *Examples:* Pay your rent; two good reasons; more than you know; zest for living

> ❏ Level II: Five- to Seven-Syllable Phrases and Sentences
> *Examples:* What are you doing? The laundry is downstairs. Mail a postcard to Dallas. Always expect the best.

◢ Level III: Eight-Syllable or More Phrases and Sentences
Examples: Winter brought snow to the mountains. Tell her the directions one more time. He treated everybody to dinner. Void where prohibited by law.

◢ Level IV: Oral Reading of Paragraphs
Stimuli: paragraphs from newspaper or magazine articles, passages from a book

◢ Level V: Structured Conversation
Stimuli: Tell three things about your favorite city. Give me the directions from your home to the nearest hospital. Describe the best birthday present you ever received.

◢ Level VI: Spontaneous and Extended Conversation
Stimuli: Help another member of the group understand how to take care of the stoma. What are some ways to earn extra money? How do you like to spend your free time?

The Activity Score Sheet for Teaching Combined Methods of Esophageal Speech

Figure 16.2 shows an activity score sheet designed for use when the methods of esophageal speech are combined within one activity. For each activity, the clinician selects the following:

- the phase (number of goals for the activity; see "Phases for Teaching All Methods of Esophageal Speech," earlier in this chapter)
- goal(s) for the activity
- level of production (length of stimuli)
- monitoring (clinician only, client–clinician, or client only)

SUMMARY

This chapter has provided information about a wide range of issues pertaining to esophageal speech rehabilitation. The advantages and disadvantages of using esophageal speech, procedures for candidate selection, and prognosis for acquisition of esophageal speech have been discussed. A review of the literature has supported a hierarchical approach to esophageal speech training. Three specific techniques for insufflating the esophagus—the injection method for obstruents, the injection method for sonorants and vowels, and the inhalation method—have been detailed. Goals and therapeutic activities that subscribe to a systematic

ACTIVITY SCORE SHEET
FOR TEACHING COMBINED METHODS
OF ESOPHAGEAL SPEECH

Name _____ Date _____

Phase: ❑ Initial (one goal)
                ❑ Intermediate (two goals)
                ❑ Advanced (multiple goals)

Goal(s):   ❑ Articulation   ❑ Loudness
                ❑ Rate and phrasing   ❑ Nonverbal behaviors
                ❑ Pitch control, intonation, and stress

Level of   Unrestricted phonetic context:
Production: ❑ I.   Two- to four-syllable phrases and sentences
                ❑ II.   Five- to seven-syllable phrases and sentences
                ❑ III. Eight-syllable or more phrases and sentences
                ❑ IV.   Oral reading of paragraphs
                ❑ V.   Structured conversation
                ❑ VI.   Spontaneous and extended conversation

Monitoring: ❑ Clinician
                ❑ Client/clinician
                ❑ Client

	Stimuli	Accuracy	Comments
1			
2			
3			
4			
5			
6			
7			
8			
9			
10			
	Total Correct		
	Percent Correct		

FIGURE 16.2. Example of an activity score sheet for teaching combined methods of esophageal speech. *Note.* Adapted from *The Clinician's Guide to Alaryngeal Speech Therapy* (p. 131), by M. S. Graham, 1997, Boston: Butterworth–Heinemann. Copyright 1997 by Butterworth–Heinemann. Adapted with permission.

approach to esophageal speech training have been identified and accompanied by discussions of potential problems and their resolution. Finally, goals and activities relevant to the advanced esophageal speaker have been presented.

REFERENCES

Atkinson, M., Kramer, P., Wyman, S. M., & Inglefinger, F. J. (1957). The dynamics of swallowing: I. Normal pharyngeal mechanisms. *Journal of Clinical Investigation, 36,* 581–588.

Baken, R. J. (1987). *Clinical measurement of speech and voice.* San Diego, CA: College-Hill Press.

Bennett, S., & Weinberg, B. (1973). Acceptability ratings of normal, esophageal, and artificial laryngeal speech. *Journal of Speech and Hearing Research, 16,* 608–615.

Berlin, C. I. (1963). Clinical measurement of esophageal speech: I. Methodology and curves of skill acquisition. *Journal of Speech and Hearing Disorders, 28,* 42–51.

Berry, W. R. (1978). Indications for the use of artificial larynx devices. In S. J. Salmon & L. P. Goldstein (Eds.), *The artificial larynx handbook* (pp. 17–23). New York: Grune & Stratton.

Blitzer, A., Komisar, A., Baredes, S., Brin, M. F., & Stewart, C. (1995). Voice failure after tracheo-esophageal puncture: Management with botulinum toxin. *Otolaryngology—Head and Neck Surgery, 113,* 668–679.

Blom, E. D., Singer, M. I., & Hamaker, R. C. (1985). An improved esophageal insufflation test. *Archives of Otolaryngology, 111,* 211–212.

Carpenter, M. A. (1991). Clinical application of alaryngeal speech judgments. In S. J. Salmon & K. H. Mount (Eds.), *Alaryngeal speech rehabilitation: For clinicians by clinicians* (pp. 161–191). Austin, TX: PRO-ED.

Casper, J. K., & Colton, R. H. (1998). *Clinical manual for laryngectomy and head/neck cancer rehabilitation* (2nd ed.). San Diego, CA: Singular.

Christensen, J. M., Weinberg, B., & Alfonso, P. J. (1978). Productive voice onset time characteristics of esophageal speech. *Journal of Speech and Hearing Research, 21,* 56–62.

Clayton, S. (1976). *Relationships among word and sentence intelligibility: Global ratings of esophageal speech skill.* Unpublished master's thesis, Michigan State University, East Lansing.

Damsté, P. H. (1994). Some obstacles in learning esophageal speech. In R. L. Keith & F. L. Darley (Eds.), *Laryngectomee rehabilitation* (3rd ed., pp. 235–242). Austin, TX: PRO-ED.

Dey, F. L., & Kirchner, J. A. (1961). The upper esophageal sphincter after laryngectomy. *Laryngoscope, 71,* 99–115.

DiCarlo, L. M., Amster, W., & Herer, G. (1955). *Speech after laryngectomy.* Syracuse, NY: Syracuse University Press.

Diedrich, W. M. (1999). Anatomy and physiology of esophageal speech. In S. J. Salmon (Ed.), *Alaryngeal speech rehabilitation: For clinicians by clinicians* (2nd ed., pp. 1–28). Austin, TX: PRO-ED.

Diedrich, W. M., & Youngstrom, K. A. (1966). *Alaryngeal speech.* Springfield, IL: Thomas.

Doyle, P. C. (1994). *Foundations of voice and speech rehabilitation following laryngeal cancer.* San Diego, CA: Singular.

Doyle, P. C., Danhauer, J. L., & Reed, C. G. (1988). Listeners' perceptions of consonants produced by esophageal and tracheoesophageal talkers. *Journal of Speech and Hearing Disorders, 53,* 400–407.

Duguay, M. J. (1999). Esophageal speech training: The initial phase. In S. J. Salmon (Ed.), *Alaryngeal speech rehabilitation: For clinicians by clinicians* (2nd ed., pp. 165–201). Austin, TX: PRO-ED.

Edels, Y. (1983). Pseudo-voice—Its theory and practice. In Y. Edels (Ed.), *Laryngectomy: Diagnosis to rehabilitation* (pp. 107–141). Rockville, MD: Aspen.

Eksteen, E. C., Rieger, J., Nesbitt, M., & Seikaly, H. (2003). Comparison of voice characteristics following three different methods of treatment for laryngeal cancer. *Journal of Otolaryngology, 32,* 250–253.

Emerson, H., & Witteman, B. (1995). *Progressive steps to a new voice.* (Available from The Bill Wilkerson Hearing and Speech Center, 1114-19th Avenue South, Nashville, TN 37213)

Gardner, W. N. (1971). *Laryngectomee speech and rehabilitation.* Springfield, IL: Thomas.

Gardner, W. N., & Harris, H. E. (1961). Aids and devices for laryngectomees. *Archives of Otolaryngology, 73,* 145–152.

Gates, G. A., Ryan, W., Cooper, J. C., Lawlis, G. F., Cantu, E., Hayashi, T., Lauder, E., Welch, R. W., & Hearne, E. (1982). Current status of laryngectomee rehabilitation: I. Results of therapy. *American Journal of Otolaryngology, 3,* 1–7.

Gilmore, S. I. (1999). Failure in acquiring esophageal speech. In S. J. Salmon (Ed.), *Alaryngeal speech rehabilitation: For clinicians by clinicians* (2nd ed., pp. 221–268). Austin, TX: PRO-ED.

Graham, M. S. (1997). *The clinician's guide to alaryngeal speech therapy.* Boston: Butterworth-Heinemann.

Gress, C. D. (2000, January 27–28). *Trouble-shooting guide* [Laryngectomy Rehabilitation Course], University of California–San Francisco Cancer Center, The Voice Center, San Francisco.

Hoops, H. R., & Curtis, J. F. (1971). Intelligibility of the esophageal speaker. *Archives of Otolaryngology, 93,* 300–303.

Hoops, H. R., & Noll, J. D. (1969). Relationship of selected acoustic variables to judgments of esophageal speech. *Journal of Communication Disorders, 2,* 1–13.

Horii, Y., & Weinberg, B. (1975). Intelligibility characteristics of superior esophageal speech presented under various levels of masking noise. *Journal of Speech and Hearing Research, 18,* 413–419.

Hyman, M. (1955). An experimental study of artificial larynx and esophageal speech. *Journal of Speech and Hearing Disorders, 20,* 291–299.

Hyman, M. (1994a). Factors influencing the intelligibility of alaryngeal speech. In R. L. Keith & F. L. Darley (Eds.), *Laryngectomee rehabilitation* (3rd ed., pp. 253–261). Austin, TX: PRO-ED.

Hyman, M. (1994b). The intermediate stage of teaching alaryngeal speech. In R. L. Keith & F. L. Darley (Eds.), *Laryngectomee rehabilitation* (3rd ed., pp. 309–321). Austin, TX: PRO-ED.

Kahane, J. C., & Irwin, J. A. (1975, November). *Comparison of hearing sensitivity and stoma noise in 90 esophageal speakers.* Paper presented at the annual convention of the American Speech-Language-Hearing Association, Washington, DC.

Kalb, M. B., & Carpenter, M. A. (1981). Individual speaker influence on relative intelligibility of esophageal and artificial larynx speech. *Journal of Speech and Hearing Disorders, 46,* 77–80.

Keith, R. L. (1977). Teaching of esophageal speech. *Journal of the National Student Speech and Hearing Association, 7,* 8–12.

Keith, R. L., & Thomas, J. E. (1989). *Speech practice manual for dysarthria, apraxia, and other disorders of articulation: Compare and contrast.* Chicago: Mosby Year Book.

Keith, R. L., & Thomas, J. E. (1996). *A handbook for the laryngectomee* (4th ed.). Austin, TX: PRO-ED.

King, P. S., Fowlks, E. W., & Pierson, G. A. (1968). Rehabilitation and adaptation of laryngectomy patients. *American Journal of Physical Medicine, 47,* 192–203.

Lauder, E. (1999). *Self-help for the laryngectomee.* San Antonio, TX: Lauder Enterprises.

Lewin, J. S. (1998, August). *Botulinum toxin to facilitate TE and esophageal speech production.* Paper presented at the annual meeting and voice institute, International Association of Laryngectomees, Indianapolis, IN.

Lewin, J. S. (1999). *Overview of laryngectomy: From surgery to rehabilitation.* Paper presented at the annual conference of the Texas Laryngectomee Association, Austin, TX.

Martin, D. E. (1994a). Evaluating esophageal speech development and proficiency. In R. L. Keith & F. L. Darley (Eds.), *Laryngectomee rehabilitation* (3rd ed., pp. 331–349). Austin, TX: PRO-ED.

Martin, D. E. (1994b). Pre- and postoperative anatomical and physiological observations in laryngectomy. In R. L. Keith & F. L. Darley (Eds.), *Laryngectomee rehabilitation* (3rd ed., pp. 77–89). Austin, TX: PRO-ED.

Martin, H. (1963). Rehabilitation of the laryngectomee. *Cancer, 16,* 823–841.

McIvor, J., Evans, P. F., Perry, A., & Cheesman, A. D. (1990). Radiological assessment of post laryngectomy speech. *Clinical Radiology, 41,* 312–316.

Moolenaar-Bijl, A. (1953). Connection between consonant articulation and the intake of air in oesophageal speech. *Folia Phoniatrica, 5,* 212-216.

Nichols, A. C. (1976). Confusions in recognizing phonemes spoken by esophageal speakers: I. Initial consonants and clusters. *Journal of Communication Disorders, 9,* 27–41.

Nichols, A. C. (1977). Confusions in recognizing phonemes spoken by esophageal speakers: III. Terminal consonants and clusters. *Journal of Communication Disorders, 10,* 285–299.

Nicolosi, L., Harryman, E., & Kresheck, J. (1983). *Terminology of communication disorders: Speech–language–hearing* (2nd ed., p. 259). Baltimore: Williams & Wilkins.

Palmer, A. D., & Graham, M. S. (2004). The relationship between communication and quality of life in alaryngeal speakers. *Journal of Speech–Language Pathology and Audiology, 28,* 3–24.

Putney, E. J. (1958). Rehabilitation of the post-laryngectomized patient. *Annals of Otology, Rhinology and Laryngology, 67,* 544–549.

Robbins, J. (1984). Acoustic differentiation of laryngeal, esophageal, and tracheoesophageal speech. *Journal of Speech and Hearing Research, 27,* 577–585.

Robbins, J., Fisher, H. B., Blom, E. D., & Singer, M. I. (1984). A comparative acoustic study of normal, esophageal, and tracheoesophageal speech production. *Journal of Speech and Hearing Disorders, 49,* 202–210.

Sacco, P. R., Mann, M. B., & Schulz, M. C. (1967). Perceptual confusions among selected phonemes in esophageal speech. *Journal of the Indiana Speech and Hearing Association, 26,* 19–33.

Salmon, S. J. (1983). Artificial larynx speech: A viable means of alaryngeal communication. In Y. Edels (Ed.), *Laryngectomy: Diagnosis to rehabilitation* (pp. 142–162). Rockville, MD: Aspen.

Salmon, S. J. (1994). Methods of air intake and associated problems. In R. L. Keith & F. L. Darley (Eds.), *Laryngectomee rehabilitation* (3rd ed., pp. 219–234). Austin, TX: PRO-ED.

Shames, G. H., Font, J., & Matthews, J. (1963). Factors related to speech proficiency of the laryngectomized. *Journal of Speech and Hearing Disorders, 28,* 273–287.

Shanks, J. C. (1986). Evoking esophageal voice. *Seminars in Speech and Language, 7,* 1–11.

Shanks, J. C. (1994a). Developing esophageal communication. In R. L. Keith & F. L. Darley (Eds.), *Laryngectomee rehabilitation* (3rd ed., pp. 205–217). Austin, TX: PRO-ED.

Shanks, J. C. (1994b). Development of the feminine voice and refinement of esophageal voice. In R. L. Keith & F. L. Darley (Eds.), *Laryngectomee rehabilitation* (3rd ed., pp. 323–329). Austin, TX: PRO-ED.

Shanks, J. C. (1996, October). *Esophageal speech, a yardstick.* Paper presented at the annual meeting of the California Association of Laryngectomees, Stockton, CA.

Shipp, T. (1967). Frequency, duration, and perceptual measures in relation to judgments of alaryngeal speech acceptability. *Journal of Speech and Hearing Research, 10,* 417–427.

Singer, M. I. (1988). The upper esophageal sphincter: Role in alaryngeal speech acquisition. *Head and Neck Surgery* (Suppl. 2), S118–S123.

Singer, M. I. (2004). The development of successful tracheoesophageal voice restoration. *Otolaryngology Clinics of North America, 37,* 507–517.

Singer, M. I., & Blom, E. D. (1981). Selective myotomy for voice restoration after total laryngectomy. *Archives of Otolaryngology, 107,* 670–673.

Singer, M. I., Blom, E. D., & Hamaker, R. C. (1986). Pharyngeal plexus neurectomy for alaryngeal speech rehabilitation. *Laryngoscope, 96,* 50–54.

Snidecor, J. C. (1974). *Speech rehabilitation of the laryngectomized* (2nd ed.). Springfield, IL: Thomas.

Snidecor, J. C. (1978). Speech therapy for those with total laryngectomy. In J. C. Snidecor (Ed.), *Speech rehabilitation of the laryngectomized* (2nd ed., pp. 180–193). Springfield, IL: Thomas.

Snidecor, J. C., & Curry, E. T. (1959). Temporal and pitch aspects of superior esophageal speech. *Annals of Otology, Rhinology and Laryngology, 68,* 623–636.

Snidecor, J. C., & Curry, E. T. (1960). How effectively can the laryngectomee expect to speak? *Laryngoscope, 70,* 62–67.

Snidecor, J. C., & Isshiki, N. (1965). Air volume and air flow relationships of six esophageal speakers. *Journal of Speech and Hearing Disorders, 30,* 205–216.

Terrell, J. E., Lewin, J. S., & Esclamado, R. (1995). Botulinum toxin injection for postlaryngectomy tracheoesophageal speech failure. *Otolaryngology—Head and Neck Surgery, 113,* 788–791.

Tikofsky, R. S. (1965). A comparison of the intelligibility of esophageal and normal speakers. *Folia Phoniatrica, 17,* 19–32.

Till, J. A., England, K. E., & Law-Till, C. B. (1987). Effects of auditory feedback and phonetic context on stomal noise in laryngectomized speakers. *Journal of Speech and Hearing Disorders, 52,* 243–250.

Weinberg, B. (1983). Voice and speech restoration following total laryngectomy. In W. H. Perkins (Ed.), *Voice disorders* (pp. 109–125). New York: Thieme-Stratton.

Weinberg, B., & Bennett, S. (1972a). A study of talker sex recognition of esophageal voices. *Journal of Speech and Hearing Research, 14,* 391–395.

Weinberg, B., & Bennett, S. (1972b). Selected acoustic characteristics of esophageal speech produced by female laryngectomees. *Journal of Speech and Hearing Research, 15,* 211–216.

Weinberg, B., & Bosma, J. F. (1970). Similarities between glossopharyngeal breathing and injection methods of air intake for esophageal speech. *Journal of Speech and Hearing Disorders, 35,* 25–32.

Weinberg, B., Horii, Y., & Smith, B. E. (1980). Long time spectral and intensity characteristics of esophageal speech. *Journal of the Acoustical Society of America, 67,* 1781–1784.

Weinberg, B., & Westerhouse, J. (1973). A study of pharyngeal speech. *Journal of Speech and Hearing Disorders, 38,* 111–118.

Weiss, C. E., Gordon, M. E., & Lillywhite, H. S. (1987). *Clinical management of articulatory and phonologic disorders* (2nd ed.). Baltimore: Williams & Wilkins.

Williams, S., & Watson, J. B. (1985). Differences in speaking proficiencies in three laryngectomy groups. *Archives of Otolaryngology, 111,* 216–219.

Zemlin, W. R. (1998). *Speech and hearing science* (4th ed.). Boston: Allyn & Bacon.

Chapter 17

Tracheoesophageal Voice Restoration

Carla DeLassus Gress and Mark I. Singer

The critical need to retain or restore vocal capabilities following the surgical treatment of laryngeal cancer has been recognized since the first successful total laryngectomy was performed by Billroth over a century ago (Güssenbauer, 1874). Numerous pneumatic and electronic artificial larynxes have been introduced over the years (see Chapter 2 in this text) to provide an artificial sound source for the alaryngeal speaker, but these devices may suffer from reduced intelligibility, naturalness, and acceptability (Blom, Singer, & Hamaker, 1986; Clements, Rassekh, Seikaly, Hokansen, & Calhoun, 1997; Merwin, Goldstein, & Rothman, 1985; see also Chapter 6 in this text). Despite rigorous scientific study of the mechanism of esophageal speech and associated teaching methods (Diedrich & Youngstrom, 1966), acquisition rates have generally been low, estimated at less than 30% in some series (Gates et al., 1982). Therefore, researchers and clinicians across the globe have worked toward improving communication for the individual who undergoes total laryngectomy and seeks to acquire alaryngeal speech.

The chapter begins with an overview of the tracheoesophageal puncture (TEP) voice restoration method. This overview is intended to provide a broad introduction to TEP and some of the more common issues confronted in clinical practice, including complications associated with TEP voice restoration. Following this introduction, topics include a discussion of patient selection and candidacy, esophageal insufflation testing, the types and selection of TEP voice prostheses, the fitting process, information on the time of prosthesis placement and patient instruction and training in the use and maintenance of the TEP voice prosthesis. Finally, we present a general discussion related to TEP speech production, including information on acoustics and speech intelligibility. Through coverage of these topic areas, we seek to offer the reader essential information on some of the more common issues confronted in clinical practice.

AN OVERVIEW OF TRACHEOESOPHAGEAL PUNCTURE VOICE RESTORATION

In the last 50 years, surgical efforts have focused on voice preservation by developing techniques to conserve portions of the voice producing mechanism (i.e., conservation laryngectomy) without jeopardizing cancer control (Biller, 1987; Pearson, Woods, & Hartman, 1980; see also Chapter 11 in this text). Nevertheless, voice conservation procedures do vary within and across surgical methods, as well as in the voice quality achieved (Doyle, 1997). These conservation laryngectomy procedures are based on understanding the routes of tumor spread (Biller, 1987; Ogura & Sessions, 1975). Other surgical attempts have been directed toward the construction of a shunting mechanism that allows pulmonary air to drive the tissues of the pharyngoesophagus; this compensatory vibration of tissue may be used for sound production in those who undergo total laryngectomy (Amatsu, 1978; Asai, 1972; Conley, DeAmesti, & Pierce, 1958; Komorn, 1974; Staffieri, 1980; Taub & Spiro, 1972). These procedures, however, have generally been limited to a small subpopulation of those treated for laryngeal cancer using total laryngectomy. Although initially promising, the results have not always been universally replicable. In many instances, such procedures have met with failures due to chronic aspiration and stenosis of the shunt. Thus, new approaches to postlaryngectomy voice restoration with reduced associated complications continued to be explored. The most promising of these methods was the TEP voice restoration procedure introduced by Singer and Blom (1980).

In the TEP procedure, a small puncture is surgically created through the posterior tracheal wall into the esophagus. A small (1.4- to 3.6-cm) one-way valved voice prosthesis is inserted into the puncture to prevent spontaneous closure of the puncture and to prevent the aspiration of pharyngoesophageal contents into the trachea. The voice prosthesis allows for the one-way flow of air from the trachea into the region below the pharyngoesophageal (PE) segment. Thus, this puncture permits diversion of pulmonary air to drive pharyngoesophageal vibration for the production of tracheoesophageal (TE) voice and speech.

To produce TE sound, the laryngectomized individual inhales, then exhales as the tracheostoma is occluded. Pulmonary air then enters the prosthesis, opens the one-way valve, and is released into the pharyngoesophagus, setting these tissues into vibration for sound generation. As the sound enters the oral and nasopharyngeal cavities, articulation and resonance shape the sounds and words in the typical fashion. Coordination of digital (i.e., finger) occlusion of the tracheostoma and associated release to meet the alternating respiratory (inhalation) and phonatory (exhalation) requirements is usually learned quickly by the TE speaker. Alternately, stoma occlusion may be achieved through the use of a tracheostoma valve for hands–free speech (see Blom, Singer, & Hamaker, 1982; see also Chapter 19 in this text). An illustration of TE speech production is shown in Figure 17.1.

The surgical creation of the puncture tract may be performed at the time of laryngectomy (primary puncture) in uncomplicated cases of total laryngectomy (Hamaker, Singer, Blom, & Daniels, 1985; Singer, 2004) or delayed until sufficient healing has occurred (secondary puncture), usually at least 6 weeks after surgery or completion of radiotherapy. To maintain patency of the surgically created TE puncture site, a catheter (or, in the case of primary puncture, a feeding tube) is placed through the puncture downward into the esophagus. The catheter is subsequently replaced by the voice prosthesis after sufficient healing has occurred. In some facilities, the surgeon places the extended-wear prosthesis as part of the operative procedure.

COMPLICATIONS ASSOCIATED WITH TEP VOICE RESTORATION

Although complications following TEP voice restoration have been reported, the majority are self-limited and minor (Andrews, Mickel, Ward, Hanson, & Monahan, 1987; Karlen & Maisel, 2001). The most significant surgical complication involves esophageal perforation with secondary mediastinal infection and cervical osteomyelitis. Perforation occurs as a result of esophagoscopy, due to trapping of the mucosa, resulting in a tear. Early management of the perforation requires drainage and antibiotic therapy.

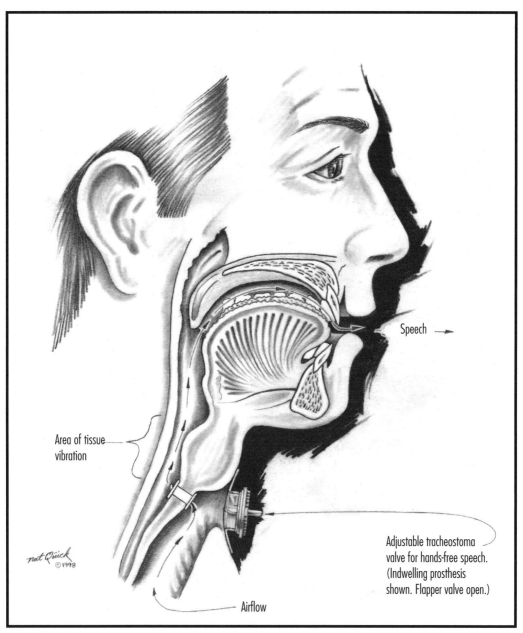

Speech →

Area of tissue
vibration

Airflow

Adjustable tracheostoma
valve for hands-free speech.
(Indwelling prosthesis
shown. Flapper valve open.)

nat Quick
©1998

FIGURE 17.1. The mechanism of tracheoesophageal (TE) voice production (adjustable tracheostoma valve is shown in place). (Courtesy of Nat Quick.)

In a small number of cases, myotomy to reduce pharyngeal constrictor hypertonicity may result in a pharyngocutaneous leakage (fistula) and neck infection (Singer & Blom, 1981). This is also managed by drainage and antibiotics, but may require reconstructive flap surgery. Although rare, this complication is not considered minor.

The most common tracheal complication is inflammation, which is usually self-limiting. Chronic peritracheal inflammation may sometimes lead to tracheal stenosis, which can be managed with the use of a silicone laryngectomy tube or stomaplasty (Ho, Wei, Lam, & Lau, 1991; Singer, Hamaker, Blom, & Yoshida, 1989). A small number of TE speakers develop circumferential granulation formation (referred to as a "doughnut") at the tracheal side of the puncture. This is believed to be a foreign body reaction to the prosthesis and is usually managed in the surgeon's office by cautery. Infrequently, tracheal necrosis can develop in the posterior wall at the site of the puncture. If confined to a small area, the preferred management strategy is to rest the stoma, avoiding the use of the prosthesis and digital pressure for a period of time. The TEP voice prosthesis should be properly sized so that the esophageal retention collar sits firmly against the anterior esophageal wall, serving as a gasket to seal the leak. Extensive tracheal necrosis with aspiration is managed by placement of a cuffed tracheostomy tube and nonoral feedings until reconstructive surgery can correct the defect (Singer, Hamaker, & Blom, 1989).

ASSESSMENT AND CANDIDACY FOR TEP VOICE RESTORATION

There are relatively few contraindications to TEP voice restoration. An individual who is under consideration for TEP, either prior to or following total laryngectomy, must be motivated to speak again, as well as willing to undergo the surgical procedure and the necessary training in the use and maintenance of the prosthetic device. An important consideration, therefore, is the patient's cognitive state. The laryngectomized individual must learn to coordinate stoma occlusion (either by manual occlusion or the use of an attached hands-free tracheostoma valve) with respiration and articulation, and be capable of learning routine daily maintenance procedures for care of the prosthetic device. There must be an awareness of potential problems that indicate device failure or require urgent medical attention (e.g., uncontrolled leakage, infection, device dislodgment). If the individual has cognitive impairments or limitations of vision or manual dexterity, the maintenance functions associated with the TEP voice prosthesis are performed by a designated caregiver who has agreed to serve in this capacity. The advent of extended-wear (indwelling) voice prostheses, however, has significantly reduced the patient's responsibilities for prosthesis maintenance. Nevertheless, those who use the extended-wear TEP voice prosthesis still require that adequately trained medical personnel are accessible for device replacement when necessary.

For some individuals, chronic alcoholism is a contraindication to TEP voice restoration, particularly if the severity of the condition limits the individual's ability to perform routine self-care and maintenance of the tracheostoma and the prosthetic device, or to return for periodic follow-up appointments. Such issues must be addressed on an individual basis, and consideration of the individual's candidacy for TEP voice restoration must involve assessment of other factors (e.g., access to a family member who can assume responsibility if problems arise).

Radiation therapy is usually not a limiting factor to use of a TEP voice prosthesis unless the dose to the treatment area has exceeded 70 Gy. Healing may be compromised in tissue that has been heavily irradiated, causing a failure of the tissue surrounding the TEP site to stenose around the voice prosthesis. If this occurs, it may result in leakage around the voice prosthesis and the potential for accidental dislodgment. Other medical conditions that contribute to reduced healing properties of the tissue surrounding the TEP include uncontrolled diabetes, thyroid dysfunction, malnutrition, and persistent or recurrent (including distant) malignant disease.

Surgical procedures that extend beyond a standard total laryngectomy, such as those requiring reconstruction of the pharynx or esophagus with local or free flaps, are not a contraindication to TEP in most instances (Bleach, Perry, & Cheesman, 1991; Deschler, Doherty, Reed, Anthony, & Singer, 1998; Deschler, Doherty, Reed, & Singer, 1998, 1999; Deschler & Gray, 2004; Haughey, Frederickson, Sessions, & Fuller, 1995; Juarbe et al., 1989; Maniglia, Leder, Goodwin, Sawyer, & Sasaki, 1989; Ziesmann, Boyd, Manktelow, & Rosen, 1989; see also Chapter 12 in this text). The TEP is performed as a secondary procedure in reconstruction procedures utilizing gastric interposition or when a lengthy or problematic postoperative recovery is anticipated. The resultant voice quality following extensive reconstructions is dependent on the vibratory capabilities of the reconstructed pharyngoesophagus, and may be suboptimal in some cases due to excessive breathiness, inadequate volume, or a strained vocal quality.

Stoma size also is an important consideration in secondary TEP. Specifically, if the tracheostoma is too small, prosthesis insertion or airway limitations may occur. A minimum tracheostomal diameter of 1.5 cm is recommended to allow for ease of insertion of the prosthesis, adequate hygiene, and a sufficient airway for respiratory exchange. An example of a TEP voice prosthesis (the Provox device) in situ is shown in Figure 17.2. In patients with smaller stomas, stomaplasty can be performed at the time of secondary TEP, or the microstoma can be managed by use of a silicone laryngectomy tube that has been fenestrated to permit the flow of air into the prosthesis. Lewin (2004) recently presented information related to nonsurgical management of the tracheostoma to maximize TE speech.

ESOPHAGEAL INSUFFLATION TESTING

Esophageal air insufflation testing is often helpful in predicting the adequacy of the PE segment for sound generation in the situation of secondary TEP voice

FIGURE 17.2. Tracheoesophageal puncture voice prosthesis (the Provox device) in the tracheostoma.

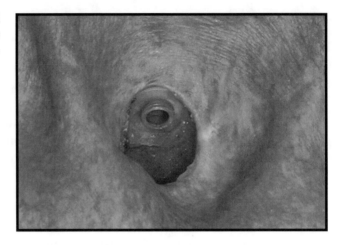

restoration (Blom et al., 1985). In this procedure, a rubber catheter is inserted transnasally approximately 25 cm past the pharyngoesophageal juncture. An airstream is then introduced via the catheter to stimulate vibration of the PE segment. Easy, fluent sound production that is greater than 8 seconds in duration is indicative of a viable vibratory mechanism. A high-pitched, strained vocal quality or reduced or intermittent fluency is regarded as an insufflation test failure and suggests that post-TEP speech will be suboptimal. The use of intraesophageal pressure monitoring in conjunction with insufflation (Lewin, Baugh, & Baker, 1987) may provide a more objective assessment of the vibratory capability of the PE segment. The causes of insufflation failure are varied, and include improper placement of the catheter, stricture, fibrosis, radiation-induced edema, tumor recurrence, hyper- or hypotonicity of the PE segment, or excessive strain or tension on the part of the patient. Confirmation of hypertonicity by means of videofluoroscopy (Sloane, Griffin, & O'Dwyer, 1991) and/or a lidocaine injection for pharyngeal plexus nerve block suggests the need for a pharyngeal constrictor relaxation procedure, such as myotomy, neurectomy, or chemical denervation, in order to achieve fluent TEP speech (Blitzer, Komisar, Baredes, Brin, & Stewart, 1995; Hamaker & Blom, 2003; Singer & Blom, 1981; Singer, Blom, & Hamaker, 1986; Terrell, Lewin, & Esclamado, 1995; see also Chapter 6 in this text). The method of esophageal insufflation testing is shown in Figure 17.3.

TYPES OF TEP VOICE PROSTHESES

The original, commercially available prostheses designed by Singer and Blom (1980) incorporated a slit-type valve; these were referred to as duckbill style devices. Many of the prostheses developed subsequently feature an internalized hinged valve with a lower opening pressure. This design requires less respiratory effort for sound generation than the duckbill style devices (Pauloski, 1998). These hinged-type TEP voice prostheses are referred to as low-pressure or low-

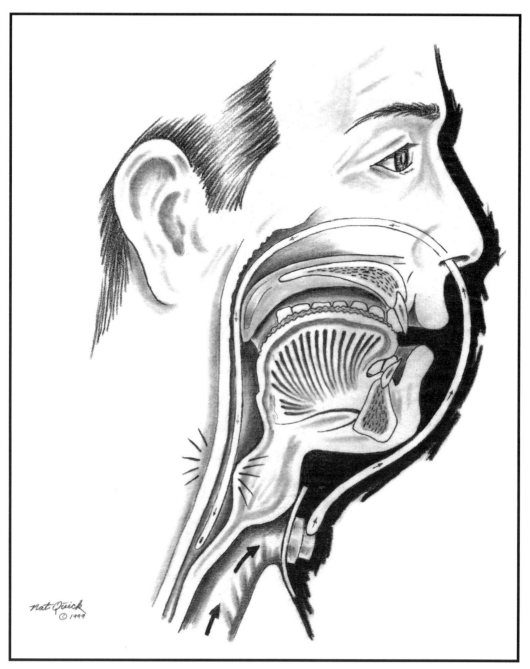

FIGURE 17.3. The method of esophageal insufflation testing. (Courtesy of Nat Quick.)

resistance prostheses. The larger diameter of some devices (20 Fr or greater) generally allows for increased airflow through the prosthesis (Pauloski, 1998). In recent years several types of extended-wear or indwelling prostheses have been developed to accommodate the demand for simplicity of maintenance and reduced patient responsibility (see Chapter 18 in this text). These devices incorporate the use of larger retention collars to avoid accidental dislodgment. During insertion, however, such devices induce slightly more trauma to the tissue surrounding the TEP than do standard prostheses. Increased trauma may occur because of the difficulty inserting the larger diameter retention collars through the puncture site. Consequently, it is recommended that extended-wear prostheses should be inserted and removed only by an experienced medical professional.

Prosthesis lengths and the method of sizing vary by manufacturer. Recently, there has been an attempt to standardize the process by measuring the interflange distance in millimeters; identifying and using the distance between the tracheal and esophageal retention collars may provide a means of standardizing fitting with different TEP voice prostheses. This measurement corresponds to the thickness of the tracheoesophageal wall. Product literature from the manufacturer should be consulted to determine the aerodynamic characteristics, sizing, and other specifications of each device. A variety of TEP voice prostheses are shown in Figures 17.4 through 17.8.

FIGURE 17.4. Bivona duckbill voice prosthesis and insertion device.

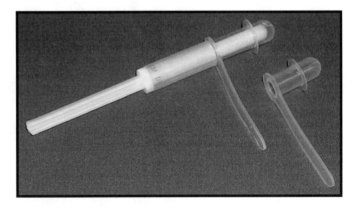

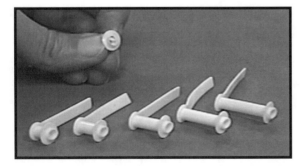

FIGURE 17.5. InHealth Technologies low-pressure TEP voice prostheses and insertion devices (note differences in diameter of prostheses according to French sizing).

FITTING THE VOICE PROSTHESIS

The TEP voice prosthesis is a small tubed device, usually of medical-grade silicone, which incorporates a one-way valve (either a slit, hinge, or ball) at the distal (esophageal) end. The diameter of the voice prosthesis varies from 16 to 24 French (Fr), depending on the brand and style. A collar or flange at the distal end aids in its retention within the esophagus. When the tracheostoma is sealed, pulmonary air enters the lumen of the prosthesis anteriorly, opens the valve, fills the esophageal reservoir, and then exits to drive vibration of the PE segment. Air pressures required to open the valve range between 2 and 100 cm H_2O and depend on the rate of airflow from the lungs and the device design (Heaton, Sanderson, Dunsmore, & Parker, 1996; Weinberg & Moon, 1984).

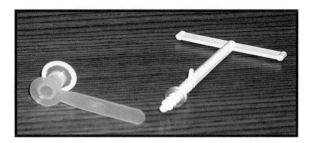

FIGURE 17.6. InHealth Technologies indwelling voice prosthesis and insertion device.

FIGURE 17.7. ATOS Medical Provox 2 TEP voice prosthesis.

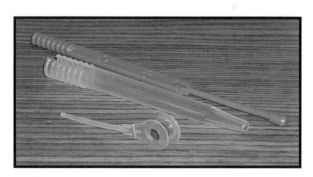

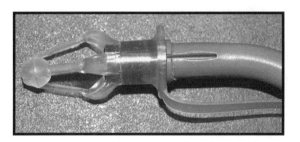

FIGURE 17.8. Entermed Voicemaster TEP voice prosthesis attached to insertion probe.

TEP VOICE PROSTHESIS SELECTION

The selection of a TE prosthetic device requires careful consideration of several important factors (Gress, 1998; see also Chapter 19 in this text). The primary concerns relate to maintaining the patency of the TEP tract, ensuring healthy TE wall tissue, and preventing aspiration of liquids either around or through the TEP voice prosthesis. If the laryngectomized individual is unable or unwilling to replace the voice prosthesis, or there is a concern regarding accidental dislodgment, an extended-wear prosthesis may be preferable. If an extended wear device is used, however, the patient must have access to trained medical personnel should the device malfunction or when other needs arise (e.g., fitting, changing the prosthesis). In contrast, the duckbill style devices may be unsuitable for individuals with a narrow esophagus because the extended distal portion may impinge on the posterior esophageal wall. Also, consideration should be given to aerodynamic properties of the various prostheses to ensure optimal voice production with minimal respiratory effort. Typically, larger diameter and low-resistance prostheses permit increased airflow and may result in louder, less effortful voice and speech production; however, a lower resistance valve also may open inadvertently during quiet respiration and may cause excess stomach gas in some individuals. Familiarity with a variety of devices will assist the clinician in selecting the optimal device for a given patient.

TIME OF PROSTHESIS PLACEMENT

The voice prosthesis can be placed in the TEP site once sufficient healing of the tissue has occurred. In some settings an extended-wear device is placed at the time of puncture, or fitting of the prosthesis can be delayed for anywhere from 2 days to 3 weeks. If prosthesis fitting is delayed, a small-diameter stenting catheter will be placed in the TEP to maintain its patency. After the catheter is removed, the TEP is then serially dilated with catheters of increasing diameter until the puncture is one size greater than that of the selected TEP voice prosthesis. This helps to decrease tissue trauma upon device insertion. Using a measuring device available from the prosthesis manufacturer, the depth of the TE party wall is assessed. An accurate measurement is critical for determining the proper length for the voice prosthesis. A prosthesis that is too short will not bridge the TEP wall sufficiently and will result in stenosis of the posterior portion of the puncture tract, whereas a prosthesis that is too long will piston in the tract and cause dilation of the puncture and tissue irritation (see Chapters 19 and 24 in this text).

Typically, the prosthesis is inserted from the tracheal side using a standard insertion tool supplied by the manufacturer. For the non–extended-wear prosthesis, a "pop" will be felt on insertion as the esophageal retention collar opens on entering the esophagus. Folding the esophageal retention collar into half of a gelatin capsule can ease insertion of the blunt-ended low-resistance devices. In contrast, some prostheses use a retrograde insertion method (Hilgers & Schouwenburg, 1990), whereby a guidewire is inserted through the TEP tract, coursed anteriorly through the pharynx and out the mouth to accept attachment of the prosthesis, and then retracted until the device is situated in the puncture. Antero-grade (from the front) insertion, however, is the most common practice currently reported by clinicians worldwide. Irrespective of the placement method, the voice prosthesis should rotate freely in the tract, confirming opening of the esophageal retention collar and suggesting proper stenting of the TEP tract through its entire depth.

PATIENT INSTRUCTION AND TRAINING

The individual who is laryngectomized and chooses to pursue TE speech must understand the method of TEP voice production, the use and care of the voice prosthesis, and the necessary procedures in the event of an emergency. Such in-formation is critical to successful voice restoration. This will require clear and careful explanation using diagrams and demonstrations, and opportunity for the patient to continually practice these developing skills (Gress, 2004). Most impor-tant, in the event of accidental dislodgment of the TEP voice prosthesis, the pa-tient needs to understand the necessity of maintaining the patency of the TEP tract at all times through placement of a properly sized prosthesis, stent, or catheter to prevent stenosis of the puncture. For users of the non–extended-wear prosthesis, instruction in device insertion is an integral part of the training and may require more than a single session with direct, independent, hands-on prac-tice (see Chapter 19 in this text).

For all TEP voice prosthesis types, the patient is alerted to the indications for device failure, such as leakage through the prosthesis or increased strain dur-ing vocal production. The typical device life for the extended-wear prosthesis is approximately 15 weeks (Delsuphe, Zink, Lejaergere, & Delaere, 1998). The most common cause of device failure is *Candida albicans* deposits that interfere with complete closure of the valve mechanism and result in leakage of liquids through the prosthesis (Mahieu, van Saene, Rosingh, & Schutte, 1986). The use of prophy-lactic antifungal medications is usually successful in increasing device life (Mahieu, van Saene, den Besten, & van Saene, 1986). The prosthesis may sometimes become occluded with secretions, which may result in a strained vocal quality. As part of the instructional program, information regarding the preferred method of clean-ing the prosthesis should be provided, as well as information on the procedure for obtaining necessary supplies, either through local or mail order vendors.

TRACHEOSTOMA BREATHING VALVE AND TEP VOICE PROSTHESIS USE

As noted, the hands-free tracheostoma breathing valve eliminates the need for manual occlusion of the stoma for speech production; the breathing valve also of-fers significant hygienic benefits (Blom et al., 1982; Hilgers et al., 2003). The valve consists of a thin, pressure-sensitive diaphragm that remains open at rest (i.e., during quiet breathing) for easy respiration. The increase in exhalatory air pressure associated with speech production causes the valve to shut, thus diverting air through the TEP voice prosthesis into the esophageal reservoir. At the end of an utterance, air pressure is naturally relaxed, and the pressure-sensitive diaphragm assembly returns to its open state. The attachment of the hands-free tracheostoma valve is achieved by use of a flexible housing attached to the peristomal area by means of adhesives or alternately by the placement and use of a special silicone tracheostomal tube that has been developed for this purpose (Lewin et al., 2000). An example of the hands-free tracheostoma breathing valve is shown in Figure 17.9.

It is estimated that less than 50% of TEP speakers are successful with the hands-free tracheostoma valve (Gress, 1998). Individuals with significant respiratory compromise may not be suitable candidates for use of the device. The most frequently encountered problem, however, is insufficient adherence of the valve housing to the skin (usually defined as less than 8 hours) due to irregularity of the peristomal area, copious tracheal secretions, or excessive exhalatory air pressure ("back pressure") during speech (Blom et al., 1982; Crum, 1996). To maximize the chances of success, the individual who is laryngectomized and receives TEP voice restoration should first master fluent TE speech using digital occlusion. The use of a

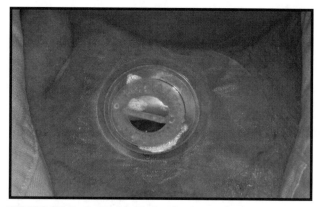

FIGURE 17.9. InHealth Technologies tracheostoma valve for hands-free speech.

prosthesis with larger diameter, lowered resistance, or both will often assist in reducing excessive respiratory effort and improve TE speech production (Grolman, Grolman, van Steenwijk, & Schouwenburg, 1998).

Once efficient respiratory control for TEP speech has developed using digital stoma occlusion, it is beneficial to help focus treatment efforts solely on achieving a housing seal of sufficient duration, without use of the hands-free tracheostoma valve in place. This will afford an opportunity to identify and alleviate the specific cause of adherence problems before attempting to learn the respiratory control needed for operation of the valve itself. Attachment of the external housing device requires meticulous technique to ensure a proper seal of adequate duration; it also requires practice to ensure consistency in the attachment procedure. The patient may need to try various combinations of housings and adhesives to achieve a sufficient seal (Canady & Martinez, 1996). The use of a heat and moisture exchange (HME) system is beneficial in reducing excess tracheal secretions that lead to premature loss of the housing seal (Hilgers, Aaronson, Ackerstaff, Schouwenburg, & van Zanwijk, 1991; see also Chapter 20 in this text). A custom housing molded from prosthodontic material, while relatively expensive, will usually alleviate the problem of an irregular peristomal contour (Cantu, Shagets, Andres, Fifer, & Newton, 1986). Additionally, successful modification to customize a standard housing to increase seal duration has been reported (Doyle, Grantmyre, & Myers, 1989).

After the patient is consistently able to maintain an adequate seal of sufficient duration, the operation of a hands-free valve is usually mastered quite quickly. The patient is instructed in placement of the pressure-sensitive valve into the housing, as well as the necessity of quickly removing the valve in anticipation of a cough. Activation of valve closure for speech is achieved by starting with a quick exhalation. Tracheostoma valves are supplied in a variety of different closure sensitivities, or have an adjustment mechanism to alter the closure sensitivity relative to the respiratory workload (Grolman et al., 1998). A trial-and-error process is always required to determine the optimal setting that allows for easy quiet respiration, minimal effort for closure during speech, and avoidance of inadvertent closure during routine physical activity, such as brisk walking and climbing stairs.

HEAT AND MOISTURE EXCHANGE

Normal upper airway filtration and humidification help to maintain the usually thin viscosity of mucus and allow it to be transported outward by cilia of the epithelial cells. The surgical procedure of laryngectomy creates a tracheostoma for respiration and the resultant bypass of the upper airways, causing thickened and increased mucus secretions and drying of the respiratory tract. Various HMEs have been developed to assist with restoration of pulmonary functions (Hilgers et al., 2003; see Chapter 20 in this text). These devices work on the principle that during exhalation, heat and moisture will be absorbed by the filtering mechanism and transferred back to the incoming air on inhalation (Hilgers et al., 1991). These products vary in design, airflow resistance, and efficiency. When the HME device is initially applied, it is not uncommon for the laryngectomized individual to complain of an interference in breathing, due to the sudden increase in resistance to the flow of air. Although these devices typically do not exceed the normal physiologic upper airway resistance, their use may require a period of adjustment, and consistent application over a period of several days is necessary to achieve the demonstrated effects. The continued use of the HME device is highly recommended for those TE speakers who wish to successfully progress to hands-free speech with the tracheostoma breathing valve. Several types of heat and moisture exchange systems are shown in Figures 17.10, 17.11, and 17.12.

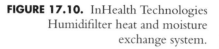

FIGURE 17.10. InHealth Technologies Humidifilter heat and moisture exchange system.

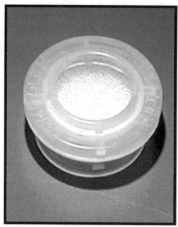

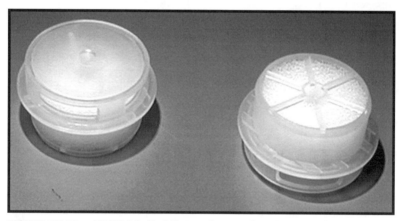

FIGURE 17.11. ATOS Medical Provox heat and moisture exchange system.

TEP SPEECH PRODUCTION

After the proper insertion, placement, and functioning of the voice prosthesis have been verified, the patient is instructed in the method of stoma occlusion and voice production. Manual (digital) tracheostoma occlusion requires a trial-and-error approach to determine the best finger and proper placement angle to prevent air escape from the stoma, while simultaneously maintaining gentle digital contact. When aspects of hygiene are considered, manual occlusion of the tracheostoma ideally should be accomplished with the nondominant hand over a stoma cover or filter. For irregular or large stomas, various implements such as a baby bottle nipple or cosmetic sponge can be of assistance in covering the stoma more effectively. The valve housing from a standard hands-free tracheostoma breathing valve may also be attached to offer a small round opening over which digital stoma occlusion can be accomplished.

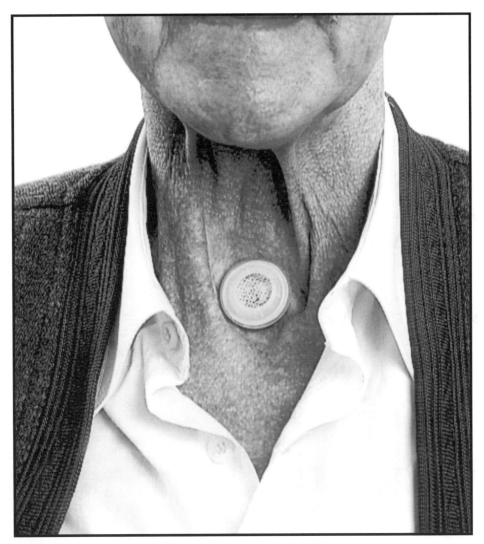

FIGURE 17.12. Kapitex Trachinaze heat and moisture exchange system.

With practice and clinician direction and feedback, the TEP speaker will master the coordination of respiratory requirements and tracheostoma occlusion for speech purposes. Refinement of TEP voice employs standard speech pathology treatment techniques while emphasizing maximum intelligibility and naturalness (Blom et al., 1986). Although the mechanism is not well understood, vocal pitch can be controlled to some degree in many TEP speakers (Deschler, Doherty, Reed, & Singer, 1998, 1999; van As, Hilgers, Verdonck-de Leeuw, & Koopmans-van Beinum, 1996). The low pitch associated with TE (as well as esophageal) speech can be socially debilitating, especially for females (Brown & Doyle, 1999; Eadie & Doyle, 2004; Trudeau & Qi, 1990). For this reason, the laryngectomized individual is encouraged to use the most natural pitch that can be achieved. Vocal loudness associated with TE speech may often exceed that of the normal speaker (Robbins, Fisher, Blom, & Singer, 1984). If loudness is a problem, the use of larger diameter and lowered resistance prostheses can assist in attaining an optimal loudness level. The person who is laryngectomized also may present with compromised articulation due to loss of dentition or as a consequence of surgical extension that involves the base of the tongue and hypoglossal nerve. The use of a reduced speaking rate and emphasis on precise articulation will usually offer satisfactory compensation for reductions in intelligibility. Phrasing should be consistent with the individual's pulmonary and phonatory capabilities, as well as the grammatical requirements of the utterance.

ACOUSTIC CHARACTERISTICS AND INTELLIGIBILITY OF TEP SPEECH

Various acoustic studies have shown that the intensity of TE speech approximates normal laryngeal speech levels (Robbins et al., 1984; Trudeau & Qi, 1990). The average fundamental frequency of TE speech is close to that of normal male speakers, but considerably less than that for normal female speakers (Robbins et al., 1984; Trudeau & Qi, 1990). Rate of speech (during oral reading) for TEP speakers has been reported as near normal compared to laryngeal speakers, with a mean duration of 128 versus 173 words per minute, respectively (Robbins et al., 1984). Intelligibility of TE speech is considerably high (Blom et al., 1986), although variability can be substantial due to individual differences in the extent of surgery that may impact articulation and the consistency of the vibratory mechanism. The typical articulation errors that have been identified for TE speakers include voicing errors and problems with fricatives and affricates (Doyle, Danhauer, & Reed, 1988). Patient satisfaction with speech quality and the ability to communicate over the telephone is generally high for TEP speakers, and they report limited interference in their interactions with others (Clements et al., 1997; Eadie & Doyle, 2004). It is generally agreed that many TE speakers do very well at the conversational level of communication. Although more detailed investigations of listener judgments of TE speaker proficiency are lacking (see Chapter 6 in this text), the access to pulmonary air in these individuals does appear to be advantageous.

SUMMARY

Tracheoesophageal puncture voice restoration and the subsequent acquisition of TE speech can provide rapid restoration of near-normal oral communication for a large number of laryngectomized individuals. Very high success rates (85%–95%) have been reported (Maniglia, Lundy, Casiano, & Swim, 1989; McEwan et al., 1996) and complications are few (Andrews et al., 1987). Although initially targeted for individuals who failed to develop or were dissatisfied with esophageal speech or use of the artificial larynx, TEP voice restoration appears to have wide applicability and has gained worldwide acceptance. As experience with the TEP technique continues to develop and as further modifications and refinements in the prosthetic devices evolve, wider application of this voice restoration method will occur. Research should be directed toward improving understanding of the physiologic mechanisms involved in PE segment sound production (see Chapter 21 in this text), with an eye toward maximizing phonatory capabilities through better methods of surgical reconstruction of this alaryngeal voice source without compromise of cancer control.

REFERENCES

Amatsu, M. (1978). A new one-stage surgical technique for postlaryngectomy speech. *Archives of Otology, Rhinology and Laryngology, 220,* 149–152.

Andrews, J. C., Mickel, R. A., Ward, P. F. L., Hanson, D. G., & Monahan, G. P. (1987). Major complications following tracheoesophageal puncture for voice rehabilitation. *Laryngoscope, 97,* 562–567.

Asai, R. (1972). Laryngoplasty after total laryngectomy. *Annals of Otology, Rhinology and Laryngology, 95,* 114–119.

Biller, H. (1987). Conservation surgery past, present, and future. *Laryngoscope, 97,* 38–41.

Bleach, N., Perry, A., & Cheesman, A. D. (1991). Surgical voice restoration with the Blom–Singer procedure following laryngo-pharyngo-esophagectomy and pharyngo-gastric anastomosis. *Annals of Otology, Rhinology and Laryngology, 100,* 142–147.

Blitzer, A., Komisar, A., Baredes, S., Brin, J. F., & Stewart, C. (1995). Voice failure after tracheoesophageal puncture: Management with botulinum toxin. *Otolaryngology—Head and Neck Surgery, 113,* 668–670.

Blom, E. D., Singer, M. I., & Hamaker, R. C. (1982). Tracheostoma valve for postlaryngectomy voice rehabilitation. *Annals of Otology, Rhinology and Laryngology, 91,* 576–578.

Blom, E. D., Singer, M. I., & Hamaker, R. C. (1985). An improved esophageal insufflation test. *Archives of Otolaryngology—Head and Neck Surgery, 111,* 211–212.

Blom, E. D., Singer, M. I., & Hamaker, R. C. (1986). A prospective study of tracheoesophageal speech. *Archives of Otolaryngology—Head and Neck Surgery, 112,* 440–447.

Brown, S. I., & Doyle, P. C. (1999). The woman who is laryngectomized: Parallels, perspectives, and a reevaluation of practice. *Journal of Speech–Language Pathology and Audiology, 23,* 10–15.

Canady, C. J., & Martinez, J. A. (1996). Increased tracheostoma valve seal duration in patients with recessed or irregular stoma using a modified application method. *American Journal of Speech–Language Pathology, 5,* 31–36.

Cantu, E., Shagets, F. W., Andres, C. J., Fifer, R. C., & Newton, A. D. (1986). Customized valve housing. *Laryngoscope, 96,* 1159–1163.

Clements, K. S., Rassekh, C. H., Seikaly, H., Hokanson, J. A., & Calhoun, K. H. (1997). Communication after laryngectomy: An assessment of patient satisfaction. *Archives of Otolaryngology—Head and Neck Surgery, 123,* 493–496.

Conley, J. J., DeAmesti, F., & Pierce, J. K. (1958). A new surgical technique for the vocal rehabilitation of the laryngectomized patient. *Annals of Otology, Rhinology and Laryngology, 67,* 655–664.

Crum, R. (1996). Attachment of the adjustable tracheostoma valve and housing from the view of a laryngectomee. *ORL—Head and Neck Nursing, 14*(1) 15–16.

Delsuphe, K., Zink, I., Lejaergere, M., & Delaere, P. (1998). Prospective randomised comparative study of tracheoesophageal voice prosthesis: Blom–Singer versus Provox. *Laryngoscope, 108,* 1561–1565.

Deschler, D. G., Doherty, E. T., Reed, C. G., Anthony, J. P., & Singer, M. I. (1998). Tracheoesophageal voice following tubed free radial forearm flap reconstruction of the neopharynx. *Annals of Otology, Rhinology and Laryngology, 103,* 929–936.

Deschler, D. G., Doherty, E. T., Reed, C. G., & Singer, M. I. (1998). Quantitative and qualitative analysis of tracheoesophageal voice after pectoralis major flap reconstruction of the neopharynx. *Otolaryngology—Head and Neck Surgery, 118,* 771–776.

Deschler, D. G., Doherty, E. T., Reed, C. G., & Singer M. I. (1999). Effects of sound pressure levels on fundamental frequency in tracheoesophageal speakers. *Otolaryngology—Head and Neck Surgery, 121,* 23–26.

Deschler, D. G., & Gray, S. T. (2004). Tracheoesophageal speech following laryngopharyngectomy and pharyngeal reconstruction. *Otolaryngology Clinics of North America, 37,* 567–583.

Diedrich, W. M., & Youngstrom, K. A. (1966). *Alaryngeal speech.* Springfield, IL: Thomas.

Doyle, P. C. (1997). Voice refinement following conservation surgery for carcinoma of the larynx: A conceptual model for therapeutic intervention. *American Journal of Speech–Language Pathology, 6,* 27–35.

Doyle, P. C., Danhauer, J. L., & Reed, C. G. (1988). Listeners' perception of consonants produced by esophageal and tracheoesophageal talkers. *Journal of Speech and Hearing Disorders, 53,* 400–407.

Doyle, P. C., Grantmyre, A., & Myers, C. (1989). Clinical modification of the tracheostoma breathing valve for voice restoration. *Journal of Speech and Hearing Disorders, 54,* 189–193.

Eadie, T. L., & Doyle, P. C. (2004). Auditory–perceptual scaling and quality of life in tracheoesophageal speakers. *Laryngoscope, 114,* 753–759.

Gates, G. A., Ryan, W., Cooper, J. C., Jr, Lawlis, G. F., Cantu, E., Hayashi, T., Lauder, E., Welch, R. W., & Hearne, E. (1982). Current status of laryngectomee rehabilitation: I. Results of therapy. *American Journal of Otolaryngology, 3,* 1–7.

Gress, C. D. (1998). Tracheoesophageal speech. In J. K. Casper, & R. H. Colton (Eds.), *Clinical manual for laryngectomy and head/neck cancer rehabilitation* (2nd ed.). San Diego: Singular.

Gress, C. D. (2004). Preoperative evaluation for tracheoesophageal voice restoration. *Otolaryngology Clinics of North America, 37,* 519–530.

Grolman, W., Grolman, E., van Steenwijk, R. P., & Schouwenburg, P. F. (1998). Airflow and pressure characteristics of three different tracheostoma valves. *Annals of Otology, Rhinology and Laryngology, 107,* 312–318.

Güssenbauer, T. (1874). Ueber die erste durch T. Billroth an menschen ge fuhrte kehldopfextstripation, und die anwendung eines kunstlichen kehlkopfes. *Verheul Deutsch Chirgurie.*

Hamaker, R. C., & Blom, E. D. (2003). Botulinum neurotoxin for pharyngeal constrictor muscle spasm in tracheoesophageal voice restoration. *Laryngoscope, 113,* 1479–1482.

Hamaker, R. C., Singer, M. I., Blom, E. D., & Daniels, H. A. (1985). Primary voice restoration at laryngectomy. *Archives of Otolaryngology, 111,* 182–186.

Haughey, B. H., Frederickson, J. M., Sessions, D. G., & Fuller, D. (1995). Vibratory segment function after free flap reconstruction of the pharyngoesophagus. *Laryngoscope, 105,* 487–490.

Heaton, J. M., Sanderson, D., Dunsmore, I. R., & Parker, A. J. (1996). In vivo measurements of indwelling tracheo-oesophageal prostheses in alaryngeal speech. *Clinical Otolaryngology, 21,* 292–296.

Hilgers, F. J. M., Aaronson, N. K., Ackerstaff, A. H., Schouwenburg, P. F., & van Zanwijk, N. (1991). The influence of a heat and moisture exchanger (HME) on the respiratory symptoms after total laryngectomy. *Clinical Otolaryngology, 16,* 152–156.

Hilgers, F. J., Ackerstaff, A. H., van As, C. J., Balm, A. J., van den Brekel, M. W., & Tan, I. B. (2003). Development and clinical assessment of a heat and moisture exchanger with a multi-magnet automatic tracheostoma valve (Provox FreeHands HME) for vocal and pulmonary rehabilitation after total laryngectomy. *Acta Otolaryngologica, 123,* 91–99.

Hilgers, F. J. M. & Schouwenburg, P. F. (1990). A new low-resistance, self-retaining prosthesis (Provox®) for voice rehabilitation after total laryngectomy. *Laryngoscope, 100,* 1202–1207.

Ho, C. M., Wei, W. I., Lam, K. H., & Lau, W. F. (1991). Tracheostomal stenosis after immediate tracheoesophageal puncture. *Archives of Otolaryngology—Head and Neck Surgery, 117,* 662–665.

Juarbe, C., Shemen, L., Wang, R., Anand, V., Eberle, R., Sirovatka, A., Malanaphy, K., & Klatsky, I. (1989). Tracheoesophageal puncture for voice restoration after extended laryngopharyngectomy. *Archives of Otolaryngology—Head and Neck Surgery, 115,* 356–359.

Karlen, R. G., & Maisel, R. H. (2001). Does primary tracheoesophageal puncture reduce complications after laryngectomy and improve patient communication? *American Journal of Otolaryngology, 22,* 324–328.

Komorn, R. M. (1974). Vocal rehabilitation in the laryngectomized patient with a tracheoesophageal shunt. *Annals of Otology, Rhinology and Laryngology, 83,* 445–451.

Lewin, J. S. (2004). Nonsurgical management of the stoma to maximize tracheoesophageal speech. *Otolaryngologic Clinics of North America, 37,* 585–596.

Lewin, J. S., Baugh, R. F., & Baker, S. R. (1987). An objective method for prediction of tracheoesophageal speech production. *Journal of Speech and Hearing Disorders, 52,* 212–217.

Lewin, J. S., Lemon, J., Bishop-Leone, J. K., Leyk, S., Martin, J. W., & Gillenwater, A. M. (2000). Experience with Barton button and peristomal breathing valve attachments for hands-free tracheoesophageal speech. *Head & Neck, 22,* 142–148.

Mahieu, H. F., van Saene, J. J. M., den Besten, J., & van Saene, H. K. F. (1986). Oropharynx decontamination preventing Candida vegetation on voice prostheses. *Archives of Otolaryngology—Head and Neck Surgery, 112,* 1090–1092.

Mahieu, H. F., van Saene, H. K. F., Rosingh, H. J., & Schutte, H. K. (1986). Candida vegetations on silicone valve prostheses. *Archives of Otolaryngology—Head and Neck Surgery, 112,* 321–325.

Maniglia, A. J., Leder, S. B., Goodwin, W. J., Sawyer, R., & Sasaki, C. T. (1989). Tracheogastric puncture for vocal rehabilitation following total pharyngolaryngoesophagectomy. *Head & Neck, 11,* 524–527.

Maniglia, A. J., Lundy, D. S., Casiano, R. C., & Swim, S. C. (1989). Speech restoration and complications of primary vs. secondary tracheoesophageal puncture following total laryngectomy. *Laryngoscope, 99,* 489–491.

McEwan, J., Perry, A., Frosh, A. C., Cheeseman, A. D., McIvor, J., & Djazaeri, B. (1996). Surgical voice restoration: 15 years experience. In J. Algaba (Ed.), *Surgery and prosthetic voice restoration after total and subtotal laryngectomy.* Amsterdam: Elsevier.

Merwin, G., Goldstein, L., & Rothman, H. (1985). A comparison of speech using artificial larynx and tracheoesophageal puncture with valve in the same speaker. *Laryngoscope, 95,* 730–734.

Ogura, J. H., & Sessions, D. G. (1975). Cancer of the larynx and hypopharynx. In J. E. Hoopes (Ed.), *Symposium on cancer of the head and neck.* St. Louis, MO: Mosby.

Pauloski, B. R. (1998). Acoustic and aerodynamic characteristics of tracheoesophageal voice. In E. D. Blom, M. I. Singer, & R. C. Hamaker (Eds.), *Tracheoesophageal voice restoration following total laryngectomy* (pp. 123–141). San Diego: Singular.

Pearson, B. W., Woods, R. D., & Hartman, D. E. (1980). Extended hemilaryngectomy for T3 glottic carcinoma with preservation of speech and swallowing. *Laryngoscope, 40*(12), 1950–1961.

Robbins, J., Fisher, H. B., Blom, E. D., & Singer, M. I. (1984). A comparative acoustic study of normal, esophageal, and tracheoesophageal speech production. *Journal of Speech and Hearing Disorders, 49,* 202–210.

Singer, M. I. (2004). The development of successful tracheoesophageal voice restoration. *Otolaryngology Clinics of North America, 37,* 507–517.

Singer, M. I., & Blom, E. D. (1980). An endoscopic technique for restoration of voice after laryngectomy. *Annals of Otology, Rhinology and Laryngology, 89,* 529–533.

Singer, M. I., & Blom, E. D. (1981). Selective myotomy for voice restoration after total laryngectomy. *Archives of Otolaryngology, 107,* 670–673.

Singer, M. I., Blom, E. D., & Hamaker, R. C. (1986). Pharyngeal plexus neurectomy for alaryngeal speech rehabilitation. *Laryngoscope, 96,* 50–53.

Singer, M. I., Hamaker, R. C., & Blom, E. D. (1989). Revision procedure for tracheoesophageal puncture. *Laryngoscope, 99,* 761–763.

Singer, M. I., Hamaker, R. C., Blom, E. D., & Yoshida, G. Y. (1989). Applications of the voice prosthesis during laryngectomy. *Annals of Otology and Laryngology, 98,* 921–925.

Sloane, P. M., Griffin, J. M., & O'Dwyer, T. P. (1991). Esophageal insufflation and videofluoroscopy for evaluation of esophageal speech in laryngectomy patients: Clinical implications. *Radiology, 181,* 433–437.

Staffieri, M. (1980). New surgical approaches for speech rehabilitation after total laryngectomy. In D. P. Shedd & B. Weinberg (Eds.), *Surgical and prosthetic approaches to speech rehabilitation* (pp. 77–117). Boston: G. K. Hall Medical.

Taub, S., & Spiro, R. H. (1972). Vocal rehabilitation of laryngectomees: Preliminary report of new technique. *American Journal of Surgery, 124,* 87–90.

Terrell, E., Lewin, J. S., & Esclamado, R. (1995). Botulinum toxin injection for postlaryngectomy tracheoesophageal speech failure. *Otolaryngology—Head and Neck Surgery, 113,* 788–791.

Trudeau, M. D., & Qi, Y. Y. (1990). Acoustic characteristics of female tracheoesophageal speech. *Journal of Speech and Hearing Disorders, 55,* 244–250.

van As, C. J., Hilgers, F. J. M., Verdonck-de Leeuw, I. M., & Koopmans-van Beinum, F. J. (1996). Acoustical and perceptual analysis of postlaryngectomy prosthetic voice (Provox®). In J. Algaba (Ed.), *Surgery and prosthetic voice restoration after total and subtotal laryngectomy.* Amsterdam: Elsevier.

Weinberg, B., & Moon, J. D. (1984). Aerodynamic properties of four tracheoesophageal puncture prostheses. *Archives of Otolaryngology—Head and Neck Surgery, 110,* 673–675.

Ziesmann, M., Boyd, B., Manktelow, R. T., & Rosen, I. B. (1989). Speaking jejunum after laryngopharyngectomy with neoglottic and neopharyngeal reconstruction. *American Journal of Surgery, 158,* 321–323.

Chapter 18

Postlaryngectomy Voice Rehabilitation with the Consistent Use of Indwelling Voice Prostheses

Frans J. M. Hilgers and Corina J. van As

oice rehabilitation after total laryngectomy has shown considerable progress over the last two decades, mainly triggered by the development of well-functioning and reliable tracheoesophageal (TE) voice prostheses. The first practical prosthetic device was the non-indwelling TE voice prosthesis, introduced in 1980 by Singer and Blom. Since their pioneering work, several other useful devices have been developed, some non-indwelling (Henley-Cohn, Hausfeld, & Jakubczak, 1984; Panje, 1981) and some indwelling (Blom, 1995; Hilgers et al., 1997; Hilgers, Cornelissen, & Balm, 1993; Hilgers & Schouwen-burg, 1990; Jebria et al., 1987; Nijdam, Annyas, Schutte, & Leever, 1982; Singer, 2004). The distinction between these two categories is based on their replacement procedure, the former being carried out by the patient, the latter by a medical professional.

In the first decade of surgical–prosthetic vocal rehabilitation, research focused on its clinical applicability (Singer, Blom, & Hamaker, 1981); safety of the TE puncture technique, both as a primary and as a secondary procedure (Annyas, Nijdam, Escajadillo, Mahieu, & Leever, 1984; Hamaker, Singer, Blom, & Daniels, 1985); long-term success rates (Manni, van den Broek, de Groot, & Berends, 1984); establishing the superiority of surgical–prosthetic (i.e., TE) over esophageal voice (Robbins, Fisher, Blom, & Singer, 1984); the importance of optimal tonicity of the pharyngoesophageal (PE) segment or neoglottis (Doyle, 1994; Singer, 1988; Singer & Blom, 1981; Singer, Blom, & Hamaker, 1986); and the inevitable, but mostly well-controllable adverse events associated with the use of a prosthetic device at this vulnerable location in the human body (Manni & van den Broek, 1990). Also, device life of the indwelling voice prostheses, which is limited by the deterioration of the silicone material by candida overgrowth (Mahieu, van Saene, Rosingh, & Schutte, 1986), has received special attention since early on.

The purpose of this chapter is to present an overview of the different surgical, clinical, and speech therapy aspects of vocal rehabilitation after total laryngectomy, based on a single institution's experience with the consistent use of indwelling TE voice prostheses since 1995.

INDWELLING VERSUS NON-INDWELLING PROSTHESES

In general, two types of TE voice prostheses can be distinguished, non-indwelling and indwelling devices. The non-indwelling TE voice prostheses can be removed and replaced by the patient. The indwelling TE voice prostheses stay in place permanently and have to be removed and replaced by a clinician experienced in the method. The need for prosthesis replacement occurs at the end of the device life, which most often is recognized by leakage of fluids through the prosthesis into the airway or increased airflow resistance. Because indwelling devices may have a more robust construction, their device life is generally longer than that of their non-indwelling counterparts. Furthermore, indwelling devices have a definite advantage in that the patient's dexterity plays a lesser role in the daily maintenance of the device, which mainly consists of internal cleaning with a brush or flushing device without the need of regularly replacing the prosthesis. Even with increasing age or decreasing general health status, a useful voice can be preserved with the indwelling prosthesis (Graville, Gross, Andersen, Everts, & Cohen, 1999; Hilgers & Balm, 1993).

The obvious disadvantage of indwelling prosthesis is that patients need a clinician for the replacement, so hospital or clinic visits remain necessary. Furthermore, as with non-indwelling devices, a regular checkup of the fistula and stoma region is necessary, because of the need for early detection of possible adverse side effects (e.g., hypertrophy, infection, widening of the TE fistula). From the beginning of our prosthetic rehabilitation program in 1980, we have had a strong preference for indwelling devices (Hilgers et al., 1997; Hilgers et al., 2003; Hilgers & Balm, 1993; Hilgers & Schouwenburg, 1990; Hilgers, Schouwenburg, & Scholtens, 1988). Our clinical and rehabilitation experiences with the indwelling Provox prostheses are the basis for the remainder of this chapter.[1] The retrograde Provox voice prosthesis system and the anterograde Provox 2 voice prosthesis system are shown in Figures 18.1 and 18.2, respectively.

FACTORS FOR SUCCESSFUL PROSTHETIC VOICE ACQUISITION

There are four dominant factors for successful prosthetic speech acquisition. First, as Singer and Blom (1981) noted, optimal tonicity of the PE segment is essential (see Chapter 21 in this text). In general, the status of the PE segment is described in five qualifications: hypotonicity, good tonicity, hypertonicity, spasm, and stricture (McIvor, Evans, Perry, & Cheesman, 1990). Tonicity refers to the muscular tension of the inferior and medial constrictor pharyngeus muscles and the cricopharyngeus muscle or upper esophageal sphincter, and can be judged best with videofluoroscopy (McIvor et al., 1990). The best voice quality is achieved with good tonicity and in slightly hypertonic PE segments.

Second, the timing of surgical prosthetic voice restoration also has some relevance to successful prosthetic speech acquisition. Primary (at time of laryngectomy) application of a voice prosthesis has been shown to result in a higher success rate than application in a secondary (postlaryngectomy) approach (Annyas et al., 1984). The most likely explanation for this is that patients are still used to pulmonary driven speech and, despite the laryngectomy, have no problem using this type of speech shortly after the surgery (Singer, 2004). Pulmonary driven speech is probably more difficult after a period of failed esophageal voice training, in which a disconnection between voicing and breathing may occur. Because Annyas et al.'s study dates from the early 1980s, when the importance of the PE segment tonicity was less well understood, another explanation for this obser-

---

[1]Provox is a trademark owned by Atos Medical AB, P.O. Box 182, S-242 00 Hörby, Sweden. This company is also the manufacturer of the Provox voice rehabilitation system.

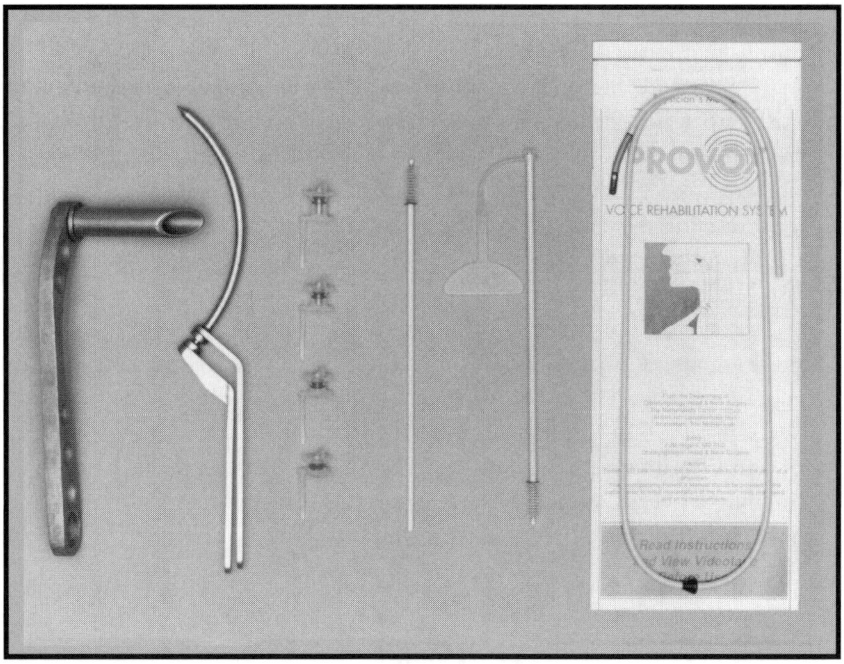

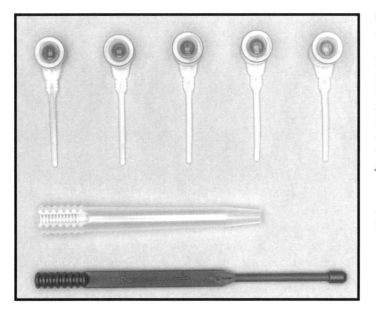

FIGURE 18.1. The Provox voice rehabilitation system with, from left to right, a pharynx protector for use during a primary TEP procedure, the trocar and cannula for primary and secondary TEP, the voice prostheses in 4 sizes (4.5, 6, 8, and 10 mm shaft length), a brush for internal cleaning, a plug for temporary occlusion of the prosthesis in case of leakage through the prosthesis, and a disposable guide wire for retrograde insertion during TEP procedure or for prosthesis replacement.

FIGURE 18.2. The Provox 2 anterograde replacement system, with five different shaft lengths (4.5, 6, 8, 10, and 12.5 mm), and the loading tube with inserter. *Note.* From "Multi-institutional Assessment of the Provox 2 Voice Prosthesis," by A. H. Ackerstaff, F. J. M. Hilgers, et al., 1999. *Archives of Otolaryngology—Head and Neck Surgery, 125,* pp. 167–173. Copyright 1999 by American Medical Association. Reprinted with permission.

vation could be the more likely suboptimal tonicity of the PE segment in failed esophageal speakers (see Chapter 21 in this text).

The third factor is the motivation of the patient and the clinician. Obviously, a patient needs to be motivated for prosthetic vocal rehabilitation, and although limited, some manual dexterity is still needed with indwelling devices. Furthermore, because prosthetic voice rehabilitation after total laryngectomy is a multidisciplinary team effort, the motivation of the clinicians involved is mandatory to obtain optimal patient results with this alaryngeal speech method. The last, but least important factor is the type of voice prosthesis used.

Any voice prosthesis nowadays gives better, more rapid, and more consistent results than esophageal voice rehabilitation (Doyle, Danhauer, & Reed, 1988; Robbins et al., 1984; Tardy-Mitzell, Andrews, & Bowman, 1985; Williams & Watson, 1985). In summary, optimal tonicity of the PE segment, early application of an indwelling or non-indwelling TE voice prosthesis, and a motivated multidisciplinary team are the key elements to successful surgical prosthetic vocal rehabilitation of laryngectomized individuals (see Chapters 17, 19, and 24 in this text).

PREOPERATIVE COUNSELING

In all clinics in The Netherlands that serve laryngectomized patients, preoperative counseling by the speech pathologist is customary. Basic preoperative counseling involves explaining the basic principles of vocal rehabilitation, as well as related aspects. For example, possible interfering factors such as problems with hearing, reading, writing, and visual acuity are addressed. The patient's manual dexterity is assessed. Also, in most clinics, it is common to involve a laryngectomized visitor in the counseling of the patient prior to the laryngectomy; this is often done to familiarize the patient with the postoperative situation and to demonstrate the possibilities of voice rehabilitation and other aspects of postlaryngectomy life (see Chapter 15 in this text). Several authors have stressed the relevance of this approach in laryngectomy rehabilitation (Doyle, 1994; Gress, 2004; Mohide, Archibald, Tew, Young, & Haines, 1992; Stam, Koopmans, & Methieson, 1991).

SURGICAL ASPECTS

After standard wide field total laryngectomy, primary tracheoesophageal puncture (TEP) is presently the method of choice for many clinicians dealing with postlaryngectomy rehabilitation. This choice is often selected because it allows for early and rapid acquisition of pulmonary driven speech. Some interesting differences can be noted, however, in the technique and timing of primary TEP. Unlike the situation in many clinics using non-indwelling systems, we have from the beginning adopted the custom of inserting the indwelling voice prosthesis immediately at the time of surgery (see Table 18.1), thus avoiding the need for

TABLE 18.1

Pros and Cons of Immediate Insertion of Voice Prosthesis
Following Tracheoesophageal Puncture (TEP)

Pros

- The retrograde insertion technique, using the Provox trocar and cannula and guide wire, diminishes the risk of separation of the tracheoesophageal party wall, and to some extent, the device stabilizes this wall.
- The tracheal and esophageal flanges of the device give optimal protection of the tracheoesophageal fistula against leakage of saliva and gastric fluids.
- There is less irritation of the tracheostoma and less pressure on the fistula tract compared to a feeding tube taped to the skin of the neck.
- There is no postoperative interference with a cannula or a heat and moisture exchanger.
- Early postoperatively, patients can become familiarized with the care for their voice prosthesis by the nurses or other professionals (speech–language pathologists, surgeon, etc.).
- There is no need for early postoperative prosthesis fitting at a time when the stoma often is not yet healed completely and may still be sore, and the patient's mental and physical status is not yet optimal.
- Around the 10th postoperative day, there can be immediate focus on voicing itself, which can give a tremendous psychological boost to the patient.
- Postoperative radiotherapy is not a contraindication, and most patients develop a useful voice prior to the start of treatment.
- The first TEP prosthesis replacement is usually months down the road when wound healing is completed, surgical edema has subsided, and patients are generally in much better condition, both physically and mentally.
- This approach may be parsimonious with the leading role of the speech–language pathologist in many multidisciplinary rehabilitation team efforts.

Cons

- The presence of a (nasogastric) feeding tube in the nose and throat is necessary during the first 10 days.
- The voice temporarily deteriorates during postoperative radiotherapy.

temporary stenting of the fistula tract with a feeding tube (Hilgers & Balm, 1993; Hilgers & Schouwenburg, 1990).

The feasibility of this technique was first described by Annyas et al. (1984) and has proven to be a reliable procedure ever since. Obviously, it is important to use a TE prosthesis of sufficient length to allow for the development of some surgical edema in the postoperative period. With some practice (there is often a rapid learning curve), the thickness of the tracheoesophageal party wall can be judged easily by palpation. In most patients, an 8- or 10-mm prosthesis length is appropriate. In case of doubt, a longer prosthesis should be inserted, because a prosthesis that is too long causes less trouble than a device that is too short (see Chapter 19 in this text).

The actual insertion of the prosthesis is a simple surgical procedure (see Figure 18.3) in which a TE fistula is created with a special Provox trocar and cannula, and a disposable guide wire is used for the retrograde introduction of the prosthetic device (Hilgers & Balm, 1993). By using a retrograde insertion route, the tracheoesophageal party wall does not separate easily, because the wall can be supported better on the tracheal than on the esophageal side, and the flanges of the indwelling voice prosthesis stabilize the party wall.

Furthermore, with an indwelling prosthesis, there is less irritation to the tissues compared to a constantly moving nasogastric tube, and leakage of saliva is prevented. Because the indwelling voice prosthesis is positioned flush against the back wall of the trachea, there is no irritation to the stoma and no interference with a cannula, if one is needed. Also, the early postoperative use of heat and moisture exchangers (see Chapter 20 in this text), as is customary now in many clinics in The Netherlands, is not hampered by a feeding tube protruding from the stoma.

Closure of the pharynx is carried out in a T shape. This T-shaped closure is a low-tension closure, tailored to the size of the pharyngeal defect, and avoids the development of a ridge at the base of tongue (i.e., the formation of a "neoepiglottis"). Before closure of the pharynx, a nasogastric feeding tube is brought into position. The mucosa is then closed with running atraumatic vicryl sutures. Tissue surplus caudally is closed with a purse string suture. A second submucosal layer is also closed with running sutures. Finally, the pharyngeal constrictor muscles are closed with running or with mattress sutures. This layer should not be closed too tightly, to prevent strictures.

Even in patients with a more extensive pharyngeal resection and reconstruction (see Chapter 12 in this text), primary TEP and insertion of the in-

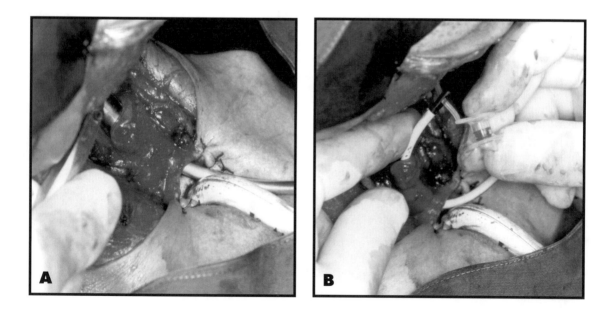

dwelling voice prosthesis can be carried out, as long as the reconstruction is located cranially of the stoma (Hilgers et al., 1995). In cases using the gastric pull-up procedure, however, we delay the TEP for 4 to 6 weeks to allow for the trachea and the stomach tube to heal together.

SPHINCTER TONICITY AND CONTROL OF THE PHARYNGOESOPHAGEAL SEGMENT

As already mentioned, optimal tonicity of the PE segment is important for fluent TE voice acquisition. A posterior myotomy with or without a plexus pharyngeus neurectomy and a non–muscle closure are recommended to achieve fluent voice (Singer & Blom, 1981; Singer et al., 1986; see also Chapters 17, 19, and 24 in this text). Because most of our patients are radiation failures and, thus, more prone to postoperative complications, we prefer to close the pharyngeal muscles to reinforce the suture line, and combine a pharyngeal plexus neurectomy with a short myotomy of the cricopharyngeus muscle (Op de Coul et al., 2003). The neurectomy procedure is carried out unilaterally, preferably on the side of the hemithyroidectomy and/or neck dissection.

If the patient develops PE segment hypertonicity or spasm despite these procedures, and speech therapy does not solve this problem, a secondary long myotomy of the constrictor pharyngeus muscles has been undertaken with success (Mahieu, Annyas, Schutte, & van der Jagt, 1987). More recently, chemical denervation with use of botulinum toxin (Botox) has proved to be an excellent method of resolving this problem (Hoffman et al., 1997; see also Chapter 21 in this text).

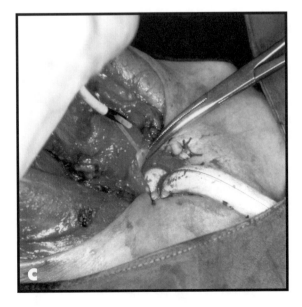

FIGURE 18.3. Primary TEP procedure. (A) The Provox trocar and cannula are used to create the fistula tract, and the pharynx protector is inserted in the esophagus to support the tracheoesophageal party wall and to prevent damage to pharyngoesophageal mucosa. (B) The voice prosthesis is anchored to the disposable guide wire for retrograde insertion into the TE fistula. (C) The Provox voice prosthesis is rotated into position with the guide wire and a hemostat.

TRACHEOSTOMA CONSTRUCTION

Special attention should be given to the stoma during total laryngectomy. The tracheostoma should be wide enough to allow comfortable, unobstructed breathing, without the need to use a tracheostomy cannula, as well as to provide easy access to the voice prosthesis, without being too wide to allow easy, airtight finger closure for TE speech. Good results are obtained with the stoma within the inferior skin flap, using a separate fenestra in the skin (see Figure 18.4) (Verschuur, Gregor, Hilgers, & Balm, 1996). The sutures should ensure that there is skin cover over the bare edges of the trachea to avoid cartilage exposure. Exposed cartilage may lead to perichondritis, infection, granulations, and eventually stenosis.

In the same way, the postoperative use of a cannula, button, or tracheostomy tube should be minimized if possible, because each causes friction to the mucocutaneous anastomosis with the same end result (i.e., stenosis). If excessive edema of the skin flaps causes obstruction or if excessive secretions occur, a temporary cannula may be used to aid in decreasing trauma to the tracheal mucosa caused by suction catheters.

Once a stoma has started to form fibrous tissue, as in the case of tracheal stenosis, it is extremely difficult to arrest the process, and such a patient may be condemned to the use of a cannula for all or much of the time. Surgical revision might be needed in some of these narrow stomas and this also poses special problems in patients with a voice prosthesis (Verschuur et al., 1996).

An additional point of interest is the area around the stoma. If the sternal heads of the sternocleidomastoid muscles are transected, which has no functional consequences, the stoma area will become more flattened and the application of stoma valves and HMEs is easier, therefore increasing the patient's compliance (see Chapter 20 in this text).

SECONDARY TEP VOICE RESTORATION

Because most patients today receive primary TEP, the frequency of secondary TEP has decreased considerably. Most secondary TEPs occur after gastric pull-up procedures and in cases where the TE fistula closes spontaneously or is closed surgically due to complications. Again, as in primary TEP, the immediate insertion of an indwelling device has clear advantages. As long as the surgeon chooses a device that is long enough to compensate for the slight edema of the TE fistula (for which the perioperative use of prophylactic antibiotics is also recommended), the TE puncture with a Provox trocar and the retrograde insertion of the indwelling device with the special guide wire (see Figure 18.5) is a safe and speedy procedure (Hilgers & Balm, 1993); this allows for the earliest possible start with voicing—that is, on the same day as the surgery.

(text continues on p. 465)

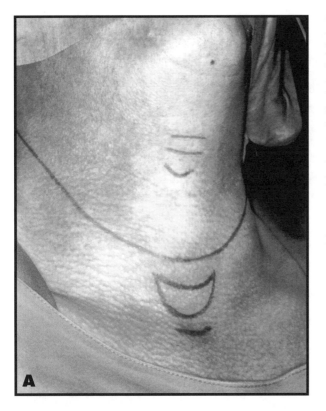

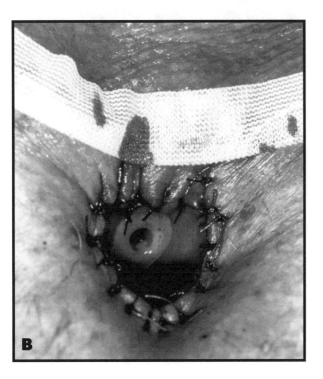

FIGURE 18.4. (A) Preoperative view of the neck with indication of the incision lines and the position of the stoma. The skin island will be removed. (B) Immediate postoperative view of the stoma and the inferior skin flap, with the primary inserted indwelling Provox voice prosthesis in situ near the mucocutaneous border of the tracheoesophageal party wall. *Note.* From "The Tracheostoma in Relation to Prosthetic Voice Rehabilitation—How We Do It," by H. P. Verschuur, R. T. Gregor, F. J. M. Hilgers, and A. J. M. Balm, 1996, *Laryngoscope, 106,* pp. 111–115. Copyright 1996 by Lippincott Williams Wilkins. Reprinted with permission.

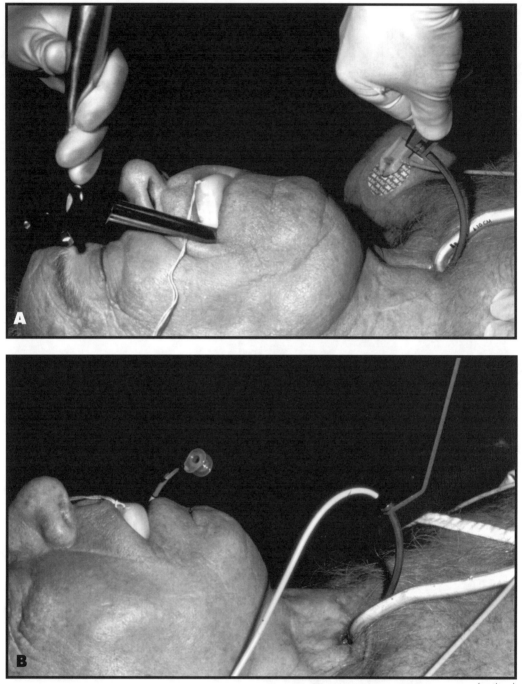

(continues)

FIGURE 18.5. Secondary TEP procedure. (A) The Provox trocar and cannula are used to create the fistula tract, and a rigid esophagoscope is used to support the tracheoesophageal party wall and to prevent damage to pharyngoesophageal mucosa. (B) The voice prosthesis is anchored to the disposable guide wire for retrograde insertion into the TE fistula. (C) The Provox voice prosthesis is rotated into position with the guide wire and a hemostat. (D) This immediate postoperative view of the stoma shows the inserted indwelling Provox voice prosthesis in situ near the mucocutaneous border of the tracheoesophageal party wall.

INDICATIONS FOR REPLACEMENT OF INDWELLING VOICE PROSTHESES, ADVERSE EVENTS, AND SOLUTIONS

Indwelling voice prostheses are semipermanent implants that require periodic replacement. Replacement of the Provox 2 voice prosthesis is presently an easy anterograde outpatient office procedure (see Figure 18.6), with the original retrograde replacement technique of Provox as a backup method (Hilgers et al., 1997). Patient discomfort is minimal, and both otolaryngologists and speech pathologists are comfortable with this procedure (Ackerstaff et al., 1999).

Both device-related and fistula-related indications occur. The two device-related indications are (a) leakage of fluids through the prosthesis caused by incomplete closure of the hinged valve and (b) obstruction of the device causing too much airflow resistance for comfortable production of speech. The main indication for replacement of the Provox voice prostheses is leakage through the valve (73% of all replacements), whereas blockage of the device occurs infrequently (4%). The fistula-related indications for replacement are leakage around the prosthesis (13%), infection or granulation formation of the fistula tract (7%), or spontaneous loss (extrusion) of the device (<1%) (Op de Coul et al., 2000). All of these fistula-related indications are considered to be adverse events except leakage around the device, as this can be solved easily by downsizing the prosthesis (Eerenstein, Grolman, & Schouwenburg, 2002). Leakage around the prosthesis is usually related to the subsiding of surgical edema, leading to a pistoning of the prosthesis, which is now too long. This phenomenon can be observed with all TEP voice prostheses presently used, and because it merely reflects a gradual improvement of the tissues, it should not be considered a real adverse event. Conversion from one TEP voice prosthesis to another is possible (Vlantis, Gregor, Elliot, & Oudes, 2003).

It has to be stressed at this point that there should be no automatism in replacing voice prostheses with an identical sized version in all instances. Proper

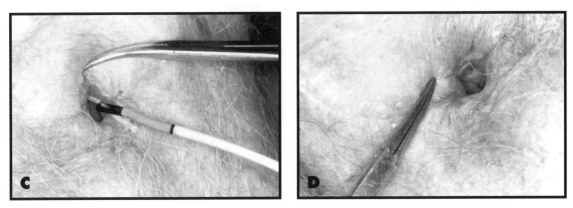

FIGURE 18.5. *Continued.*

FIGURE 18.6. Anterograde replacement procedure of Provox 2 voice prosthesis. (A) Securing the prosthesis in and onto the inserter. (B) Forward folding of the esophageal flange into the loading tube. (C) Start of the anterograde insertion. *Note.* Figure 18.6C is from "Comprehensive Rehabilitation After Total Laryngectomy Is More Than Voice Alone," by F. J. M. Hilgers and A. H. Ackerstaff, 2000, *Folia Phoniatrica et Logopaedica, 52,* pp. 65–73. Copyright 2000 by Karger. Reprinted with permission. (D) End result of the anterograde insertion. Figure 18.6D is from "Development and Clinical Evaluation of a Second-Generation Voice Prosthesis (Provox®2), Designed for Anterograde and Retrograde Insertion," by F. J. M. Hilgers et al., 1997, *Acta Otolaryngologica (Stockholm), 117,* pp. 889–896. Copyright 1997 by Taylor & Francis. Reprinted with permission.

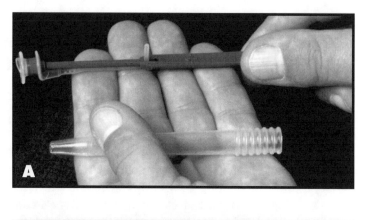
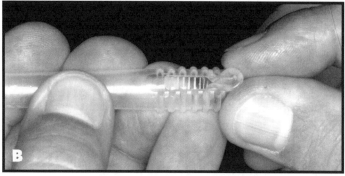
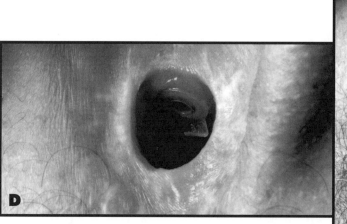
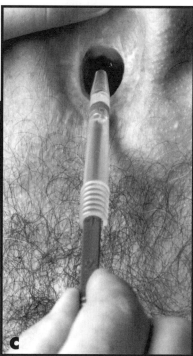

sizing remains important, although there is a good tolerance for a device that is slightly too long in the case of the indwelling Provox devices. In a recent survey of 2,700 replacements in 318 patients over a 10-year period, with a follow-up of 364.3 days (1,000 patient years), only 65% of the replaced prostheses were of the same size (Op de Coul et al., 2000).

With the use of a prosthetic device at this vulnerable spot in the human body, some adverse events have to be expected, and special attention has to be given to this concern (Manni & van den Broek, 1990). Proper patient instruction about the possible adverse events is important to encourage the patient to seek the advice of the clinician early on when problems are typically still minor and treatment is generally not difficult. As a rule of thumb, it can be stated that two thirds of patients have no problems whatsoever and that they consume approximately one third of the total time spent on prosthetic voice rehabilitation (Hilgers & Balm, 1993). These patients come into the clinic only infrequently for an easy and quick anterograde replacement of the prosthesis, usually after the TEP prosthesis has become incompetent and shows mild leakage of fluids (Ackerstaff et al., 1999; Hilgers et al., 1997). The other one third of patients occasionally have problems in a small percentage of their replacements, and these patients will need special attention, which consumes a majority of the total time spent on prosthetic voice rehabilitation. If these patients are treated properly, success rates up to 90% can be expected (Hilgers & Balm, 1993; Op de Coul et al., 2000; van Weissenbruch & Albers, 1993).

It should be noted that the influence of radiotherapy on the final outcome of TE voice rehabilitation seems to be minor, except for the temporary deterioration of the voice during postoperative irradiation. The device life of Provox prostheses appears to be significantly longer in nonirradiated patients, and there is a slight but significant increase in fistula-related indications for replacement in patients who have undergone radiotherapy on the larynx preceding their laryngectomy (Mendenhall et al., 2004; Op de Coul et al., 2000).

Device-Related Indications for Replacement

Leakage through the prosthesis signals the end of device life and occurs mainly in association with candida overgrowth (Mahieu, van Saene, Rosingh, & Schutte, 1986). Sometimes, mucus or food remnants may interfere with valve closure or obstruct the device, therefore increasing the airflow resistance of the prosthesis. Endoscopic examination and cleaning of the TEP prosthesis with suction or a brush might be attempted. If cleaning does not solve the problem, prosthesis replacement is indicated. Candida overgrowth occurs in almost all patients. A typical example of such overgrowth is shown in Figure 18.7.

The mere presence of candida by itself is no reason for prosthesis replacement. In cases where frequent prosthesis replacements are needed due to candida overgrowth, however, some form of treatment with antifungal agents might be considered (Mahieu, van Saene, den Besten, & van Saene, 1986; van Weissenbruch et al., 1997). We prefer a Nystatin oral solution, which can be used orally by

FIGURE 18.7. Typical appearance of Provox voice prosthesis with candida infestations after removal.

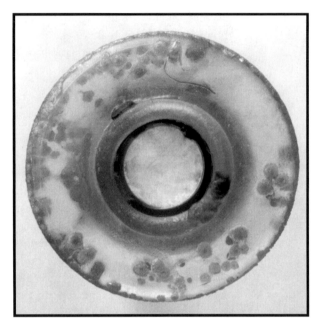

swishing and swallowing or can be applied (topically) directly into the prosthesis with the cleaning brush. In some patients an improved device life was observed with this treatment. A rather inexpensive alternative is the treatment with a .5% iodine solution in saline (without alcohol), applied directly into the prosthesis with a brush two or three times daily; this local treatment appears to be beneficial for prolonging device life in some patients as well. Another option is the treatment with 50 mg of Diflucan suspension once a day, used both orally (swish and swallow) and locally applied into the prosthesis with a brush. The advantage of this drug is its long half-life, requiring only once-daily application, which increases patient compliance. In a recent multi-institutional study, some form of antifungal treatment was deemed to be necessary in 29% of the 239 consecutive patients assessed (Ackerstaff et al., 1999).

Fistula-Related Indications for Replacement

Leakage Around the Prosthesis

Leakage around the prosthesis is an indication of a discrepancy between the size of the device and the length or diameter of the fistula tract. A prosthesis that is too long might cause leakage due to a pistoning effect, thus squeezing fluids around the device. Simple downsizing of prosthesis length often solves this problem, which might occur over time due to subsiding of postoperative tissue edema and healing of the party wall. As already mentioned, if simple downsizing does not solve the problem of leakage around the prosthesis, we consider this to be an adverse event. Temporary removal of the prosthesis and insertion of a cuffed tracheal cannula or nasogastric feeding tube to allow for shrinkage of the fistula may be necessary to solve this problem. Some success has been reported from injection of collagen to thicken the fistula tract and party wall (Remacle & Declaye, 1988).

Another solution, which we prefer, is the application of a purse-string suture around the fistula tract, using an atraumatic, absorbable 3 × 0 vicryl suture. The procedure is schematically shown in Figure 18.8. After the new prosthesis is inserted, the suture is carefully and gently tied, causing the fistula wall to be tightened around the prosthesis. The suture should not be removed, but left to be absorbed spontaneously. This suture often will cause thickening of the fistula tract, curing the problem. A short course of broad-spectrum antibiotics should be given to prevent local infection. If leakage around the prosthesis is intractable to this relatively conservative measure, surgical closure of the fistula and subsequent repuncture may be necessary.

Infection or Granulation of the TE Fistula

Infection or formation of granulation tissue around the TE fistula is always considered to be an adverse event. This problem occurs at a reported rate of between

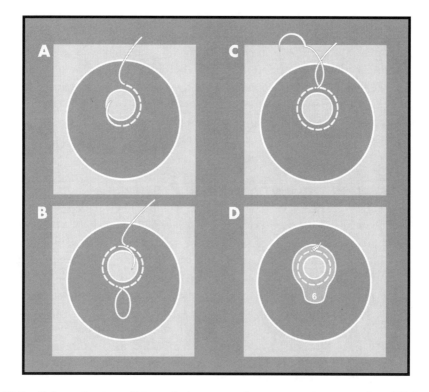

FIGURE 18.8. Schematic view of the technique to apply a purse-string suture for a TE fistula that is too wide, to treat leakage around the voice prosthesis. (A) A 3 × 0 atraumatic vicryl suture is inserted at 12 o'clock at a distance of 1 to 2 mm from the fistula edge and curved clockwise submucosally to 6 o'clock. (B) The needle is reinserted at 6 o'clock and curved clockwise submucosally to return to 12 o'clock. (C) The situation is shown before anterograde insertion of the voice prosthesis. (D) After the voice prosthesis is inserted, the suture is gently and carefully tied, closing the gap between the fistula wall and the prosthesis shaft.

5% and 10% of prosthesis replacements (Hilgers & Balm, 1993; Manni & van den Broek, 1990; Op de Coul et al., 2000). If only granulation tissue is present, some form of cauterization (electro-, chemo-, or laser cauterization) of the area of the granulation may be considered. Sometimes there can be slight bleeding caused by this granulation tissue, mostly during removal of the TEP prosthesis (Ackerstaff et al., 1999), but this is seldom a problem. A phenomenon in the same category is hypertrophic scarring, which sometimes occurs when the prosthesis is relatively short in length, leading to bulging of the tracheal mucosa over the tracheal flange. This excess tissue can be removed by using a carbon dioxide (CO_2) laser or neodymium: yttrium–aluminum–garnet (NdYAG) *without having to remove the voice prosthesis*. Alternatively, a longer prosthesis can be used.

In case of infection around the prosthesis with granulation formation or edema, the fistula tract may become longer, causing the prosthesis to be pulled inward and under the tracheal mucosa. Conversely, the prosthesis may be extruded from the fistula tract due to infection and overgrowth of the mucosa on the esophageal side of the TE fistula. When this problem occurs, the best solution is replacement of the prosthesis with a longer one. Treatment with broad-spectrum antibiotics might be added to control infection. Removal of the device is rarely necessary and should be avoided, because this often leads to a spontaneous closure of the fistula tract, requiring secondary puncture for reinsertion of a new prosthesis at a later date. An exception to this recommendation is overt protrusion of the prosthesis and its potential spontaneous extrusion caused by an infection of the TE fistula. In this case, removal of the prosthesis is mandatory to avoid accidental dislodgment into the trachea. Spontaneous closure of the fistula tract is common in these cases, and secondary puncture is then necessary to reestablish prosthetic speech.

Disappearance of the Voice Prosthesis

If the TEP prosthesis visually disappears, it should be verified whether the device has been ingested or extruded and not merely hidden under the mucosa. If the TEP prosthesis is not found in the fistula tract, it may have been ingested. As with any other foreign body, the symptoms caused by ingestion depend largely on the item's size and location, the degree of obstruction (if any), and the length of time since ingestion. If the ingested component lies in the lower esophagus, it may be removed by esophagoscopy or observed for a short period of time. In this situation, the object may pass spontaneously into the stomach and pass through the intestinal tract. Surgical removal of foreign bodies in the intestinal tract must be considered if bowel obstruction or perforation occurs, bleeding is present, or the object fails to pass through the intestinal tract.

The other possibility is disappearance due to aspiration of the prosthesis. In case of accidental aspiration of a voice prosthesis or other device used for maintenance, acute symptoms may include gagging, coughing, choking, and wheezing. As with any other foreign body, complications from aspiration of a prosthetic component may be caused by an obstruction or related infection (e.g., pneumonia, atelectasis, bronchitis, lung abscess, bronchopulmonary fistula, asthma). If the patient can speak or breathe, coughing may dislodge the foreign body without the need for emergency action. Also, the Heimlich maneuver might be attempted. Partial or complete airway obstruction requires immediate intervention for removal of the object. This will typically involve retrieval of the component via flexible or, preferably, rigid bronchoscopy.

In the majority of cases, adverse events can be solved with relatively simple measures. Infection or granulation formation and hypertrophic scarring are easily manageable with conservative or minor surgical procedures. Leakage around the prosthesis that does not resolve with downsizing can be managed easily with a purse-string suture; this is the first and mostly successful option. Ultimately, surgical closure of the TEP tract may be necessary, but this option is seldom needed. These adverse events do occur, however, in approximately 11% of all replacements (Op de Coul et al., 2000). These events emphasize the fact that surgical–prosthetic vocal rehabilitation is a multidisciplinary team effort in which the speech pathologist and the otolaryngologist need to cooperate and communicate closely. Ideally, both professionals will have direct and immediate access to each other's expertise when needed.

VOICE AND SPEECH THERAPY[2]

Tracheoesophageal and esophageal voice production have in common that the PE segment is the sound source, but they differ in the air supply to this source. Conventional esophageal voice is obtained by injecting relatively small amounts of air (60–80 ml) from the mouth into the esophagus and redirecting this column of air upward through the PE segment. Prosthetic voice production, however, is like normal laryngeal voicing; it is pulmonary driven. Much like the vocal fold mucosa in laryngeal voicing, the PE segment mucosa is vibrating and mucosal waves can be seen with high-speed digital imaging during such voicing (van As et al., 1999). Speech and voice therapy in TEP prosthetic speakers, therefore, resembles normal laryngeal voice training.

Voice training can start approximately 10 days after primary surgery when the esophagus and the surrounding tissues, especially the tracheostoma, are sufficiently healed and the nasogastric tube has been removed, or the same day in the case of secondary TEP puncture. Because the indwelling voice prosthesis is already in place, no time is lost by fitting of the device. The first therapy session begins with a short recapitulation of the preoperative information (e.g., explanation of the changes in the anatomy and the basic principles of the vocal rehabilitation) and an inspection of the prosthesis to make sure it is not obstructed.

---

[2]This section is adapted from Hilgers et al. (1999).

Next, the patient is instructed to breathe in gently and to open the mouth and produce a /ha/ sound. In these first voicing attempts, the speech pathologist should digitally occlude the stoma for the patient. In most cases, the voice will come through after one or several attempts.

Normally, we believe it is best to start with exclamations such as "ha" and "hi." It is easier to start the airflow with the fricative /h/ than with an isolated vowel, which is mostly used by others. If the voice does not occur easily, the patient is asked to shout. A stronger airflow in this situation helps to initiate the voice. After the first several voicing attempts, the patient can be encouraged to lengthen the vowels and to start with short statements or two- or three-syllable phrases or sentences (e.g., "Hello," "Hi there," "How are you?"). Furthermore, the laryngectomized patient can begin trying to occlude the stoma together with the speech pathologist, and then by him- or herself (see Chapters 17 and 19 in this text).

In the beginning, voice therapy should focus on four general issues:

1. The acquisition of an *airtight occlusion of the tracheostoma* during phonation is important. In case the stoma is not yet well healed or is too large in relation to the patient's finger size, airtight digital occlusion might pose a problem at this stage. The availability of special, valved HMEs may eliminate this problem to a great extent (Ackerstaff, Hilgers, Balm, & Tan, 1998; van As, Hilgers, Koopmans-van Beinum, & Ackerstaff, 1998). These devices are often provided to patients shortly after surgery. As a reaction to nonairtight stoma occlusion, the patient may exert too much pressure on the stoma, hence forcing the prosthesis against the posterior pharyngeal wall and obstructing airflow. Another unfavorable side effect of nonairtight stoma closure is the occurrence of disturbing stoma noise. To obtain a good occlusion with only light pressure on the stoma, the patient is advised to bring the stoma or the body weight toward the finger, instead of pressing the finger onto the stoma. An additional advantage of using a valved HME is that the pressure placed on the stoma is more evenly distributed.

2. An *upright, relaxed body position* is important for good breath support. The back should be straight and the head bent forward just a little to avoid tension in the neck region around the stoma. Therefore, practicing while seated on a chair is preferred over sitting in bed early in therapy.

3. A *calm abdominal breathing pattern*—that is, gentle abdominal inhalation before phonation and an easy, unforced expiration—is necessary to obtain a good and relaxed voice. We observe the patient's breathing pattern before starting breathing exercises because some patients already use a good abdominal breathing pattern. In these patients, the therapist's role is to make them aware of their abdominal breathing, whereas in those with a thoracic breathing pattern, breathing exercises should be integrated into the speech therapy program.

4. Good *breath–voice coordination and timing of stoma occlusion* are important factors, because stoma noise may occur when the patient (a) closes the stoma too late at the beginning of a sentence or (b) releases finger pressure too early at the end of a sentence.

When short sentences are formed easily and fluently, exercises can be extended by trying longer phrases starting with any initial vowel or consonant.

Speech becomes more fluent by using meaningful sentences, instead of by reading a list of words.

When the patient has acquired easy phonation, more specific exercises addressing fluency, loudness, intonation, stress and pitch modulation, articulation, and speech rate are provided, to work on a more natural voice and intelligible speech (Eadie & Doyle, 2004; van As, Koopmans-van Beinum, Pols, & Hilgers, 2003; see also Chapters 5, 6, and 24 in this text). In general, functional speech is obtained within a very short time, often during the first therapy session, and most patients will leave the hospital with intelligible speech after only a few days of practice. After discharge from the hospital, voice and speech therapy is continued on an outpatient basis until an optimal result has been achieved.

GENERAL ASPECTS OF PATIENT INSTRUCTION

Instruction should be given to patients about daily cleaning of the TEP voice prosthesis with a brush or flushing unit. Cleaning of the TEP voice prosthesis also can be done by occluding the stoma and producing a loud sound. The patient should be aware that the prosthesis will stay cleaner by speaking regularly. The speech–language pathologist should explain that the valve of the prosthesis eventually will become incompetent and leakage of liquids can occur. The patient should properly clean the prosthesis with a brush. If this does not solve the problem, replacement probably is indicated. If the patient is unable or unwilling to make an appointment with the clinician (e.g., during weekends or holidays), temporary control of leakage through the prosthesis can be obtained by using a special plug. The patient also should be instructed how to use this plug during the consumption of liquids (solid food rarely causes problems).

Prosthesis users are always given the opportunity and are encouraged to learn esophageal speech as well. Unlike in the United States, in The Netherlands electrolarynx use is limited to patients unable to use either prosthetic or esophageal voice. (For more information on the use of an electrolarynx as an alternative alaryngeal communication method, see Chapters 4, 5, 22, and 23 in this text.) In our institute, the use of an automatic speaking valve for hands-free speech is encouraged only after the patient has mastered all daily practical aspects of prosthetic speech and has developed a fluent, not too strained voice. It appears to be important that the patient has enough manual dexterity to handle these devices comfortably (van den Hoogen, Meeuwis, Oudes, Janssen, & Manni, 1996). In daily practice, success rates are still relatively low, with less than a quarter of the patients achieving a full-day unrestricted use, which is comparable to the results reported by van den Hoogen et al. (1996).

PROBLEM SOLVING

Unsatisfactory voice rehabilitation results may occur due to one or more problems on several different levels (i.e., oral structures, PE segment, voice prosthesis, tracheostoma, trachea). Therefore, such factors should always be considered in a comprehensive program of postlaryngectomy rehabilitation and communication outcomes (see Chapters 3, 4, and 5 in this text). Furthermore, the patient may have problems with respiration or posture. Two other specific kinds of problems are (a) combined or intermittent use of esophageal along with TE speech and (b) voice problems during radiotherapy. Diagnostic videofluoroscopy of speech and swallowing is an excellent tool for visualization of the anatomy and function of the PE segment (McIvor et al., 1990). Table 18.2 presents an overview of the different problems, the levels or areas at which they exist, and possible solutions.

FUTURE DEVELOPMENTS

Present-day indwelling voice prostheses are much more comfortable to use than older generation devices (Ackerstaff et al., 1999; Hilgers et al., 1997; Leder & Erskine, 1997). This improvement is primarily due to their anterograde replacement technique. Although a device life of several months is generally obtained, the limited lifespan of indwelling voice prostheses in some patients might discourage some clinicians from using them more widely. At The Netherlands Cancer Institute, we have used indwelling voice prostheses exclusively for the last two decades, since the first indwelling (Groningen) device became available (Ackerstaff et al., 2003; Ackerstaff et al., 1999; Hilgers et al., 1997; Hilgers & Balm, 1993; Hilgers & Schouwenburg, 1990; Hilgers et al., 1988; Op de Coul et al., 2000). In view of the reported success rates of almost 90% with the Provox and Provox 2, it is our opinion that if the candida problem, and thus the issue of device life, can be solved, and replacements can be limited to regular medical follow-up visits, indwelling voice prostheses are the more promising devices (Hotz, Baumann, Schaller, & Zbären, 2002; van den Hoogen, van den Berg, Oudes, & Manni, 1998). Projects seeking to solve the problem of candida growth on the TE valve are currently in progress.

SUMMARY

This chapter has addressed a variety of issues related to surgical prosthetic voice rehabilitation, as practiced in a multidisciplinary cancer institute. Topics included the pros and cons of indwelling versus non-indwelling devices, the surgical aspects of TEP, the advantages of the immediate insertion of the voice prosthesis at the time of surgery, the different factors for successful speech acquisition, and the long-term results and the handling of adverse events. Finally, an overview is given of the most important aspects of the necessary voice and speech treatment to achieve the best verbal communication possible.

TABLE 18.2

Problems Encountered in Prosthetic Voice and Speech Rehabilitation

Level or Area	Problem	Possible Solutions
Oral structures	• Decreased intelligibility	• Do articulation exercises
Pharyngoesophageal segment	• Strained voice due to stricture or hypertonicity	• If speech therapy fails, discuss with otorhinolaryngologist the need for dilation, myotomy, Botox, etc.
	• Breathy voice due to hypo-tonicity or reconstruction	• Apply digital pressure on the neck, adjust head position, decrease airflow, lower pitch
Voice prosthesis	• Internal obstruction	• Clean with brush, flush, or suction
	• External obstruction due to overgrowth of mucosa	• Increase length of device
	• External obstruction by esophageal back wall	• Shorten device, exert less digital pressure, use heat and moisture exchange system (HME)
Stoma	• Difficult occlusion due to irregular, still painful, or too large stoma	• Use small balloon covered with gauze, or valved HME
	• Difficulty in finding the stoma with the finger	• Practice in front of mirror
Trachea	• Excessive phlegm production, interfering with voicing	• Do inhalation therapy, apply HME
Respiration	• Forced, too strong, or too weak an expiration causing voicing problems	• Do abdominal respiration exercises, train with chant-talk technique (Boone & McFarlane, 2000)
Posture	• A collapsed body position, causing poor voice and a short phonation time	• Correct body position or posture
	• Incorrect head position, caus-ing muscular tension and a strained voice	• Do relaxation exercises, cor-rect head position
Confusing esophageal and tracheoesopha-geal voice	• Short phonation time, iden-tical with or without stoma occlusion	• Explain problem to patient, lengthen the vowels, use chant-talk technique, do breathing exercises
Radiotherapy	• Decrease in voice quality during radiotherapy	• Reassure patient and continue speech therapy

REFERENCES

Ackerstaff, A. H., Fuller, D., Irvin, M., Maccracken, E., Gaziano, J., & Stachowiak, L. (2003). Multi-center study assessing effects of heat and moisture exchanger use on respiratory symptoms and voice quality in laryngectomized individuals. *Otolaryngology—Head and Neck Surgery, 129*, 705–712.

Ackerstaff, A. H., Hilgers, F. J. M. (1999). Multi-institutional assessment of the Provox® 2 voice prosthesis. *Archives of Otolaryngology—Head and Neck Surgery, 125,* 167–173.

Ackerstaff, A. H., Hilgers, F. J. M., Balm, A. J. M., & Tan, I. B. (1998). Long term compliance of laryngectomized patients with a specialized pulmonary rehabilitation device, Provox® Stoma-filter. *Laryngoscope, 108*, 257–260.

Ackerstaff, A. H., Hilgers, F. J. M., Meeuwis, C. A., van der Velden, L. A., van den Hoogen, F. J. A., Marres, H. A. M., Vreeburg, G. C. M., & Manni, J. J. (1999). Multi-institutional assessment of the Provox®2 voice prosthesis. *Archives of Otolaryngology—Head and Neck Surgery, 125*, 167–173.

Annyas, A. A., Nijdam, H. F., Escajadillo, J. R., Mahieu, H. F., & Leever, H. (1984). Groningen prosthesis for voice rehabilitation after laryngectomy. *Clinical Otolaryngology, 9*, 51–54.

Blom, E. D. (1995). Tracheoesophageal speech. *Seminars in Speech and Language, 16* (pp. 191–205). New York: Thieme Medical.

Boone, D. R., & McFarlane, S. C. (2000). *The voice and voice therapy* (6th ed.). Boston: Allyn & Bacon.

Doyle, P. C. (1994). *Foundations of voice and speech rehabilitation following laryngeal cancer*. San Diego: Singular.

Doyle, P. C., Danhauer, J. L., & Reed, C. G. (1988). Listeners' perceptions of consonants produced by esophageal and tracheoesophageal talkers. *Journal of Speech and Hearing Disorders, 53*, 400–407.

Eadie, T. L., & Doyle, P. C. (2004). Auditory–perceptual scaling and quality of life in tracheoesophageal speakers. *Laryngoscope, 114*, 753–759.

Eerenstein, S. E. J., Grolman, W., & Schouwenburg, P. F. (2002). Downsizing of voice prosthesis diameter in patients with laryngectomy: An in vitro study. *Archives of Otolaryngology—Head and Neck Surgery, 128*, 838–841.

Graville, D., Gross, N., Andersen, P., Everts, E., & Cohen, J. (1999). The long-term indwelling tracheoesophageal prosthesis for alaryngeal voice rehabilitation. *Archives of Otolaryngology—Head and Neck Surgery, 125*, 288–292.

Gress, C. D. (2004). Preoperative evaluation for tracheoesophageal voice restoration. *Otolaryngology Clinics of North Ameica, 37*, 519–530.

Hamaker, R. C., Singer, M. I., Blom, E. D., & Daniels, A. (1985). Primary voice restoration at laryngectomy. *Archives of Otolaryngology, 111*, 182–186.

Henley-Cohn, J., Hausfeld, J. N., & Jakubczak, G. (1984). Artificial larynx prosthesis: Comparative clinical evaluation. *Laryngoscope, 94*, 43–45.

Hilgers, F. J. M., & Ackerstaff, A. H. (2000). Comprehensive rehabilitation after total laryngectomy is more than voice alone. *Folia Phoniatrica et Logopaedica, 52*, 65–73.

Hilgers, F. J. M., Ackerstaff, A. H., Balm, A. J. M., Tan, I. B., Aaronson, N. K., & Persson, J. O. (1997). Development and clinical evaluation of a second-generation voice prosthesis (Provox®2), designed for anterograde and retrograde insertion. *Acta Otolaryngologica (Stockholm), 117*, 889–896.

Hilgers, F. J., Ackerstaff, A. H., Balm, A. J., van den Brekel, M. W., Tan, B., & Persson, J. O. (2003). A new problem-solving indwelling voice prosthesis, eliminating the need for frequent Candida- and "underpressure"-related replacements: Provox ActiValve. *Acta Otolaryngologica, 123*, 972–979.

Hilgers, F. J. M., & Balm, A. J. M. (1993). Long-term results of vocal rehabilitation after total laryngectomy with the low-resistance, indwelling Provox® voice prosthesis system. *Clinical Otolaryngology, 18*, 517–523.

Hilgers, F. J. M., Balm, A. J. M., Gregor, R. T., Tan I. B., Scholtens, B. E. G. M., van As, C. J., & Ackerstaff, A. H. (1999). *The Provox® system: A practical guide to post-laryngectomy vocal and pulmonary rehabilitation* [CD-ROM]. Amsterdam: The Netherlands Cancer Institute.

Hilgers, F. J. M., Cornelissen, M. W., & Balm, A. J. M. (1993). Aerodynamic characteristics of the low-resistance, indwelling Provox® voice prosthesis. *European Archives of Otorhinolaryngology, 250*, 375–378.

Hilgers, F. J. M., Hoorweg, J. J., Kroon, B. B. R., Schaeffer, B., de Boer, J. B., & Balm, A. J. M. (1995). Prosthetic voice rehabilitation with the Provox® system after extensive pharyngeal resection and reconstruction. In J. Algaba (Ed.), *6th International Congress on Surgical and Prosthetic Voice Restoration after Total Laryngectomy* (Vol. 1112, pp. 111–120). San Sebastian, Puerto Rico: Exerpta Medica International Congress Series.

Hilgers, F. J. M., & Schouwenburg, P. F. (1990). A new low-resistance, self-retaining prosthesis (Provox®) for voice rehabilitation after total laryngectomy. *Laryngoscope, 100*, 1202–1207.

Hilgers, F. J. M., Schouwenburg, P. F., & Scholtens, B. (1988). Long term results of prosthetic voice rehabilitation after total laryngectomy. *Clinical Otolaryngology, 14*, 365–366.

Hoffman, H. T., Fischer, H., VanDenmark, D., Peterson, K. L., McCulloch, T. M., Hynds Karnell, L., & Funk, G. F. (1997). Botulinum neurotoxin injection after total laryngectomy. *Head & Neck, 3*, 92–97.

Hotz, M. A., Baumann, A., Schaller, I., & Zbären, P. (2002). Success and predictability of Provox prosthesis voice rehabilitation. *Archives of Otolaryngology—Head and Neck Surgery, 128*, 687–691.

Jebria, A. B., Henry, C., Petit, J., Gioux, M., Devars, F., & Traissac, L. (1987). Physical and aerodynamic features of the Bordeaux voice prosthesis. *Artificial Organs, 11*, 383–387.

Leder, S. B., & Erskine, M. C. (1997). Voice restoration after laryngectomy: Experience with the Blom–Singer extended-wear indwelling tracheoesophageal voice prosthesis. *Head & Neck, 19*, 487–493.

Mahieu, H. F., Annyas, A. A., Schutte, H. K., & van der Jagt, E. J. (1987). Pharyngoesophageal myotomy for vocal rehabilitation of laryngectomees. *Laryngoscope, 97*, 451–457.

Mahieu, H. F., van Saene, H. K. F., Rosingh, H. J., & Schutte, H. K. (1986). Candida vegetations on silicone voice prostheses. *Archives of Otolaryngology—Head and Neck Surgery, 112*, 321–325.

Mahieu, H. F., van Saene, J. J. M., den Besten, J., & van Saene, H. K. F. (1986). Oropharynx decontamination preventing Candida vegetations on voice prostheses. *Archives of Otolaryngology—Head and Neck Surgery, 112*, 1090–1092.

Manni, J. J., & van den Broek, P. (1990). Surgical and prosthesis related complications using the Groningen button voice prosthesis. *Clinical Otolaryngology, 15*, 515–523.

Manni, J. J., van den Broek, P., de Groot, A. H., & Berends, E. (1984). Voice rehabilitation after laryngectomy with the Groningen prosthesis. *Journal of Otolaryngology, 13*, 333–336.

McIvor, J., Evans, P. F., Perry, A., & Cheesman, D. (1990). Radiological assessment of post laryngectomy speech. *Clinical Radiology, 41*, 312–316.

Mendenhall, W. M., Morris, C. G., Stringer, S. P., Amdur, R. J., Hinerman, R. W., Villaret, D. B., & Robbins, K. T. (2004). Voice rehabilitation after total laryngectomy and postoperative radiation therapy. *Journal of Clinical Oncology, 15,* 2500–2505.

Mohide, E. A., Archibald, S. D., Tew, M., Young, J. E., & Haines, T. (1992). Postlaryngectomy quality-of-life dimensions identified by patients and health care professionals. *American Journal of Surgery, 164*, 619–622.

Nijdam, H. F., Annyas, A. A., Schutte, H. K., & Leever, H. (1982). A new prosthesis for voice rehabilitation after laryngectomy. *Archives of Otorhinolaryngology, 237*, 27–33.

Op de Coul, B. M. R., Hilgers, F. J. M., Balm, A. J. M., Tan, I. B., van den Hoogen, F. J. A., & van Tinteren, H. (2000). A decade of postlaryngectomy vocal rehabilitation in 318 patients: A single institution's experience with consistent application of Provox indwelling voice prostheses. *Archives of Otolaryngology—Head and Neck Surgery, 126,* 1320–1328.

Op de Coul, B. M. R., van den Hoogen, F. J. A., van As, C. J., Marres, H. A. M., Joosten, F. B. M., Manni, J. J., & Hilgers, F. J. M. (2003). Evaluation of the effects of primary myotomy in total laryngectomy on the neoglottis with the use of quantitative videofluoroscopy. *Archives of Otolaryngology—Head and Neck Surgery, 129,* 1000–1005.

Panje, W. R. (1981). Prosthetic vocal rehabilitation following laryngectomy. *Annals of Otology, Rhinology and Laryngology, 90,* 116–120.

Remacle, M. J., & Declaye, X. J. (1988). Gax-collagen injection to correct an enlarged tracheoesophageal fistula for a vocal prosthesis. *Laryngoscope, 98,* 1350–1352.

Robbins, J., Fisher, H. B., Blom, E. D., & Singer, M. I. (1984). A comparative acoustic study of normal, esophageal, and tracheoesophageal speech production. *Journal of Speech and Hearing Disorders, 49,* 202–210.

Singer, M. I. (1988). The upper esophageal sphincter: Role in alaryngeal speech acquisition. *Head & Neck Surgery, 10,* 118–123.

Singer, M. I. (2004). The development of successful tracheoesophageal voice restoration. *Otolaryngology Clinics of North America, 37,* 507–517.

Singer, M. I., & Blom, E. D. (1980). An endoscopic technique for restoration of voice after laryngectomy. *Annals of Otology, Rhinology and Laryngology, 89,* 529–533.

Singer, M. I., & Blom, E. D. (1981). Selective myotomy for voice restoration after total laryngectomy. *Archives of Otolaryngology, 107,* 670–673.

Singer, M. I., Blom, E. D., & Hamaker, R. C. (1981). Further experience with voice restoration after total laryngectomy. *Annals of Otology, Rhinology and Laryngology, 90,* 498–502.

Singer, M. I., Blom, E. D., & Hamaker, R. C. (1986). Pharyngeal plexus neurectomy for alaryngeal speech rehabilitation. *Laryngoscope, 96,* 50–53.

Stam, H. J., Koopmans, J. P., & Methieson, C. M. (1991). The psychosocial impact of laryngectomy: A comprehensive assessment. *Journal of Psychosocial Oncology, 9,* 37–58.

Tardy-Mitzell, S., Andrews, M. L., & Bowman, S. A. (1985). Acceptability and intelligibility of tracheoesophageal speech. *Archives of Otolaryngology, 111,* 213–215.

van As, C. J., Hilgers, F. J. M., Koopmans-van Beinum, F. J., & Ackerstaff, A. H. (1998). The influence of stoma occlusion on aspects of tracheoesophageal voice. *Acta Otolaryngologica (Stockholm), 118,* 732–738.

van As, C. J., Koopmans-van Beinum, F. J., Pols, L. C., & Hilgers, F. J. (2003). Perceptual evaluation of tracheoesophageal speech by naive and experienced judges through the use of semantic differential scales. *Journal of Speech-Language-Hearing Research, 46,* 947–959.

van As, C. J., Tigges, M., Wittenberg, T., Op de Coul, B. M. R., Eysholdt, U., & Hilgers, F. J. M. (1999). High-speed digital imaging of neoglottic vibration after total laryngectomy. *Archives of Otolaryngology—Head and Neck Surgery, 125,* 891–897.

van den Hoogen, F. J. A., Meeuwis, C., Oudes, M. J., Janssen, P., & Manni, J. J. (1996). The Blom–Singer tracheostoma valve as a valuable addition in the rehabilitation of the laryngectomized patient. *European Archives of Otorhinolaryngology, 253,* 126–129.

van den Hoogen, F. J., van den Berg, R. J., Oudes, M. J., & Manni, J. J. (1998). A prospective study of speech and voice rehabilitation after total laryngectomy with the low-resistance Groningen, Nijdam and Provox voice prostheses. *Clinical Otolaryngology, 23,* 425–431.

van Weissenbruch, R., & Albers, F. W. J. (1993). Vocal rehabilitation after total laryngectomy using the Provox® voice prosthesis. *Clinical Otolaryngology, 18,* 359–364.

van Weissenbruch, R., Bouckaert, S., Remon, J.-P., Nelis, H. J., Aerts, R., & Albers, F. W. J. (1997). Chemoprophylaxis of fungal deterioration of the Provox® silicone tracheoesophageal prosthesis in postlaryngectomy patients. *Annals of Otology, Rhinology and Laryngology, 106,* 329–337.

Verschuur, H. P., Gregor, R. T., Hilgers, F. J. M., & Balm, A. J. M. (1996). The tracheostoma in relation to prosthetic voice rehabilitation—How we do it. *Laryngoscope, 106,* 111–115.

Vlantis, A. C., Gregor, R. T., Elliot, H., & Oudes, M. (2003). Conversion from a non-indwelling to a Provox2 indwelling voice prosthesis for speech rehabilitation: comparison of voice quality and patient preference. *Journal of Laryngology & Otology, 117,* 815–820.

Williams, S., & Watson, J. B. (1985). Differences in speaking proficiencies in three laryngectomy groups. *Archives of Otolaryngology, 111,* 216–219.

Chapter 19

Clinical Troubleshooting with Tracheoesophageal Puncture Voice Prostheses

Gail Monahan

Voice restoration using a tracheoesophageal fistula has become a widely used method of postlaryngectomy speech rehabilitation since the introduction of the Blom–Singer tracheoesophageal (TE) voice prosthesis in 1980 (Singer & Blom, 1980). Studies evaluating the tracheoesophageal puncture (TEP) procedure and TE speech rehabilitation by its developers (Blom, Singer, & Hamaker, 1986; Singer, 1983; Singer & Blom, 1981a) and others (Geraghty, Smith, Wenig, & Portugal, 1996; Kao, Mohr, Kimmel, Getch, & Silverman, 1994; Leder & Erskine, 1997; Singer, 2004) have shown both the procedure and the prosthesis to be a reliable method of voice restoration. As a result, TEP voice restoration has rapidly gained universal acceptance because of its simplicity, reproducibility, and relatively high rate of success (see Chapter 24 in this text).

Based on 20 years of clinical experience, however, it has become clear that the TEP voice restoration procedure can be deceivingly simple and is seldom problem free. The follow-up care required for many TEP patients can be extremely time consuming and challenging to both the patient and the voice restoration team. Some patients who have a TEP voice prosthesis in place have no knowledge of its purpose, use, or maintenance. In some instances, those who were unsuccessful with the TEP procedure were never good candidates for its application (Stafford, 2003). Although the majority of individuals who undergo total laryngectomy can benefit from TEP voice restoration, this is not true of all patients. Success with this procedure requires careful candidate selection, adequate patient education (both pre-TEP and post-TEP), and careful follow-up patient training. Successful voice restoration requires the combined expertise of the otolaryngologist and the speech–language pathologist as a team to achieve optimal patient care. A new team with minimal clinical experience in this area should not hesitate to contact colleagues who are experienced in TEP voice restoration.[1] Regardless of the time, energy, and work involved, TEP voice restoration can be some of the most gratifying work experienced by a clinician. Therefore, the primary purpose of this chapter is to provide information on how to identify potential problems with the TEP procedure, specify the causes of such problems, and offer various solutions for clinically addressing the problem.

Various voice prostheses have been employed over the past 25 years to restore postlaryngectomy speech. Currently, the most commonly used types of voice prostheses are the Blom–Singer indwelling (clinician assisted) and the Provox extended-wear devices (see Chapters 17 and 18 in this text). A comparative study of two more recent indwelling types of voice prostheses (Delsuphe, Zink, Lajaegere, & Delaere, 1998) concluded that there were equal and positive results in terms of voice quality for both devices. However, nonindwelling TE puncture voice prostheses continue to be used. Therefore, a secondary purpose of this chapter is to provide a brief discussion of the various types of TEP voice prostheses that are in current use.

---

[1]A list of experienced clinicians can be found in *Clinical Insights,* a quarterly newsletter published by the International Center for Post-Laryngectomy Voice Restoration, 7440 Shadeland, Suite 200, Indianapolis, IN 42650 (phone 800/283-1056). This newsletter is a valuable resource to both beginning and experienced clinicians.

Troubleshooting for the speech–language pathologist and otolaryngologist working as a team actually begins at the time of patient selection. Appropriate selection of potential candidates for TEP, as either a primary or secondary procedure, is an important concern. Thus, to begin, a brief review of selection criterion is necessary as a precursor to formal troubleshooting procedures.

PATIENT SELECTION AND CANDIDACY FOR TRACHEOESOPHAGEAL PUNCTURE

A patient who presents for secondary voice restoration should be assessed for anatomical, physiological, psychological, social, and learning factors. A comprehensive table of candidacy criteria, as provided by Doyle (1994), is presented in Table 19.1.

With the advent of the indwelling or extended-wear voice prosthesis, adequate manual dexterity has become less important because the indwelling voice prosthesis is removed and replaced by a physician or trained speech–language pathologist, not the patient (Hilgers et al., 2003; see also Chapter 18 in this text). Manual dexterity is still a desirable factor, however, for ease of cleaning and care of the tracheostoma and voice prosthesis in situ.

In addition to meeting standard selection criteria, patients who are considered for secondary TEP and voice prosthesis placement also benefit from videofluoroscopic assessment whenever possible. Such assessment is performed to evaluate postlaryngectomy reconstructive changes and general aspects of PE segment physiology. A comprehensive radiographic study for this purpose should

TABLE 19.1

Criteria for Candidacy: Tracheoesophageal Puncture Voice Restoration Procedure

1. Patient must be motivated.
2. Patient must have adequate understanding of post-surgical anatomy.
3. Patient must have basic understanding of function of the TE voice prosthesis.
4. Patient must demonstrate adequate manual dexterity to manage prosthesis.
5. Visual acuity must be sufficient for purpose of managing tracheostoma and voice prosthesis.
6. Patient must exhibit ability to care for prosthesis.
7. Patient should have no significant hypopharyngeal stenosis.
8. Patient should demonstrate positive results following esophageal insufflation test.
9. Patient must have adequate pulmonary support for prosthesis use.
10. Patient should have stoma of adequate depth and diameter for prosthesis to avoid airway occlusion.
11. Patient should be mentally stable.

Note. From *Foundations of Voice and Speech Rehabilitation Following Laryngeal Cancer* (p. 194), by P. C. Doyle, 1994, San Diego: Singular. Copyright 1994 by Singular Publishing Group. Reprinted with permission.

include a modified barium swallow, attempted phonation, and esophageal in-sufflation. The intent of the study is to rule out the presence of a PE segment stricture, or a fistula, and to view the PE segment tonicity (Cheesman, Knight, McIvor, & Perry, 1986; McIvor, Evans, Perry, & Cheesman, 1990; Perry & Edels, 1985; Sloan, Griffin, & O'Dwyer, 1991; see also Chapter 21 in this text). If primary TE voice restoration is to be performed, the surgeon has control over the pha-ryngeal closure and, thus, the tonicity of the PE segment. In this case, there is no need to undertake radiographic study or insufflation testing as long as the princi-ples of pharyngeal closure have been followed (Hamaker, Singer, Blom, & Daniels, 1985; Singer & Blom, 1981b).

Although assessment of a patient's physical status relative to PE segment tonicity is of great importance in TEP voice restoration, so too are psychological and social factors. These factors include the patient's ability to understand, care for, and use his or her voice prosthesis. These concerns are equally important for both primary and secondary voice restoration candidates if such procedures are to be successful. Careful patient selection helps prevent future problems and com-plications, some of which may be serious.

PROBLEM IDENTIFICATION AND CLINICAL ASSESSMENT

Once the patient has met the standard selection criteria, undergone either pri-mary or secondary TEP, and had the selected voice prosthesis placed into the TEP site, postoperative troubleshooting begins. When attempting to solve a TE voic-ing system problem, the clinician should assess and eliminate problems related to (a) the TEP itself, (b) the status of the TEP voice prosthesis in combination with that of the TEP tract, and (c) the muscular capacity of the PE segment. To assist the reader in quick referencing, a comprehensive categorical summary of prob-lems and solutions discussed in this chapter is provided in Table 19.2.

Immediate Postfitting Aphonia, Dysphonia, or Effortful Phonation

Postradiation tissue edema, which may occur with both primary and early sec-ondary TEPs, may result in forced and effortful TE phonation. If this problem en-sues, the clinician should replace the stent or catheter and allow the edema to sub-side before attempting further TEP tract sizing and voice prosthesis replacement.

To eliminate the voice prosthesis itself as a causative factor of immediate postfitting aphonia or difficulty initiating TE voice production, the clinician should have the patient attempt voicing through the open TEP (i.e., without a prosthesis in place). If effortless and fluent voice is produced but is again lost once the voice prosthesis is reinserted, then the prosthesis requires closer examination.

(text continues on p. 489)

TABLE 19.2

Troubleshooting Guide for Tracheoesophageal Speech: Problems, Causes, and Solutions

Problem	Possible Cause	Solution
Difficulty inserting prosthesis	• Puncture closing • Low-pressure voice prosthesis • Angled puncture • Puncture difficult to visualize • Resistance	• Dilate with stent or catheter • Use duckbill or gel cap • Use catheter to check angle, direct inferiorly; repuncture • Pull up skin to visualize; re-cline patient • Dilate; use lubricant
Painful insertion	• Voice prosthesis not fully inserted • Tracheoesophageal tract stenosis • Gastroesophageal reflux • Granulation tissue, irritation	• Remove, dilate, and reinsert • Dilate and reinsert • Use antireflux protocol • Dilate one to two sizes larger than prosthesis, then insert; cauterize
Immediate postfitting aphonia or effortful phonation	• Voice prosthesis too long (overfitting) • Valve tip is closed • Forceful stoma occlusion • Postradiation edema (primary and early secondary punctures) • Pharyngeal constrictor hypertonicity or spasm • Excessive resistance • Gel cap has not dissolved	• Remove voice prosthesis and resize • Flush voice prosthesis in situ with pipette; remove voice prosthesis, inspect, squeeze end • Use light finger contact with downward pressure • Replace catheter, allow edema to subside (up to 4 weeks), refit • Assess voicing "open tract"; perform transtracheal insufflation via 18 Fr (French) catheter; do pharyngeal plexus nerve block; insufflate under fluoroscopy; if confirmed, consider myotomy or Botox injection • Change to low-pressure or 20 Fr voice prosthesis • Drink water; wait 4 minutes
Delayed postfitting aphonia	• Valve tip is closed • Puncture tract closure due to underfitting • Voice prosthesis is not fully inserted • False tract creation associated with reinsertion of voice prosthesis	• Flush voice prosthesis in situ with pipette; remove voice prosthesis, inspect, squeeze end • Dilate, resize, insert longer voice prosthesis, repuncture • Dilate and reinsert; confirm with endoscopy or radio-graphic study • Replace catheter and reinsert, confirm with endoscopy or radiographic study

(continues)

TABLE 19.2 *Continued.*

Troubleshooting Guide for Tracheoesophageal Speech: Problems, Causes, and Solutions

Problem	Possible Cause	Solution
Leakage through prosthesis	• Valve deterioration • Candida deposits	• Replace prosthesis • Disinfect voice prosthesis with hydrogen peroxide; Nystatin suspension
	• Duckbill tip against posterior pharyngeal wall	• Resize; replace with correct size voice prosthesis; replace with low-pressure voice prosthesis
	• Valve is stuck in the open position due to food or saliva • Valve is stuck in the open position immediately post-insertion • Postinsertion kinking of prosthesis causing valve to stay in the open position • Resistance of flap valve too low	• Perform repeated dry swallows • Use wooden tip of cotton applicator to gently release the valve • Dilate for longer period of time before voice prosthesis insertion • Place duckbill or high-resistance voice prosthesis
Leakage around prosthesis	• Overfitting; voice prosthesis pistons in tract	• Resize, replace with correct size voice prosthesis; consider retention collar for between sizes
	• Tract dilation due to stiffness of voice prosthesis • Tract dilation in irradiated tissue	• Replace with non-indwelling voice prosthesis • Place smaller catheter (14–16 Fr) for 3 to 4 weeks, then place non-indwelling voice prosthesis; perform flap re-construction
	• Tract dilation due to plaque deposits (indwelling prosthesis) • Superior migration of tract, resulting in vertical position-ing of voice prosthesis • Insufficient party wall thickness	• Replace voice prosthesis more frequently • Replace catheter and direct inferiorly; allow tract to close and repuncture • Reconstruct with muscle flap
Microstoma	• Stenosis	• Fenestrated laryngectomy tube; perform surgical revision
Macrostoma	• Natural tracheal size; tracheo-malacia	• Perform surgical revision
Insufficient duration of tracheostoma valve seal	• Excessive "back pressure"	• Assess with pressure meter during speech; change to 20 Fr voice prosthesis; reduce loudness and effort, consider change to Barton-Mayo button

(continues)

TABLE 19.2 *Continued.*

Troubleshooting Guide for Tracheoesophageal Speech: Problems, Causes, and Solutions

Problem	Possible Cause	Solution
Insufficient duration (*continued*)	• Inadequate cleansing of skin prior to application	• Remove old adhesive completely with Remove; use SkinPrep or alcohol to prepare area
	• Failure to allow adhesive to set	• Wait for minutes for liquid adhesive to dry before applying housing; use self-adhering housing
	• Careless application of tape and foam discs to housing	• Retrain application procedures to remove air bubbles; use self-adhering housings
	• Irregular peristomal area	• Retrain application method, with extra care to irregular area; pull up and smooth skin before application; use larger self-adhering housings; attempt use of skin barrier products to form more regular area; use custom housing for tracheostoma valve; consider change to Barton-Mayo button
	• Break in seal due to secretions	• Remove valve prior to cough, wipe secretions carefully from inside surface of housing chimney; consider heat and moisture exchange system; use prescription medications (e.g., Ponaris)
Granulation tissue	• Irritation associated with presence of foreign body	• Surgically remove tissue; cauterize
	• Inflammation from infrequent removal of voice prosthesis	• Retrain; regularly rotate voice prosthesis in tract
Inability to digitally occlude stoma	• Irregular stoma configuration	• Create custom adaptive devices; fit with tracheostoma valve; surgically revise
	• Upper extremity dysfunction	• Fit with adaptive devices; fit with tracheostoma valve
Poor quality speech	• Voice prosthesis not fully inserted	• Remove, resize, and replace with correct voice prosthesis
	• Loose segment, especially with pharyngoesophageal reconstructions	• Change to pressure band; manually occlude instead of using tracheostoma valve
	• Tight segment, poor elasticity of segment	• Reduce effort; change to low-pressure or 20 Fr voice prosthesis; increase moisture

(continues)

TABLE 19.2 *Continued.*

Troubleshooting Guide for Tracheoesophageal Speech: Problems, Causes, and Solutions

Problem	Possible Cause	Solution
Poor quality speech (*continued*)	• Poor vibratory activity	• Change to low-pressure or 20 Fr voice prosthesis; alter tone focus; retrain stoma occlusion
	• Air leakage around stoma	• Retrain stoma occlusion; use adaptive devices; fit with tracheostoma breathing valve
	• Short phrases	• Reduce effort; change to 20 Fr or low-pressure voice prosthesis; retrain respiratory effort
	• Strained high pitch	• Alter tone focus to lower in throat; evaluate for hypertonicity or spasm
	• Excessively low pitch	• Alter tone focus higher in throat

Note. Sources for this table are Blom (1986, 1988) and Gress (2000).

Two possible problems may be occurring if such an observation is made. First, the duckbill or flap valve of the voice prosthesis should be inspected to see if it is stuck in the closed position. If so, the voice prosthesis may require manual manipulation by the clinician to open the duckbill or flap valve. Occasionally, when a gel-cap insertion method is used, the gel cap itself may not have completely melted. If this problem is suspected, a sip of warm water usually dissolves the remaining capsule particle and resolves the problem in a few minutes. Second, if the voice prosthesis appears to be functioning well, then "overfitting" (use of a voice prosthesis that is too long) may be the problem and further assessment is necessary. When overfitting is the suspected problem, the proximal end of the voice prosthesis may be impinging on the posterior wall of the esophagus, thereby restricting or preventing airflow through the valve. In other words, a voice prosthesis that is too long may be pushed into the posterior esophageal wall and restrict opening of the prosthesis. The solution for this problem is to remove the voice prosthesis and resize and downsize as indicated. If a duckbill prosthesis is being used, the clinician should replace it with a low-pressure or low-profile voice prosthesis (i.e., replace an 8-mm duckbill valve tip with the shorter 2-mm valve tip).

Another possible cause of immediate postfitting aphonia or effortful phonation is overly forceful digital stoma occlusion. In this case, the clinician should explain the potential problem to the patient, demonstrate the appropriate combination of light digital contact with downward pressure for adequate occlusion, and encourage relaxed respiratory and phonatory effort for the best level of voice production. Next, the clinician should guide the patient to do the same. Three to four sessions are usually required to teach the patient the correct method and to establish consistent carryover into daily communication situations. Once the status of the voice prosthesis, the degree of digital occlusion, and potential associated forceful phonation have been addressed and ruled out as a cause of post-fitting voice difficulties, the clinician again checks to see if voicing can be achieved with an open TEP tract. If TE vocal quality still does not approximate open-tract production, the clinician should evaluate the type of voice prosthesis being used. If the patient is using a duckbill voice prosthesis, a change to a low-pressure (16-Fr) voice prosthesis might work. If vocal quality improves but still does not improve relative to open-tract voice quality, gradually dilate the TE fistula with a 22-Fr dilator or in graduated steps using 18-, 20-, 22-Fr catheters and insert a 20-Fr low-pressure prosthesis.

If the patient's voice remains effortful or inconsistent, or the patient can only voice in short phrases with both an open TE tract and with the optimal prosthesis in place, and forceful finger occlusion is not an issue, then the problem is most likely related to pharyngeal constriction, muscle spasm, or hypertonicity. Complete spasm or hypertonicity of the pharyngeal constrictor muscles can be diagnosed by fluoroscopic evaluation while the patient attempts phonation or through its temporary elimination using a percutaneous pharyngeal plexus nerve block with 2% lidocaine (Singer & Blom, 1981a, 1981b; see also Chapter 17 in this text). Also, because hypertonicity or spasm is a dynamic action elicited by airflow-induced distention of the cervical esophagus (Doyle, 1985), swallowing function is usually unaffected.

One solution to PE or cricopharyngeal spasm is unilateral pharyngeal constrictor muscle myotomy, which has commonly been employed with positive results (Singer & Blom, 1981a). The drawbacks of myotomy are that the procedure requires an anesthetic and is associated with possible complications, including pharyngocutaneous fistula (Izdebski, Reed, Ross, & Hilsinger, 1994). Another option is the pharyngeal plexus neurectomy, which surgically denervates the constrictor muscles to prevent spasm of the PE segment (Singer, Blom, & Hamaker, 1986). This approach has a much smaller chance of causing a pharyngocutaneous fistula than does myotomy, but the procedure still requires surgery and a general anesthetic and is not without risk. A third alternative is botulinum neurotoxin (Botox) injection (Blitzer, Komisar, Baredes, Brin, & Stewart, 1995; Hamaker & Blom, 2003; Hoffman et al., 1997; Ramachandran, Arunachalam, Hurren, Marsh, & Samuel, 2003; Terrel, Lewin, & Esclamado, 1995). This relatively recent development of chemical denervation of the PE segment through injection of Botox offers an invasive, yet nonsurgical approach to solving the problem of PE spasm. Early results indicate that Botox injection may not only relieve constrictor spasm but also facilitate a learned volitional relaxation of the constrictor musculature, thereby reducing and eventually doing away with the need for regular reinjection (see Chapter 21 in this text).

If the patient displays initial effortful phonation, both through an open TE tract and through a prosthesis, and also complains of reduced swallowing function, PE stricture may be the problem. This is a static narrowing at or near the PE segment junction above the level of the voice prosthesis. If a stricture exists, it can result in restricted airflow and phonation. Stricture normally responds well to dilation with only severe cases needing surgical reconstruction. Diagnosis of stricture can be achieved with a radiographic evaluation that includes both modified barium swallow and attempts at TEP phonation.

Delayed Aphonia or Dysphonia

Occasionally, a patient may experience increased phonatory effort, decreased duration of voicing, or complete aphonia following weeks, months, or years of successful voice prosthesis use. Again, the clinician should first rule out the voice prosthesis as the problem. To determine whether the valve tip is closed, stuck, or clogged, the clinician can flush the voice prosthesis in situ with a pipette if the prosthesis is a Blom–Singer device (see Chapter 17 in this text), or clean it with the appropriate brush if it is a Bivona or Provox prosthesis (see Chapter 18). If voice production does not improve, the clinician should remove the voice prosthesis, inspect the valve, and clean it of any secretions. If no structural problems are found with the voice prosthesis, the clinician should reinsert the device and have the client try voicing again. Once the voice prosthesis is ruled out as the cause of the dysphonia, TEP tract closure or partial stenosis of the tract should be considered as a possible cause. Stenosis or complete tract closure of the proximal aspect of the TEP may occur if

1. the voice prosthesis is too short to reach into the esophagus and maintain the patency of the TEP tract,
2. the tract has been elongated due to granuloma formation at the tracheal aspect of the TEP, thereby rendering the prosthesis too short,
3. the patient has removed the prosthesis for cleaning and failed to correctly reinsert it through the TEP into the esophageal lumen, or
4. a "false" puncture tract is created during reinsertion of the prosthesis.

Complete closure of a TEP tract can be determined if no voicing can be produced with an open tract or if liquids are not observed to flow through the puncture and penetrate the trachea on swallowing. In this case, the TEP procedure needs to be performed once again. If, however, a weak voice can still be produced through the open tract or if liquids penetrate, then at least some opening of the tract remains. The puncture tract can then be carefully and serially dilated using soft urethral catheters (sizes 8 Fr through 22 Fr). Rigid instruments and force *should never be used* to avoid dissecting the tracheoesophageal party wall and creating a false passage or causing an esophageal tear. If the clinician has difficulty with initial catheter placement, the team physician should be consulted immediately. Once dilated, the tract should be stented with an 18 Fr or 22 Fr catheter for at least 24 hours, remeasured, and then refitted with a voice prosthesis of appropriate length and diameter (Blom, Singer, & Hamaker, 1998; see also Chapters 17, 18, and 24 in this text). To rule out further problems after dilation and refitting, the clinician should confirm positioning (seating) of the voice prosthesis with endoscopy or radiographic study. During the radiographic study, the clinician should include a lateral view with TEP during voicing and an anterior–posterior view for verification that the retention collar of the voice prosthesis is opened fully within the esophagus.

Leakage Through the Prosthesis

If the patient complains of leakage through the prosthesis, it is important to illuminate the stoma with a bright light and observe the voice prosthesis in situ. As the patient drinks small amounts of liquid, the clinician can confirm whether the leakage is through or around the prosthesis. Leakage through the voice prosthesis will indicate problems with the prosthesis itself. The simplest cause may be a defective valve or one stuck in the open position, perhaps by a piece of food or, if a new voice prosthesis, from undissolved gel-cap debris. Upon questioning, a patient often will indicate that the leakage is transient and only occurs occasionally during meals. To determine if it is a transient problem, the clinician should first flush out the voice prosthesis or clean it with the appropriate cleaning instrument and have the patient drink again. If the problem is solved, the patient needs to be instructed again on appropriate cleaning techniques. If the problem is not solved, the clinician should remove the voice prosthesis and inspect the valve mechanism for debris and adequacy of closure, then reinsert and reevaluate the voice prosthesis as the patient sips water. If the voice prosthesis still leaks, the problem is probably due to a faulty valve or valve deterioration.

Leakage Around the Prosthesis

Leakage around a prosthesis is a problem that may lead to aspiration pneumonia. Leakage results when the puncture dilates or when the party wall tissues fail to naturally tighten around the shaft of the prosthesis. Factors that may affect tissue viability include prior radiation therapy exceeding 6,500 rads, uncontrolled diabetes, significant nutritional imbalance, and recurrent metastatic or new disease (Blom et al., 1998). If a comprehensive medical evaluation determines that the problem is not the result of recurrent, metastatic, or new disease, but instead is caused by radiation necrosis or a very thin party wall, a number of solutions are possible.

Overfitting occurs if the voice prosthesis is too long for the puncture tract. Because the device is too long, the prosthesis pistons in the tract and eventually causes a mechanical dilation. In this case, the original voice prosthesis should be replaced with a voice prosthesis of the correct size. This change will often reduce the friction and allow the tract to tighten down to the voice prosthesis. Complete cessation of leakage may occur within 24 hours but in some instances may require up to 3 or 4 days, depending on the extent of the dilation.

Although many sizes and types of voice prostheses are now available, occasionally a patient will require an "in-between" size. In this case the clinician may consider attaching a 2-mm silicone washer or "shim" (InHealth Technologies) securely onto the external shaft of the prosthesis to shorten its length. This addition prevents the pistoning of the prosthesis and achieves a firm fit of the retention flange against the anterior esophageal wall mucosa (Blom et al., 1998).

Dilation of a thin TEP party wall may also occur secondary to the presence of a stiff, large-diameter, unforgiving indwelling voice prosthesis. Replacement of the prosthesis with a non-indwelling model will often solve the problem. If tract dilation is considered the result of thin irradiated tissue, the clinician may gradually downsize the puncture to 14 Fr or 16 Fr with catheters, and then place a non-indwelling voice prosthesis in the puncture. This procedure is not always successful, but when it is, it rules out the need for corrective surgery. If it is eventually determined that the party wall is of insufficient thickness to tolerate a puncture, a surgical solution for repair, or if necessary closure of the TEP, may be warranted (Singer, Hamaker, & Blom, 1989). A third possible solution to the problem is the use of injectable Gax-Collagen to eliminate leakage around the voice prosthesis (Blom et al., 1998). This procedure is easily performed by the physician at his or her office. It also can be repeated if necessary and does not compromise subsequent use of other corrective procedures.

Deterioration of the TEP Voice Prosthesis

Normal valve deterioration varies with each patient and depends on the amount of voice prosthesis usage and how frequently and carefully the patient cleans the prosthesis. The average prosthesis can last anywhere from 3 to 9 months. When cleaning a voice prosthesis, the manufacturer's instructions should be stringently followed to maximize voice prosthesis life span. The clinician should review these instructions with the patient and assist with clarification when needed. Once a voice prosthesis is no longer functioning properly, whether from a faulty valve or due to normal deterioration, the voice prosthesis should be replaced with a new one as soon as possible.

If the voice prosthesis begins to leak after only several weeks of use, the possibility of yeast colonization should be considered (Busscher & van der Mei, 1998; Izdebski, Ross, & Lee, 1987; Mahieu, van Saene, den Besten, & van Saene, 1986; Mahieu, van Saene, Rosingh, & Schutte, 1986). One cause of deterioration is proliferation of *Candida albicans,* a flora common to the oropharyngeal region. Once colonization occurs, it is not reversible and the voice prosthesis must be replaced. Various methods of minimizing or preventing colonization should be considered. The first method involves the use of the non-indwelling voice prosthesis that is cleaned and changed regularly by the patient, not the clinician. If the patient has been using an indwelling model, he or she should switch to a 20-Fr non-indwelling self-changing prosthesis. The patient should alternate use of two voice prostheses every other day, soaking the device that is not in use in a solution of 3% hydrogen peroxide after thorough cleaning.

If the patient chooses to continue using an indwelling or extended-care voice prosthesis (see Chapters 17 and 18 in this text), the fungal colonization can be eliminated or significantly diminished through use of nystatin oral suspension. The patient should swish 1 teaspoon of the solution in the mouth for not less than 4 minutes twice daily, followed by expectoration or swallowing. The clinician should impress upon the patient that following these instructions to the letter is mandatory for successful control of colonization (Blom & Hamaker, 1996; Leder & Erskine, 1997).

Another possible cause of leakage through the voice prosthesis is when the tip of a duckbill device impinges against the posterior esophageal wall, forcing the valve tip open. This increases wear and tear on the valve, thus reducing its one-way flow capacity. Converting to a lower profile voice prosthesis with a protected internal valve should solve the problem.

Cyclical valve opening will sometimes occur as a result of a decrease in negative pressure within the esophagus during the inhalation phase of respiration. When voice prosthesis flap opening coincides with a swallow of liquid, leakage and aspiration may occur. Switching to a higher resistance voice prosthesis, such as the duckbill device or a special order high-resistance prosthesis, usually solves this problem.

Indwelling or extended-wear voice prosthesis users depend on their speech–language pathologists or physicians to remove and replace a prosthesis when it fails. In cases when a prosthesis begins to leak and patients are unable to get to a speech clinician or physician immediately, a temporary insert or plug is available to stop leakage and potential aspiration. Two companies (InHealth Technologies, Carpenteria, California, and Bivona, Gary, Indiana) commercially market these plug inserts for this purpose. The InHealth model is a one-way valve that inserts into the open end of the prosthesis and is attached to a neck strap for safety. It can be used with the Blom–Singer indwelling voice prostheses (sizes 1.8–3.3). This plug temporarily prevents leakage through the voice prosthesis while permitting continued speech until the voice prosthesis is replaced. A 1.4-mm indwelling voice prosthesis requires the use of a nonvalved plug insert secondary to the shortness of the prosthesis. The Provox model also has a nonvalving plug that effectively stops leakage, but does not allow voicing (see Chapter 18 in this text).

Microstoma

A patient's tracheostoma should be no smaller than 2.0 cm in diameter to safely and adequately accommodate a voice prosthesis. Prior to TEP, a small tracheostoma should be either serially dilated to accept a size 10 silicone laryngectomy tube, or the stoma can be surgically revised (enlarged) with tracheoplasty. When using a laryngectomy tube with a voice prosthesis, the posterior wall of the tube that corresponds to the distal opening in the voice prosthesis requires fenestration in the midline to allow airflow through the fenestration into the voice prosthesis. Tubes available commercially (Bivona and InHealth Technologies) are marked for fenestration or are already fenestrated for use. The two devices should be disarticulated with the voice prosthesis positioned behind the silicone laryngectomy tube.

Although some patients can wear a combined device (e.g., the Bivona Colorado voice prosthesis), disarticulation of the two components is generally favored over the bonding of a silicone voice prosthesis to a silicone laryngectomy tube. Unibody construction transfers movement from the laryngectomy tube to the voice prosthesis during coughing and head movement and can cause TEP dilation and leakage; that is, when the voice prosthesis and laryngectomy tube exist as a unit, as the laryngectomy tube moves within the TEP, the prosthesis moves as well. Additionally, maintaining separation of the two devices permits removal of the laryngectomy tube for routine cleaning without disturbing the intact voice prosthesis. To prevent dislodgement or aspiration of the voice prosthesis during the removal and replacement of the laryngectomy tube, the safety strap of the voice prosthesis may be left in place and taped to the neck. The patient also is instructed to slightly rotate the laryngectomy tube prior to removal to prevent catching the retention collar on the fenestrated edge of the tube. Most patients who wear a laryngectomy tube for stomal stenosis can be gradually "weaned" to nighttime use only, whereas those with more significant acute stenosis may require constant use.

Macrostoma

In some patients, the tracheostoma may be naturally large (macrostoma) or it may be caused by tracheomalacia. If macrostoma exists, the tracheostoma may be too large for the patient to achieve airtight occlusion for speech production with a finger or thumb. Surgical stoma reduction is one solution to this problem. Another involves a tracheostoma breathing valve housing used with a hands-free valve or with digital occlusion. In 1982, Blom, Singer, and Hamaker introduced the tracheostoma breathing valve to be used for hands-free TE voice production. The patient is taught to attach the TE breathing valve housing to the peristomal skin with adhesive, occlude the entrance of the housing with a thumb or finger, or insert and use a hands-free tracheostoma valve.

Insufficient Duration of Tracheostoma Valve Seal

When placed over the tracheostoma, the tracheostoma breathing valve closes with forced expiration, causing occlusion of the tracheostoma, and thus eliminating the need for the patient to use digital tracheostoma occlusion. A decade after the introduction of the original breathing valve, the adjustable tracheostoma valve (ATV) was introduced (see Blom, 1998). This newer valve may be adjusted for relaxed quiet breathing, normal phonation, or routine physical exercise, thus eliminating the need to change pressure-sensitive diaphragms of different thicknesses (and varied pressure sensitivities). The adjustment for the newer ATV is achieved by rotating the faceplate of the valve assembly, which incorporates a cam that pushes the valve diaphragm to varying degrees of closure.

The ATV consists of two components: (a) the tracheostoma housing that attaches to the peristomal skin with adhesive and two-sided tape and (b) the valve body, which inserts into and is easily removed from the housing when necessary. A similar device marketed by Bivona uses interchangeable springs of varying resistances to provide the user with a preselected sensitivity for valve diaphragm closure. This device also utilizes a tracheostomal tape housing. Unfortunately, not all laryngectomized individuals who attempt to use a tracheostoma valve on a regular basis are successful (Doyle, 1994). Success has been defined as continuous use of the tracheostoma valve during a 12- to 15-hour day. Failure of the hands-free device is almost always due to the premature failure of the adhesive seal that attaches the device to the peristomal skin and subsequent leakage. Deterrents to a durable seal are numerous and can occur alone or in any combination (Grolman et al., 1995).

Failure of the Tracheostoma Breathing Valve

Once careless application of the adhesive is ruled out, the most common cause for failure of the adhesive seal is excessive intratracheal pressure. This problem is a result of resistance to airflow through a valved voice prosthesis, the TE vocal tract, or a combination of both (Blom et al., 1998; Weinberg, Horii, Blom, & Singer, 1982). This back pressure pushes the tracheostoma housing adhesive loose from behind the seal, causing air leakage that can only be repaired durably by completely replacing the seal from the start.

Initially, the majority of TE speakers may attempt to speak too loudly and with unnecessary effort, which contributes to the problem of shortened valve seal duration. In therapy, patients can be instructed on how to reduce vocal effort and loudness through variation of production. With direction and practice, they eventually learn to recognize how just the right amount of pressure "sounds" and "feels" to maintain a durable seal and generate voicing (Doyle, 1994).

Direct assessment during TE speech production using a pressure meter is also an option. A manometer reading of 25 to 40 cm H_2O is considered acceptable, with higher levels contributing to a proportionally shorter seal duration because of this excessive back pressure. The patient may also use the meter as a biofeedback tool to ascertain correct vocal intensity and pressure (Blom et al., 1998).

Other Variables Influencing Tracheostoma Breathing Valve Use

Prosthetic variables must also be considered when dealing with tracheostoma breathing valve back pressure. If a patient is using a Blom–Singer duckbill voice prosthesis, switching to a low-pressure model may reduce resistance. This, in turn, may help to reduce back pressure. Similarly, the use of a 20-Fr voice prosthesis instead of a 16-Fr device may also reduce resistance and effort. One can determine whether a 20-Fr voice prosthesis would be beneficial in reducing back pressure by simply removing the smaller diameter voice prosthesis and having the patient voice with an open tract, which simulates the wider diameter pathway. Pharyngeal constrictor muscle hypertonicity may also contribute to reducing seal duration. This problem and its solutions have been discussed previously in this chapter.

Mucus production is also an important issue in the success of tracheostoma valve use. Bypassing of the upper airway places the burden of humidification on the lower airway. The increase in phlegm production is a response of the pulmonary system in an effort to compensate for the loss of heat, moisture, and filtration associated with tracheostomal breathing (see Chapter 20 in this text). This copious mucus production makes use of the tracheostoma breathing valve more inconvenient and difficult. When phlegm is inadequately wiped away from the tracheostoma after coughing, it can rapidly dissolve the adhesive seal of the TE breathing valve housing. Thus, the clinician should instruct the patient to remove the valve prior to coughing whenever possible, and then wipe the secretions carefully from the inside surface of the valve housing before reinserting the valve.

A final cause of failure of a durable tracheostoma valve seal is a tracheostoma that is deeply recessed by the sternocleidomastoid muscle. This last problem can be eliminated with a custom housing for the tracheostoma breathing valve (Cantu, Shagets, Fifer, Andres, & Newton, 1986; Doyle, Grantmyre, & Myers, 1989), nonsurgical management (Lewin, 2004), or a bilateral division of the sternocleidomastoid muscle on nonirradiated patients (Blom & Hamaker, 1996). Heat and moisture exchange (HME) systems specifically designed for use by laryngectomized individuals to reduce excessive mucus are commercially available (see Chapter 20 in this text). These devices include the Blom–Singer Humidifilter and the Provox Stomafilter System. A minimum trial use of 7 days is usually necessary for the patient to experience the benefits of an HME system (Grolman, Blom, Branson, Schouwenburg, & Hamaker, 1997; Hilgers, Aaronson, Ackerstaff, Schouwenburg, & Zandwijk, 1989; Hilgers, Ackerstaff, Balm, & Gregor, 1996).

Granuloma

Granuloma formation is generally believed to be a foreign body response to the presence of the voice prosthesis in the tracheostoma region and is most often seen at the tracheal entrance of the TEP site. It has the appearance of a circumferential thickening, or "doughnut." If the granuloma becomes thick enough, it can make insertion of the voice prosthesis painful and difficult. Granulation tissue thickness may also increase the length of the TE tract, and a longer voice prosthesis may be required to keep the tract open. Failure to resize the voice prosthesis usually results in effortful phonation or dysphonia as the unstented esophageal side of the TEP tract slowly closes and may eventually close completely. Another possible cause of granulation tissue formation is inflammation from infrequent removal of the voice prosthesis. If the patient is wearing an indwelling voice prosthesis, he or she should change it more frequently or wear a self-changing model.

Removal of the granulation tissue is often done by the physician as an office procedure. The granuloma is removed by first injecting it circumferentially with 1% lidocaine with epinephrine. After adequate time for hemostasis, the prosthesis is removed, and a red rubber catheter is inserted to prevent aspiration. The granuloma is then grasped with a hemostat and removed circumferentially with sharp scissors. Silver nitrate or electrocautery is used to cauterize the excision area. The catheter remains in place for 24 to 48 hours, after which the TEP tract is resized and a new voice prosthesis is inserted (Blom & Hamaker, 1996).

Excessive Gastric Air

The most common cause of excessive gastric air, an infrequent but nevertheless irritating problem, is air being drawn through a low-pressure voice prosthesis during inspiration. Increased negative pressure within the esophagus during inspiration creates a vacuum that opens the flap valve, allowing air to enter the esophagus. The problem may be confirmed by looking directly into the prosthesis in situ with a bright light while the patient breathes. The solution is to replace the low-pressure voice prosthesis with one of higher resistance, such as a duckbill device. If the patient's esophagus is too narrow to accommodate a duckbill model, a custom-modified, high-resistance flap valve can be ordered from the prosthesis manufacturer.

Another possible cause of excessive gastric air is pharyngeal constrictor muscle hypertonicity. Airflow distention of the esophagus during TE voice production may cause contraction of the pharyngeal constrictor muscles. This contraction results in increased resistance of the PE segment, with air being driven in the reverse direction into the stomach during attempts at voicing, as well as leading to effortful voice production. If a related problem of flatulence or increased phonatory effort is significant, unilateral pharyngeal constrictor myotomy or Botox injection into the constrictor muscles may eliminate the problem (see Chapter 21 in this text).

A hypotonic PE segment may also produce excessive flatulence. In this case, air is unintentionally exchanged in and out of the esophagus simultaneously with each respiratory cycle. As a result, the patient's TE voice quality is breathy and weak. An elastic band worn around the neck directly above the stoma will slightly constrict the PE segment tissue and simultaneously improve voice quality, while also decreasing air ingestion.

Finally, marked esophageal stricture above the level of the voice prosthesis may also restrict and reverse airflow into the stomach. Stricture is managed by mechanical dilation or surgical reconstruction. If none of these causes is found to be present, the patient may suffer from some form of gastrointestinal dysfunction and should be referred to a gastroenterologist for evaluation.

Poor Speech Quality

If the patient has undergone pharyngoesophageal reconstruction with gastric pull-up or jejunal interposition (see Chapter 12 in this text), the PE segment may be hypotonic and the TE voice weak and breathy. Vocal quality may be improved by slightly constricting the pharyngeal muscles of the neck directly above the stoma. There are various methods of accomplishing this goal. First, the patient could wear a comfortably tight elastic band around the neck directly above the stoma. Another alternative would be to forego use of the tracheostoma breathing valve and use manual stomal occlusion, with a slight increase in digital coverage of the stoma and associated closure pressure. Lowering the chin or slightly altering the head position to either side may also increase vocal quality.

If the PE segment is hypertonic or has poor vibratory elasticity, TE voice can sound strained or forced, or be of short duration. In this case, the clinician should work with the patient to reduce effort during voice production. If the patient is using a duckbill or 16-Fr voice prosthesis, he or she should change to a low-pressure 20-Fr prosthesis to reduce resistance and increase airflow. The patient should be retrained to use light stomal occlusion, to alter muscle tone, and to focus production "lower in the throat." If vocal quality improves but speech production remains short in phrase level, the patient needs to reduce respiratory effort. Finally, if the patient continues to produce a strained, high-pitch voice of limited duration, the clinician should provide further evaluation for possible PE segment hypertonicity or spasm.

SUMMARY

The purpose of this chapter has been to address the most common problems encountered by clinicians working with TEP voice restoration. Although TEP voice restoration has proven to be an important rehabilitation option following total laryngectomy, problems with its use still arise. The solutions to such problems are varied and often require the combined cooperation of the speech–language pathologist, the physician, and the patient to achieve maximum success. In most instances, however, careful, systematic evaluation of the problem is best guided by a thorough knowledge of the surgical procedure, anatomy and physiology, the design and structure of the voice prosthesis and its use, and an understanding of the patient's needs.

REFERENCES

Blitzer, A., Komisar, A., Baredes, S., Brin J. F., & Stewart, C. (1995). Voice failure after tracheoesophageal puncture: Management with botulinum toxin. *Otolaryngology—Head and Neck Surgery, 113,* 668–670.

Blom, E. D. (1986, November). *Tracheoesophageal puncture: Problems and solutions.* Paper presented at the annual meeting of the American-Speech-Language-Hearing Association, Detroit, MI.

Blom, E. D. (1988). Tracheoesophageal valves: Problems, solutions, and directions for the future. *Head and Neck Surgery, 10* (Suppl. 2), 142–145.

Blom, E. D. (1998). Tracheostoma valve fitting and instruction. In E. D. Blom, M. I. Singer, & R. C. Hamaker (Eds.), *Tracheoesophageal voice restoration following total laryngectomy* (pp. 103–108). San Diego, CA: Singular.

Blom, E. D., & Hamaker, R. C. (1996). Tracheoesophageal voice restoration following total laryngectomy. In E. N. Myers & J. Suen (Eds.), *Cancer of head and neck* (pp. 839–852). Philadelphia: Saunders.

Blom, E. D., Singer, M. I., & Hamaker, R. C. (1982). Tracheostoma valve for postlaryngectomy voice rehabilitation. *Annals of Otology, Rhinology and Laryngology, 91,* 576–578.

Blom, E. D., Singer, M. I., & Hamaker, R. C. (1986). A prospective study of tracheoesophageal speech. *Archives of Otolaryngology—Head and Neck Surgery, 112,* 440–447.

Blom, E. D., Singer, M. I., & Hamaker, R. C. (1998). *Tracheoesophageal voice restoration following total laryngectomy.* San Diego, CA: Singular.

Busscher, H. J., & van der Mei, H. C. (1998). Biofilm formation and its prevention on silicone rubber voice prostheses. In E. D. Blom, M. I. Singer, & R. C. Hamaker (Eds.), *Tracheoesophageal voice restoration following total laryngectomy* (pp. 89–102). San Diego, CA: Singular.

Cantu, E., Shagets, F. W., Fifer, R. C., Andres, C. J., & Newton, A. D. (1986). Customized valve housing. *Laryngoscope, 96,* 1159–1163.

Cheesman, A. D., Knight, J., McIvor, J., & Perry, A. (1986). Tracheoesophageal "puncture speech" an assessment technique for failed esophageal speakers. *Journal of Laryngology and Otology, 100,* 191–199.

Delsuphe, K., Zink, I., Lajaegere, M., & Delaere, P. (1998). Prospective randomized comparative study of tracheoesophageal voice prosthesis: Blom–Singer versus Provox. *Laryngoscope, 108,* 1561–1565.

Doyle, P. C. (1985). Another perspective on esophageal insufflation testing. *Journal of Speech and Hearing Disorders, 50,* 408–409.

Doyle, P. C. (1994). *Foundations of voice and speech rehabilitation following laryngeal cancer.* San Diego, CA: Singular.

Doyle, P. C., Grantmyre, A., & Myers, C. (1989). Clinical modification of the tracheostoma breathing valve for voice restoration. *Journal of Speech and Hearing Disorders, 54,* 189–192.

Geraghty, J. A., Smith, B. E., Wenig, B. L., & Portugal, L. G. (1996). Long-term follow-up of tracheoesophageal puncture results. *Annals of Otology, Rhinology and Laryngology, 105,* 501–503.

Gress, C. D. (2000, January 27–28). *Trouble-shooting guide,* [Laryngectomy Rehabilitation Course], University of California–San Francisco Cancer Center, The Voice Center, San Francisco.

Grolman, W., Blom, E. D., Branson, R. D., Schouwenburg, P. F., & Hamaker, R. C. (1997). An efficiency comparison of four heat and moisture exchanges in the laryngectomized patient. *Laryngoscope, 107,* 814–820.

Grolman, W., Schouwenburg, P. F., de Boer, M. F., Knegt, P. P., Spoelstra, H. A. A., & Meeuwis, C. A. (1995). First results with the Blom–Singer adjustable tracheostoma valve. *ORL—Head and Neck Nursing, 57,* 165–170.

Hamaker, R. C., & Blom, E. D. (2003). Botulinum neurotoxin for pharyngeal constrictor muscle spasm in tracheoesophageal voice restoration. *Laryngoscope, 113,* 1479–1482.

Hamaker, R. C., Singer, M. I., Blom, E. D., & Daniels, H. A. (1985). Primary voice restoration at laryngectomy. *Archives of Otolaryngology, 111,* 182–186.

Hilgers, F. J. M., Aaronson, N. K., Ackerstaff, A. H., Schouwenburg, P. F., & Zandwijk, N. V. (1989). The influence of a heat and moisture exchanger (HME) on the respiratory symptoms after total laryngectomy. *Clinical Otolaryngology, 16,* 152–156.

Hilgers, F. J. M., Ackerstaff, A. H., Balm, A. J. M., & Gregor, R. T. (1996). A new heat and moisture exchanger with speech valve (Provox stomafilter). *Clinical Otolaryngology, 21,* 414–418.

Hilgers, F. J. M., Ackerstaff, A. H., van As, C. J., Balm, A. J., van den Brekel, M. W., & Tan, I. B. (2003). Development and clinical assessment of a heat and moisture exchanger with a multi-magnet automatic tracheostoma valve (Provox FreeHands HME) for vocal and pulmonary rehabilitation after total laryngectomy. *Acta Otolaryngologica, 123,* 91–99.

Hoffman, H. T., Fischer, H., Van Demark, D., Peterson, K. L., McCullough, T. M., Karnell, L. H., & Funk, G. F. (1997). Botulinum neurotoxin injection after total laryngectomy. *Head & Neck, 19,* 92–97.

Izdebski, K., Reed, C. G, Ross, J. C., & Hilsinger, R. L. (1994). Problems with tracheoesophageal fistula voice restoration in totally laryngectomized patients. *Archives of Otolaryngology—Head and Neck Surgery, 120,* 840–845.

Izdebski, K., Ross, J. C., & Lee, S. (1987). Fungal colonization of tracheoesophageal voice prostheses. *Laryngoscope, 97,* 594–597.

Kao, W. F., Mohr, R. M., Kimmel, C. A., Getch, C., & Silverman, C. (1994). The outcome and techniques of primary and secondary tracheoesophageal puncture. *Archives of Otolaryngology—Head and Neck Surgery, 120,* 301–307.

Leder, S. B., & Erskine, M. C. (1997). Voice restoration after laryngectomy: Experience with the Blom–Singer extended-wear indwelling tracheoesophageal voice prosthesis. *Head & Neck, 19,* 487–493.

Lewin, J. S. (2004). Nonsurgical management of the stoma to maximize tracheoesophageal speech. *Otolaryngology Clinics of North America, 37,* 585–596.

Mahieu, H. F., van Saene, J. J. M., den Besten, J., & van Saene, H. K. F. (1986). Oropharynx decontamination preventing Candida vegetation on voice prostheses. *Archives of Otolaryngology—Head and Neck Surgery, 112,* 1090–1092.

Mahieu, H. F., van Saene, H. K. F., Rosingh, H. J., & Schutte, H. K. (1986). Candida vegetations on silicone voice prostheses. *Archives of Otolaryngology—Head and Neck Surgery, 112,* 321–325.

McIvor, J., Evans, P. F., Perry, A., & Cheesman, A. D. (1990). Radiological assessment of post-laryngectomy speech. *Clinical Radiology, 41,* 312–316.

Perry, A., & Edels, Y. (1985). Recent advances in the assessment of failed esophageal speakers. *British Journal of Disorders of Communication, 20,* 229–236.

Ramachandran, K., Arunachalam, P. S., Hurren, A., Marsh, R. L., & Samuel, P. R. (2003). Botulinum toxin injection for failed tracheo-oesophageal voice in laryngectomees: The Sunderland experience. *Journal of Laryngology and Otology, 117,* 544–548.

Singer, M. I. (1983). Tracheoesophageal speech: Voice rehabilitation after total laryngectomy. *Laryngoscope, 93,* 1454–1465

Singer, M. I. (2004). The development of successful tracheoesophageal voice restoration. *Otolaryngology Clinics of North America, 37,* 507–517.

Singer, M. I., & Blom, E. D. (1980). An endoscopic technique for restoration of voice after laryngectomy. *Annals of Otology, Rhinology and Laryngology, 89,* 529–533.

Singer, M. I., & Blom, E. D. (1981a). Further experience with voice restoration after total laryngectomy. *Annals of Otology, Rhinology and Laryngology, 90,* 498–502.

Singer, M. I., & Blom, E. D. (1981b). Selective myotomy for voice restoration after total laryngectomy. *Archives of Otolaryngology, 107,* 670–673.

Singer, M. I., Blom, E. D., & Hamaker, R. C. (1986). Pharyngeal plexus neurectomy for alaryngeal speech rehabilitation. *Laryngoscope, 96,* 50–53.

Singer, M. I., Hamaker, R. C., & Blom, E. D. (1989). Revision procedure for tracheoesophageal puncture. *Laryngoscope, 99,* 761–763.

Sloan, P. M., Griffin, J. M., & O'Dwyer, T. P. (1991). Esophageal insufflation and videofluoroscopy for evaluation of esophageal speech in laryngectomy patients: Clinical implications. *Radiology, 181,* 433–437.

Stafford, F. W. (2003). Current indications and complications of tracheoesophageal puncture for voice restoration after laryngectomy. *Current Opinion in Otolaryngology—Head and Neck Surgery, 11,* 89–95.

Terrel, J. E., Lewin, J. S., & Esclamado, R. (1995). Botulinum injection for postlaryngectomy tracheoesophageal speech failure. *Otolaryngology—Head and Neck Surgery, 113,* 788–791.

Weinberg, B., Horii, Y., Blom, E. D., & Singer, M. I. (1982). Airway resistance during esophageal phonation. *Journal of Speech and Hearing Disorders, 47,* 194–199.

Chapter 20

Respiratory Consequences of Total Laryngectomy and the Need for Pulmonary Protection and Rehabilitation

Frans J. M. Hilgers and Annemieke H. Ackerstaff

Total laryngectomy not only results in the loss of the normal voice, but also causes a wide range of physical and psychosocial changes, including respiratory complaints, sleep disturbances, feelings of fatigue and malaise, and diminished social contacts (Ackerstaff, Hilgers, Aaronson, & Balm, 1994; Hilgers, Ackerstaff, Aaronson, Schouwenburg, & van Zandwijk, 1990; see also Chapter 28 in this text). In contrast to the impact on voicing (Schuster et al., 2004; Stafford, 2003), the changes in pulmonary physiology after laryngectomy have been given relatively little attention in the literature. Due to the elimination of the air-conditioning functions (warming, humidifying, and filtering of inhaled air) of the upper airway, many laryngectomized patients suffer from respiratory symptoms, including coughing, excessive sputum production, crusting, and short-ness of breath (Harris & Jonson, 1974; Natvig, 1984b; Todisco, Maurizi, Paludetti, Dottorini, & Merante, 1984; Togawa, Konno, & Hoshino, 1980; Torjussen, 1968; Usui, 1979). Natvig (1984a) pointed to seasonal fluctuations in the prevalence of these problems; laryngectomized patients have fewer respiratory problems during the summer than during the winter period. Sputum production tends to increase during the first half year following surgery and then seems to stabilize (Harris & Jonson, 1974). An additional aspect of excessive sputum production is that it may impair vocalization (Mendelsohn, Morris, & Gallagher, 1993).

To clear the airway of secretions and sputum, effective coughing is vital. The laryngectomized patient has to acquire a technique to improve the effect of his or her coughing. Due to the loss of the function of the glottis, the effectiveness of coughing is considerably decreased (Harris & Jonson, 1974). Murty, Smith, and Lancaster (1991) stated that the explosive initial "spike," referred to as a supra-maximal expiratory flow, is absent in the laryngectomized patient. In a study by Jay, Ruddy, and Cullen (1991), 54% of patients complained of an increased fre-quency of chest infections, probably due to direct exposure of the lower respira-tory tract to infective agents that normally result in infection of the upper res-piratory tract. As a result, a statistically significant impairment of the overall pulmonary function parameters of laryngectomized patients was observed 1 year after total laryngectomy (Todisco et al., 1984). Additional common complaints after total laryngectomy are shortness of breath (Gilchrist, 1973; Jones, Lund, Howard, Greenberg, & McCarthy, 1992; Stell & McCormick, 1985; Torjussen, 1968) and nasal discharge (Jay et al., 1991; Moore-Gillon, 1985).

THE TRACHEOSTOMA: THE DOMINATING PROBLEM

Patients often have different views on the impact and disadvantages of a surgical procedure than those expected by medical professionals. A striking example of this phenomenon comes from the study by Mohide, Archibald, Tew, Young, and Haines (1992). These authors described a study in which rankings were applied to the severity of the various side effects of total laryngectomy. The actual rank-ings given by patients were compared to the rankings that clinicians thought the patients would apply. Several striking, significant differences were observed. Whereas clinicians expected that patients would judge the loss of the normal voice as the most severe consequence of the surgery, patients ranked the physical consequences—that is, the frequent sputum and phlegm production from the stoma and the interference of this with their social activities—as the two most important negative consequences of the total laryngectomy. Thus, changes to the airway are judged to pose significant limitations to these patients.

PHYSIOLOGICAL AND MORPHOLOGICAL EFFECTS OF STOMA BREATHING

The removal of the larynx has obvious and significant repercussions for the respiratory system (schematically shown in Figure 20.1) and the individual. Due to the separation of the upper and lower airways, the breathing air no longer passes through the upper respiratory tract, precluding its normal warming, humidifying, and filtering (Harris & Jonson, 1974; Todisco et al., 1984; Togawa et al., 1980; Torjussen, 1968; Usui, 1979). Obviously, this change will have unfavorable effects on the lower airways, such as irritation of the tracheobronchial mucosa, excessive sputum production, crusting, and coughing (Hilgers et al., 1990; Pruyn et al., 1986).

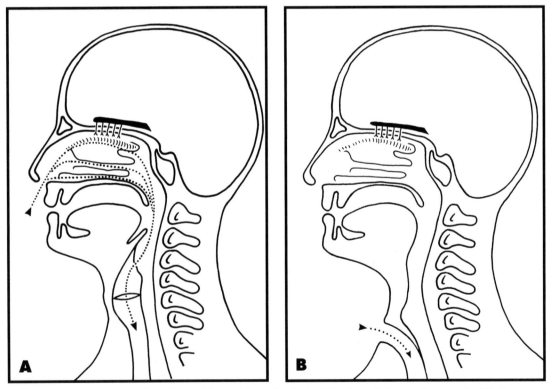

FIGURE 20.1. (A) Normal nasal breathing with optimal conditioning of the respiratory air. (B) Stoma breathing with loss of upper respiratory tract air conditioning, filtering, and airflow resistance.

Extensive histologic changes, such as squamous metaplasia of the respiratory ciliary epithelium and chronic inflammatory changes of the lamina propria, have been observed after total laryngectomy in the trachea at the level of the carina (Griffith & Friedberg, 1964; Roessler, Grossenbacher, & Walt, 1988). Furthermore, in a small series of patients, a progressive bronchial obstruction and bacteriological infection of the tracheobronchial tree during the first postoperative year was demonstrated (Todisco et al., 1984), eventually causing permanent disturbances in pulmonary function (Ackerstaff, Hilgers, Balm, & van Zandwijk, 1995; Ackerstaff, Hilgers, Meeuwis, Knegt, & Weenink, 1999; Hess, Schwenk, Frank, & Loddenkemper, 1999). In addition, changes in the pulmonary physiology have also been reported, with a decrease of the pressure gradient between the alveoli and the trachea. A change in pressure gradient leads to a shift of the equal pressure point toward the more peripheral, smaller airway region, resulting in suboptimal intrapulmonary gas exchange (Togawa et al., 1980). Consequently, many laryngectomized patients suffer from respiratory problems, including coughing, excessive sputum production, and shortness of breath (Hilgers et al., 1990).

As already mentioned, these symptoms develop and increase during the first 6 to 12 months postoperatively and tend to stabilize over the next year (Ackerstaff, Hilgers, Aaronson, et al., 1995; Ackerstaff, Hilgers, Balm, & van Zandwijk, 1995; Harris & Jonson, 1974). An objective impairment of the pulmonary function of the laryngectomized patient can also be expected (Ackerstaff, Hilgers, Balm, & van Zandwijk, 1995). The already mentioned seasonal fluctuations in symptoms, with patients reporting fewer respiratory problems during the summer than during the winter months (Natvig, 1984b), were confirmed in several of our studies (Ackerstaff, Hilgers, Aaronson, Balm, & van Zandwijk, 1993; Hilgers et al., 1990). Moreover, significant correlations were found between respiratory symptoms and the perceived quality of voice, aspects of daily life, and anxiety and depression (Hilgers et al., 1990; see also Chapters 5 and 28 in this text).

With regard to respiratory complaints, coughing was significantly related only to fatigue, whereas sputum production and breathlessness were found to be associated with a much wider range of physical and psychosocial problems, including voice quality, fatigue, sleeping problems, and depression. With regard to voice quality, there was a significant correlation with fatigue, depression, and social contacts. Significant correlations between stoma size and respiratory symptoms have not been noted in the literature (Gregor & Hassman, 1984; Natvig, 1984b).

PULMONARY FUNCTION ASSESSMENT

In the literature, objective information on the respiratory condition in the person who has been laryngectomized, as assessed in the pulmonary function laboratory, is scarce (Davidson, Hayward, Pounsford, & Saunders, 1986; Gardner & Meah,

1989; Gregor & Hassman, 1984; Harris & Jonson, 1974; Todisco et al., 1984; Togawa et al., 1980). Traditionally, the assessment of pulmonary function in these patients has been performed by means of a cuffed trachea cannula (see Figure 20.2), connected to a pulmonary function analyzer (Harris & Jonson, 1974; Todisco et al., 1984). The use of a cannula, however, is troublesome for two reasons. First, its insertion is often an unpleasant experience for the patient and leads to uncomfortable coughing, sometimes lasting for several minutes. Spraying of a local anesthetic does not completely solve this problem, as it often initiates a coughing fit. More important, the use of a cuffed cannula is considered to have a negative influence on the results of forced expiration and inspiration tests by decreasing the actual diameter of the trachea (Togawa et al., 1980). Some authors have used extratracheal devices, such as specially constructed "mouthpieces" to avoid this problem (Davidson et al., 1986; Gardner & Meah, 1989; Gregor & Hassman, 1984). Also, trachea masks, manually placed over the stoma, have been used for this reason (Togawa et al., 1980).

Easy, comfortable, and standardized pulmonary function assessment can be achieved with an extratracheal connection of the patient with the pulmonary function equipment by means of a commercially available base holder of a heat and moisture exchanger (HME) (see Figure 20.3) (Ackerstaff, Souren, van Zandwijk, Balm, & Hilgers, 1993). For this purpose, other extratracheal base holders (e.g., for tracheostoma valves) can be used. The test results obtained using the HME base holder give a more accurate representation of the actual lung function of these patients. An example of the differences in the flow–volume

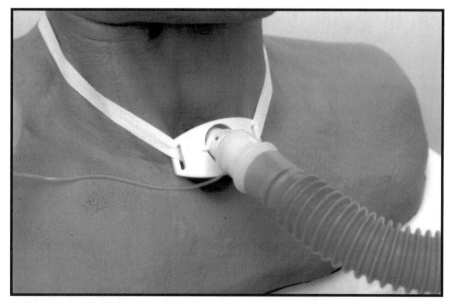

FIGURE 20.2. Traditional method of postlaryngectomy pulmonary function assessment with cuffed trachea cannula (here demonstrated in a dummy).

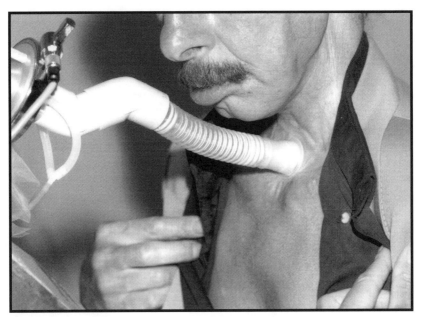

FIGURE 20.3. Postlaryngectomy pulmonary function assessment, as it should be carried out, by means of an extratracheal device, such as the easily obtainable commercial base holders of heat and moisture exchangers or tracheostoma valves.

loops between the extratracheal device and a cuffed cannula clearly shows the inadequacy of the latter method (see Figure 20.4).

HEAT AND MOISTURE EXCHANGERS AND PULMONARY REHABILITATION

HMEs have been in clinical use for many years (UK Departments of Health and Social Security, 1987). The principle on which HMEs are based is the exchange of heat and moisture between a gas and a surface over which it flows. Expired gas may be assumed to be saturated with water vapor at the temperature at which it leaves the respiratory tract. If the humid gas then comes into contact with a surface at a lower temperature, the gas is cooled, the surface is warmed, and condensation of some of the vapor onto the surface occurs. The extent of deposition depends on the magnitude of the fall in gas temperature. After exhalation has ceased and inspiration begins once again, gas at an ambient temperature comes into contact with the same surface and, being dry by comparison, is able to take up as vapor some of the water previously deposited. Air is also warmed as it passes over the surface of the HME. Hence, a proportion of both the heat and the water from the exhaled air has been transferred to the inspired gas, thereby reducing the extent to which water would otherwise be drawn from the mucosa of

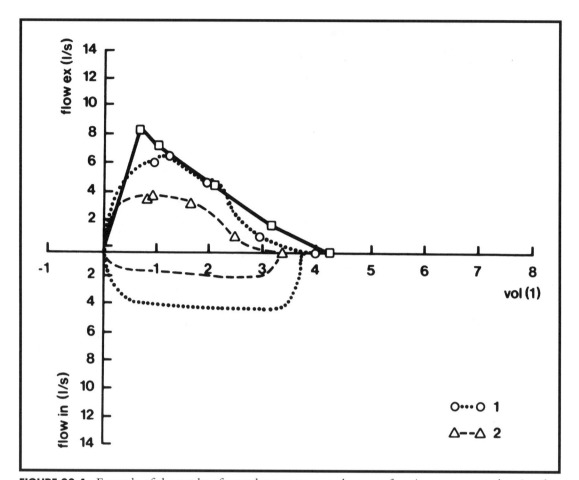

FIGURE 20.4. Example of the results of a postlaryngectomy pulmonary function assessment, showing the flow–volume loops obtained with a cuffed trachea cannula (inner curves, dotted lines) and with an extra-tracheal base holder (outer curves, dashed lines). The continuous line above the *x*-axis represents the expected expiratory flow (matched for age, gender, height, and ethnic group). The values obtained with a cuffed cannula are significantly low. *Note.* From "Improvements in the Assessment of Pulmonary Function in Laryngectomized Patients," by A. H. Ackerstaff, T. Souren, N. van Zandwijk, A. J. M. Balm, and F. J. M. Hilgers, 1993, *Laryngoscope, 103,* pp. 1391–1394. Copyright 1993 by Lippincott, Williams & Wilkins. Reprinted with permission.

the respiratory tract. In this way, the tendency toward drying of the respiratory mucosa is reduced and, in turn, because of the reduced need for vaporization at the mucosal surface, less heat is lost. The use of an HME also restores, to some extent, the airway resistance (Ogura & Harvey, 1971), which is needed for adequate pulmonary function; that is, by adding the HME at the tracheostoma, a "resistance" to airflow is provided, and this permits increased inhalatory volume. Additionally, hands-free devices continue to be modified with good success (Hilgers, Ackerstaff, van As, et al., 2003).

These HME properties seem useful in the (partial) restoration of the loss of the air conditioning and resistance function of the upper respiratory tract in laryngectomized patients. It also can be shown that HMEs form an effective, nonpharmaceutical treatment option for pulmonary problems experienced by laryngectomized patients. In several studies the positive influence of regular HME use was clearly demonstrated subjectively and objectively (Ackerstaff, Hilgers, et al., 1993; Ackerstaff, Hilgers, Aaronson, et al., 1995; Hilgers, Aaronson, Ackerstaff, Schouwenburg, & van Zandwijk, 1991). After a trial period of only 6 weeks, respiratory problems diminished, indicating recovery of the tracheobronchial mucosa. In addition, several related physical and psychosocial factors were noted to improve. Significant reductions in the incidence of coughing, mean daily frequency of sputum production, forced expectoration, and stoma cleaning were observed. Significant reductions were also found in the perception of shortness of breath, feelings of fatigue and malaise, sleep problems, and levels of anxiety and depression.

Interestingly, the decrease in sputum production was also correlated with positive changes in the quality of voice as reported by the patients, and this was found to be statistically significant (Ackerstaff, Hilgers, et al., 1993; Ackerstaff, Hilgers, Balm, & Tan, 1998). Additionally, an early postoperative start (i.e., as soon as wounds were healed sufficiently, in general after 2 weeks) using an HME to some extent appeared to prevent the development of pulmonary complaints by patients (Ackerstaff, Hilgers, Aaronson, et al., 1995). Pulmonary rehabilitation could be objectively demonstrated by a significant increase in inspiratory flow–volume values (Ackerstaff, Hilgers, et al., 1993), which is consistent with the recovery of the tracheobronchial mucosa. Other research of importance in this respect is that of McRae, Young, Hamilton, and Jones (1996), who showed that with use of an HME, the temperature and relative humidity in the trachea significantly increase; this increase is schematically shown in Figure 20.5. Furthermore, tissue oxygenation was shown to improve.

Another important figure to keep in mind is that laryngectomized patients lose in excess of approximately 500 ml of water by breathing through the stoma in comparison with normal nasal breathing. By using an HME, it is possible to retain 250 to 300 ml of this excessive water loss in the respiratory system (Toremalm, 1960). This finding alone serves to explain much of the decrease in sputum and coughing problems reported.

The results of these research projects indicate the benefits of starting HME use on the first postoperative day (see Figure 20.6). An early start has several important advantages, such as early airway protection and unobtrusive stoma coverage, easy adjustment to the airflow resistance of the filter, retention of substantial volumes of water, and the elimination of the need for a noisy external humidifier. Also, early familiarization with this device for pulmonary rehabilitation enables easier voicing despite the possibility of suboptimal healing of the tracheostoma.

Although HME use offers considerable advantages, the HMEs used in the previously mentioned studies also present some distinct problems. First, problems related to the adhesive, such as skin irritation, insufficient adhesion to the skin, loosening of the adhesive by coughing, forced expectoration, mucus production, and perspiration have been observed. Second, problems related to voicing

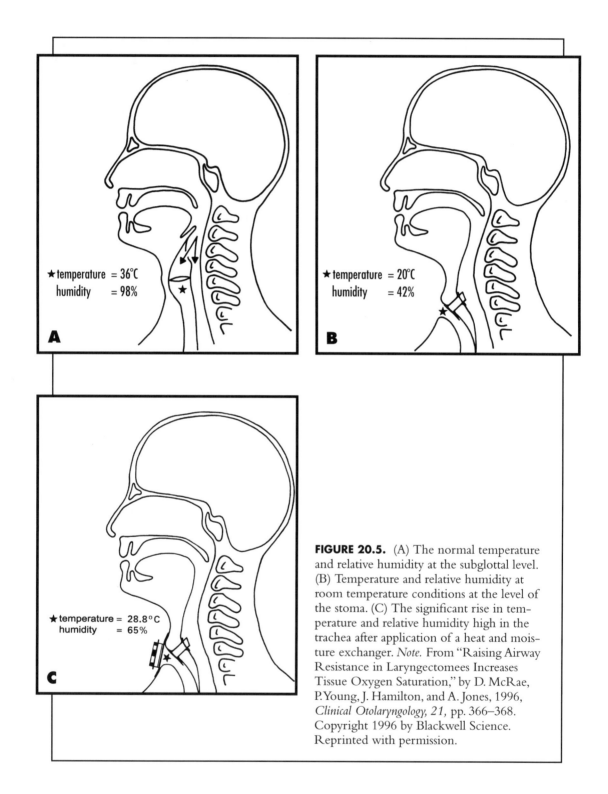

★ temperature = 36°C
humidity   = 98%

A

★ temperature = 20°C
humidity   = 42%

B

★ temperature = 28.8°C
humidity   = 65%

C

FIGURE 20.5. (A) The normal temperature and relative humidity at the subglottal level. (B) Temperature and relative humidity at room temperature conditions at the level of the stoma. (C) The significant rise in temperature and relative humidity high in the trachea after application of a heat and moisture exchanger. *Note.* From "Raising Airway Resistance in Laryngectomees Increases Tissue Oxygen Saturation," by D. McRae, P. Young, J. Hamilton, and A. Jones, 1996, *Clinical Otolaryngology, 21,* pp. 366–368. Copyright 1996 by Blackwell Science. Reprinted with permission.

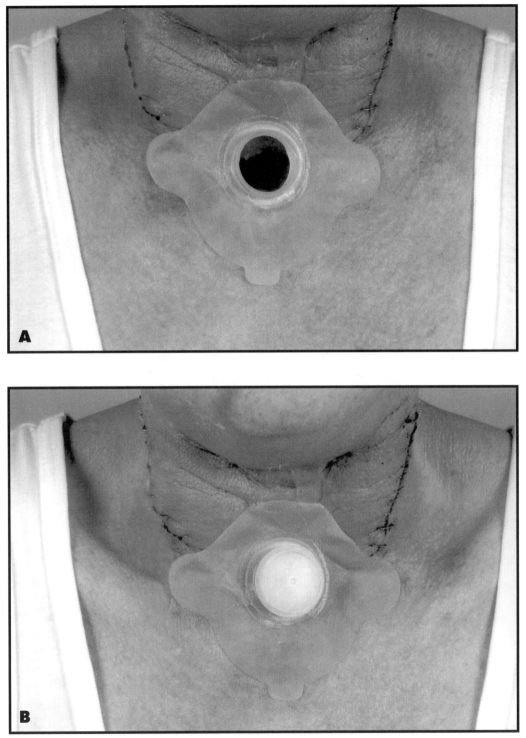

FIGURE 20.6. Early postoperative application of a heat and moisture exchanger. (A) The base holder has been applied over the stoma and the fresh suture line. (B) The cassette with the heat and moisture exchanger has been inserted. The availability of a colloid adhesive permits early postoperative use.

sometimes occur, as these early HMEs were developed before the widespread use of TE puncture voice prostheses. The design of these HMEs made airtight closure of the stoma difficult, therefore resulting in voicing problems (see Chapters 17 annd 19 in this text). Confronted with the choice between adequate pulmonary protection and optimal voicing, patients invariably choose the latter. In an attempt to solve these problems and consequently enhance the patient's compliance, a specialized valved HME, the Provox HME, was designed (Ackerstaff et al., 1998; Hilgers, Ackerstaff, Balm, & Gregor, 1996).[1]

The Provox HME device (Figure 20.7) has a disposable plastic housing, which is glued to the skin around the stoma by means of adhesive tape. The adhesion problems reported are diminished with the availability of three different types of adhesives in two sizes, which accommodate different skin types and anatomical situations. The actual HME filter-cassette, which is also disposable, contains a heat and moisture exchanging foam that is impregnated with $CaCl_2$. The device also contains a speech valve with a spring for airtight digital closure of the HME and, thus, the tracheostoma. The spring is intended to open the valve after release of finger pressure (see Figure 20.8).

The long-term compliance for patients using this Provox HME clearly improved relative to older devices (Ackerstaff et al., 1998). Patients were particularly positive about the special spring valve to facilitate airtight digital occlusion of the stoma for voicing. In 55% of the patients, Ackerstaff et al. noted that patients reported speech intelligibility to be improved. Problems observed with the earlier devices, such as skin adhesion difficulties, irritation, and handling of the device, were clearly diminished. As already mentioned, objectively measured improvement in voice characteristics could be demonstrated by a statistically significant increase in maximum phonation time and dynamic (intensity) range, and benefited 75% of patients (van As, Hilgers, Koopmans-van Beinum, & Ackerstaff, 1998). This means that, with the use of this dedicated HME system, voicing is improved not only by the earlier established reduction in respiratory problems experienced by the patient, but also by optimizing the stoma occlusion.

The hygienic handling of the stoma with these devices is another benefit. It is also likely that the efficiency of coughing for mucus clearance from the trachea is improved by deliberately closing and releasing the valve while coughing, thus imitating the explosive initial "spike" that is absent in laryngectomized patients (Murty et al., 1991). In this regard, counseling of the patient to improve understanding of the physiological effects and the practical aspects of these medical devices is of importance for optimal compliance; such counseling by the speech–language pathologist should be integrated in the pulmonary rehabilitation training program. Also, the use of HMEs on stoma valves, such as the Blom–Singer adjustable tracheostoma breathing valve (van den Hoogen, Meeuwis,

[1]Provox is a trademark owned by Atos Medical AB, P.O. Box 183, S-242 00 Hörby, Sweden. This company is also the manufacturer of the Provox HME system.

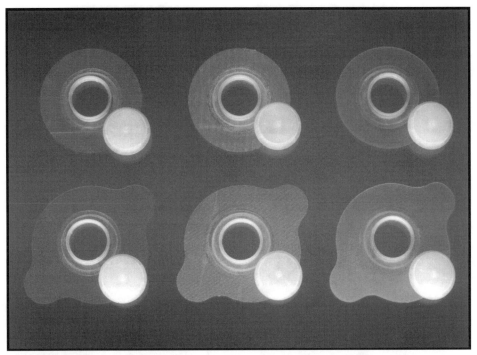

FIGURE 20.7. The Provox HME system, with three different adhesives in two sizes, to accommodate different skin types and stoma anatomy. *Note.* From "A New Heat and Moisture Exchanger with Speech Valve (Provox Stomafilter)," by F. J. M. Hilgers, A. H. Ackerstaff, A. J. M. Balm, and R. T. Gregor, 1996, *Clinical Otolaryngology, 21,* pp. 414–418. Copyright 1996 by Elsevier Science. Reprinted with permission.

Oudes, Janssen, & Manni, 1996), should be encouraged. From our own research data and those of others, we can conclude that pulmonary rehabilitation deserves special attention by those professionals who provide service to laryngectomized individuals, should be an integral part of the patient's rehabilitation program, and ultimately is seen to optimize total rehabilitation (Hilgers & Ackerstaff, 2000).

MEDICAL TREATMENT

Besides the application of HMEs to normalize (in part) the individual's pulmonary physiology, and thus treat postlaryngectomy respiratory problems, the observed decrease in pulmonary function values suggests that medical treatment also might be of benefit for a subgroup of laryngectomized patients. Several recent reports confirm this observation. Hess et al. (1999) suggested that 42% of the 59 laryngectomized individuals tested in their study might benefit from further medical treatment. As demonstrated by Hess et al. (1999) and in one of our earlier studies (Ackerstaff, Hilgers, Balm, & van Zandwijk, 1995), a positive effect of

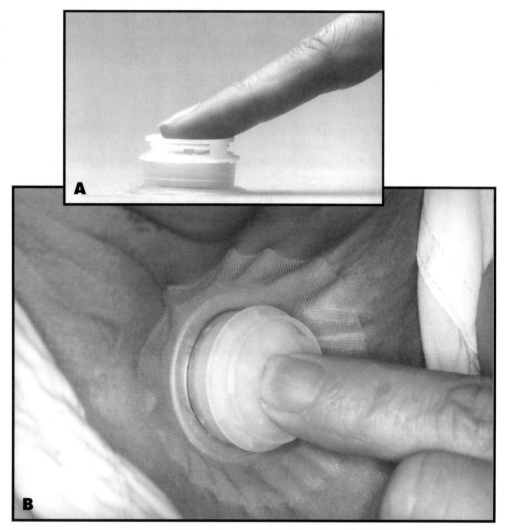

FIGURE 20.8. (A) The Provox HME with a speaking valve for easy digital occlusion of the stoma. A spring opens the valve after release of the finger pressure. (B) The Provox HME in position and closed with a finger. *Note.* Figure 20.8B is from "Comprehensive Rehabilitation After Total Laryngectomy Is More Than Voice Alone," by F. J. Hilgers and A. H. Ackerstaff, 2000, *Folia Phoniatrica and Logopaedia, 52,* pp. 65–73. Copyright 2000 by Karger. Reprinted with permission.

bronchodilator medication on the pulmonary function values was found for some patients.

Regular treatment with bronchodilators or anti-inflammatory medications, however, is only infrequently provided for our patient population. Furthermore, the optimal mode of application of the regularly prescribed inhalation drugs is not known. For example, metered dose inhalers, which deliver the aerosol particles in such a size and flow that oropharyngeal deposition is limited, probably are not optimal for direct tracheal inhalation. The use of a spacer might overcome this problem to some extent (see Figure 20.9) (Nakhla, 1997; Webber & Brown,

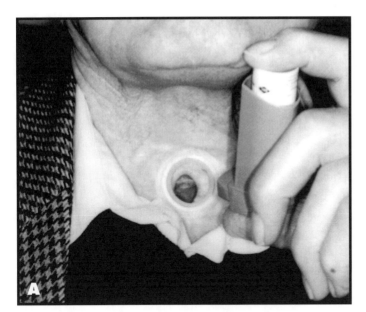

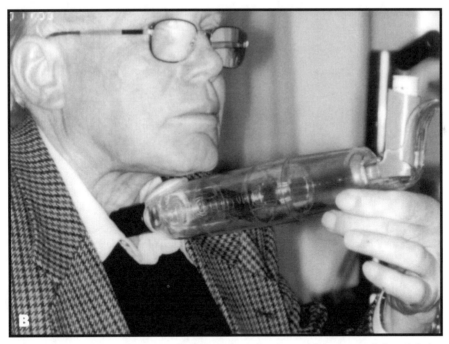

FIGURE 20.9. (A) Application of inhalation medication with a metered-dose inhalor directly in front of the stoma. (B) Application of inhalation medication with a spacer (Babyhaler, GlaxoWellcome) connected to the stoma by means of an adapter and an HME base holder.

1984). Further research into the role of medical treatment on the pulmonary complaints of the laryngectomized individual is clearly warranted in view of the aforementioned and frequently encountered impaired pulmonary function and the negative effects of these problems on quality of life. Studies on these topics continue in our institute (Hilgers et al., 2002; Op de Coul et al., 2000).

FUTURE DEVELOPMENTS

The effectiveness of HMEs for the reduction of respiratory problems of laryngectomized patients has been clearly established. If respiratory problems can be reduced, other physical and psychosocial problems may also be influenced in a positive manner. Hence, it is of utmost importance that patients have unrestricted access to these devices. For this to occur, full reimbursement by medical insurance is a prerequisite. At present, and based on the available clinical studies, it is encouraging that this has been achieved in several European countries, such as The Netherlands, Belgium, Germany, Scandinavia, Switzerland, and the United Kingdom. Not only are improvements in the availability of these devices encouraged, but further development related to the physical properties of the actual heat and moisture exchanging materials is also needed. According to McRae et al. (1996), the patient's airflow resistance cannot be fully restored; that is, patients tolerate only approximately 75% of the prelaryngectomy upper airway resistance (McRae et al., 1996). Thus, the size of these devices has some obvious limitations relative to airway resistance offered, as well as on decreasing their humidification effectiveness. Finally, as already mentioned, more insight in the role of additional medical treatment for the pulmonary rehabilitation of this patient population is needed, so that comprehensive postlaryngectomy rehabilitation can be achieved.

REFERENCES

Ackerstaff, A. H., Hilgers, F. J. M., Aaronson, N. K., & Balm, A. J. M. (1994). Communication, functional disorders and lifestyle changes after total laryngectomy. *Clinical Otolaryngology, 19,* 295–300.

Ackerstaff, A. H., Hilgers, F. J. M., Aaronson, N. K., Balm, A. J. M., & van Zandwijk, N. (1993). Improvements in respiratory and psychosocial functioning following total laryngectomy by the use of a heat and moisture exchanger. *Annals of Otology, Rhinology and Laryngology, 102,* 878–883.

Ackerstaff, A. H., Hilgers, F. J. M., Aaronson, N. K., de Boer, M. F., Meeuwis, C. A., Knegt, P. P. M., Spoelstra, H. A. A., van Zandwijk, N., & Balm, A. J. M. (1995). Heat and moisture exchangers as a treatment option in the post-operative rehabilitation of laryngectomized patients. *Clinical Otolaryngology, 20,* 504–509.

Ackerstaff, A. H., Hilgers, F. J. M., Balm, A. J. M., & Tan, I. B. (1998). Long-term compliance of laryngectomized patients with a specialized pulmonary rehabilitation device: Provox Stomafilter. *Laryngoscope, 108,* 257–260.

Ackerstaff, A. H., Hilgers, F. J. M., Balm, A. J. M., & van Zandwijk, N. (1995). Long-term pulmonary function after total laryngectomy. *Clinical Otolaryngology, 20,* 547–551.

Ackerstaff, A. H., Hilgers, F. J. M., Meeuwis, C. A., Knegt, P. P. M., & Weenink, C. (1999). Pulmonary function pre- and post-total laryngectomy. *Clinical Otolaryngology, 24,* 491–494.

Ackerstaff, A. H., Souren, T., van Zandwijk, N., Balm, A. J. M., & Hilgers, F. J. M. (1993). Improvements in the assessment of pulmonary function in laryngectomized patients. *Laryngoscope, 103,* 1391–1394.

Davidson, R. N., Hayward, L., Pounsford, J. C., & Saunders, K. B. (1986). Lung function and within-breath changes in resistance in patients who have had a laryngectomy. *Quarterly Journal of Medicine, 60,* 753–762.

Gardner, W. N., & Meah, M. S. (1989). Respiration during exercise in conscious laryngectomized humans. *Journal of Applied Physiology, 66,* 2071–2078.

Gilchrist, A. G. (1973). Rehabilitation after laryngectomy. *Acta Otolaryngologica, 75,* 511–518.

Gregor, R. T., & Hassman, E. (1984). Respiratory function in postlaryngectomy patients related to stomal size. *Acta Otolaryngologica (Stockholm), 97,* 177–183.

Griffith, T. E., & Friedberg, S. A. (1964). Histologic changes in the trachea following total laryngectomy. *Annals of Otology, 73,* 883–892.

Harris, S., & Jonson, B. (1974). Lung function before and after laryngectomy. *Acta Otolaryngologica (Stockholm), 78,* 287–294.

Hess, M. M., Schwenk, R. A., Frank, W., & Loddenkemper, R. (1999). Pulmonary function after total laryngectomy. *Laryngoscope, 109,* 988–994.

Hilgers, F. J. M., Aaronson, N. K., Ackerstaff, A. H., Schouwenburg, P. F., & van Zandwijk, N. (1991). The influence of a heat and moisture exchanger (HME) on the respiratory symptoms after total laryngectomy. *Clinical Otolaryngology, 16,* 152–156.

Hilgers, F. J. M., & Ackerstaff, A. H. (2000). Comprehensive rehabilitation after total laryngectomy is more than voice alone. *Folia Phoniatrica and Logopaedia, 52,* 65–73.

Hilgers, F. J. M., Ackerstaff, A. H., Aaronson, N. K., Schouwenburg, P. F., & van Zandwijk, N. (1990). Physical and psychosocial consequences of total laryngectomy. *Clinical Otolaryngology, 15,* 421–425.

Hilgers, F. J. M., Ackerstaff, A. H., Balm, A. J. M., & Gregor, R. T. (1996). A new heat and moisture exchanger with speech valve (Provox® Stomafilter). *Clinical Otolaryngology, 21,* 414–418.

Hilgers, F. J. M., Ackerstaff, A. H., van As, C. J., Balm, A. J., van den Brekel, M. W., & Tan, I. B. (2003). Development and clinical assessment of a heat and moisture exchanger with a multi-magnet automatic tracheostoma valve (Provox FreeHands HME) for vocal and pulmonary rehabilitation after total laryngectomy. *Acta Otolaryngologica, 123,* 91–99.

Hilgers, F. J. M., Jansen, H. A., van As, C. J., Polak, M. F., Muller, M. J., & van Dam, F. S. (2002). Long-term results of olfaction rehabilitation using the nasal airflow-inducing ("polite yawning") maneuver after total laryngectomy. *Archives of Otolaryngology—Head and Neck Surgery, 128,* 648–654.

Jay, S., Ruddy, J., & Cullen, R. J. (1991). Laryngectomy: The patient's view. *The Journal of Laryngology and Otology, 105,* 934–938.

Jones, E., Lund, V. J., Howard, D. J., Greenberg, M. P., & McCarthy, M. (1992). Quality of life of patients treated surgically for head and neck cancer. *The Journal of Laryngology and Otology, 106,* 238–242.

McRae, D., Young, P., Hamilton, J., & Jones, A. (1996). Raising airway resistance in laryngectomees increases tissue oxygen saturation. *Clinical Otolaryngology, 21,* 366–368.

Mendelsohn, M., Morris, M., & Gallagher, R. (1993). A comparative study of speech after total laryngectomy and total laryngopharyngectomy. *Archives of Otolaryngology—Head and Neck Surgery, 119,* 508–510.

Mohide, E. A., Archibald, S. D., Tew, M., Young, J. E., & Haines, T. (1992). Postlaryngectomy quality-of-life dimensions identified by patients and health care professionals. *American Journal of Surgery, 164,* 619–622.

Moore-Gillon, V. (1985). The nose after laryngectomy. *Journal of the Royal Society of Medicine, 78,* 435–439.

Murty, G. E., Smith, M. C. F., & Lancaster, P. (1991). Cough intensity in the laryngectomee. *Clinical Otolaryngology, 16,* 25–28.

Nakhla, V. (1997). A homemade modification of a spacer device for delivery of bronchodilator or steroid therapy in patients with tracheostomies. *The Journal of Laryngology and Otology, 111,* 363–365.

Natvig, K. (1984a). Influence of different climates on the peak expiratory flow in laryngectomees. *The Journal of Laryngology and Otology, 98,* 53–58.

Natvig, K. (1984b). Study No. 5: Problems of everyday life. *The Journal of Otolaryngology, 13,* 15–22.

Ogura, J. H., & Harvey, J. E. (1971). Nasopulmonary mechanics—Experimental evidence of the influence of the upper airway upon the lower. *Acta Otolaryngologica (Stockholm), 17,* 123–132.

Op de Coul, B. M., Hilgers, F. J. M., Balm, A. J., Tan, I. B., van den Hoogen, F. J., & van Tinteren, H. (2000). A decade of postlaryngectomy vocal rehabilitation in 318 patients: A single institution's experience with consistent application of Provox indwelling voice prostheses. *Archives of Otolaryngology—Head and Neck Surgery, 126,* 1320–1328.

Pruyn, J. F. A., de Jong, P. C., Bosman, L. J., van Poppel, J. W. M. J., van den Borne, H. W., Ryckman, R. M., & de Meij, K. (1986). Psychosocial aspects of head and neck cancer—A review of the literature. *Clinical Otolaryngology, 11,* 469–474.

Roessler, F., Grossenbacher, R., & Walt, H. (1988). Die tracheobronciale schleimhautbeschaffenheit bei patienten mit langzeit-tracheostoma. *Laryngologie, Rhinologie und Otologie, 67,* 66–71.

Schuster, M., Lohscheller, J., Hoppe, U., Kummer, P., Eysholdt, U., & Rosanowski, F. (2004). Voice handicap of laryngectomees with tracheoesophageal speech. *Folia Phoniatrica and Logopaedia, 56,* 62–67.

Stafford, F. W. (2003). Current indications and complications of tracheoesophageal puncture for voice restoration after laryngectomy. *Current Opinion in Otolaryngology—Head and Neck Surgery, 11,* 89–95.

Stell, P. M., & McCormick, M. S. (1985). Cancer of the head and neck: Are we doing any better? *The Lancet, 2,* 1127.

Todisco, T., Maurizi, M., Paludetti, G., Dottorini, M., & Merante, F. (1984). Laryngeal cancer: Long-term follow-up of respiratory functions after laryngectomy. *Respiration, 45,* 303–315.

Togawa, K., Konno, A., & Hoshino, T. (1980). A physiologic study on respiratory handicap of the laryngectomized. *Archives of Otorhinolaryngology, 223,* 69–79.

Toremalm, N. G. (1960). Heat and moisture exchange for post-tracheotomy care. *Acta Otolaryngologica (Stockholm), 52,* 1–12.

Torjussen, W. (1968). Airway obstructions in laryngectomized patients. *Acta Otolaryngologica (Stockholm), 66,* 161–170.

UK Departments of Health and Social Security. (1987). Evaluation report: Heat and moisture exchangers. *Journal of Medical Engineering Technique, 11,* 117–127.

Usui, N. (1979). Ventilatory function in laryngectomized patients. *Auris Nasis Larynx, 6,* 87–96.

van As, C. J., Hilgers, F. J. M., Koopmans-van Beinum, F. J., & Ackerstaff, A. H. (1998). The influence of stoma occlusion on aspects of tracheoesophageal voice. *Acta Otolaryngologica (Stockholm), 118,* 732–738.

van den Hoogen, F. J. A., Meeuwis, C., Oudes, M. J., Janssen, P., & Manni, J. J. (1996). The Blom–Singer tracheostoma valve as a valuable addition in the rehabilitation of the laryngectomized patient. *European Archives of Otorhinolaryngology, 253,* 126–129.

Webber, P. A., & Brown, A. R. (1984). The use of a conical spacer after laryngectomy. *British Medical Journal, 288,* 1537.

Chapter 21

Pharyngoesophageal Segment Function
A Review and Reconsideration

Philip C. Doyle and Tanya L. Eadie

Since the late 1950s, considerable information related to the role of the pharyngoesophageal (PE) segment on intrinsic methods of alaryngeal speech production has appeared in the literature. The information reported has largely centered on the anatomical composition of this structure and its vibratory capacity during traditional "esophageal" phonation. Over the past 25 years, however, an improved understanding of this vicarious alaryngeal voicing mechanism has emerged. More complete understanding of the PE segment clearly has been facilitated by a viable contemporary method of surgical–prosthetic voice restoration, tracheoesophageal (TE) speech (Blom, Singer, & Hamaker, 1986). Understanding has also been increased as a direct result of clinical observations of speech failure following TE puncture (TEP) voice restoration and pre– and post–TE puncture assessment of the PE segment following air insufflation, or what is more commonly referred to as "esophageal insufflation testing" (Blom, Singer, & Hamaker, 1985; Taub, 1980). The purpose of this chapter is to review historical information about the PE segment and its sphincteric function as an alaryngeal voice source. In addition to a review of classic literature addressing the PE sphincter and its function in alaryngeal speech, contemporary knowledge that has emerged with increased refinements and understanding of the TE speech method is outlined.

The purpose of reviewing information related to use of the PE segment as an alaryngeal voicing source following total laryngectomy has important and direct clinical implications. Specifically, although commonalities from both historic and contemporary literature exist, information provided since the early 1980s suggests that past interpretations of why some individuals successfully acquired esophageal speech and others did not, in some instances, may have been unwarranted. Thus, information on three distinct but overlapping areas that have an impact on voice reacquisition following laryngectomy is presented. First, information on normal and postlaryngectomy esophageal function is provided in an attempt to outline critical variables that must be considered by clinicians. Second, the basis of what has been termed "cricopharyngeal spasm," including anatomical, physiological, and neurophysiological components of this response, is described. Third, a discussion regarding the clinical evaluation of postlaryngectomy esophageal function using esophageal insufflation testing is presented. This information provides a framework for a discussion of issues that may serve to enhance understanding of potential factors influencing use of the PE segment as an alaryngeal voicing source. Careful consideration of contemporary data related to the PE segment may permit clinicians to (a) reevaluate the viability of intrinsic postlaryngectomy speech rehabilitation options, (b) seek to gather current information on the acquisition and refinement of esophageal voice production, (c) reassess potential "causal" factors that influence failure to acquire esophageal speech or TE speech, and (d) make more informed rehabilitation decisions that will affect the individual who undergoes total laryngectomy for laryngeal malignancy.

ALARYNGEAL VOICE GENERATION

Esophageal voice production has a long history in the literature on postlaryngectomy rehabilitation. Esophageal voice is generated by forcing air into the esophageal reservoir located inferior to the PE segment. Once insufflation occurs, this air is pushed through the sphincter, creating oscillation of this tissue. The esophageal signal then moves into the vocal tract, where speech is articulated (Diedrich, 1968). The role of myoelastic and aerodynamic influences on (tracheo) esophageal voice production has been reported (Moon & Weinberg, 1987). Although different methods of air insufflation exist (e.g., injection vs. inhalation), charging the esophageal reservoir is a prerequisite to the generation of PE segment vibration, and an esophageal site of vibration is essential for functional esophageal speech (Weinberg & Westerhouse, 1973).

Tissue oscillation for esophageal voicing is created through vibration of anatomical structures comprising the region that merges muscular tissues of the lower pharynx and of the upper esophagus. Both pharyngeal and esophageal muscular structures make up a region identified as the upper esophageal sphincter. From a strict anatomical perspective, the cricopharyngeus muscle has been implicated for many years as a primary vibratory structure for alaryngeal speech (Diedrich & Youngstrom, 1966; Snidecor, 1978); however, it might be best to view composite structures comprising the pharynx and esophagus in discussions of esophageal phonation. Therefore, because esophageal voicing may be identified best as the result of contributions of the PE segment (Diedrich, 1968), we refer to this region as the PE segment or PE sphincter in the remainder of this chapter.

BASIC CONSIDERATIONS OF PE SEGMENT STRUCTURE AND FUNCTION

The literature suggests that the PE segment exhibits considerable variability in its form (Damsté, 1958; Levin, 1962; Robe, Moore, Andrews, & Holinger, 1956; van den Berg & Moolenaar-Bijl, 1959; Vrticka & Svoboda, 1961). The PE segment may be found in a variety of locations (Diedrich & Youngstrom, 1966), and the esophageal pseudoglottis "can vary from wide to narrow, from long to short, and its shape can be flat, round, and prominent" (Damsté, 1979, p. 55). Reconstruction and subsequent tissue healing following laryngectomy also may correspond to variations in the location of the esophageal pseudoglottis (Damsté, 1986; Diedrich & Youngstrom, 1966; Welch, Gates, Luckmann, Ricks, & Drake, 1979), with multiple postsurgical vibratory sources suggested by some authors (Brewer, Gould, & Casper, 1974; Damsté & Lerman, 1969; Daou, Schultz, Remy, Chan, & Attia, 1984, Kirchner, Scatliff, Dey, & Shedd, 1963). Furthermore, the basic neurophysiology of the postlaryngectomy PE segment is somewhat poorly understood, and therefore our understanding of neurologic control mechanisms governing function for alaryngeal speech is necessarily limited.

It is likely that the lack of knowledge about neurological influences on postlaryngectomy PE segment function has culminated in clinical difficulty in resolving the underlying causes of failure, either partial or complete, in those individuals who meet with limited success with esophageal voice reacquisition. Doyle (1994) suggested that the clinical difficulty in identifying factors responsible for esophageal speech failure may be due in part to the reluctance of speech–language pathologists to seek and evaluate information from sources external to speech pathology and communication sciences and disorders. At times, speech clinicians have failed to evaluate the literature from different disciplines (e.g., anatomy, physiology, gastroenterology), which has significantly restricted their ability to appreciate the degree of anatomical and physiological change that may impact the speech system. Doyle (1994) also stated that when speech acquisition failures were observed, clinicians at times viewed these difficulties in an incomplete manner, which led to what he described as a de facto diagnosis of the problem. Rather than directly acknowledging that the reason for esophageal speech acquisition failure was unknown, clinicians found it easier to point to suspicions of poor motivation or compliance on the part of the individual patient. As one carefully evaluates a broader literature, however, many questions continue as to why esophageal speech has met with such high failure rates historically (Gates, Ryan, Cantu, & Hearne, 1982; Gates, Ryan, Cooper, et al., 1982; Schaefer & Johns, 1982).

Regardless of what structures comprise the PE segment, a combined, systemic view of this sphincter is required (Doyle, 1994). Because the sphincter seems to function in a rather synergistic fashion (Henderson, 1976; Logemann, 1983), the ability to assess response characteristics of the cricopharyngeus as an "isolated sphincter" may not be possible (Lund & Ardran, 1964). Mu and Sanders (1996) provided information that clarifies understanding of the complex neurological innervation of the upper esophageal sphincter. In addition to identifying that each muscular component of the upper esophageal sphincter differs, Mu and Sanders also observed neural connections between the recurrent laryngeal nerve and the pharyngeal plexus serving these structures. Hence, functional relationships between muscular structures forming the upper esophageal sphincter (or the PE segment) also may be dependent on interactive neural relationships. When these connections are disrupted as a result of surgery and subsequent reconstruction, atypical and varied response of the sphincter may be exhibited. This adds support to the hypothesis that inability to achieve functionally serviceable use of the PE segment as a postlaryngectomy alaryngeal voicing source, whether for esophageal or TE speech, may find its causal roots at the level of neurological control of the sphincter.

In reality, assessment of the PE segment used for esophageal voice is likely to result in a combined response that includes isolated, complementary, and agonist–antagonist control mechanisms at the physiological level. This suggests not only that those who are laryngectomized may experience the consequences of obvious changes in the anatomy of this region and subsequent physiological changes, but also that neurological control may be disrupted (Doyle, 1985, 1994). Changes in the neurological control mechanisms of the esophagus and pharynx contribute substantially to this complexity (e.g., Blom, Pauloski, & Hamaker, 1995; Chodosh, Giancarlo, & Goldstein, 1984; Code, 1981; Dey & Kirchner, 1961; Mu & Sanders, 1996). Because the control mechanisms are essentially poorly understood in many cases, the system and its function must be carefully reconsidered when "abnormal" function (i.e., failure to acquire esophageal voicing) is observed. This consideration is primary in our desire to reconsider what many clinicians have observed clinically but not extended intellectually. We believe that, in many instances, the failure to successfully acquire esophageal speech may find its causal underpinnings in a disrupted neural control mechanism rather than a simple gross anatomical change. One of the most critical and unfortunately often overlooked aspects of this control pertains to the differential response of the sphincter to varied stimuli (air vs. fluid distention, chemoresponsiveness, etc.) and subsequent interaction or responses in the PE sphincter (Creamer & Schlagel, 1957).

In considering the responsive nature of the esophagus to varied stimuli, several important issues emerge. First, the introduction of air into the esophageal reservoir and the resulting distention of this structure may culminate in a response that differs from that associated with introduction of fluid (Henderson, 1976). Thus, swallowing liquids and solids differs from "swallowing" air. Second, mediation of a specific sphincteric response (normal or abnormal) is a consequence of innervation influences and the nature of various receptors in this region. A more complete presentation of innervation is required, however, to understand the significance of these differences on use of the PE segment as an alaryngeal voicing source. Kirchner et al. (1963) concluded that no significant relationship existed between good esophageal speakers and anatomical morphology in the postlaryngectomy pharynx and that the size of the "hypopharyngeal lumen" contributed little to one's ultimate speech ability. Manometric data have indicated that pressures vary by region in the esophageal lumen, with anterior and posterior pressures almost three times greater than pressure observed in lateral regions (Gerhardt, Shuck, Bordeaux, & Winship, 1978; Winans, 1972). These data suggest that postlaryngectomy alterations in anatomy may further disrupt regional pressure characteristics of the PE segment. Hence, reconstruction following laryngectomy has a critical influence on physiology (Conley, 1964; Dey & Kirchner, 1961; Doyle, 1985; Gates, 1980; Kallen, 1934; Robe et al., 1956; Simpson, Smith, & Gordon, 1972; Singer, 1988; Singer & Blom, 1980, 1981; Singer, Blom, & Hamaker, 1986). Furthermore, Welch et al. (1979) noted that "partial sensory denervation due to section of the superior laryngeal nerves may impair the coordination of sphincter relaxation" (p. 808). Consequently, changes throughout the PE sphincter, whether caused by anatomical, physiological or neurophysiological factors (or a combination thereof), require consideration as an objective culprit underlying one's ability to generate or fail to generate continuous air-driven oscillation of the sphincter.

Based on intraluminal (esophageal) manometric measures, Winans, Reichback, and Waldrop (1974) found reduced cricopharyngeal sphincter resting pressures in laryngectomized participants who had acquired fluent, sustained esophageal voicing when compared with those who had failed to acquire esophageal voice. Mean intraluminal resting pressures were more than twice as great in those who could not produce esophageal voicing (30 mm Hg vs. 13 mm Hg). Although this information has suggested that pressure within the esophagus may influence the individual's ability to generate (tracheo)esophageal voicing, what is not known is what factors underlie intraluminal pressure reductions. These data would appear to collectively support the notion that when pressures become too great, the utility of the PE segment may diminish in part or in its entirety. Once again, however, information on why such changes are present remains unresolved. Information presented by Hoffman et al. (1997) suggests that changes in pressures within the trachea, and inferentially within the esophageal reservoir, do result in changes in the functional ability of the PE segment. Specifically, Hoffman et al. graphically presented data from a single patient who exhibited loss of TE voice generation and who could be seen to demonstrate increased tracheal pressure. This finding suggests that if pressures are increased and airflow concurrently transfers to the esophageal reservoir, then intrinsic pressure receptors may respond with subsequent changes in one's ability to drive the PE sphincter for alaryngeal voicing. Such concerns are most important relative to tracheoesophageal speech (Oh, Meleca, Simpson, & Dworkin, 2002).

NEUROLOGICAL CONTROL OF THE PHARYNGOESOPHAGEAL SEGMENT

The pharynx in general and the cricopharyngeus muscle in specific have been reported to receive direct parasympathetic and sympathetic nervous system input (Henderson, 1976). Parasympathetic innervation arises from several cranial nerves, the glossopharyngeus (IX), the vagus (X), and the spinal accessory (XI). Sympathetic input to these structures is provided by branches of the cervical sympathetic ganglia (Henderson, 1983). It has been suggested that the resting tone of the sphincter and its normal relaxation may be mediated via input from the sympathetic system. Normal tone for the region is reportedly mediated via the cervical sympathetic chain, with the motor response mediated via the vagus nerve (Henderson, 1976; Henderson, Boszko, & van Nostrand, 1974) and possibly trigeminal fibers (Chodosh et al., 1984). Therefore, muscular structures forming the sphincter have the capacity to respond to specific stimuli and relative changes in internal pressure via proprioceptive fibers. It appears, however, that innervation to the cricopharyngeus and the pharynx are separate (Palmer, 1976). Function of the PE sphincter requires interaction of both afferent and efferent components of the nervous system; a disturbance to either control mechanism can result in dysfunction, and in the postlaryngectomized individual, this disruption may account for deficits in his or her ability to produce esophageal voicing despite successful charging of the reservoir. The confirmation of such disruption has been suggested by numerous authors who observed sphincteric "spasm" when substantial levels of air charging were provided via access to the pulmonary air supply in tracheoesophageal voice restoration (Schneider, Thumfart, Potoschnig, & Eckel, 1994; Sellin, 1981; Singer & Blom, 1980, 1981). Support for communication between neural structures also has emerged through the work of Mu and Sanders (1996), which was discussed previously.

Welch et al. (1979) stated, "It appears that residual sphincter tension after laryngectomy plays no role in the acquisition of esophageal speech" (p. 808). Unfortunately, this makes it unlikely that a simple procedure such as myotomy of the sphincter muscle would be of benefit for patients with high pressures who are unable to master esophageal air charging. However, if neurophysiological control is disrupted or modified to some extent, the ability to oscillate the PE segment in response to airflow may be facilitated. Regarding electromyographic activity of the sphincter in esophageal speakers, Shipp (1970) suggested that "each individual utilizes a method of alaryngeal phonation that is most efficient for him consistent with his post-operative anatomy and physiology" (pp. 191–192). Shipp further suggested that a speaker's voluntary "control" of muscles (particularly the cricopharygeus) may underlie and differentiate proficiency levels. Thus, Shipp believed that more proficient esophageal speakers demonstrated greater control over the "velocity and magnitude of pharyngoesophageal muscle contraction" (p. 192). Total laryngectomy may then result in an inability to volitionally control contractile resistance following air insufflation (Diedrich & Youngstrom, 1966; Shanks, 1986). Similarly, Damsté and Lerman's (1969) belief that "different forms of the pharyngo-esophageal junction" (p. 347) are a consequence of "selective activation" of the musculature associated with esophageal voice may not account for one's inability to achieve esophageal voicing. Although differences do indeed exist within the structures and functional capabilities of the PE segment, Damsté and Lerman's implication of selective activation applies specifically to one's ability to achieve more proficient esophageal speech from the perspective of controlling output. Pharyngoesophageal "spasm" is typically observed as an "onset" phenomenon once proprioception responses occur, rather than one that is triggered as an inconsistently intermittent process; that is, while some muscles comprising the reconstructed PE segment may indeed be more active in voicing, their utility is likely guided more by innervation of that muscular complex rather than through structural capacity alone.

Spasm of the PE segment is likely reflexive rather than volitional; hence, selective activation of musculature may not be an influencing factor. This information may erroneously lead one to assume that when proficiency levels are poor or nonexistent in those seeking to acquire esophageal voicing, a volitional incapacity exists. The contrasting hypothesis would suggest that under such circumstance, loss of volitional control may evolve from an involuntary, neurologically mediated response of the PE segment following air distension.

A NEW ERA OF SURGICAL–PROSTHETIC VOICE RESTORATION

The introduction of the tracheoesophageal puncture (TEP) voice restoration technique by Singer and Blom in 1980 clearly revolutionized voice and speech rehabilitation following total laryngectomy. Without question, postlaryngectomy voice and speech rehabilitation moved into a new era with this clinical advance and the numerous modifications that have occurred since its introduction. Until Singer and Blom's pioneering efforts, individuals who had undergone laryngectomy for management of laryngeal cancer were provided only with the postsurgical speech alternatives of esophageal speech or electrolaryngeal speech. Although use of the electrolarynx should remain an important and essential rehabilitative option today (see Chapter 22 in this text), considerable controversy regarding the use of the artificial larynx, much of it without cause, has persisted historically in the postlaryngectomy speech rehabilitation literature.

Prior to the TEP voice restoration technique, the negative bias toward artificial laryngeal speech typically led to complementary biases toward esophageal speech. Those who criticized the electrolarynx were often staunch advocates of esophageal speech, and vice versa. Although in most instances, the use of esophageal speech may indeed offer many advantages to the alaryngeal speaker even in the new era of postlarygectomy speech rehabilitation, esophageal speech is fraught with its own problems. Foremost among these concerns is the poor rate of acquisition for esophageal speech (e.g., Schaefer & Johns, 1982). Further limitations from a larger communicative perspective include reductions in acoustical characteristics (Robbins, Fisher, Blom, & Singer, 1984; Smith, Weinberg, Feth, & Horii, 1978; Snidecor & Curry, 1959); changes in temporal aspects of phoneme production, which alter perceptual judgments of voicing contrasts (Christensen, Weinberg, & Alphonso, 1978; Doyle, 1999; Gomyo & Doyle, 1989; MacKnight & Doyle, 1992); reduced prominence of the esophageal signal in situations of competing noise (Horii & Weinberg, 1975); and altered speech intelligibility (Doyle, Danhauer, & Reed, 1988; Tardy-Mitzell, Andrews, & Bowman, 1985). Collectively, these types of changes also may influence global judgments by listeners, as well as overall communication effectiveness (see Chapter 6 in this text). Perhaps primary among the limitations was the rather clear indication that acquiring esophageal speech was problematic for some, if not in fact many, individuals. To further complicate this matter, clinical data on success in acquiring esophageal speech have been replete with controversy relative to the minimal level of acquisition for functional verbal communication purposes (see Chapter 5 in this text).

ESOPHAGEAL SPEECH ACQUISITION

When the dogma of both the esophageal and artificial laryngeal camps is put aside and evaluated as objectively as possible, the reality of postsurgical speech rehabilitation prior to the advent of TEP voice restoration (Singer & Blom, 1980) cannot discount the fact that for many who underwent total laryngectomy, the acquisition of esophageal speech was not always possible. One of the seminal works in the area of alaryngeal speech rehabilitation suggested that those individuals who ultimately would learn esophageal speech that could meet communicative demands could often be identified quite early in the course of training (Berlin, 1963). In fact, early work by Wepman, MacGahan, Rickard, and Shelton (1953) was directed at developing the first method of rating esophageal speech capability. This 7-point equal-appearing interval scale sought to merge levels of esophageal sound acquisition with a perceived level of esophageal speech "proficiency." Three of seven of Wepman et al.'s speech proficiency descriptors (*no, involuntary,* or *intermittent esophageal speech production*) were assessed as "no speech."

The remaining four levels of the scale were applied if esophageal speech was produced *voluntarily most of the time, at will, at will with continuity,* and *automatically.* The correlated levels of speech proficiency varied from differentiated vowels and monosyllables to full esophageal speech. Thus, Wepman et al. realized that the acquisition of esophageal speech would be met with varied levels of success. The descriptors used, however, imply a distinct binary approach to classifying speech acquisitions. Namely, the transition between *intermittent* and *voluntary most of the time* appears to be very distinct in that a demarcation of failure is implied.

The important issue to understand relative to Wepman et al.'s (1953) scale is that the authors clearly acknowledged that acquisition capacity differs from individual to individual. Additionally, although subjectively evaluated, success or failure could be inferred according to their scale. Specifically, three of seven rating categories identified a capacity that indicated no speech proficiency. In hindsight, this early contribution to the esophageal speech literature provided an early method for assessing an individual's status relative to a short- or long-term course of alaryngeal speech treatment. Clinical data prior to Wepman et al.'s report suggested that variability would be observed in the degree of progress in acquiring esophageal speech, as well as in the ultimate level of acquisition (voluntary or involuntary) and subsequent speech proficiency. When one considers data provided by Berlin (1963), it seems clear that if a patient were to be successful in acquiring esophageal voice, he or she would likely be identified fairly early on in the clinical process. However, the ability to define specific characteristics of early success in one's acquisition profile may have influenced the simple, discrete need for evaluation of overall success or failure, which might then have been reflected in varied success–failure rates reported in the literature (see Table 21.1). This variable trend was observed throughout the early period of esophageal speech training.

At a glance, data presented in Table 21.1 reveal that the ability to acquire esophageal speech has ranged from a low of approximately 25% to a high of approximately 60%. Additional reports in the literature until the early 1980s continued to document problems associated with the success of esophageal speech acquisition (Gates, Ryan, Cantu, & Hearne, 1982; Gates, Ryan, Cooper, et al., 1982). When these data are merged with the clinical report provided by Berlin (1963), some very unusual observations and inferential assumptions emerge. First, and perhaps most obviously, some factor or set of factors most certainly appears to influence the individual's ability to acquire esophageal speech. Second, many "causes" for failed acquisition were directed at the individual patient. Among these causative factors, motivation was frequently identified. Therefore, in many instances the burden of failure to acquire esophageal speech was unjustifiably placed at the proverbial doorstep of many laryngectomized individuals. Additional information in the literature suggests that other factors associated with esophageal speech difficulties should be considered.

Sloane, Griffin, and O'Dwyer (1991) studied 75 laryngectomized patients using videolaryngoscopy during swallowing, phonation, and transnasal insufflation of the esophagus. Twenty-four individuals (32%) exhibited fluent esophageal speech, with all speakers demonstrating good vibratory function of the PE seg-

TABLE 21.1

Rates of Acquisition for Esophageal Speech

Study	Type	Rate of Success/ % Users
Hunt (1964); Johnson (1960); King, Fowlks, & Pierson (1968)	Retrospective	38%–97%
Gates, Ryan, Cooper, et al. (1982)	Retrospective	62%
Gates, Ryan, Cooper, et al. (1982)	Prospective	26%
Schaefer & Johns (1982)	Prospective	12%
St. Guily et al. (1992)	Prospective	5%
Hillman, Walsh, Wolf, Fisher, & Hong (1998)	Prospective	6%
Anderson (2000)	Prospective	20%

ment. This number is higher than the success rates reported in more recent studies (e.g., the 6% success rate reported by Hillman, Walsh, Wolf, Fisher, & Hong, 1998). Sloane et al. (1991) found hypotonicity in 21 of 75 subjects (28%), stricture in 3 (4%), and hypertonicity or spasm in 28 (37%) of those studied. These data indicate that difficulties exhibited with the PE segment and noted with the advent of TEP voice restoration (Singer & Blom, 1981) are also indicated in esophageal speech. Therefore, the past practice of attributing one's failure to acquire esophageal speech to "motivational" or "learned" factors is not supported based on physiological data.

Personal factors such as positive attitude, psychosocial adjustment difficulty, and family support issues have been associated with the successful acquisition of esophageal speech, whereas the failure to acquire esophageal speech has been associated with lack of motivation and limited physical strength (Gates, Ryan, Cantu, & Hearne, 1982; Gates, Ryan, & Lauder, 1982; Richardson & Bourque, 1985; Volin, 1980). Although other, more biological explanations have been posited, such as extent of surgery and the effects of dysphagia (see Chapter 14 in this text) and radiation therapy on the tissues associated with esophageal speech production, these factors have often been overlooked. So, too, has the cause of many difficulties associated with TEP speech—that is, the pharyngoesophageal spasm—been ignored in esophageal speech acquisition (Singer & Blom, 1980). One question that arises in this context is that if psychological factors such as motivation influence one's ability to use the PE segment, why do alterations in the system as a result of myotomy, neurectomy, or use of Botox facilitate function of the system?

Chodosh et al. (1984) provided another explanation that did not focus on psychological or personal factors. They stated, "It would appear that laryngectomy repair subsequently can interfere with the orderly contraction and relaxation of the pharyngeal constrictors as well as the cricopharyngeus. This may produce a functional block to inspired and regurgitated air interfering with esophageal speech" (p. 55). More recently, Hammarberg, Lundstrom, and Nord

(1996) emphasized the influences of surgical procedures and radiotherapy on esophageal voice acquisition. Thus, a neurologically mediated or structural impedence block to transmission of air across the PE sphincter for its use as an alaryngeal voice source in either esophageal or TE speech may be responsible for some esophageal speech failures. Had one looked carefully at Berlin's (1963) data, as well as attended to information provided anecdotally by clinicians, some unique suspicions concerning a physiological explanation for esophageal voicing failure would have been raised. Namely, Berlin found that "good" speakers achieved 100% levels of "successful (esophageal) phonation" in 10 to 14 therapy days, whereas "poor" speakers seemed to cease substantial improvements at approximately 16 sessions, and averaged around 68% phonation over 20 trials. When the latency between esophageal air insufflation and phonation was assessed, good speakers showed dramatic reductions in mean latencies at six sessions, whereas poorer rated speakers continued to exhibit substantial difficulty with this task. Finally, good speakers exhibited a rapid growth in ability to sustain esophageal phonatory duration, whereas the poor speakers plateaued at approximately 16 therapy sessions, with mean durations well below 1.8 seconds. Thus, those who failed to acquire esophageal voicing essentially did so from the start, and those who acquired the skills did so very rapidly. Thus, physiological explanations may account for a majority of esophageal speech acquisition failures.

The information suggesting a physiological limitation strongly suggested that something about Snidecor's (1978) adage of "get air in and get air out" was at the root of the problem; the question that was never addressed in a systematic fashion was why some individuals were more prone than others to achieving successful esophageal speech. This information should have led clinicians to assume that some individuals were esophageal "naturals," whereas others were not (Gates, Ryan, Cantu, Hearne, 1982; Gates, Ryan, & Lauder, 1982). Substantial data in the literature suggested that something related to the structure and function of the postsurgical PE remnant may have held the key (Chodosh et al., 1984; Singer & Blom, 1981; Singer et al., 1986). Those who acquired esophageal speech were ultimately those who had all the necessary anatomical and physiological "tools" that increased their chance of success. Similarly, those who failed did so not because of personal factors such as poor motivation, cognitive limitations, the inability to follow instructions, and so on, but because they were quite simply unable due to limitations in the anatomical and physiological systems, which included neurological control mechanisms. Those who met with success exhibited the capacity to produce esophageal voicing. In fact, in the same year that Blom and Singer introduced TEP voice restoration to the world, Weinberg (1980) wrote in an introduction to a compendium of articles on intrinsic methods of alaryngeal speech "that the relationships between speech or vocal proficiency and morphological or physiological characteristics of the PE segment or esophagus remain unspecified" (p. 40). Weinberg was indeed correct, although research conducted to date had in essence disregarded the extreme variability of the postlaryngeal PE segment. Although variability was noted in many of the classic publications in this area (Diedrich & Youngstrom, 1966; Gardner, 1971; Snidecor, 1978), it was usually regarded as "noise" in the data pool rather than the primary data of interest. Thus, the TEP voice restoration method held not only a new option for the laryngectomized, but it held the key to discover why many had failed to acquire esophageal speech in the past. With the formal introduction of TEP voice restoration as an additional postlaryngectomy communication option in 1980, however, the focus of alaryngeal speech rehabilitation certainly shifted.

In some respects, information presented by Schaefer and Johns (1982) likely led many clinicians to vanquish consideration of esophageal speech as an alaryngeal option. Schaefer and Johns provided evidence that the success of esophageal speech acquisition may have been less than 25%. Nevertheless, regardless of method, the major controversy concerning alaryngeal speech training over many years of research may in part be a function of how "success" was defined. Clearly, learning to oscillate tissues of the upper esophageal region or PE segment did not always culminate in alaryngeal verbal communication that met communicative needs (Berlin, 1963; Wepman et al., 1953). Regardless of the reason, introduction of the TE voice restoration method and data supporting its viability decreased long-standing concerns about the failure of esophageal speech training. If TEP became the method of choice for postsurgical alaryngeal speech, concerns about failure with esophageal speech would no longer need to be considered.

Clinical data on TE voice restoration are now prominent in the literature. A theme that appeared in the first 10 years following Singer and Blom's (1980) report centered on the success of the method. TE speech was generally judged to have been successfully acquired if speech was "fluent" (e.g., Blom et al., 1985; Singer & Blom, 1980, 1981; Singer et al., 1986), and success based on this criterion was often high. The most frequently reported problem associated with TE speech acquisition in the early stages of the procedure centered on the presence of the observation of a "spasm" of the PE segment in response to esophageal air insufflation; the problem was termed "cricopharyngeal spasm." It may be fair to say, at least within the first 10 years that the procedure was available, that when TEP voice restoration culminated in failure, approximately 80% of these failures could be attributed to PE segment spasm (e.g., Baugh, Lewin, & Baker, 1990; see also Chapter 24 in this text). This problem had not been observed previously in postlaryngectomized speakers; hence, the report of this phenomenon in the TEP population raised questions about the functional capacity of the PE segment as a postlarygectomy voicing source. Although Taub's (1980) "air blowing" test served as the impetus for esophageal insufflation testing, it was the information presented by Blom and Singer and their colleagues that ultimately drove the need to reevaluate potential "treatments" for PE segment spasm.

Literature reports of cricopharyngeal spasm subsequent to TEP voice restoration probably offered one of the most important "potential" windows into understanding (or lack thereof) of the success or failure in esophageal voice production, yet it also may be argued that this window was never opened at the applied or basic levels of inquiry. Valuable insights into why esophageal speech acquisition was problematic for so many seemed to be supported by clinical observations on a regular basis; however, concerns about PE segment pressure and physiological function in those individuals who exhibit functional limitations in this system without laryngectomy have also been noted (Blom et al., 1995; Hoffman et al., 1997; Koybasioglu et al., 2003). In this regard, Mendelsohn and McConnel (1987) indicated that, although not always acknowledged, "cricopharyngeal and inferior constrictor muscle tone does not solely control the sphincter action in the PE segment" (p. 485).

In their first report of TE puncture voice restoration, Singer and Blom (1980) noted one particular problem that affected a small percentage of their patients. This problem was reported to be the result of an "airflow-induced cricopharyngeal spasm." In essence, Singer and Blom observed that some individuals appeared to demonstrate an unusual response to esophageal insufflation related to TE voice production. This "occlusive spasm" (Singer & Blom, 1980, 1981) was believed to be consistent with an abnormal response termed "pharyngoesophageal spasm." Blom et al. (1985) reported that pharyngoesophageal spasm was characterized by "elevated tonicity with incomplete or uncoordinated failure to relax during attempted esophageal phonation" (p. 211). Singer and Blom (1981) had previously demonstrated that this behavior could be eliminated with infiltration of anesthetic into the parapharyngeal space, which served as direct evidence that if control of the sphincter could be disrupted artificially, then tonicity and coordination would be optimized so that the PE sphincter could be used as a (tracheo)esophageal voice source. Thus, their clinical observations indicated that some individuals exhibited considerable difficulty maintaining "fluent" TE speech production because of an apparently abnormal response of the PE sphincter.

Additionally, in a prospective study, Blom, Singer, and Hamaker (1986) evaluated 47 individuals who had undergone laryngectomy. Of this study group, 25 were reported to have undergone esophageal speech training without success. Prospective assessment included an esophageal insufflation test. It was interesting to note that of the initial 47 subjects, 26 failed insufflation testing; that is, these individuals were incapable of sustaining esophageal vibration upon direct air insufflation. When durational data on insufflation for those individuals who required pharyngeal constrictor myotomy were examined, it was clear that voicing was facilitated. Based on the numbers of subjects evaluated and those who were reported to have failed esophageal speech acquisition, along with the temporal data on voicing, it would seem clear that some alteration in the response of the esophagus to airflow does result in a system that has been optimized in respect to use of the PE segment as an alaryngeal voice source.

The observation of this spasm of the PE segment continued to be reported by many authors in later clinical literature addressing endoscopic voice restoration and TE puncture (Blom et al., 1995; Singer & Blom, 1981; Singer et al., 1986; Terrell et al., 1995). Although similar responses had been noted in those who had not undergone laryngectomy and were identified by varied nomenclature (cricopharyngeal dysphagia, PE dysfunction, cervical block dysphagia, and cricopharyngeal achalasia), controversy regarding the causal factors and pathophysiological mechanism(s) remained (e. g., Ingelfinger, 1958; Robe et al., 1956; Ross, Green, Auslander, & Biller, 1982).

A BRIEF DESCRIPTION OF CRICOPHARYNGEAL SPASM DURING TE VOICING

Although some difficulties encountered with esophageal voicing are due to anatomical changes, such as scar tissue or contracture, data from assessment of the PE segment relative to response changes following anesthesia indicate other reasons. For example, if a cervical nerve block can disrupt airtight closure of the sphincter, one cannot assume that "structural" abnormalities are causal. That is not to say that in some instances anatomical variance due to these or multiple factors may exist and that such change(s) may alter one's ability to functionally use the PE segment as an alaryngeal voicing source. The findings, however, that structural observations are altered when the general physiological capability of the sphincter is altered lend credence to the belief that PE segment spasm is a consequence of changes in the response of this system. This altered reaction may be the result of either air insufflation, luminal distention, or altered neurophysiological response (e.g., stretch, chemoreception) that directly affects motility of this system.

Changes in the motility of the sphincter are reported to be substantially influenced by increased resistance to airflow during TE voicing. This implies that a speaker is unable to modulate or regulate flow through the vicarious voicing mechanism when spasm occurs. In fact, when one assesses the more simplistic index of TE speech ability, Singer et al. (1986) have characterized it best; they stated that TE speech is effective when "effortless, fluent, and intelligible" (p. 50). This simple definition implies that for efficient voicing and its inherent physical properties of frequency and intensity, air must flow easily and continuously through the sphincteric structure(s) used for "esophageal" oscillation (Deschler, Doherty, Reed, & Singer, 1999). This goal was achieved by Singer et al. (1986) through selective denervation of the neurologic control of the region comprising the upper esophageal sphincter via neurectomy. It is now clinically accepted that if a speaker can achieve continuous voicing for 8 seconds or longer during esophageal insufflation, no spasm is present. This would suggest that one component of assessment is found in one's ability to achieve adequate and continuous esophageal reservoir insufflation. Thus, both response to distention and the ultimate triggering of reflex mechanisms may induce spasm. If the neurologic responses can be reduced or eliminated, this negative response can no longer interfere with the smooth flow of air across the sphincter. Altering the system in that manner, however, cannot be done without considering other consequences, such as those related to swallowing. Thus, care must be taken and a selective approach to treating PE segment spasm is necessary.

SURGICAL AND MEDICAL TREATMENTS FOR PE SPASM AND VOICE FAILURE

Because of the observations of PE segment spasm in those who had undergone TEP voice restoration (Singer & Blom, 1980), new avenues of treatment were undertaken, including unilateral myotomy, neurectomy, and the combined approaches of myotomy and neurectomy. More recently, the use of botulinum toxin (Botox) has emerged as a potential method of reducing PE segment spasm. Hamaker and Cheesman (1998) provided an excellent overview of the surgical management of PE segment hypertonicity. Although the specific details of these procedures are beyond the scope of this chapter, brief descriptions of these treatment methods are provided.

Myotomy of the pharyngeal constrictor muscles was first introduced as a treatment for TEP voice restoration failure by Singer and Blom (1981). This procedure was in direct response to their observations of excessive airflow-induced hyperfunction (closure) during attempts at TE voicing. The procedure was further elaborated upon by Singer et al. (1986). Initially, this procedure was typically performed as a secondary procedure following TE speech failure due to spasm. In this procedure, the pharyngeal constrictors are disrupted unilaterally via surgical incision. The musculature is not, however, incised completely, but rather to the level of the submucosa. Unilateral pharyngeal constrictor myotomy is believed to disrupt the reflex arc of the constrictors (Chodosh et al., 1984), thereby reducing the reflexive ability of these muscles enough so that spasm is reduced or eliminated completely. The depth and length of the myotomy is critical in that insufficient incisions may result in continued problems with spasm (Hamaker & Cheesman, 1998). As more was learned about this procedure and its effect on the musculature of the upper pharynx, it was introduced as a primary method of treatment at the time of laryngectomy. This procedure is seen as equally effective and perhaps more cost and time effective. Currently, most surgeons seek to modify the pharyngeal constrictor muscles via myotomy as part of the total laryngectomy procedure (see Chapter 14 in this text).

Although disrupting the reflex arc of the constrictor muscles proved effective for treating PE segment spasm, pharyngeal plexus neurectomy has been shown to be very effective at eliminating PE spasm. In this procedure, nerve branches serving the constrictor muscles are electrically stimulated. When a muscle response is observed, the neural branches are then disrupted via sectioning and electrocautery. This permits disruption of the neural innervation to specific muscles. The selective disruption of neural innervation to the sphincter must be done with extreme care. Furthermore, this procedure is done on a unilateral basis similar to myotomy as bilateral disruption would directly alter swallowing (Hamaker & Cheesman, 1998).

Although myotomy and pharyngeal plexus neurectomy have been employed with successful results, they also have been associated with complications such as pharyngocutaneous fisutulas and leakage, as well as longer hospitalization (Izdebski, Reed, Ross, & Hilsinger, 1994; P. M. Scott, Bleach, Perry, & Cheesman, 1993). The recent application of Botox to chemically denervate the PE segment has introduced a nonsurgical method to possibly aid those patients affected by PE spasm and voice failure (Hamaker & Blom, 2003; Hoffman et al., 1997; Ramachandran, Arunachalam, Hurren, Marsh, & Samuel, 2003).

Botulinum neurotoxin type A, synthesized by the bacillus *Clostridium botulinum,* is commonly employed in the treatment of a variety of neuromuscular dis-

TABLE 21.2

Studies Demonstrating Benefit from Botox Injection on Tracheoesophageal
Puncture (TEP) Speech Production for Patients with PE Segment Spasm

Study	Subjects	Subjects Showing Benefit
Blitzer, Komisar, Baredes, Brin, & Stewart (1995)	6 subjects, 55–75 years	6 of 6 showed improvement; 20% to 60% improvement on self-rated ability to speak
Hoffman et al. (1997)	8 subjects	7 of 8 showed improved TEP speech
Terrell, Lewin, & Esclamado (1995)	1 subject, 70 years, male	At 9 months, still "ongoing benefit"
Crary & Glowasky (1996)	8 subjects	6 of 8 showed benefit from lidocaine, 5 of 8 showed improved voice
Zormeier et al. (1999)	8 subjects, all male	7 of 8 showed significant voice quality improvement

orders characterized by excessive or inappropriate muscular contraction. For example, Botox has been used to treat opthalmologic disorders of strabismus and blepharospasm (A. B. Scott, Kennedy, & Stubbs, 1984), as well as disorders of the head and neck, such as laryngeal dystonia (Blitzer & Brin, 1991), oromandibular dystonia (Blitzer, Brin, & Fahn, 1989), and spasmodic torticollis (Jankovic & Orman, 1987). Botox acts by impairing the release of acetylcholine at the presynaptic neuromuscular junction, thereby producing a dose-related weakness of the affected muscle (called "chemical denervation") (Sellin, 1981). The clinical effect of Botox is transient, and has been reported to last from several weeks up to 9 months or more (Jankovic & Orman, 1987). Recently, Botox has been used to address spasm of the PE segment in individuals undergoing total laryngectomy who undergo both problems with swallowing or speech production (e.g., Hamaker & Blom, 2003; Schneider et al., 1994). Table 21.2 exhibits a number of studies that have demonstrated the benefits of Botox to treat voice problems due to PE spasm.

Although success rates were reportedly high in the studies outlined in Table 21.2, "success" was usually measured by self-rated or experimenter-rated scales of generalized and ill-defined dimensions (e.g., "fluent," "ability to speak") or durational measures. Thus, future studies should include more specified perceptual and acoustic measurements to examine the usefulness of this promising technique (e.g., Zormeier et al., 1999).

THEN, NOW, AND LATER: A NEED FOR RESEARCH

TEP voice restoration has revolutionized postlaryngectomy speech rehabilitation. Although no method of alaryngeal speech is perfect and problem free, the

TE method does offer substantial advantages from many perspectives. Based on the literature of both successes and failures using this method, however, a cause for reevaluation of esophageal speech failures emerges. The data generated as a result of continuing developments in TEP voice restoration has led to a much improved understanding of the PE segment and its function after laryngectomy. Clinicians and researchers alike have been remiss in their neglect of further exploring the nature of "esophageal" voicing. We do not suggest that TE speech is unnecessary; it is without question a viable method of communication for many. We do, however, suggest that when retrospective examination of data is conducted, researchers may discover a much more justifiable explanation for why esophageal speech acquisition was characterized by such poor success rates. The ultimate advantage of such findings would be that "blame" for such failures could be withdrawn from the individual in many instances. Many clinicians in the initial stages of esophageal speech training can confirm the efforts of their patients during this endeavor: Although many of these patients exerted considerable effort in attempts to generate voicing, many could not achieve proficiency.

The postlaryngectomy PE segment today is likely much different from that of the past. Alterations in reconstruction, as well as preemptive treatment strategies, such as myotomy, neurectomy, Botox, or combined procedures, may now provide for increased facilitation of esophageal voicing. Further research efforts that focus on comprehensive assessment of the PE segment and esophageal reservoir will no doubt provide a more complete and perhaps more important, more equitable method of explaining esophageal speech failures of the past. Consequently, esophageal speech should be retained as a method of alaryngeal speech rehabilitation along with TEP voice restoration and the use of electrolaryngeal devices. If researchers reexplore use of esophageal speech secondary to the current understanding and treatments of the PE segment, a more comprehensive program of rehabilitation with the greatest opportunity for options to those who undergo surgical treatment for laryngeal malignancy will emerge.

SUMMARY

This chapter has provided information on issues underlying the structure and function of the PE segment. The specific issue raised and discussed has pertained to continuing questions regarding use of the PE segment as a postlaryngectomy alaryngeal voicing source. Over the history of postlaryngectomy speech rehabilitation, clinical data indicate that the ability to acquire serviceable esophageal speech may be quite limited. Although many reasons for such failure have been postulated in the literature, it seems that the impact of anatomical and physiological changes in the postlaryngectomized system were seldom considered. With the advent of TEP voice restoration in 1980, early problems with consistent voice production were encountered. These problems were addressed through use of several procedures that altered the functional capacity of the PE segment through disruption of the tonicity of this sphincteric system. Because of the outcome of these procedures on the patient's ability to produce TE voice, incidental questions about similar influences emerged. In many instances, however, the consideration of inherent structural or functional causes for esophageal failure may have been overlooked, with "causal" factors focusing more on those areas broadly defined as motivational, psychological, or psychosocial in origin. In this chapter, we have sought to raise awareness of the obvious influence of anatomy and physiology on the individual's ability to successfully acquire esophageal voice. Although many questions remain relative to this important area of inquiry, we hope that information provided in this chapter will prompt a reevaluation of the cause of esophageal speech failure. Such reconsideration may assist in furthering understanding of the esophageal voicing mechanism in both traditional esophageal and TE speech production.

REFERENCES

Anderson, C. (2000). *Information and service provision preferences of laryngectomized individuals.* Unpublished master's thesis, University of Western Ontario, London, Ontario, Canada.

Baugh, R. F., Lewin, J. S., & Baker, S. R. (1990). Vocal rehabilitation of tracheoesophageal speech failures. *Head & Neck, 12,* 69–73.

Berlin, C. I. (1963). Clinical measurement of esophageal speech: I. Methodology and curves of skill acquisition. *Journal of Speech and Hearing Disorders, 28,* 42–51.

Blitzer, A., & Brin, M. F. (1991). Laryngeal dystonia: A series with botulinum toxin therapy. *Annals of Otology, Rhinology and Laryngology, 100,* 85–90.

Blitzer, A., Brin, M. F., & Fahn, S. (1989). Botulinum toxin injection for the treatment of oromandibular dystonia. *Annals of Otology, Rhinology and Laryngology, 98,* 93–97.

Blitzer, A., Komisar, A., Baredes, S., Brin, M. F., & Stewart, C. (1995). Voice failure after tracheoesophageal puncture: Management with botulinum toxin. *Otolaryngology—Head and Neck Surgery, 113,* 668–670.

Blom, E. D., Pauloski, B. R., & Hamaker, R. C. (1995). Functional outcome after surgery for prevention of pharyngospasm in tracheoesophageal speakers. Part I: Speech characteristics. *Laryngoscope, 105,* 1093–1103.

Blom, E. D., Singer, M. I., & Hamaker, R. C. (1985). An improved esophageal insufflation test. *Archives of Otolaryngology—Head and Neck Surgery, 111,* 211–212.

Blom, E. D., Singer, M. I., & Hamaker, R. C., (1986). A prospective study of tracheoesophageal speech. *Archives of Otolaryngology—Head and Neck Surgery, 112,* 440–447.

Brewer, D. W., Gould, L. V., & Casper, J. (1974). Fiber-optic study of the post-laryngectomized voice. *Laryngoscope, 84,* 666–670.

Chodosh, P. L., Giancarlo, H. R., & Goldstein, J. (1984). Pharyngeal myotomy for vocal rehabilitation postlaryngectomy. *Laryngoscope, 94,* 52–57.

Christensen, J. M., Weinberg, B., & Alphonso, P. J. (1978). Productive voice onset time characteristics of esophageal speech. *Journal of Speech and Hearing Research, 21,* 56–62.

Code, C. F. (1981). Normal esophageal function. In S. Stipa, R. H. R. Belsey, & A. Moraldi (Eds.), *Medical and surgical problems of the esophagus* (pp. 4–6). New York: Academic Press.

Conley, J. J. (1964). Swallowing dysfunction associated with radical surgery of the head and neck. *Archives of Surgery, 80,* 602–612.

Crary, M. A., & Glowasky, A. L. (1996). Using botulinum toxin A to improve speech and swallowing function following total laryngectomy. *Archives of Otolaryngology—Head and Neck Surgery, 122,* 760–763.

Creamer, B., & Schlagel, J. (1957). Motor responses of the esophagus to distention. *Journal of Applied Physiology, 10,* 498–504.

Damsté, P. H. (1958). *Oesophageal speech after laryngectomy.* Groningen, The Netherlands: Hoitsema.

Damsté, P. H. (1979). Some obstacles in learning esophageal speech. In R. L. Keith & F. L. Darley (Eds.), *Laryngectomee rehabilitation* (pp. 49–61). San Diego, CA: College-Hill Press.

Damsté, P. H. (1986). Some obstacles to learning esophageal speech. In R. L. Keith & F. L. Darley (Eds.), *Laryngectomee rehabilitation* (2nd ed., pp. 85–92). San Diego, CA: College-Hill Press.

Damsté, P. H., & Lerman, J. W. (1969). Configuration of the neoglottis: An X-ray study. *Folia Phoniatrica, 21,* 347–358.

Daou, R. A., Schultz, J. R., Remy, H., Chan, N. T., & Attia, E. L. (1984). Laryngectomee study: Clinical and radiologic correlates of esophageal voice. *Otolaryngology—Head and Neck Surgery, 92,* 628–634.

Deschler, D. G., Doherty, E. T., Reed, C. G., & Singer, M. I. (1999). Effects of sound pressure levels on fundamental frequency in tracheoesophageal speakers. *Otolaryngology—Head and Neck Surgery, 121,* 23–26.

Dey, F. L., & Kirchner, J. A. (1961). The upper esophageal sphincter after laryngectomy. *Laryngoscope, 7,* 99–115.

Diedrich, W. M. (1968). The mechanism of esophageal speech. *Annals of the New York Academy of the Sciences, 155,* 303–317.

Diedrich, W. M., & Youngstrom, K. A. (1966). *Alaryngeal speech.* Springfield, IL: Thomas.

Doyle, P. C. (1985). Another perspective on esophageal insufflation testing. *Journal of Speech and Hearing Disorders, 50,* 408–409.

Doyle, P. C. (1994). *Foundations of voice and speech rehabilitation following laryngeal cancer.* San Diego, CA: Singular.

Doyle, P. C. (1999). Postlaryngectomy speech rehabilitation: Contemporary considerations in clinical care. *Journal of Speech–Language Pathology and Audiology, 23,* 109–116.

Doyle, P. C., Danhauer, J. L., & Reed, C. G. (1988). Listeners' perceptions of consonants produced by esophageal and tracheo-esophageal talkers. *Journal of Speech and Hearing Disorders, 53,* 400–407.

Gardner, W. H. (1971). *Laryngectomee speech and rehabilitation.* Springfield, IL: Thomas.

Gates, G. A. (1980). Upper esophageal sphincter: Pre and post-laryngectomy—A normative study. *Laryngoscope, 90,* 454–464.

Gates, G. A., Ryan, W., Cantu, E., & Hearne, E. (1982). Current status of laryngectomy rehabilitation: II. Causes of failure. *American Journal of Otolaryngology, 3,* 8–14.

Gates, G. A., Ryan, W., Cooper, J. C., Lawlis, G. F., Cantu, E., Hayashi, T., Lauder, E., Welch, R. W., & Hearne, E. (1982). Current status of laryngectomee rehabilitation: I. Results of therapy. *American Journal of Otolaryngology, 3,* 1–7.

Gates, G. A., Ryan, W., & Lauder, E. (1982). Current status of laryngectomee rehabilitation: IV. Attitudes about laryngectomy rehabilitation should change. *American Journal of Otolaryngology, 3,* 97–103.

Gerhardt, D. C., Shuck, T. J., Bordeaux, R. A., & Winship, D. H. (1978). Human upper esophageal sphincter: Response to volume, osmotic, and acid stimuli. *Gastroenterology, 75,* 268–274.

Gomyo, Y., & Doyle, P. C. (1989). Perception of stop consonants produced by esophageal and tracheoesophageal speakers. *Journal of Otolaryngology, 18,* 184–188.

Hamaker, R. C., & Blom, E. D. (2003). Botulinum neurotoxin for pharyngeal constrictor muscle spasm in tracheoesophageal voice restoration. *Laryngoscope, 113,* 1479–1482.

Hamaker, R. C., & Cheesman, A. D. (1998). Surgical management of pharyngeal constrictor muscle hypertonicity. In E. D. Blom, M. I. Singer, & R. C. Hamaker (Eds.), *Tracheoesophageal voice restoration following total laryngectomy* (pp. 33–39). San Diego, CA: Singular.

Hammarberg, B., Lundstrom, E., & Nord, L. (1996). Detailed observations of laryngectomee voice source characteristics from videofluoroscopy and perceptual–acoustic assessment. *Speech, Music and Hearing Quarterly Progress and Status Report* (pp. 63–66). Stockholm: KTH Royal Institute of Technology.

Henderson, R. D. (1976). *Motor disorders of the esophagus.* Baltimore: Williams & Wilkins.

Henderson, R. D. (1983). *Esophageal manometry in clinical investigation.* New York: Praeger.

Henderson, R. D., Boszko, A., & van Nostrand, A. W. P. (1974). Pharyngoesophageal dysphagia and recurrent laryngeal nerve palsy. *Journal of Thoracic and Cardiovascular Surgery, 68,* 507–511.

Hillman, R. E., Walsh, M. J., Wolf, G. T., Fisher, S. G., & Hong, W. K. (1998). Functional outcomes following treatment for advanced laryngeal cancer. *Annals of Otology, Rhinology and Laryngology, 107,* 2–27.

Hoffman, H.T., Fischer, H., Van Denmark, D., Peterson, K. L., McCulloch, T. M., Hynds Karnell, L. H., & Funk, G. F. (1997). Botulinum neurotoxin A injection after total laryngectomy. *Head & Neck, 19,* 92–97.

Horii, Y., & Weinberg, B. (1975). Intelligibility characteristics of superior esophageal speech presented under various levels of masking noise. *Journal of Speech and Hearing Research, 18,* 413–419.

Hunt, R. B. (1964). Rehabilitation of the laryngectomee. *Laryngoscope, 74,* 382–395.

Ingelfinger, F. (1958). Esophageal motility. *Physiology Review, 35,* 533–584.

Izdebski, K., Reed, C. G., Ross, J. C., & Hilsinger, R. L. (1994). Problems with tracheoesophageal fistula voice restoration in totally laryngectomized patients. *Archives of Otolaryngology—Head and Neck Surgery, 120,* 840–845.

Jankovic, J., & Orman, J. (1987). Botulinum A toxin for cranial–cervical dystonia. *Neurology, 37,* 616–623.

Johnson, C. (1960). A survey of laryngectomee patients in Veterans Administration hospitals. *Archives of Otolaryngology, 72,* 768–773.

Kallen, L. A. (1934). Vicarious vocal mechanisms. *Archives of Otolaryngology, 20,* 460–503.

King, P., Fowlks, E., & Pierson, G. (1968). Rehabilitation and adaptation of laryngectomy patients. *American Journal of Physical Medicine, 47,* 192–203.

Kirchner, J. A., Scatliff, J., Dey, F. L., & Shedd, D. P. (1963). The pharynx after laryngectomy. *Laryngoscope, 73,* 18–33.

Koybasioglu, A., Oz, O., Uslu, S., Ileri, F., Inal, E., & Unal, S. (2003). Comparison of pharyngo-esophageal segment pressure in total laryngectomy patients with and without pharyngeal neurectomy. *Head & Neck, 25,* 617–623.

Levin, N. M. (1962). *Voice and speech disorders: Medical aspects.* Springfield, IL: Thomas.

Logemann, J. (1983). *Evaluation and treatment of swallowing disorders.* Austin, TX: PRO-ED.

Lund, W. S., & Ardran, G. M. (1964). The motor nerve supply of the cricopharyngeal sphincter. *Annals of Otology, Rhinology and Laryngology, 73,* 599–617.

MacKnight, C. A., & Doyle, P. C. (1992, November). *Idiosyncratic patterns of voice onset time in superior tracheoesophageal speakers.* Paper presented at the annual convention of the American Speech-Language-Hearing Association, San Antonio, TX.

Mendelsohn, M. S., & McConnel, F. M. S. (1987). Function in the pharyngoesophageal segment. *Laryngoscope, 97,* 483–489.

Moon, J. B., & Weinberg, B. (1987). Aerodynamic and myoelastic contributions to tracheoesopha-geal voice production. *Journal of Speech and Hearing Research, 30,* 387–395.

Mu, L., & Sanders, I. (1996). The innervation of the human upper esophageal sphincter. *Dysphagia, 11,* 234–238.

Oh, C. K., Meleca, R. J., Simpson, M. L., & Dworkin, J. P. (2002). Fiberoptic examination of the pharyngoesophageal segment in tracheoesophageal speakers. *Archives of Otolaryngology—Head and Neck Surgery, 128,* 692–697.

Palmer, E. D. (1976). Disorders of the cricopharyngeus muscle: A review. *Progress in Gastroenterology, 71,* 510–519.

Ramachandran, K., Arunachalam, P. S., Hurren, A., Marsh, R. L., & Samuel, P. R. (2003). Botulinum toxin injection for failed tracheo-oesophageal voice in laryngectomees: The Sunderland experience. *Journal of Laryngology & Otology, 117,* 544–548.

Richardson, J., & Bourque, L. (1985). Communication after laryngectomy. *Journal of Psychosocial Oncology, 3,* 83–97.

Robbins, J., Fisher, H. B., Blom, E. D., & Singer, M. L. (1984). A comparative acoustic study of normal, esophageal, and tracheoesophageal speech production. *Journal of Speech and Hearing Disorders, 49,* 202–210.

Robe, E. Y., Moore, P., Andrews, A. H., & Holinger, P. H. (1956). A study of the role of certain factors in the development of speech after laryngectomy: Site of pseudoglottis. *Laryngoscope, 66,* 382–401.

Ross, E. R., Green, R., Auslander, M. O., & Biller, H. F. (1982). Cricopharyngeal myotomy: Management of cervical dysphagia. *Otolaryngology—Head and Neck Surgery, 90,* 434–441.

Schaefer, S., & Johns, D. (1982). Attaining esophageal speech. *Archives of Otolaryngology, 108,* 647–649.

Schneider, I., Thumfart, W. F., Potoschnig, C., & Eckel, H. E. (1994). Treatment of dysfunction of the cricopharyngeal muscle with botulinum A toxin: Introduction of a new, noninvasive method. *Annals of Otology, Rhinology and Laryngology, 103,* 31–35.

Scott, A. B., Kennedy, R. A., & Stubbs, H. A. (1984). Botulinum toxin A injection is a treatment for blepharospasm. *Archives of Opthalmology, 103,* 347–350.

Scott, P. M, Bleach, N. R., Perry, A. R., & Cheesman, A. D. (1993). Complication of pharyngeal myotomy for laryngeal rehabilitation. *Journal of Laryngology and Otology, 197,* 430–433.

Sellin, L. C. (1981). The action of botulinum toxin at the neuromuscular junction. *Medical Biology, 59,* 11–20.

Shanks, J. C. (1986). Essentials for alaryngeal speech: Psychology and physiology. In R. L. Keith & F. L. Darley (Eds.), *Laryngectomee rehabiliation* (pp. 337–349). San Diego: College-Hill Press.

Shipp, T. (1970). EMG of pharygoesophageal musculature during alaryngeal voice production. *Journal of Speech and Hearing Research, 13,* 184–192.

Simpson, I. C., Smith, J. C. S., & Gordon, M. T. (1972). Laryngectomy: The influence of muscle reconstruction on the mechanism of esophageal voice production. *Journal of Laryngology and Otology, 86,* 961–989.

Singer, M. I. (1988). The upper esophageal sphincter: Role in alaryngeal speech acquisition. *Head and Neck Surgery* (Suppl. II), S118–S123.

Singer, M. I., & Blom, E. D. (1980). An endoscopic technique for restoration of voice after laryngectomy. *Annals of Otology, Rhinology and Laryngology, 89,* 529–533.

Singer, M. I., & Blom, E. D. (1981). Selective myotomy for voice restoration after total laryngectomy. *Archives of Otolaryngology, 107,* 670–673.

Singer, M. I., Blom, E. D., & Hamaker, R. C. (1986). Pharyngeal plexus neurectomy for alaryngeal speech rehabilitation. *Laryngoscope, 96,* 50–54.

Sloane, P. M., Griffin, J. M., & O'Dwyer, T. P. (1991). Esophageal insufflation and videofluoroscopy for evaluation of esophageal speech in laryngectomy patients: Clinical implications. *Radiology, 181,* 433–437.

Smith, B. E., Weinberg, B., Feth, L. L, & Horii, Y. (1978). Vocal roughness and jitter characteristics of vowels produced by esophageal speakers. *Journal of Speech and Hearing Research, 21,* 240–249.

Snidecor, J. C. (1978). Speech therapy for those with total laryngectomy. In J. C. Snidecor (Ed.), *Speech rehabilitation of the laryngectomized* (2nd ed., pp. 180–193). Springfield, IL: Thomas.

Snidecor, J. C., & Curry, E. T. (1959). Temporal and pitch aspects of superior esophageal speech. *Annals of Otology, Rhinology and Laryngology, 68,* 1–14.

St. Guily, J. L., Angelard, B., El-Bez, M., Julien, N., Debry, C., Fichaux, P., & Gondret, R. (1992). Postlaryngectomy voice restoration: A prospective study of 83 patients. *Archives of Otolaryngology, 118,* 252–255.

Tardy-Mitzell, S., Andrews, M. L., & Bowman, S. A. (1985). Acceptability and intelligibility of tracheoesophageal speech. *Archives of Otolaryngology, 111,* 213–215.

Taub, S. (1980). Air bypass voice prosthesis: An 8 year experience. In D. P. Shedd & B. Weinberg (Eds.), *Surgical and prosthetic approaches to speech rehabilitation* (pp. 17–26). Boston: G.K. Hall.

Terrell, J. E., Lewin, J. S., & Esclamado, R. (1995). Botulinum toxin injection for postlaryngectomy tracheoesophageal speech failure. *Otolaryngology—Head and Neck Surgery, 113,* 788–791.

van den Berg, J., & Moolenaar-Bijl, A. J. (1959). Cricopharyngeal sphincter, pitch, intensity, and fluency in esophageal speech. *Practical Otorhinolaryngology, 21,* 298–315.

Volin, R. (1980). Predicting failure to speak after laryngectomy. *Laryngoscope, 90,* 1727–1736.

Vrticka, K., & Svoboda, M. (1961). A clinical and X-ray study of 100 laryngectomized speakers. *Folia Phoniatrica, 13,* 174–186.

Weinberg, B. (1980). Intrinsic forms of alaryngeal voice and speech: Esophageal speech. In B. Weinberg (Ed.), *Readings in speech following total laryngectomy* (pp. 35–43). Baltimore: University Park Press.

Weinberg, B., & Westerhouse, J. (1973). A study of pharyngeal speech. *Journal of Speech and Hearing Disorders, 38,* 111–118.

Welch, R. W., Gates, G. A., Luckmann, K. F., Ricks, P. M., & Drake, S. T. (1979). Change in the force-summed pressure measurements of the upper esophageal sphincter prelaryngectomy and postlaryngectomy. *Annals of Otolaryngology, 88,* 804–808.

Wepman, J. P., MacGahan, J. A., Rickard, J. C., & Shelton, N. W. (1953). The objective measure of progressive esophageal speech development. *Journal of Speech and Hearing Disorders, 18,* 247–251.

Winans, C. S. (1972). The pharyngoesophageal closure mechanism: A manometric study. *Gastroenterology, 63,* 768–777.

Winans, C. S., Reichback, E. J., & Waldrop, W. F. (1974). Esophageal determinants of alaryngeal speech. *Archives of Otolaryngology, 99,* 10–14.

Zormeier, M. M., Meleca, R. J., Simpson, M. L., Dworkin, J. P., Klein, R., Gross, M., & Mathog, R. H. (1999). Botulinum toxin injection to improve tracheoesophageal speech after total laryngectomy. *Otolaryngology—Head and Neck Surgery, 120,* 314–319.

Chapter 22

Clinical Procedures for Training Use of the Electronic Artificial Larynx

Philip C. Doyle

Use of the artificial larynx has a long history in the clinical literature on postlaryngectomy speech rehabilitation. The evolution of the artificial larynx, both in pneumatic and electronic formats, also has an extensive and rich history (Lebrun, 1976; Lowry, 1981; see also Chapter 2 in this text). Despite the importance and success of surgical prosthetic approaches to postlaryngectomy voice restoration over the past two decades (Blom, Singer, & Hamaker, 1998; see also Chapter 17 in this text), clinical information on use of the electronic artificial larynx (more widely used than the pneumatic larynx) remains essential. Programs that do not provide the electrolarynx as an alaryngeal speech option are likely not meeting the needs of individuals who undergo laryngectomy or of their family members (Hillman, Walsh, Wolf, Fisher, & Hong, 1998). Because the artificial larynx remains an important and viable method of postlaryngectomy speech rehabilitation, interest in refining the "end product" of the artificial larynx—the speech signal produced—continues today. Information on clinical training procedures for use of the electrolarynx has been offered by many authors in several well-recognized textbooks addressing laryngectomy and alaryngeal speech (e.g., Diedrich & Youngstrom, 1966; Doyle, 1994; Edels, 1983; Goldstein, 1982; Keith & Shanks, 1994; Salmon & Goldstein, 1978; Salmon & Mount, 1991; Snidecor, 1978).

In addition to the useful information on the variety of electronic artificial larynxes, the availability of such devices, and the clinical training to use them, there is also a secondary literature that suggests that the artificial larynx, regardless of type, may be an inferior method of postlaryngectomy speech rehabilitation. This assumption has no merit even in the current era of postlaryngectomy rehabilitation in which surgical–prosthetic methods are widely used. Salmon (1983) explicitly acknowledged that, even though considerable criticism has been leveled against use of artificial larynxes as a postsurgical method of alaryngeal communication, such criticism is "rarely directed toward their facility for providing a means of communication" (p. 142). As with all methods of postlaryngectomy voice and speech rehabilitation, no "perfect" method exists. Rather, each method has unique advantages and disadvantages relative to the other options (Doyle, 1994). Although electrolaryngeal speech does not compare with that of normal speech, neither does esophageal speech or tracheoesophageal (TE) voice restoration. The details and refutation of such a negative bias against the electronic artificial larynx have been addressed in several sources (Doyle, 1994; Duguay, 1978; Gates, Ryan, & Lauder, 1982; Goldstein, 1978). Careful evaluation of the clinical literature, however, will show that the electronic artificial larynx is a valuable option for those who are laryngectomized. In fact, in most clinical circles, the electrolarynx continues to be viewed as an essential component of comprehensive postlaryngectomy clinical care throughout the rehabilitation process (Hillman et al., 1998; see also Chapter 4 in this text).

Although other alaryngeal speech options exist (esophageal and tracheoesophageal speech), the various methods and their particular commonalities must be acknowledged by both patient and clinician (see Chapter 3 in this text). Because of such commonalities, the electronic artificial larynx should never be excluded from clinical consideration. Therefore, this chapter focuses on issues related to training use of the electronic artificial larynx. Topics include information related to the common types of artificial larynxes used clinically, the basic design components of neck-type and intraoral electronic artificial laryngeal devices, the associated utility of these devices for postlaryngectomy speech rehabilitation, a description of speech rehabilitation methods using the artificial larynx, early methods of therapeutic intervention, a discussion of ongoing refinements of artificial larynx speech, and the value of the artificial larynx in restoring functional communication.

CLINICAL APPLICATION OF THE ELECTRONIC ARTIFICIAL LARYNX

A careful review of the literature will reveal that the value of the electrolarynx can be seen in both short- and long-term rehabilitative efforts (see Chapter 5 in this text). From a practical point of view, the electrolarynx is likely to be the only functional method of verbal communication in the early postoperative period. Additionally, many individuals will ultimately rely on this method of alaryngeal communication throughout their postsurgical lives. Contemporary data suggest that when longer term outcomes are assessed, the electrolarynx may garner sufficient usage as a primary and quite satisfactory method of postlaryngectomy verbal communication (see Chapter 4 in this text). Culton and Gerwin (1998) reported that 39% of alaryngeal speakers they surveyed relied on the electrolarynx over the 5-year period postlaryngectomy; usage increased to 43% in the period 10 years postlaryngectomy. These data clearly indicate that the electrolarynx should not be viewed as an inadequate or inefficient method of postlaryngectomy voice and speech rehabilitation. Because of this, the electrolarynx should be viewed by clinicians as far more than a temporary or interim method of postlaryngectomy alaryngeal speech. As noted by Salmon (1983), "Acceptance of artificial larynx devices by patient and family members can best be achieved by the projection of an accepting attitude by members of the rehabilitation staff" (p. 153).

If the clinician is open to the use of an electrolarynx, he or she might then foster a positive attitude toward its use and value by others. Fair assessments of the importance of an artificial larynx as a postlaryngectomy option cannot be made if bias exists. This potential bias against the artificial larynx may be avoided through the open exchange of information between professionals involved in postlaryngectomy care. Clinicians must fight the urge to dismiss any of the postlaryngectomy communicative options presently available (esophageal, TE, and artificial laryngeal speech) without adequate cause. The early goal of postlaryngectomy speech rehabilitation efforts should be directed toward facilitating verbal communication. Given the good success rates that are usually achieved with the artificial larynx, its utility for functional communication purposes cannot be justifiably questioned or overlooked. Although distinct disadvantages exist for electrolarynxes (as for other methods of alaryngeal voice and speech), these disadvantages are far outweighed by the advantages. The most critical advantage is that in most circumstances the electrolarynx will facilitate a relatively rapid and efficient opportunity for verbal communication.

The ability to verbally communicate, particularly in the early postoperative period, is deemed to be a critical component of recovery and successful rehabilitation (Doyle, 1994). Leuders (1956) was one of the first authors to point out the "psychological importance" of facilitating artificial laryngeal speech in the early postoperative period, as well as to stress the key role that speech plays in the "social" functions of individuals. The ability to verbally communicate at a time of a health crisis may decrease fear and anxiety, thus reducing the vulnerability of the individual to depression and withdrawal. Therefore, all individuals who undergo total laryngectomy, including those who undergo primary TE puncture voice restoration, should be trained to efficiently and effectively use the electrolarynx. Establishing a prompt and functional method of verbal communication must be a fundamental component of postlaryngectomy patient care.

THE ARTIFICIAL LARYNX DEFINED

The artificial larynx has taken many forms over the years. In fact, *artificial larynx* may be viewed as an omnibus term. Substantial efforts to improve the artificial larynx have existed over many years and have taken many forms. In fact, the search for the prosthetic restoration of voice following laryngectomy has existed since the first total laryngectomy was undertaken in the mid–18th century (see Chapter 2 in this text). Efforts to refine and improve the artificial larynx have persisted into the modern era of postlaryngectomy clinical efforts. For example, in the early 1970s, considerable efforts were directed toward developing a "reed–fistula" method of alaryngeal speech (e.g., Shedd et al., 1972; Taub & Spiro, 1972). This method of postlaryngectomy speech rehabilitation involved "interposing an external air-bypass and pseudolaryngeal mechanism between the laryngectomized patient's tracheal stoma and a surgically created pharyngeal fistula" (Weinberg, Shedd, & Horii, 1978, p. 402). Similar methods were reported by several others as this approach to voice restoration was pursued vigorously in the early 1970s (Sisson, McConnel, Logemann, & Yeh, 1975; Taub & Bergner, 1973). The use of electrolarynxes, however, remained a viable, valuable, and preferred option for postlaryngectomy speech rehabilitation when problems with air-bypass devices were confronted.

Regardless of the method employed, the ultimate goal of the artificial larynx is to restore, through some "external" method, a vibratory source for speech production. Electronically driven devices remain a prominent fixture of contemporary postlaryngectomy patient care, and the importance of such devices is supported through recent reports in the literature (Hillman et al., 1998; see also Chapter 4 in this text). The extent of development over many years has been rich (Salmon & Goldstein, 1978; see also Chapter 2 in this text) and has continued into the modern era with the pioneering work conducted at the Massachusetts

Eye and Ear Infirmary in Boston (see Chapter 23 in this text). For purposes of the present discussion, electronic artificial laryngeal devices—those that provide an external, battery-driven vibratory source that will be used for speech articulation—will be the sole and central theme.[1] In many clinical settings throughout the world, in at least some form, the electrolarynx remains a prominent and widely used method of communication in postlaryngectomy voice and speech rehabilitation programs.

Design Considerations

From the simple standpoint of design, Barney (1958) suggested that two acoustic factors should be considered when seeking to develop an ideal electronic artificial larynx: (a) the ideal artificial larynx should generate a vocal intensity that is equivalent to that of a normal speaker, and (b) the "speech quality" and extent of pitch variability (e.g., inflection) should be similar to that of the normal laryngeal speaker. These two considerations are critical in that they permit the alaryngeal signal generated through use of the artificial larynx to be perceivable to the listener (relative to the loudness of the signal) and to sound as natural as possible. Normal intensity and improved speech quality serve both general aspects related to speech intelligibility (strictly speaking) and reduce potential difficulties associated with identification of the electrolaryngeal signal as being highly abnormal or unnatural to the listener.

Barney (1958) also noted that several other factors should be considered in designing the ideal electrolarynx. He suggested that the artificial larynx should be (a) small and unobtrusive, (b) reliable and trouble-free to the user, (c) acceptable to the user from the standpoint of hygiene, and (d) affordable. Though unstated, the underlying goal of most of these collective ideals seems to focus on naturalizing the speech process and improving its overall acceptability within the context of social communication and interaction. Thus, use of an electrolarynx must be evaluated fairly relative to its advantages and disadvantages as a postlaryngectomy communication option.[2]

Speech Acceptability

Bennett and Weinberg (1973) showed that, relative to normal speakers and those using esophageal speech, speakers using the electrolarynx suffer reductions in ratings of acceptability by listeners. Given the nature of the sound source, this finding is not unexpected. In fact, based on Bennett and Weinberg's study, listeners

---

[1]This is not to suggest that nonelectronic devices, such as those that are pneumatic (e.g., the Tokyo artificial speech aid), are less valuable or of inferior quality.

[2]Goldstein (1978) provided a succinct summary of the pros and cons of artificial larynx use.

identified that the most troublesome aspect of the electrolarynx used (a Bell 5A) was the "mechanical" nature of the signal produced and associated monotony. Although the "effectiveness" of communication should in some fashion form a basis for judgments of the success or failure of postlaryngectomy communication, an "effective" signal is ultimately insufficient if the listener finds him- or herself uncomfortable because the signal is deemed unacceptable by others. Hence, the communication dyad must form the primary matrix from which alaryngeal speech success is derived. By doing so, both the speaker and the listener are considered. From the standpoint of communication effectiveness and potential limitations to the individual who is laryngectomized, these more expansive issues and the influence of signal characteristics on auditory–perceptual judgments of the signal always must be considered (see Chapter 6 in this text).

One additional factor that may be implied from the concerns expressed by Barney (1958) is that such devices should be easy to use. Ease of use is likely an important design feature of devices available today. In fact, the majority of individuals undergoing total laryngectomy can easily be taught to use an artificial larynx at a very basic, functional level of proficiency (i.e., for expressing basic wants, needs, and desires) with a relatively minimal level of instruction. The occasional individuals who are unable to use the electrolarynx at all are those with, for example, cognitive limitations, associated motor impairment, and extensive head and neck resection. Instruction in electrolarynx use always should be systematic and sensitive to related factors that may have an impact on communication in a larger sense.

Clinicians must always consider the potential social impact of using any method of postlaryngectomy alaryngeal communication. Such considerations may involve not only the quality of the signal produced for verbal communication purposes, but also the visual nature of the device. When an external device is used, it may draw attention to itself and, as a result, alter some dimension(s) of the communication process. This concern has far-reaching and important considerations for the individual user of any type of artificial larynx. In an era when clinicians are acknowledging more global aspects of therapeutic and rehabilitative outcomes, an effort to understand more about the effect of alaryngeal speech in general, and of artificial laryngeal speech in particular, on the communicative process (Beaudin, Doyle, and Eadie, 2004) and social participation is essential (Doyle, 1999; Eadie, 2001; see also Chapter 6 in this text).

DEVICES IN COMMON CLINICAL USE

Two general types of electronic artificial laryngeal devices are used today: (a) the *neck-type* or *transcervical* device and (b) the *intraoral* or *transoral* device. These two types are distinguished by how the artificial voicing source is transmitted to the vocal tract for articulation to occur. Both types have direct and widespread clinical application in North America and abroad, and the primary decision to use one or the other type of device is usually related to when in the postlaryngectomy period the device is used. Factors related to surgery, possible complications in healing, extended resectioning and reconstruction, and so on, may require the clinician to defer use of a particular device in some instances.

Neck-type devices are often not of great utility in the early postoperative period because direct contact of the vibratory head of a transcervical device on neck tissues may cause discomfort. In contrast, an intraoral device often can be used without causing discomfort for the patient. Therefore, intraoral devices are ideal in the early period of recovery and rehabilitation. In this regard, it is important to point out that many neck-type devices can be easily modified to become intraoral devices. Such adaptations have been presented early on in the clinical literature by Blom (1978) and Zwitman and colleagues (Zwitman & Disinger, 1975; Zwitman, Knorr, & Sonderman, 1978). Several chapters of *The Artificial Larynx Handbook* (Salmon & Goldstein, 1978) provide excellent reviews of the varied types of artificial laryngeal devices in use, as well as details of clinical modification of such devices.

Neck-Type Devices

A neck-type device is designed so that when it is placed on the neck, the external sound source generated via the electrolarynx is passed through neck tissue into the vocal tract. Because a vibratory head serves as the direct source of signal transmission, "coupling" of the neck and the device is essential for optimizing signal transmission into the vocal tract, where articulation will occur. Several commonly used neck-type electrolarynxes are shown in Figure 22.1.

A common problem confronted with neck-type devices relates to changes in the impedance of neck tissue (due either to surgery and associated tissue scarring or to radiation-induced fibrosis). In the presence of such changes, coupling of a transcervical device to the neck tissues may prove to be problematic and will require careful and comprehensive clinical assessment. Many of these devices permit adjustment of signal frequency and intensity levels, although the functional

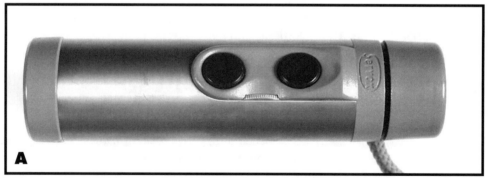

(continues)

FIGURE 22.1. Commonly used neck-type artificial laryngeal devices. (A) Servox electronic artificial larynx. (B) OptiVox electronic artificial larynx. (C) Denrick 2 electronic artificial larynx. (D) Nu-Vois electronic artificial larynx. (E) Neovox electronic artificial larynx.

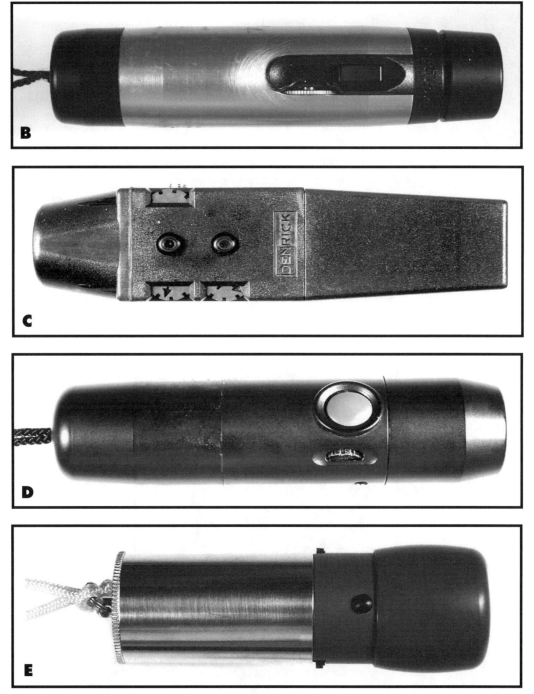

FIGURE 22.1. *Continued.*

advantage of this capacity has just begun to be explored at the acoustic or perceptual level (Beaudin, Meltzner, Doyle, & Hillman, 2004; Beaudin, Meltzner, Hillman, & Doyle, 2003; see also Chapter 23 in this text).

Intraoral Devices

An intraoral artificial larynx is designed so that the electronic voice source is passed through a small-diameter tube and introduced directly into the oral cavity. Thus, the vocal tract can be energized for articulatory purposes. As with the neck-type devices, care must be taken to ensure optimal placement of the intraoral tube—in this case within the oral cavity—for speech production to be achieved. The most frequently used intraoral devices are the Cooper-Rand artificial larynx (see Figure 22.2A) and a modified Servox (transcervical) artificial

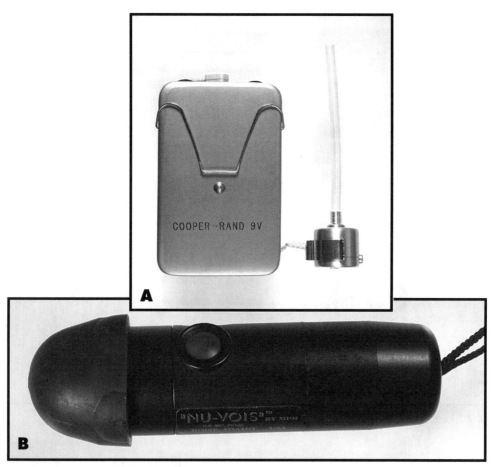

FIGURE 22.2. Intraoral artificial laryngeal devices. (A) Cooper-Rand electronic artificial larynx (with on–off switch and coupler for oral tube to right). (B) Nu-Vois electronic artificial larynx (with intraoral adapter attached and intraoral tube below).

larynx. Many of the neck-type devices mentioned previously can also be converted easily into intraoral devices by either the speech–language pathologist or the laryngectomized individual. Figure 22.2B shows an example of a neck-type artificial larynx (Nu-Vois) with the oral adapter attached to the vibratory head of the device (the intraoral tube that inserts into the adapter is shown below the device). Blom (1978) provided an excellent summary of such early modifications. Similar to some transcervical devices, the Cooper-Rand device has the capacity for adjustment of both frequency and intensity.

SELECTING AN ELECTRONIC ARTIFICIAL LARYNX

Determining which type of artificial larynx is best for any given individual involves consideration of several factors. As stated by Doyle (1994, p. 123) regarding alaryngeal rehabilitation efforts, "no alaryngeal option is free of communicative liabilities." Doyle elaborated upon this statement, however, by acknowledging that despite such liabilities, relative "strengths and weaknesses must also be viewed within the context of the patient's physical, psychological, and cognitive abilities" (p. 123), as well as his or her communicative needs. It has been suggested by several authors that the use of an artificial larynx, at a minimum, provides some level of motivation for communication and may serve to maintain the individual's morale following loss of the normal mechanism of voice and speech production (Diedrich & Youngstrom, 1966; Doyle, 1994; Duguay, 1978; Goldstein, 1978; Lauder, 1970; Salmon & Goldstein, 1978). Thus, clinicians and their patients must enter into an open discussion when alaryngeal methods of communication are presented for consideration (Gates et al., 1982). Ideally, the clinician acknowledges the positive and negative considerations associated with each device and explains each in sufficient detail using simple language so that the patient can make an informed choice. Information provided by Salmon (1978) suggested that about 43% of those individuals who chose to use an artificial larynx were not embarrassed about their decision to use such a device. Salmon explicitly suggested, however, that with better provision of information, the level of acknowledged embarrassment would likely be reduced.

Although the signal generated by each electrolarynx should be at the forefront of many decisions about which device will provide optimal communication (Happ, Roesch, & Kagan, 2004), it would not be appropriate for the clinician to choose a device that the user does not like. The clinician should clearly explain why he or she believes a given device is better than another, using simple, jargon-free language with a well-reasoned justification for such a belief. Needless to say, if the clinician encourages use of a device that is not preferred by the patient, the chance of having the individual successfully use the device will be limited. Additionally, this type of forced-choice decision may affect the patient's desire to communicate, which may have very real and serious consequences on the person's social behavior, comfort with his or her new method of verbal communication, and ultimately the individual's well-being and quality of life (Doyle, Eadie, Beaudin, & White, 2003).

GOALS OF THERAPY:
USE OF THE ARTIFICIAL LARYNX

Clinical information supports the notion that the electrolarynx will prove to be a valuable rehabilitation tool for many individuals (Hillman et al., 1998; Salmon & Mount, 1991; see also Chapter 4 in this text). Regardless of whether the artificial larynx will ultimately be used as an individual's primary or secondary method of alaryngeal communication, clinicians are obliged to offer comprehensive training and guidance to those who are laryngectomized. Initial rehabilitation efforts include careful instruction in how the device works, including simple troubleshooting strategies, as well as direct treatment, which targets optimal usage of the device.

From the standpoint of clinical management, three specific but global goals are targeted for artificial larynx training. The term *global* reflects the fact that these three goals provide the foundation for the successful use of any electrolarynx. These goals are: (a) correct and consistent placement, (b) use of a slowed speech rate or overarticulation, and (c) device on–off control during speech production (Doyle, 1994). Graham (1997) suggested that optimal use of the electrolarynx is achieved through five goals, the three noted above, as well as goals addressing (a) appropriate speech rate and phrasing and (b) clinical attention to nonverbal behaviors. Similarly, Duguay (1983) included phrasing and pitch, inflection, and stress as important components of electrolarynx training. Phrasing may fall into the more global goal focused on speech rate (see description of training sequence in the following section); addressing aspects of pitch, inflection, and stress may fall into an advanced program of training. Thus, comprehensive clinical training with the electrolarynx encompasses much more than providing a supplemental voicing source following laryngectomy.

Although other issues will arise, and these will also require attention, the three global goals are essential to developing the most proficient electrolaryngeal speech possible. Some individuals, however, will experience a variety of problems in using the artificial larynx. In many instances, these problems can be overcome with simple modifications (e.g., adjusting frequency and intensity of signal output) or through additional explanation and clinical instruction about the characteristics and correct use of the device. Any good postlaryngectomy rehabilitation program requires that the clinician and the patient communicate freely about slight adjustments, modifications, and related advantages or disadvantages of particular devices. All devices are similar, but effective communication will help to ensure the best possible clinical outcome following a systematic course of treatment. Whenever possible, early clinical efforts should explore the use of several commercially available brands of artificial larynxes. Slight changes in the specifications of a given device at times may offer substantial advantages to the user. Additionally, for any given clinical training task that is undertaken, clear advancement criterion is necessary. Establishing criterion will permit a method of clinical accountability (see Chapter 27 in this text), as well as allow the clinician to identify mid-level tasks should problems arise with a particular skill (i.e., if the user passes one program step but fails the next, the clinician is obliged to determine what intermediary step is necessary to enable the user to acquire that step).

Facilitating Correct and Consistent Placement

Practice in placement of the electrolarynx should seek to ensure that two particular behaviors become fail-safe. First, the device must be approximated to the location that results in the most resonant sound production. This selection process is usually done with the production of vowels. Second, the clinician must instruct the individual to make sure that the vibratory head of the transcervical electrolarynx is in direct and flush contact with tissues that provide the best overall resonance of the signal (often referred to as the "sweet spot"). Once the spot is identified, the individual must be able to consistently and quickly find this location.

For a neck-type device, a perpendicular orientation of the vibratory head to skin is essential. If contact is not complete, the sound source will be inefficiently transferred across tissue and into the vocal tract for articulatory purposes. In this situation, extraneous noise will also occur, which not only reduces the source being transmitted into the vocal tract but, perhaps more importantly, creates competing noise that may ultimately reduce communication efficiency and effectiveness. This problem is also possible with the intraoral artificial larynx, although extraneous noise is often more difficult to reduce because of the design of this type of speech aid. Adequate loudness of the speech signal is essential (Barney, 1958). When practicing device placement, the individual may find mirror work helpful because sensation is often impaired, which limits the tactile feedback required for necessary adjustments.

When instructing the patient in the use of an intraoral artificial larynx, the clinician needs to target correct and consistent placement of the intraoral tube within the oral cavity. The patient might see the intraoral tube as a potential limiting factor in oral articulation; however, with practice and care, the patient can minimize the tube's effect on articulation in an effort to enhance speech communication. Although some basic guidelines regarding placement have emerged in the clinical literature, experienced clinicians typically explore a variety of placements with an ongoing assessment of the speech produced. Some speakers achieve excellent degrees of articulatory precision with oral placements that would be expected to jeopardize precision (e.g., tube placement in the central portion of the oral cavity).

The point being emphasized here is that exploration with either a transcervical or intraoral type of device is essential if foundation skills are to be achieved. If a patient does not learn where the best placement is, the ability to habituate to an ideal location, regardless of electrolaryngeal device, is decreased significantly. Salmon (1983) aptly stated that "locating the spot and determining the most effective coupling for best resonance are of utmost importance since they are basic to good artificial larynx voice" (p. 155). Without attention to this critical detail, the individual speaker's chance for developing and successfully using an electrolarynx is diminished.

Identifying the Best Location for Device Placement

Regardless of the type of device used, correct and consistent placement of the electrolarynx is essential. In the case of neck-type devices, the clinician must ensure that the location on which the vibratory head is placed is the most compatible with sound transmission. The clinician and the patient must explore a variety of locations on the neck to compare the quality of signals produced. Furthermore, in the case of neck-type devices, the clinician must ensure that the vibrating head is in full contact with neck tissue. Vowel production serves as the ideal speech target for this part of training. When changes in resonance occur, it is best if they can be appreciated and distinguished by both the device user and the clinician. As suggested by Salmon (1997), when the clinician and patient find the sweet spot, they should mark it with a pen or tape to maximize its identification in further practice. For individuals who have difficulty in consistently moving to the sweet spot, mirror work should be aggressively pursued.

Distinguishing Good Productions

Regardless of whether an intraoral or transcervical device is used, the task of identifying the best location for device placement requires trial and error. The clinician should always be the person to place the artificial larynx early in training, because slight adjustments in position may result in sufficient changes in the acoustic signal. Even though the patient is not actively involved in manipulating the artificial larynx at this point, he or she must be encouraged to focus on and carefully listen to the sound produced. What the patient hears and what the clinician hears are different, but hopefully the two agree about what constitutes a "good" or a "poor" production. Although the clinician usually manipulates the device at this stage of instruction, the user simultaneously needs to be introduced to aspects of device use. Early exposure to the device will help the user to develop preliminary device manipulation skills and permit the clinician to observe potential problems that can be addressed as part of the treatment program. This early involvement often assists the user later, when transferring some basic skills to those that are more advanced (e.g., coordinating multiple skills, such as device placement and manipulating the on–off switch). If placement difficulties arise, the clinician must assume the responsibility of reinstructing the user.

Modifying Placements

For placement of intraoral devices, minimal insertion into a lateral region of the anterior oral cavity is often best. The depth of insertion usually should be less than 2.5 cm (1 in.). Exploration of a variety of locations, however, may instruct the user on how specific placements may significantly reduce the signal quality. With some individuals who absorb information and develop basic skills quickly, use of negative practice may be of value.[3]

---

[3]Negative practice allows the user to perform "bad" use behaviors, such as incorrect device placement, in an effort to firmly facilitate good ones.

For transcervical devices, a location just lateral to the midline region of the neck is often best. Other placements should be evaluated, however, because some individuals may exhibit good speech transmission from less common placement locations (e.g., directly under the chin). Duguay (1983) suggested that care be taken to avoid placements on suture lines or on those areas where a stoma cover eventually may prevent good placement of the device. Suture lines soon after surgery may be tender, and well-healed lines may not transmit the signal effectively.

Again, the goals at this early stage of training are to facilitate production of the most resonant speech signal possible and to have the user habituate to the ideal placement of the device. The user must be given adequate opportunity to use the device at this stage, with ongoing demonstration, instruction, and refinements directed by the clinician. Both positive and negative feedback regarding use should always be presented immediately in a clear manner. The clinician should also have the user manipulate the artificial larynx with greater regularity as training progresses.

Optimizing Signal Transmission

After locating the correct placement, the goal is to maintain the ideal contact between the neck tissue and the vibratory head of a transcervical device, or for the tube of an intraoral electrolarynx within the oral cavity. At this point, the individual is asked to more actively use and manipulate the artificial larynx on an almost exclusive basis. From an engineering perspective, ideal signal transmission must involve matching components of the source signal to the medium of transmission. For both intraoral and neck-type devices, this matching will be altered to some extent with changes in the frequency level of the device (i.e., the pitch level produced). The clinician, however, should identify a pitch level that is most appropriate for the individual speaker despite the clearly unusual nature of the vibratory source. In some cases, specific adjustments in frequency may result in increased or decreased signal transmission. Frequency adjustments require that the user assess the quality of the speech to ensure that he or she is comfortable with it prior to making any final decision on a specific frequency setting.

Although frequency variability is not extensive in the artificial larynx because of limitations in driving such an oscillator (see Chapter 23 in this text), an attempt should be made to make the pitch appropriate to the speaker's gender. Better pitch levels may not always result in the best resonance, but from the standpoint of user and listener acceptability, the choice to use a pitch level that is not as resonant may be necessary. Thus, consideration of both signal characteristics and vocal tract transfer function is essential for optimizing electrolaryngeal devices, and attempts at modifying existing devices to create an improved speech signal may be of value (Meltzner & Hillman, 2003; Meltzner, Kobler, & Hillman, 2003). Decisions about what is best may be based on vowel productions or simple speech tasks such as counting.

Targeting for Articulatory Precision

When the best location for signal transmission is identified, several secondary concerns must be addressed. The user of an intraoral device needs to be instructed that direct contact with the tongue or other oral structures may reduce articulatory precision. Additionally, the user cannot "bury" the tube in oral tissues, or the tube may become clogged with saliva, which may negatively influence signal transmission. An additional concern pertains to hygienic concerns should the tube become clogged with saliva.

The patient using a transcervical device must avoid pressing the vibratory head into tissues of the neck with too much effort. Doing so will restrict vibration of the device head, with subsequent reductions in the loudness, efficiency, and quality of the speech signal. Thus, correct placement of the transcervical device involves paying careful attention to both location and contact pressure. Because of neck sensitivity issues in some individuals, a demonstration on the palm of the hand or cheek may be required.

Clinicians must remember that although these early steps of training the person to use an artificial larynx may be somewhat time consuming, the individual's ability to master these skills is fundamental to his or her longer term success as an alaryngeal speaker. Therefore, clinicians should not rush through placement goals without carefully documenting that the user has consistently demonstrated correct behaviors for electrolarynx use.

Other Considerations

Regardless of which type of device is chosen for use, additional questions always arise, such as whether the individual should hold the electrolarynx with the dominant or nondominant hand, and whether the individual should place or couple the device to the neck in an ipsilateral or contralateral (i.e., crossover) fashion. These questions are not trivial relative to the individual patient's desire for flexibility in use and need to perform complementary tasks while using the artificial larynx (e.g., shaking hands, speaking on the phone). Perhaps the best approach under these circumstances is to assess an individual's use of such complementary tasks when training electrolaryngeal device use. Situations that may be unique to the individual must be addressed to make the artificial larynx as useful as possible. Addressing the individual's unique communication demands and environments will increase the likelihood that the device can be used as effectively as possible in the greatest number of situations.

Specifically, the clinician should help the individual explore use of both hands and both sides of the neck. Many individuals will identify a clear preference; however, the initial preference may be associated with the earliest "best" result with the dominant hand. As with any physical task that is new or awkward, or that requires physical adjustments and modifications due to dexterity limitations, practice is required. Learning to use the artificial larynx has a large motor skill component associated with it; therefore, sufficient practice of the required motor skill must be undertaken. Developing foundation skills that will increase the chance of successful electrolarynx use requires regular, systematic practice that is guided and monitored by the clinician, as well as direct feedback to the individual so that corrections can be made when necessary.

Most individuals will acquire and refine these manual skills in a fairly short period of time. Some individuals, however, will require considerable reinstruction in using the device with the best level of skill possible. As with most clinical endeavors, what may seem simple and straightforward to the trained clinician is likely to be new and unclear for the nonprofessional. Consequently, clinicians should strive to speak in plain language, provide written and visual materials when appropriate, provide demonstrations, and perhaps most important, directly ask the individual if he or she has understood the instructions or has any questions.

Use of a Slowed Speech Rate or Overarticulation

Attention to the speech rate of those who use an artificial larynx is necessary. First, any degraded speech signal has the potential to be further disrupted if speech rate is excessive, which would increase the burden on the listener and influence communication effectiveness. Second, many of those who communicate with the electrolarynx user are of the same older age group in which hearing loss may add to the communication difficulty. A reduced rate of speech may enhance communication to some extent in this situation. Careful monitoring of speech rate by the clinician can be helpful in achieving the best possible signal transmission. Reductions in speech rate may be achieved by increasing pause time at the phrase or sentence level, slowing articulation of sound elements in any given utterance, or a combination of both. Although a "normal" rate of speech should clearly not be exceeded, some slight reduction in speech rate through overarticulation is often beneficial to optimizing speech intelligibility.

Approaches that have been used for other classes of speech disorders (i.e., the dysarthrias and fluency disorders) may be appropriate during training with the artificial larynx. For most individuals, rate control may be habituated in a relatively short period of time, but it does require substantial drillwork. The clinician should take a systematic approach, starting at an introductory level (usually two- or three-word phrases) and then working up to longer utterances, oral reading, and conversational interactions. As a general rule, each of the following levels of treatment is appropriate for training with both the transcervical and intraoral electrolarynxes.

Introductory Level

Each clinician should develop a basic set of stimulus materials for practice with control of speech rate and overarticulation or obtain materials (for other disorders) from commercial sources. The introductory stimulus set should include a series of phrases and sentences that range in length from 3 to 8 or more syllables. I structure these materials as follows: All phrases and sentences comprise one-syllable words. Because the number of words in any given stimulus item is the same as its syllabic length, treatment monitoring is more efficient. For example,

"I won't go" has three syllables and words; "She came by the house in time for lunch" has nine syllables and words. Longer stimuli should be free of any breaks in the flow of speech; that is, materials should have simple main clauses and avoid subordinate clauses or compound objects. In such constructions, commas would require some level of pausing that is contrary to the objectives of this introductory training.

The number of items for each stimulus set (based on number of words or syllables) should range from 10 to 20. Clinical treatment involves drillwork focusing on the precise and even control of speech production throughout the length of the stimulus. During the production of each stimulus item, the clinician should carefully monitor to ensure that the speaker is not producing each word in an isolated manner (e.g., "I–won't–go"). Rather, the speaker should be encouraged to move through the phrase or sentence in a smooth, near-natural manner while briefly prolonging continuant sounds; if the task is performed adequately, it will not exceed a normal speech rate. It is important that during the initial phases of training the electrolarynx remain "on" during the entire utterance regardless of length. On–off control will be introduced in later stages of training.

In slowing speech rate, the speaker inevitably slows articulation to some extent. Therefore, the goals of slowing speech rate and of overarticulation (sound and syllable prolongation) can be worked on simultaneously in most instances. Although instrumentation may be of use (e.g., acoustic analysis software that can show results of speech production), the educated "clinical ear" may provide a very good method of monitoring appropriate speech rate. The best speech rate will often coincide with a good level of articulatory precision and speech intelligibility. If reductions in phoneme intelligibility are observed, treatment should center on specific articulation targets. The phrase and sentence stimuli described for this level do not require a priori control of phonemic elements. Although aspects of phonetic structure could be controlled and such carefully controlled stimuli could be developed, such stimuli ultimately do not mirror that observed in natural speech. Therefore, the development of stimulus materials without direct consideration of what sounds appear and in what context is recommended. If articulation difficulties are observed, a more structured program of treatment directed at improving articulation proper can be developed and employed with an individual.

Intermediate Level

The intermediate level of speech rate and overarticulation training involves oral reading tasks. Although the clinician may develop stimuli for this task, such as paragraph-length materials, a reasonable alternative is to use a newspaper or magazine. Most newspapers are written in simple language, and sentence length is generally short. What makes this task different from the introductory level of phrase and sentence production is that additional pauses due to normal juncture are required. For example, the sentence "Mike took the ball, bat, and mitt, then left home" requires some brief pauses (which also can be exaggerated as part of training). In this circumstance, the speaker must be encouraged to stop speaking completely so as to break the flow of speech, reducing the chance of rapidly moving through longer utterances without pausing. This type of task also might be of value when components of device "on–off" control are considered. In the intermediate phase of device training, however, it is often best to leave the device on throughout the utterance, even though the extraneous noise during pauses is distracting and will not be permitted in later stages of instruction.

Advanced Level

The advanced level of speech rate and overarticulation training when using the artificial larynx should take place at the conversational level. In many clinical environments, this level is often overlooked due to the demands of increasing clinical caseloads, financial constraints, and other reasons (Doyle, 2002). Nevertheless, some level of attention, even if somewhat cursory, should be given to this more natural manner of speech production. It is at this level that "fine-tuning" of the speaker's skills can take place. Advanced levels of training require the user to exhibit consistent placement (location and contact pressure), maintain an acceptable speech rate with overarticulation, and manipulate the on–off control of the artificial larynx. As a rule, this part of training should be done in a responsive mode (i.e., the clinician poses questions that will need to be answered by the user) or in conversational interactions. Performance at this level will almost always mimic that used outside of the clinical environment. If bad habits develop, they can be observed during conversation and remedied accordingly. If noted, the clinician must structure appropriate tasks to resolve a problem before it becomes habitual. If problems arise with aspects of device placement, speech rate, overarticulation, or combinations thereof, a return to earlier portions of the program is required. When this occurs, use of a more rigorous success criterion may be necessary at each level of retraining similar to that in all prior efforts of skill acquisition.

Device On–Off Control

The ability to appropriately control the onset and offset of artificial larynx vibration is not a simple skill and, if employed incorrectly, can adversely affect the transfer of information during communication. A number of factors must be considered when defining a reasonable therapeutic "target" relative to device on–off control. For example, users with reduced manual dexterity may fully appreciate the need to turn their artificial larynx "on" or "off" at a specific time, but they may not be able to do so easily. Similarly, because this task requires considerable coordination of speech, phrasing, device–neck coupling, manual manipulation of the device, and so on, the "ceiling" of performance capacity needs to be assessed on an individual basis. Likewise, some individuals may not understand why such adjustments are necessary, and the clinician's explanation may not be of value. In this type of clinical encounter, the clinician must set goals that do not require more than the individual is able to achieve. All performance goals must be individualized and realistic.

The essence of correct on–off control for artificial larynx use is twofold. First, the device must be on at all times that speech is being produced. Second, the device must be off when silence is dictated (e.g., at the termination of utterances). Failure to turn on the artificial larynx immediately prior to speech runs the risk that the initial sound(s) or word(s) will be articulated in the absence of "voice." In contrast, if the device is left on when silence is necessary, the extraneous noise may become irritating to the listener, or may detract from the listener's ability to attend to the message being communicated. On–off control is to be as close as possible to that of the normal speech process, with some slight modifications (e.g., because it is not as easy to interject single-word elements using an artificial larynx, some alterations in communication strategy may be an advanced goal of training).

Instruction for optimal on–off control should begin at the single-word level, then progress to sentence-based materials. More elaborate materials that have natural pauses (as discussed earlier for the intermediate level of speech rate control and overarticulation training) can be used for on–off control tasks. The clinician needs to provide immediate and direct feedback to the speaker if device onset is too early or too late at the start of an utterance or a given component of an utterance (i.e., following a natural pause due to juncture). Mastering this skill is not always easy and usually involves a level of progressive approximation. For example, early in the training of on–off control skills, the user is asked to initiate artificial larynx sound generation before starting to speak. The duration between device onset and speech onset can be progressively reduced so that they closely approximate one another. It is essential, however, that device onset *does not occur* after speech is initiated; it is preferable to allow a brief period of artificial larynx sound to precede the true onset of speech so as not to degrade the intended signal. Delayed onset of sound has much greater potential to disrupt communication than does onset that is too quick.

Attention to Nonverbal Behaviors

Most individuals can acquire good if not excellent skills with an electrolarynx. As with any method of postlaryngectomy alaryngeal speech, however, the clinician must carefully assess whether any unusual or distracting nonverbal behaviors exist during verbal communication. Behaviors such as unusual head positioning with use of a transcervical device or maintaining insertion of the oral tube with an intraoral device in periods when speech is not quickly required are not conducive to good communication. Many of these behaviors may be somewhat idiosyncratic and must be addressed on an individual basis.

CLINICAL PROBLEM SOLVING

All clinical endeavors have the potential for both anticipated and unanticipated problems. Training individuals to use the artificial larynx is no different. In solving problems, clinicians should consider what options may be available and gather information from other resources (textbooks and guides, manufacturer specifications, and other experienced clinicians) in an effort to expediently find solutions to the problems. When unexpected medical complications occur, the clinician may feel the need to "back off" from electrolarynx training for a period of time. When a patient is unable to verbally communicate, the opportunity for frustration and depression is increased, and these feelings may influence clinical progress. Thus, alternative methods of communication, such as a communication board, simple speech encoding system, or a writing board, must be considered.

SOME ADDITIONAL CONCERNS

Within prior sections of this chapter, specific issues pertaining to training artificial larynx use have been outlined. This chapter has strongly supported the use of the electrolarynx as a viable and essential method of speech rehabilitation for all individuals who undergo total laryngectomy. Furthermore, the artificial larynx is an asset for individuals who may not be candidates for esophageal or tracheoesophageal speech due to extensive surgical resection of the pharyngoesophageal segment or other conditions such as esophageal stenosis. The artificial larynx is also advantageous for individuals who suffer recurrence of malignant disease. In such instances, the electrolarynx can provide communication when intrinsic methods may no longer be possible because of recurrence.

Restrictions for use, however, may apply to some individuals. Those who suffer from extensive postsurgical scarring or who exhibit extensive fibrosis due to radiotherapy may not be ideal candidates for use of a transcervical device. In contrast, those individuals who have excessive saliva flow or those who have undergone additional surgery to the oral cavity may not do well with an intraoral device. The use of dentures may also pose a problem for some individuals trying to use an intraoral device. Also, substantial limitations in finger dexterity in particular and upper extremity dexterity in general may provide sufficient challenges to the successful use of the electronic artificial larynx. The clinician may need to modify a device or help the patient to work on its use despite limitations, but with appropriate adjustments in expectations for the best possible verbal communication.

Finally, any therapy program with the artificial larynx should include an instructional period on troubleshooting. The user must know how to modify the pitch level if an internal control exists (e.g., with the Servox device). Users must know how to charge batteries correctly and how to replace the batteries when necessary. Instruction on how to use a stand-alone battery charger is essential. It is also important to instruct the user in simple maintenance and cleaning to keep the device in optimal working condition. As a final issue, all users should know about the conditions of warranty and the address of the local authorized service provider.

REHABILITATION OUTCOMES

According to a substantial body of data in the literature, use of the artificial larynx can provide very good speech. From the standpoint of speech intelligibility, several authors have shown that, with proper instruction and training, artificial larynx speech is quite good (see Carpenter, 1991). Stalker, Hawk, and Smaldino (1982) suggested that the type of artificial laryngeal device used may have a direct influence on intelligibility; therefore, clinicians may wish to evaluate the use of several devices with each patient. Other research has confirmed the type of errors that are most likely to occur with those using the electrolarynx (Nascimento & Doyle, 2000; Weiss & Basili, 1985; Weiss, Yeni-Komshian, & Heinz, 1979), and these types of data may help clinicians to target particular phonemic elements in a given individual's rehabilitation program.

The collective data gathered to date, however, show that those who use an artificial larynx are faced with considerable challenges in producing voiced–voiceless distinctions. This finding is directly related to the fact that sound propagation through the vocal tract in those using the artificial larynx is done with an excited source; thus, "voicelessness" is not a characteristic of artificial laryngeal device use. In many instances, however, the nature of the speech code does permit the listener to correctly identify lexical items within the context of verbal communication. Lerman (1991) termed this approach of *not* focusing on the voiced–voiceless distinction as "context intelligibility," and this practical goal is clearly of clinical value. Although proficient communication requires that an extra burden is not placed on the listener to decipher messages, the voiced–voiceless problem may manifest in only a few circumstances (e.g., when the speaker is required to provide a response that has the potential to be problematic from the standpoint of interpreting a minimal pair).

Because the act of communication requires both a speaker and a listener, clinicians should work with individuals who have undergone laryngectomy to become more active members of the dyad. A speaker using alaryngeal speech (regardless of the method used) is obliged to optimize communication interactions. The speaker must become sensitive to whether the listener seems to be having difficulty interpreting the message. If difficulty is apparent, the speaker can help to alleviate the communicative burden by revising, restating, repeating, or emphasizing key elements of the message. The secure communicator will not be uncomfortable asking a communicative partner whether he or she understood what was said. This type of communication strategy permits the speaker to assist the listener in a situation where the code and intelligibility are not natural sounding. The value of addressing this type of broad communication therapy once basic skills are achieved is of utmost importance, especially considering that the communicative partners of many who undergo laryngectomy may exhibit hearing loss (Clark, 1985). Combining formal structured drills to increase speech intelligibility with larger scale activities that make the speaker aware of potential problems may have significant impact on communication proficiency and ultimately on rehabilitation outcome.

For example, structured therapeutic tasks that target specific phonemes or phoneme classes may have value for some patients. If such direct sound-based intervention is undertaken, the clinician needs to establish a good baseline measure of performance. This intervention may require the speaker to produce sounds in nonsense syllable format to reduce context effects on listener judgments; however, real-word stimuli may provide an excellent overview of how the speaker does with particular stimuli. Weiss and Basili (1985) created an excellent and highly usable set of stimuli that provide valuable information on speaker performance. This word list also permits the clinician to assess sound intelligibility for the majority of English consonants in both pre- and postvocalic positions. When such assessments are conducted, having one or more listeners unfamiliar with the speaker evaluate the stimuli helps to reduce listener bias. Similarly, the clinician might want to assess intelligibility based on judgments of naive as opposed to experienced (professional) listeners (Doyle, Swift, & Haaf, 1989).

SUMMARY

This chapter has provided an overview and framework for use and training of the electronic artificial larynx. Because the electronic artificial larynx provides a valuable method of postlaryngectomy verbal communication, all clinicians who work with individuals who are treated for laryngeal cancer should gain as much expertise as possible with this alaryngeal speech method. Use of the artificial larynx should be encouraged in all individuals following laryngectomy, with the goal of facilitating the best possible level of speech production. In addition to teaching the basic skills, speech clinicians should strive to improve electrolarynx user awareness so as to optimize speaker–listener communication. Through drillwork, as well as communication activities and awareness, the individual who uses the electronic artificial larynx will be better prepared to reenter society and function as effectively as possible (Doyle, 1999). As noted by Aronson (1980, p. 401) "versatility in different speaking situations" should guide clinical intervention. By becoming familiar with a wide array of electronic artificial laryngeal devices, the clinician will be better able to train, modify, and refine the speech production of users of both transcervical and intraoral-type devices. Through such efforts, speech rehabilitation may be expedited so that other aspects of the individual's care may be improved. Through the facilitation of a functional method of verbal communication, the larger issue of recovery and rehabilitation, along with the individual's overall well-being and quality of life, may be better addressed by members of the laryngectomy team.

REFERENCES

Aronson, A. (1980). *Clinical voice disorders: An interdisciplinary approach.* New York: Decker.

Barney, H. L. (1958). A discussion of some technical aspects of speech aids for postlaryngectomized patients. *Annals of Otology, Rhinology and Laryngology, 67,* 558–570.

Beaudin, P. G., Doyle, P. C., & Eadie, T. L. (2004, May). *Psychophysical evaluation of pleasantness and acceptability for electrolaryngeal speech*. Paper presented at the annual conference of the Canadian Association of Speech–Language Pathologists and Audiologists, Ottawa, Ontario.

Beaudin, P. G., Meltzner, G. S., Doyle, P. C., & Hillman, R. E. (2004, May). *Paired-comparison evaluation of listener preference for electrolaryngeal sentence stimuli*. Paper presented at the annual conference of the Canadian Association of Speech–Language Pathologists and Audiologists, Ottawa, Ontario.

Beaudin, P. G., Meltzner, G., Hillman, R. E., & Doyle, P. C. (2003, May). *A paired-comparison assessment of preference for the speech of a prototype electrolarynx*. Paper presented at the annual conference of the Canadian Association of Speech–Language Pathologists and Audiologists, St. John's, Newfoundland.

Bennett, S., & Weinberg, B. (1973). Acceptability ratings of normal, esophageal, and artificial larynx speech. *Journal of Speech and Hearing Research, 16,* 608–615.

Blom, E. D. (1978). Modification. In S. J. Salmon & H. B. Goldstein (Eds.), *The artificial larynx handbook* (pp. 57–86). New York: Grune & Stratton.

Blom, E. D., Singer, M. I., & Hamaker, R. C. (1998). *Tracheoesophageal voice restoration following total laryngectomy*. San Diego, CA: Singular.

Carpenter, M. A. (1991). Clinical application of alaryngeal speech judgments. In S. J. Salmon & K. H. Mount (Eds.), *Alaryngeal speech rehabilitation: For clinicians by clinicians* (pp. 161–192). Austin, TX: PRO-ED.

Clark, J. G. (1985). Alaryngeal speech intelligibility in the older listener. *Journal of Speech and Hearing Disorders, 50,* 60–65.

Culton, G. L., & Gerwin, J. M. (1998). Current trends in laryngectomy rehabilitation: A survey of speech–language pathologists. *Otolaryngology—Head & Neck Surgery, 118*(4), 458–463.

Diedrich, W. M., & Youngstrom, K. A. (1966). *Alaryngeal speech*. Springfield, IL: Thomas.

Doyle, P. C. (1994). *Foundations of voice and speech rehabilitation following laryngeal cancer*. San Diego, CA: Singular.

Doyle, P. C. (1999). Postlaryngectomy speech rehabilitation: Contemporary considerations in clinical care. *Journal of Speech–Language Pathology and Audiology, 23,* 109–116.

Doyle, P. C. (2002). The changing face of health care. *Journal of Speech–Language Pathology and Audiology, 26,* 3–4.

Doyle, P. C., Eadie, T. L., Beaudin, P. G., & White, H. D. (2003, November). *Voice-related quality of life in alaryngeal speakers*. Paper presented at the annual convention of the American Speech-Language-Hearing Association, Chicago.

Doyle, P. C., Swift, E. R., & Haaf, R. G. (1989). Effects of listener sophistication on judgments of tracheoesophageal talker intelligibility. *Journal of Communication Disorders, 22,* 105–113.

Duguay, M. (1978). Why not both? In S. J. Salmon & L. P. Goldstein (Eds.), *The artificial larynx handbook* (pp. 3–10). New York: Grune & Stratton.

Duguay, M. (1983). Teaching use of an artificial larynx. In W. H. Perkins (Ed.), *Current therapy of communication disorders* (pp. 127–135). New York: Thieme–Stratton.

Eadie, T. L. (2001). The ICIDH–2: Theoretical and clinical implications for speech–language pathology. *Journal of Speech–Pathology and Audiology, 25,* 193–211

Edels, Y. (1983). *Laryngectomy: Diagnosis to rehabilitation*. Rockville, MD: Aspen.

Gates, G. A., Ryan, W. J., & Lauder, E. (1982). Current status of laryngectomee rehabilitation: II. Attitudes about laryngectomee rehabilitation should change. *American Journal of Otolaryngology, 3,* 97–103.

Goldstein, L. P. (1978). The artificial larynx: Pro and con. In S. J. Salmon & L. P. Goldstein (Eds.), *The artificial larynx handbook* (pp. 11–15). New York: Grune & Stratton.

Goldstein, L. P. (1982). History and development of laryngeal prosthetic devices. In A. Sekey (Ed.), *Electroacoustic analysis and enhancement of alaryngeal speech* (pp. 137–165). Springfield, IL: Thomas.

Graham, M. S. (1997). *The clinician's guide to alaryngeal speech therapy.* Boston: Butterworth-Heinemann.

Happ, M. B., Roesch, T., & Kagan, S. H. (2004). Communication needs, methods, and perceived voice quality following head and neck surgery: A literature review. *Cancer Nursing, 27,* 1–9.

Hillman, R. E., Walsh, M. J., Wolf, G. T., Fisher, S. G., & Hong, W. K. (1998). Functional outcomes following treatment for advanced laryngeal cancer. *Annals of Otology, Rhinology and Laryngology, 107,* 2–27.

Keith, R. L., & Shanks, J. C. (1994). Historical highlights: Laryngectomee rehabilitation. In R. L. Keith & F. L. Darley (Eds.), *Laryngectomee rehabilitation* (3rd ed., pp.1–48). Austin, TX: PRO-ED.

Lauder, E. (1970). The laryngectomee and the artificial larynx—A second look. *Journal of Speech and Hearing Disorders, 35,* 62–65.

Lebrun, Y. (1976). *The artificial larynx.* Basel, Switzerland: Lea.

Leuders, O. W. (1956). Use of the electrolarynx in speech rehabilitation. *Archives of Otolaryngology, 63,* 134–137.

Lerman, J. W. (1991). The artificial larynx. In S. J. Salmon & K. H. Mount (Eds.), *Alaryngeal speech rehabilitation* (pp. 27–45). Austin, TX: PRO-ED.

Lowry, L. D. (1981). Artificial larynges: A review and development of a prototype self-contained intra-oral artificial larynx. *Laryngoscope, 91,* 1332–1355.

Meltzner, G. S., & Hillman, R. E. (2003, August). *Impact of abnormal acoustic properties on the perceived quality of electrolaryngeal speech.* Paper presented at the Conference of Voice Quality, Functions, Analysis, and Synthesis, Geneva, Switzerland.

Meltzner, G. S., Kobler, J. B., & Hillman, R. E. (2003). Measuring the neck frequency response function of laryngectomy patients: Implications for the design of electrolarynx devices. *Journal of the Acoustical Society of America, 114,* 1035–1047.

Nascimento, F. T., & Doyle, P. C. (2000). *A perceptual evaluation of fricative and stop production using two artificial larynges.* Unpublished manuscript.

Salmon, S. J. (1978). *The artificial larynx handbook.* New York: Grune & Stratton.

Salmon, S. J. (1983). Artificial larynx speech: A viable means of alaryngeal communication. In Y. Edels (Ed.), *Laryngectomy: Diagnosis to rehabilitation* (pp. 142–161). Rockville, MD: Aspen Systems.

Salmon, S. J. (1997). Using an artificial larynx. In J. Lauder (Ed.), *Self help for the laryngectomee* (pp. 31–33). San Antonio, TX: Lauder Enterprises.

Salmon, S. J., & Goldstein, H. B. (Eds.). (1978). *The artificial larynx handbook.* New York: Grune & Stratton.

Salmon, S. J., & Mount, K. H. (1991). *Alaryngeal speech rehabilitation: For clinicians by clinicians* (pp. 161–192). Austin, TX: PRO-ED.

Shedd, D., Bakamjian, V., Sako, K., Mann, M., Barba, S., & Schaaf, N. (1972). Reed–fistula method of speech rehabilitation after laryngectomy. *American Journal of Surgery, 124,* 510–524.

Sisson, G. A., McConnel, F. M. S., Logemann, J. A., & Yeh, S. (1975). Voice rehabilitation after laryngectomy: Results with the use of a hypopharyngeal prosthesis. *Archives of Otolaryngology, 101,* 178–181.

Snidecor, J. C. (1978). Speech therapy for those with total laryngectomy. In J. C. Snidecor (Ed.), *Speech rehabilitation of the laryngectomized* (2nd ed., pp. 180–193). Springfield, IL: Thomas.

Stalker, J. L., Hawk, A. M., & Smaldino, J. J. (1982). The intelligibility and acceptability of speech produced by five different electronic artificial larynx devices. *Journal of Communication Disorders, 15,* 299–307.

Taub, S., & Bergner, L. H. (1973). Air bypass voice prosthesis for vocal rehabilitation of laryngectomees. *American Journal of Surgery, 125,* 748–756.

Taub, S., & Spiro, R. H. (1972). Vocal rehabilitation of laryngectomees: Preliminary report on a new technique. *American Journal of Surgery, 124,* 87–90.

Weinberg, Shedd, & Horii, (1978). Reed-fistula speech following pharyngolaryngectomy. *Journal of Speech and Hearing Disorders, 43*(3), 401–413.

Weiss, M. S., & Basili, A. M. (1985). Electrolaryngeal speech produced by laryngectomized subjects: Perceptual characteristics. *Journal of Speech and Hearing Research, 28,* 294–300.

Weiss, M. S., Yeni-Komshian, G. H., & Heinz, J. M. (1979). Acoustical and perceptual characteristics of speech produced with an artificial larynx. *Journal of the Acoustical Society of America, 65,* 1298–1308.

Zwitman, D. H., & Disinger, J. L. (1975). Experimental modification of the Western Electric #5 electrolarynx to a mouth-type instrument. *Journal of Speech and Hearing Disorders, 40,* 35–39.

Zwitman, D. H., Knorr, S., & Sonderman, J. C. (1978). Development and testing of an intraoral artificial larynx for laryngectomee patients. *Journal of Speech and Hearing Disorders, 43,* 263–269.

Chapter 23

Electrolaryngeal Speech
The State of the Art and Future Directions for Development

Geoffrey Meltzner, Robert E. Hillman, James T. Heaton, Kenneth M. Houston, James Kobler, and Yingyong Qi

The electrolarynx (EL) is an electrically powered artificial laryngeal device that produces a sound (or buzz) that can be used to acoustically excite the vocal tract and, thereby, substitute for laryngeal voice production. The reported prevalence of EL use among individuals undergoing total laryngectomy surgery varies widely. Some studies report that a minority of total laryngectomy patients use EL speech as their primary means of communication, with estimates of EL use ranging from 11% to 34% (Diedrich & Youngstrom, 1966; Gates, Ryan, Cantu, & Hearne, 1982; Gates, Ryan, Cooper, et al., 1982; King, Fowlks, & Peirson, 1968; Kommers & Sullivan, 1979; Richardson & Bourque, 1985; Webster & Duguay, 1990). Other studies have shown that a majority of total laryngectomy patients use some type of EL to communicate, with estimates of EL use ranging from 50% to 66% (Gray & Konrad, 1976; Hillman, Walsh, Wolf, Fisher, & Hong, 1998; Morris, Smith, Van Demark, & Maves, 1992).

The disparity among reports of EL use may be attributed to a number of factors, including differences in the psychosocial or economic status of the population sampled; the relative availability of or emphasis placed on alternative options for alaryngeal communication, such as tracheoesophageal (TE) speech; and the definition of EL use employed in various studies (e.g., as a primary vs. secondary mode of communication). Even though the prevalence of EL speech may vary among subpopulations of laryngectomized individuals, EL devices continue to represent an important option for speech rehabilitation (see Chapter 22 in this text). Even for individuals who ultimately develop esophageal or TE speech, EL devices may serve early on to provide a viable and relatively rapid method of postlaryngectomy oral communication (Hillman et al., 1998). It is also not unusual for the EL device to continue to serve as a reliable backup in instances where individuals experience difficulties using esophageal or TE speech.

The purpose of this chapter is to describe the current status of electrolarynx devices for restoring oral speech communication to total laryngectomy patients. A brief review is given of the history of electrolarynx development, as well as some suggestions for approaches that might be pursued in the future to improve EL speech.

DESCRIPTION OF ELECTROLARYNGEAL DEVICES

Three different types of electrolarynxes have been developed. The first two, the *neck type* (transcervical or transcutaneous) and *mouth type* (transoral or intraoral), are readily available for use by laryngectomized patients today. The third type, *implantable* devices, have been experimental and are not available for routine clinical use. All three types of EL devices function on the same principles used in a standard loudspeaker; that is, when activated, an electromechanical driver within the EL device causes a rigid membrane (or diaphragm) to vibrate and, hence, to produce a sound. The primary difference between each type of EL centers on where and how the EL acoustically excites the vocal tract. Specifics about each type of EL device are provided in the subsequent sections.

Neck-Type EL Devices

The most commonly used EL devices likely are those that are placed against the neck. All transcervical ELs transmit sound energy through neck tissue to provide acoustic excitation of the vocal tract. The optimal location of EL placement on the neck can be highly individualized, and a trial-and-error process is necessary to find the point of maximum energy transfer, or that location on the neck that produces the loudest speech output (sometimes referred to as the "sweet spot"). Factors such as the nature of surgical reconstruction and the extent to which postsurgical radiation treatment was used may contribute to the variability in the location and transmission capacity of the sweet spot across different patients. Also, due to postsurgical- or postradiation-related changes to their neck tissue (e.g., scarring, fibrosis), some laryngectomy patients cannot transmit usable levels of sound energy into their vocal tracts with a neck-placed EL (Meltzner, Kobler, & Hillman, 2003; see also Chapter 22 in this text).

Early forms of the neck-type ELs employed an electromechanical driver, much like a standard loudspeaker, to generate the sound source. In fact, the most successful of the original neck-type ELs used a modified telephone receiver as the driver (Barney, Haworth, & Dunn, 1959; Bell Laboratories, 1959). The driver was modified by placing a small rigid disk in the center of the diaphragm that was then used to serve as the focal point for transmitting vibrations into the vocal tract. This early device used transistors to generate an electrical pulse train that was used as the driving signal for the modified telephone receiver (speaker). The pulse interval could be adjusted to approximate the average fundamental frequencies of normal adult male or female voices. This EL was marketed by the Western Electric Company (Weiss & Basili, 1985) as the Western Electric Models 5A and 5B. The difference between the two models was in the respective fundamental frequency ranges. The 5A device was designed to be the "male" version with a lower pitch range, whereas the 5B was the "female" version with a higher pitch range. Both models allowed for some pitch modulation via real-time adjustment of the voicing activation button, but there was no method for adjusting the loudness of these devices.

Since the introduction of Western Electric's EL in the late 1950s, other companies have introduced different models of neck-type EL devices. Instead of having an electromechanical transducer drive neck tissue directly, these newer models use a mechanism that operates like a piston hitting a drumhead. When the electromechanical driver is activated, it forces a small cylindrical head mounted on a diaphragm (like a piston) to strike against a rigid plastic disk (like a drumhead), thus producing a series of impulse-like excitations. This type of system is capable of producing a larger amplitude signal (louder) for vocal tract excitation, but it is essentially a nonlinear transducer, which limits the extent to which other characteristics of the excitation waveform can be controlled (e.g., wave shape, spectral properties).

Examples of neck-type EL devices that use nonlinear transducers include the Neovox by Aurex (Chicago, Illinois), Speech-Aid by Romet (Honolulu, Hawaii), Optivox by Bivona (Gary, Indiana), Nu-Vois by Mountain Precision Manufacturing (Boise, Idaho), SPKR by UNI Manufacturing Company (Ontario, Oregon), TruTone and SolaTone by Griffin Laboratories (Temecula, California), and Servox Inton by Siemens (Munich, Germany). Examples of neck-type EL devices are shown in Figure 23.1. The Servox Inton is currently one of the most widely used neck-type EL devices. Features include an internal adjustment screw for modifying the fundamental frequency of vibration to accommodate male and female users, two externally placed control buttons that provide dual pitch variation, an externally placed dial for volume adjustments, and rechargeable batteries (see Figure 23.2). Similar features can be found on the other models of neck-type ELs, but specifications vary to some extent. Although there is little objective information concerning how the different models of neck-type EL devices compare to each other in terms of performance criteria, such as sound quality or ease of use, it has been demonstrated that the intelligibility of EL speech produced by the older Western Electric devices and the newer Servox Inton are similar (Weiss & Basili, 1985). Studies are still needed to establish whether

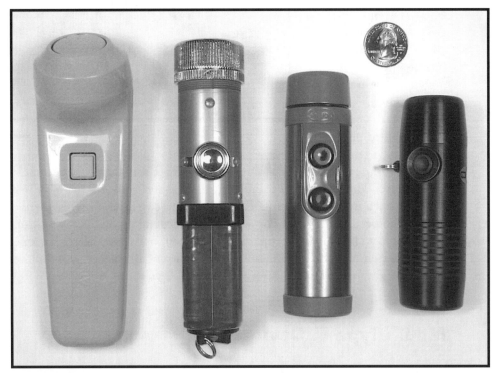

FIGURE 23.1. Examples of neck-type electrolarynxes. From left to right: the Western Electric, Neovox, Servox, and TruTone ELs.

FIGURE 23.2. The Siemens Servox Inton neck-type electrolarynx. (1) Plastic cap, (2) buttons for dual pitch variation, (3) volume control wheel, and (4) carrying strap.

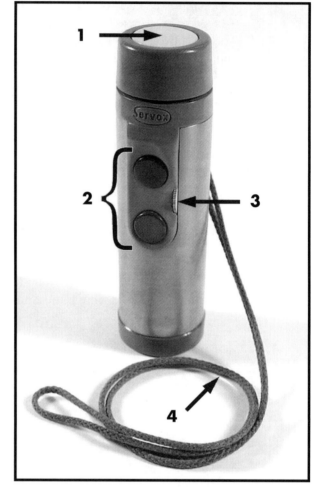

particular EL features, such as dynamic pitch modulation offered by the TruTone or the dual pitch modulation capabilities of the Servox Inton, improve EL speech quality or intelligibility.

One shortcoming common to all neck-type ELs is that, in addition to providing acoustic excitation to the vocal tract, these devices also directly radiate sound energy into the surrounding air. The resulting airborne "buzzing" sound competes with, or masks, the EL speech that is being produced via vocal tract excitation. This phenomenon, which occurs to a greater or lesser degree depending on how well a particular device can be coupled to the neck of a given individual, clearly has a negative impact on both the intelligibility and quality of EL speech and the overall communicative effectiveness when using such a device.

Mouth-Type EL Devices

Mouth-type EL devices are designed to provide acoustic excitation of the vocal tract by generating sound energy in the oral cavity of the laryngectomized patient. In some devices the sound is generated externally and coupled to the oral cavity by a tube, whereas in others the sound source is placed inside the oral cavity. The most common approach takes the sound generated by an electro-mechanical vibratory source and directs it into the mouth of the user via a translabially placed plastic tube (usually at the corner of the mouth). This type of device is useful for individuals during the immediate postlaryngectomy period when placement of a neck-type EL is not possible. This limitation may be due to insufficient healing of the surgical field or may be deferred until postsurgical radiation has been completed. Mouth-type devices are also the only EL option available for those who cannot use a neck-type EL device because of scarred or fibrotic neck tissue. Shortcomings that are specific to EL devices that use a translabial tube to deliver sound to the oral cavity include (a) the tube can interfere with the articulation of an unskilled user and (b) the tube often fills with saliva, which interferes with sound transmission and must therefore be periodically removed (see Chapter 22 in this text). The most widely used mouth-type EL is the Cooper–Rand Electronic Speech Aid by Luminaud (Mentor, Ohio), which was developed in 1959 (Lowry, 1981). An example of the Cooper–Rand is shown in Figure 23.3.

Several neck-type ELs also have oral adapters that allow them to be used as mouth-type devices (see the SolaTone with oral adapter in Figure 23.3). Modification of neck-type devices for intraoral use date back to the mid-1970s (Salmon & Goldstein, 1978) when conversion of the Western Electric EL to a mouth-type device was achieved by securing a tube over the vibrating diaphragm (Blom, 1979). The obvious advantage of an oral adapter is that the same device can be used immediately after surgery as a mouth-type EL and later as a neck-type device, thus eliminating the need to purchase two EL devices.

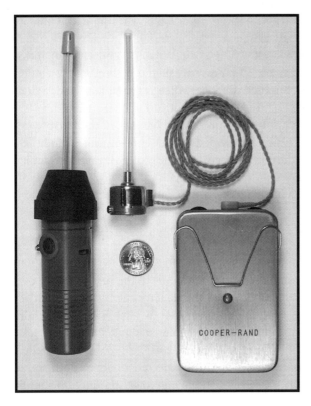

FIGURE 23.3. Example of a SolaTone neck-type EL (on left) fitted with an oral adapter for intraoral use and a Cooper–Rand intraoral EL (on right).

The second approach for providing intraoral acoustic excitation has involved attempts to place the entire sound source into the oral cavity. The earliest published reports of attempts to develop an intraoral EL describe the placement of a small electromagnetic vibrator into a denture with an external oscillator and power source connected via a wire through the mouth (Tait, 1959). This system ultimately evolved into one that was described as being entirely contained in the mouth and activated by tongue pressure (Tait, 1960). Anecdotal reporting suggests that synchronization of sound activation and articulation was difficult, but that intelligibility described as "quite satisfactory" was achieved with this early version of an intraoral EL. One obvious attraction of a self-contained intraoral device is that it would be less obtrusive. Subsequent attempts to further develop the intraoral EL have included the use of FM technology to remotely transmit (e.g., wireless transmitter worn in a shirt pocket) a driving signal to a receiver and speaker embedded in a denture (Zwitman, Knorr, & Sonderman, 1978), and the application of digital technology to produce more efficient self-contained EL devices (Lowry, 1981; Lowry, Katz, Brenman, & Schwartz, 1982).

The first intraoral EL that became commercially available was the Speech-master, produced and marketed by Xomed (Jacksonville, Florida). The Speech-master was available in two forms, as a dental plate that could be fitted to the user's real teeth or as a denture. In 1984, however, its production was halted due to complaints about its performance. User complaints focused on the low sound level output, difficulty using the tongue-activated control buttons, and difficulty articulating with the prosthesis in place. In addition, objective tests of the Speech-master revealed that, in terms of its acoustic output and speech intelligibility, it was noticeably inferior to the Cooper–Rand mouth-type EL (Bennett, Hillman, & Walsh, 1984).

More recently, a company called UltraVoice (Paoli, Pennsylvania) introduced the latest generation of intraoral EL devices called the UltraVoice (see Figure 23.4). Like the older Speechmaster, the UltraVoice is available as both a dental plate and as a denture, and is fitted with a control circuit and speaker. The UltraVoice has removed all tongue-based controls and has moved them to a wireless "control unit." Additional features provided by the control unit include settings for male, female, and whispered voice; volume control; preprogrammed pitch variation; and additional amplification of speech via a collar-mounted microphone and loudspeaker. Claims made by the manufacturer that the device is comfortable to wear and that it produces more natural-sounding and more intelligible speech have not yet been verified through objective studies (see Chapter 6 in this text).

As a final note on mouth-type ELs, over 40 years ago, Barney (1958) demonstrated that placing the source for voiced sounds in the oral cavity, instead of in the pharynx, significantly alters the acoustic characteristics of the sounds being produced. Specifically, zeros are added to the vocal tract transfer function, thereby reducing or eliminating certain source frequencies and altering the relative amplitudes of the formants (Myrick & Yantoro, 1993). Thus, on a theoretical basis, such changes in speech acoustics could be expected to affect both sound quality and speech intelligibility. For example, during vowel production the in-

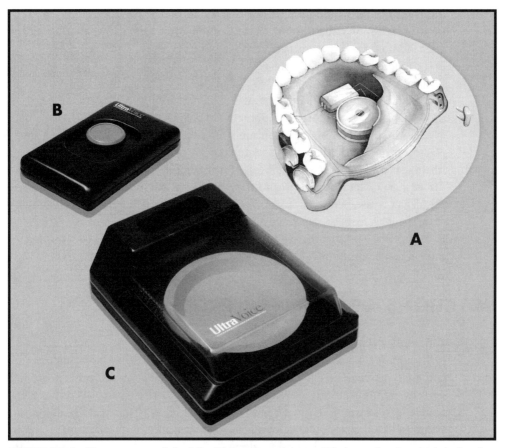

FIGURE 23.4. Components of the UltraVoice electrolarynx: (A) the oral unit, which is fitted into the user's mouth and contains a loudspeaker that generates the voicing source; (B) the control unit which provides the user with on–off control; settings for male, female, and whispered voice; volume control; preprogrammed pitch variation; and additional amplification of speech through a loudspeaker; (C) the charging unit, which recharges batteries for both the oral and control units. (Courtesy UltraVoice Company.)

troduction of antiresonances (zeroes) and the reduction of formant amplitudes might be expected to result in a more nasal-like sound.

Attempts to Develop EL Implants

To date, despite a number of serious attempts, there has not been a successful effort to develop a commercially viable EL implant. Most work in this area has focused on replacing the sound-producing function of the larynx with a sound source that can be implanted near the terminal (pharyngeal) end of the vocal tract. Such efforts have been motivated by the belief that an implanted device would be inherently superior to currently available ELs because it would be unobtrusive and would provide acoustic excitation at the appropriate vocal tract location without radiating competing sound into the surrounding air (Barney, 1958). Before such methods are feasible, however, issues concerning biocompatibility, maintenance of a sterile environment in the vicinity of the implant, and surgical invasion of tissue that has already been compromised by extensive surgery or radiation therapy must be overcome. Examples of attempts to develop an implantable EL device that have actually involved some testing in humans include (a) placement of an insert earphone transducer powered by Cooper–Rand EL electronics into a hypopharyngeal–cutaneous fistula that has been sealed with a silicone rubber tube (Goode, 1969) and (b) implantation of an electromagnetic driver in a pocket just posterior to the pharyngeal constrictor muscles, and wiring this driver to a subcutaneous receiver implanted just below the clavicle which received signals from a controller held in a pocket (Painter, Kaiser, Fredrickson, & Karzon, 1987). Unfortunately, there have been no follow-up reports that establish the clinical viability of these experimental approaches.

LIMITATIONS OF EL SPEECH PRODUCTION

Although today's commercially available neck-type and mouth-type ELs generally provide a serviceable means of communication for the laryngectomized patients who depend on them, there are a number of persistent deficits in EL speech communication. The most problematic of these deficits were highlighted in a needs assessment that we conducted as part of an effort to establish a research program that focuses on developing an improved EL communication system (VA Rehabilitation Research and Development Grant C1996DA). Seventeen postlaryngectomy EL users and 7 speech–language pathologists (experienced in laryngectomy speech rehabilitation) were asked to rank-order a randomized list of major deficits in EL speech communication that have been cited in the literature, as well as to add and rank any additional factors that they felt were problems with the use of currently available EL devices. The top five deficits identified by both groups were the same, with a slightly different rank ordering by each group. These deficits include the following, with the corresponding statements used in the needs assessment shown in parentheses:

1. reduced intelligibility ("EL speech is hard to understand")
2. lack of fine control over pitch and loudness variation, and voice onset and offset ("EL speech is monotonous")
3. unnatural, nonhuman sound quality ("EL speech sounds mechanical")
4. reduced loudness ("EL speech is too quiet")
5. inconveniences related to EL use ("EL is inconvenient to use")

These five areas of deficit are discussed briefly in the following paragraphs.

Several studies have demonstrated that EL speech has reduced intelligibility (see Chapter 4 in this text), with the amount of reduction related to the type of speech material that is used. When closed-set response paradigms are employed (i.e., listeners have to identify the target word from a limited set of options), intelligibility for EL speech has been reported to range from 80.5% to 90% (Hillman et al., 1998; Weiss, Yeni-Komshian, & Heinz, 1979). When listeners have been asked to transcribe running speech produced with an EL, however, intelligibility drops to a range of 36% to 57% (Weiss & Basili, 1985; Weiss et al., 1979). Studies that have examined the types of intelligibility errors that listeners make in evaluating EL speech have reported that the greatest source of confusion is in discriminating between voiced and unvoiced stop consonants, with more of these errors occurring when consonants are in the word-initial position than in word-final position (Weiss & Basili, 1985; Weiss et al., 1979). Weiss et al. (1979) postulated that voicing feature confusions occur more frequently for word-initial consonants because EL users are unable to exercise the fine control over voice onset time that is necessary for producing these voiced–voiceless distinctions. Furthermore, the lower incidence of voiced–voiceless confusions for word-final consonants is attributed to the additional cues for this distinction that are provided by the length of the vowel preceding the consonant (i.e., vowels preceding unvoiced consonants are of significantly shorter duration than vowels preceding voiced consonants) (Weiss & Basili, 1985).

There is evidence that the intelligibility of EL speech also varies depending on characteristics of the listener and listening environment. Clark (1985) used two groups of judges, one comprised of normally hearing young adults, and the other made up of older adults with high-frequency hearing loss. Judges evaluated the intelligibility of normal, esophageal, TE, and EL speech in quiet and with competing speech in the background at different signal-to-noise ratios. Overall, the young normal-hearing judges did better in evaluating intelligibility than the older hearing-impaired group; however, the hearing-impaired group always found artificial laryngeal speech to be more intelligible than the other modes of alaryngeal communication. In terms of performance in the presence of competing speech noise, EL speech was more intelligible than the other modes of alaryngeal communication (i.e., esophageal and TE speech) across the different signal-to-noise conditions. Furthermore, it has been reported that over telephone lines, EL speech is more intelligible than esophageal speech (Damsté, 1975); however, it should be pointed out that many EL users complain that they cannot be adequately heard in a noisy environment.

In addition to the difficulties with voiced–voiceless distinctions for EL speech associated with poor on–off control, EL devices also lack the capability to produce finely controlled, dynamic changes in pitch and loudness. The lack of such control appears to contribute to the impression that EL speech is monotonous sounding, as well as to the negative perceptions of EL speech as sounding nonhuman, mechanical, robotic, and so on (Bennett & Weinberg, 1973). Many EL users describe how the unnatural sound quality of their speech draws unwanted attention (Beaudin, Meltzner, Doyle, & Hillman, 2004; Beaudin, Meltzner, Hillman, & Doyle, 2003; Meltzner & Hillman, 2003), and can even spawn barriers to communication, such as the often heard tale of EL users being hung up on during attempts to use the telephone (see Chapters 3 and 5 in this text). In attempting to compensate for these deficits, some electrolarynxes include a finger-controlled button or switch for altering pitch or loudness. Unfortunately, finger-based control appears too cumbersome to adequately mimic the natural variation of these parameters in normal speech. The lack of adequate pitch control has been shown to be even more detrimental to the intelligibility of EL users who speak tone-based languages such as Thai and Cantonese (Gandour, Weinberg, Petty, & Dardarananda, 1988; Ng, Lerman, & Gilbert, 1998). EL speakers also often complain that EL use is inconvenient because it occupies the use of one hand. In addition, the most commonly used devices are very conspicuous because they must be held to the neck or mouth (Goode, 1969), thus attracting unwanted attention to this method of alaryngeal communication.

Although the lack of normal pitch and loudness variation appears to contribute to the unnatural sound quality of EL speech, additional acoustic characteristics of the EL sound source may also play a role. Several investigators have noted that there is significantly less sound energy below 500 Hz in EL speech as compared to normal laryngeal speech (Qi & Weinberg, 1991; Weiss et al., 1979) (see Figure 23.5). Compensating for this low-frequency deficit via a second-order filter improves the quality of EL speech (Qi & Weinberg, 1991). Furthermore, the lack of random period-to-period fluctuations in both the frequency (jitter) and amplitude (shimmer) of typical EL sound sources may also contribute to the unnatural sound quality of these devices. Supporting this possibility is evidence that a constant pitch in the voicing source of synthesized speech produces a mechanical sound quality (Klatt & Klatt, 1990). To date, however, no systematic study has been done of the effect on EL speech quality of adding such random fluctuations in pitch and amplitude to EL sound sources. Finally, the already mentioned fact that neck-type ELs directly radiate sound energy (the electronic buzz) into the surrounding air also likely contributes to the unnatural quality of speech produced with these types of devices.

CURRENT DEVELOPMENTS FOR IMPROVED EL SPEECH

Although there is much room for improving EL speech communication, until recently little effort has been made to remedy the primary deficits associated with EL speech production since the technology was introduced over 40 years ago (Barney et al., 1959). Moreover, these attempts to improve the speech have produced few, if any, clinically viable improvements. The lack of successful innovation can be at least partly attributed to the fact that there are relatively few EL users—that is, the potential commercial market is too small for mainstream industry to justify investing in EL research and design. This section describes some recent and ongoing efforts to improve EL speech communication and indicates future directions for work in this area.

An early attempt to improve the intelligibility of EL speech produced with a mouth-type device employed a simple amplification system developed by an EL user and called the Voice Volume Aid (Verdolini, Skinner, Patton, & Walker, 1985).

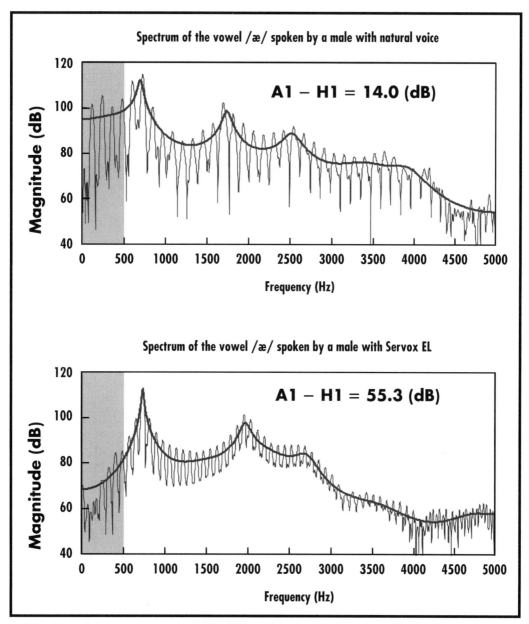

FIGURE 23.5. The spectral content of both normal (top) and electrolaryngeal (bottom) speech. The thick solid line representing the linear predictive smooth spectrum is displayed to emphasize the overall spectral shape. The spectrum below 500 Hz has been highlighted in gray to emphasize the low-frequency deficit inherent in EL speech. The difference between the amplitude of the first formant and the amplitude of the first harmonic (A1−H1) is also shown for each case. Notice that in EL speech, this difference is much greater than that in normal speech, indicating that there is little energy at low frequencies.

The amplification system, which consisted of a microphone placed close to the user's lips and attached to a powered speaker worn in a shirt pocket, sought to improve the intelligibility of EL speech by amplifying the sound produced at the lips relative to the directly radiated sound produced by the EL. It was found that the Voice Volume Aid enhanced EL speech intelligibility in quiet rooms or in rooms with moderate background noise (66 and 72 dB SPL, respectively), but was less effective in relatively high levels of background noise (76 dB SPL).

Norton and Bernstein (1993) tested a new design for an EL sound source based on an attempt to measure the sound transmission properties of neck tissue. They also attempted to minimize the sound that is directly radiated from the neck-type EL by encasing the EL in sound shielding. These proposed improvements to the EL source were implemented on a large, heavy, bench-top mini-shaker, making their prototype impractical for routine use. In addition, there is some question about whether their estimates of the neck transfer function were confounded by vocal tract formant artifacts (Meltzner, 1998). The speech produced with the newly configured sound source, however, was subjectively judged to sound better, thereby indicating that such alterations to the EL sound source could potentially improve the quality of EL speech.

In an endeavor to give EL users some degree of improved dynamic pitch control, Uemi, Ifukube, Takahashi, and Matsushima (1994) designed a device that used air pressure measurements obtained from a resistive component placed over the stoma to control the fundamental frequency of an EL. Unfortunately, only 2 of the 16 study subjects were able to master the control of the device and produce pitch contours that resembled those in normal speech. These results demonstrate that a pitch control device must not be so difficult for the user to employ that it is clinically impractical.

Some investigators have applied signal processing techniques to postprocess recorded EL speech to remove the effects of the directly radiated EL noise (i.e. sound not transmitted through the neck wall, or "self-noise"). Cole, Sridharan, Moody, and Geva (1997) demonstrated that a combination of noise reduction algorithms originally developed for the removal of noise corruption in speech signals could be used to effectively remove the EL self-noise for the recordings of EL speakers. Espy-Wilson, Chari, MacAuslan, Huang, and Walsh (1998) used a somewhat different approach to remove the EL self-noise. They simultaneously recorded the output at both the lips and the EL itself, and then employed both signals in an adaptive filtering algorithm to remove the directly radiated EL noise. Spectral analysis of the filtered speech demonstrated that the enhancement algorithm effectively removed the directly radiated EL sound during nonsonorant speech intervals with no significant impact on overall intelligibility. In addition, perceptual experiments revealed that listeners generally preferred the postprocessed enhanced speech to the unfiltered speech.

Other researchers have used postprocessing techniques to try to compensate for deficits in the EL sound source. Qi and Weinberg (1991) attempted to improve the quality of EL speech by enhancing its low-frequency content. Hypothesizing that the low-frequency roll-off of EL speech first noted by Weiss et al. (1979) was at least partially responsible for the poor quality of EL speech,

Qi and Weinberg developed an optimal second-order low-pass filter to compensate for this low-frequency deficit. Briefly, this filter was designed to provide emphasis to spectral energy below 500 Hz, without significantly altering the level of energy at higher frequencies. Perceptual experiments showed that almost all listeners preferred the EL speech with the low-frequency enhancement. In an even more ambitious approach, Ma, Demirel, Espy-Wilson, and MacAuslan (1999) used cepstral analysis of speech to replace the EL excitation signal with a normal speech excitation signal, while keeping the vocal tract information constant. Not only did the normal excitation signal contain the proper frequency content (i.e., no low-frequency deficit), but it also contained a natural pitch contour to help eliminate the monotone quality of EL speech. In formal listening experiments, most judges preferred the postprocessed speech to the original EL speech. The practical application of this enhancement technique is limited because it would require having a natural speech version of the utterances being spoken that could then be used as a basis for enhancing the EL speech. Both reports, however, demonstrate improvements in EL speech quality gained by recognizing and compensating for the differences between conventional EL sound sources and the normal laryngeal voicing source. Specifically, these postprocessing strategies demonstrate the potential for substantial improvements in EL speech quality over the telephone, and in broader contexts if these strategies can be implemented in a truly portable system that is capable of real-time processing.

A Modular Prototype EL Communication System

A comprehensive approach to developing an improved EL communication system continues to be pursued by our group in the W. M. Keck Neural Prosthesis Research Center in Boston (established in 1997). This effort includes some methodologies that are similar to those described previously in this chapter, in combination with some new innovations. The goal of this project is to provide EL users with a substantially improved EL communication system that more closely approximates normal voice and speech production. To accomplish this, we are working on the development of a three-module system that is designed to remedy the major deficits in EL speech (see Figure 23.6). The three modules are as follows:

1. ***Improved EL sound source,*** which consists of a new neck-type linear transducer (EL) with an improved frequency response to remedy the low-frequency deficit inherent in current EL speech. Measurements of the neck load impedance and frequency response function from laryngectomized patients are being used to guide the design of the EL transducer and associated driving signal. Presently, two prototype sound source modules have been fabricated and are undergoing testing and evaluation. The ultimate goal is to have a version of this transducer that can be mounted on the neck and enable hands-free operation in conjunction with the control module described next.

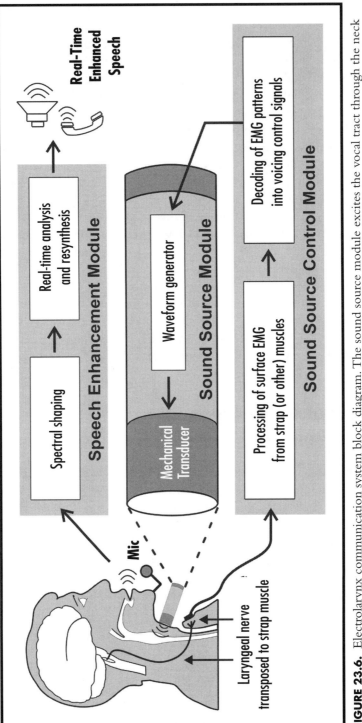

FIGURE 23.6. Electrolarynx communication system block diagram. The sound source module excites the vocal tract through the neck wall. Control of speech onset–offset, pitch, and loudness will be provided by the sound source control module. Finally, the speech enhancement module will process the signal recorded at the lips in real time to further improve EL speech.

2. ***Sound source control unit,*** which will use control signals to restore some pitch and timing control to the voicing source. The innovative concept behind this module is the plan to "reclaim" laryngeal motor control signals associated with phonation by redirecting a recurrent laryngeal nerve (RLN) to neck strap muscles that originally attached the larynx to other neck structures at the time of laryngectomy. Our preliminary results show that noninvasive electromyographic (EMG) recording from the neck surface above target strap muscles (e.g., sternohyoid, sternothyroid, and/or omohyoid) several months after redirecting the RLN provides signals that can be used for onset–offset and pitch modulation of an EL voicing source. Current users of EL devices may also be able to use this EMG-EL unit by employing other voluntary arm, trunk or neck muscles as EMG sources.

3. ***Signal processing speech enhancement device,*** which will acquire the oral EL speech signal with a microphone and digitally analyze and resynthesize it in real time. The function of this module is to correct for deficiencies in EL speech that cannot be remedied by the other two modules, including residual sound source deficits or distortions introduced into the vocal tract transfer function by laryngectomy surgery, the location of the EL on the neck, and so on. The output of this device will be an electrical speech waveform that can be used as an input signal to either a telephone or a miniature wearable speaker. Initial versions of signal processing algorithms have been developed and are currently being implemented and tested on digital signal processing (DSP)–based laboratory prototype hardware.

Because of the modular nature of the proposed EL system, we anticipate that it will be possible to apply advances in the development of individual components to improvements in the communication functioning of patients.

The Future of Artificial Larynxes

The ideal artificial larynx, whether powered electronically or by some other method (e.g., aerodynamic), would meet the following criteria: (a) completely implantable, (b) controlled by signals from residual laryngeal motor nerves, (c) capable of supplying a natural sounding voicing source for speech production (Beaudin et al., 2004; Beaudin et al., 2003; Meltzner & Hillman, 2003; see also Chapter 6 in this text), and (d) able to provide the non–speech-related functions normally served by the larynx (e.g., reconnecting the respiratory system to the upper airway or vocal tract, protection of the lower airway during swallowing). Researchers and clinicians should remain vigilant in monitoring emerging technologies that could someday be applied to developing such an implantable device. In fact, a European consortium has already begun an ambitious project to develop a totally implantable artificial larynx (Verkerke et al., 1996), but it is too early to predict their chances for success. In the meantime, and as noted earlier, there is substantial opportunity for the application of current technologies to improving the speech communication of laryngectomy patients using nonimplanted EL devices. Presently, a multidisciplinary group of researchers in Boston is working toward the design and clinical application of a hands-free electrolarynx that is controlled through a neural interface to strap muscles of the neck (Goldstein, Heaton, Kobler, Stanley, & Hillman, 2004; Heaton et al., in press). The outcome of this work has significant implications for reducing the need for the use of one's hands while using an electrolarynx. Clearly, the implication of such developments is directed at normalizing the communication process.

SUMMARY

In summary, the electrolarynx continues to represent an important option for the speech rehabilitation of laryngectomy patients, even though commercially available EL devices have obvious shortcomings that serve to limit the communication function of the users. We hope that efforts to apply state-of-the-art technology to EL design will result in the future development of devices that more closely approximate normal voice and speech production.

REFERENCES

Barney, H. L. (1958). A discussion of some technical aspects of speech aids for postlaryngectomized patients. *Annals of Otology, Rhinology and Laryngology, 67,* 558–570.

Barney, H. L., Haworth, F. E., & Dunn, H. K. (1959). An experimental transistorized artificial larynx. In B. Weinberg (Ed.), *Readings in speech following total laryngectomy* (pp. 1337–1356). Baltimore: University Park Press.

Beaudin, P. G., Meltzner, G. S., Doyle, P. C., & Hillman, R. E. (2004, May). *Paired-comparison evaluation of listener preference for electrolaryngeal sentence stimuli.* Paper presented at the annual conference of the Canadian Association of Speech–Language Pathologists and Audiologists, Ottawa, Ontario.

Beaudin, P. G., Meltzner, G. S., Hillman, R. E., & Doyle, P. C. (2003, May). *A paired-comparison assessment of preference for the speech of a prototype electrolarynx.* Paper presented at the annual meeting of the Canadian Association of Speech–Language Pathologists and Audiologists, St. John's, Newfoundland.

Bell Laboratories. (1959). New artificial larynx. *Transactions of the American Academy of Ophthalmology and Otolaryngology, 63,* 548–550.

Bennett, S., Hillman, R. E., & Walsh, M. J. (1984). Speech characteristics of a newly developed intraoral artificial larynx. *ASHA, 26*(10), 187.

Bennett, S., & Weinberg, B. (1973). Acceptability ratings of normal, esophageal, and artificial larynx speech. *Journal of Speech and Hearing Research, 16,* 608–615.

Blom, E. (1979). The artificial larynx: Types and modifications. In R. Keith & F. Darley (Eds.), *Laryngectomy rehabilitation* (pp. 63–85). Houston, TX: College-Hill Press.

Clark, J. G. (1985). Alaryngeal speech intelligibility and the older listener. *Journal of Speech and Hearing Disorders, 50,* 60–65.

Cole, D., Sridharan, S., Moody, M., & Geva, S. (1997). Application of noise reduction techniques for alaryngeal speech enhancement. *IEEE TENCON,* pp. 491–494.

Damsté, P. H. (1975). Methods of restoring the voice after laryngectomy. *Laryngoscope, 85*(4), 649–655.

Diedrich, W., & Youngstrom, K. (1966). *Alaryngeal speech.* Springfield, IL: Thomas.

Espy-Wilson, C. Y., Chari, V. R., MacAuslan, J. M., Huang, C. B., & Walsh, M. J. (1998). Enhancement of electrolaryngeal speech by adaptive filtering. *Journal of Speech–Language–Hearing Research, 41,* 1253–1264.

Gandour, J., Weinberg, B., Petty, S. H., & Dardarananda, R. (1988). Tone in Thai alaryngeal speech. *Journal of Speech and Hearing Disorders, 53,* 23–29.

Gates, G. A., Ryan, W., Cantu, E., & Hearne, E. (1982). Current status of laryngectomee rehabilitation: II. Causes of failure. *American Journal of Otolaryngology, 3,* 8–14.

Gates, G. A., Ryan, W., Cooper, J. C., Jr., Lawlis, G. F., Cantu, E., Hayashi, T., Lauder, E., Welch, R. W., & Hearne, E. (1982). Current status of laryngectomee rehabilitation: I. Results of therapy. *American Journal of Otolaryngology, 3,* 1–7.

Goldstein, E. A., Heaton, J. T., Kobler, J. B., Stanley, G. B., & Hillman, R. E. (2004). Design and implementation of a hands-free electrolarynx device controlled by neck strap muscle electromyographic activity. *IEEE Transactions on Biomedical Engineering, 51*(2), 325–332.

Goode, R. L. (1969). The development of an improved artificial larynx. *Transactions of the American Academy of Ophthalmology and Otolaryngology, 73,* 279–287.

Gray, S., & Konrad, H. R. (1976). Laryngectomy: Postsurgical rehabilitation of communication. *Archives of Physical Medicine and Rehabilitation, 57,* 140–142.

Heaton, J. T., Goldstein, E. A., Kobler, J. B., Zeitels, S. M., Randolph, G. W., Walsh, M. J., Gooey, J. E., & Hillman, R. E. (in press). Surface electromyographic activity in total laryngectomees following laryngeal nerve transfer to neck strap muscles. *Annals of Otology, Rhinology and Laryngology.*

Hillman, R. E., Walsh, M. J., Wolf, G. T., Fisher, S. G., & Hong, W. K. (1998). Functional outcomes following treatment for advanced laryngeal cancer. Part I—Voice preservation in advanced laryngeal cancer. Part II—Laryngectomy rehabilitation: The state of the art in the VA System. Research Speech–Language Pathologists. Department of Veterans Affairs Laryngeal Cancer Study Group. *Annals of Otology, Rhinology and Laryngology, 172* (Suppl.), 1–27.

King, P. S., Fowlks, E. W., & Peirson, G. A. (1968). Rehabilitation and adaptation of laryngectomy patients. *American Journal of Physical Medicine, 47,* 192–203.

Klatt, D. H., & Klatt, L. C. (1990). Analysis, synthesis, and perception of voice quality variations among female and male talkers. *Journal of the Acoustical Society of America, 87*(2), 820–857.

Kommers, M. S., & Sullivan, M. D. (1979). Wives' evaluation of problems related to laryngectomy. *Journal of Communication Disorders, 12,* 411–430.

Lowry, L. D. (1981). Artificial larynges: A review and development of a prototype self-contained intra-oral artificial larynx. *Laryngoscope, 91,* 1332–1355.

Lowry, L. D., Katz, P. A., Brenman, H. S., & Schwartz, H. L. (1982). An intraoral self-contained artificial larynx. *Otolaryngology—Head and Neck Surgery, 90,* 208–214.

Ma, K., Demirel, P., Espy-Wilson, C., & MacAuslan, J. (1999). *Improvement of electrolarynx speech by introducing normal excitation information.* Retrieved from http://formant.bu.edu

Meltzner, G. S. (1998). *Measuring the neck transfer function of layrngectomy patients.* Unpublished master's thesis, Massachusetts Institute of Technology, Cambridge.

Meltzner, G. S., & Hillman, R. E. (2003, August). *Impact of abnormal acoustic properties on the perceived quality of electrolaryngeal speech.* Paper presented at the Conference on Voice Quality, Functions, Analysis, and Synthesis, Geneva, Switzerland.

Meltzner, G. S., Kobler, J. B., & Hillman, R. E. (2003). Measuring the neck frequency response function of laryngectomy patients: Implications for the design of electrolarynx devices. *Journal of the Acoustical Society of America, 114,* 1035–1047.

Morris, H. L., Smith, A. E., Van Demark, D. R., & Maves, M. D. (1992). Communication status following laryngectomy: The Iowa experience 1984–1987. *Annals of Otology, Rhinology and Laryngology, 101,* 503–510.

Myrick, R., & Yantorno, R. (1993). Vocal tract modeling as related to the use of an artificial larynx. *Proceedings of the 19th Annual Northeastern Bioengineering Conference,* (pp. 75–77).

Ng, M. L., Lerman, J. W., & Gilbert, H. R. (1998). Perceptions of tonal changes in normal laryngeal, esophageal, and artificial laryngeal male Cantonese speakers. *Folia Phoniatrica and Logopaedia, 50*(2), 64–70.

Norton, R. L., & Bernstein, R. S. (1993). Improved LAboratory Prototype ELectrolarynx (LAPEL): Using inverse filtering of the frequency response function of the human throat. *Annals of Biomedical Engineering, 21*(2), 163–174.

Painter, C., Kaiser, T., Fredrickson, J. M., & Karzon, R. (1987). Human speech development for an implantable artificial larynx. *Annals of Otology, Rhinology and Laryngology, 96,* 573–577.

Qi, Y. Y., & Weinberg, B. (1991). Low-frequency energy deficit in electrolaryngeal speech. *Journal of Speech and Hearing Research, 34*(6), 1250–1256.

Richardson, J., & Bourque, L. (1985). Communication after laryngectomy. *Journal of Psychosocial Oncology, 3,* 83–97.

Salmon, S. J., & Goldstein, L. P. (1978). *The artificial larynx handbook.* New York: Grune & Stratton.

Tait, R. V. (1959). The oral vibrator. *British Dental Journal, 107,* 392–399.

Tait, R. V. (1960). The oral vibrator: An experimental development. *British Dental Journal, 108,* 506–508.

Uemi, N., Ifukube, T., Takahashi, M., & Matsushima, J. (1994). Design of a new electrolarynx having a pitch control function. *IEEE Workshop on Robot and Human Communication,* 198–202.

Verdolini, K., Skinner, M. W., Patton, T., & Walker, P. A. (1985). Effect of amplification on the intelligibility of speech produced with an electrolarynx. *Laryngoscope, 95,* 720–726.

Verkerke, G. J., Veenstra, A., de Vries, M. P., Schutte, H. K., Busscher, H. J., Herrmann, I. F., van der Mei, H. C., & Rakhorst, G. (1996). *Development of a totally implantable artificial larynx: Voice update.* New York: Elsevier Science.

Webster, P. M., & Duguay, M. J. (1990). Surgeons' reported attitudes and practices regarding alaryngeal speech. *Annals of Otology, Rhinology and Laryngology, 99*(3, Pt. 1), 197–200.

Weiss, M. S., & Basili, A. G. (1985). Electrolaryngeal speech produced by laryngectomized subjects: Perceptual characteristics. *Journal of Speech and Hearing Research, 28,* 294–300.

Weiss, M. S., Yeni-Komshian, G. H., & Heinz, J. M. (1979). Acoustical and perceptual characteristics of speech produced with an electronic artificial larynx. *Journal of the Acoustical Society of America, 65*(5), 1298–1308.

Zwitman, D. H., Knorr, S. G., & Sonderman, J. C. (1978). Development and testing of an intraoral electrolarynx for laryngectomy patients. *Journal of Speech and Hearing Disorders, 43,* 263–269.

PART IV

Chapter 24

Problems Associated with Alaryngeal Speech Development

Jan S. Lewin

Total laryngectomy results in a loss of human voice and postoperative changes that have many psychological, emotional, social, and economic implications. Problems often occur as a function of the cancer itself and its treatment, which interfere with the development of successful alaryngeal speech production. The goal of this chapter is to help the clinician identify, understand, and resolve those obstacles or problems that are unique to the alaryngeal speaker to help facilitate communicative success. The following are some of the changes that create problems for all laryngectomized persons, regardless of the mode of alaryngeal speech used:

- Loss of the senses of taste and smell to some degree
- Dryness and crusting associated with a respiratory tract that no longer warms, cools, moistens, or cleanses air
- Inability to laugh, sing, or whistle normally
- Psychological assault to the self-concept associated with a new body image and perceived physical attractiveness
- Probable or imagined change in roles and relationships in familial, occupational, and social worlds
- Constant hazard of immersion or drowning in water, even when washing or bathing
- Coughing and wiping mucous secretions from the tracheostoma as opposed to the mouth and nose
- Changes in the procedure for emergency resuscitation in the event of cardiac or respiratory arrest
- Dysphagia associated with radiation treatment, delayed healing, infection, fistula formation, or hypopharyngeal stricture

The speech pathologist is usually the member of the interdisciplinary team who will develop the strongest bond with the laryngectomized individual throughout the course of treatment because of the severe communicative deficit that results from removal of the larynx. The speech pathologist, therefore, plays a major role in providing support, counseling, and rehabilitation, both pre- and postoperatively (Gress, 2004; see also Chapter 15 in this text). The rehabilitative goal is to restore communication as closely as possible to that of the individual's premorbid state, keeping in mind that no person undergoing uncomplicated total laryngectomy should be without some method of functional speech production. Frequently, however, problems arise postoperatively that interfere with the process of acquiring a new method of communication. Many of the problems will be exacerbated by, or occur as a result of the surgery itself, the surgeon's technique, or the adjuvant treatments provided, such as radiation, that may be performed as part of the overall course of cancer management. Other problems might be considered a consequence of the patient's personal characteristics, such as age, cognition, and mental state. Successful alaryngeal speech rehabilitation, in part, will depend on the clinician's ability to recognize these obstacles and overcome them.

Alaryngeal speech is usually produced using one of three alternatives: the artificial larynx, esophageal speech production, or surgical–prosthetic methods (e.g., tracheoesophageal [TE] voice restoration). Problems associated with the

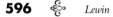

production of alaryngeal speech basically can be divided into two categories: (a) general problems, which affect the acquisition of all forms of alaryngeal speech production, and (b) specific problems, which are medically or physiologically based, but have the greatest effect on TE speech production.

GENERAL PROBLEMS

General problems that may affect the laryngectomized individual's acquisition of alaryngeal speech production include (a) the person's age, (b) the history of radiation therapy, (c) the patient's cognitive–mental status, (d) the patient's general health and medical history, (e) pulmonary health, (f) sensory changes, (g) the extent of surgery, and (h) the availability and quality of alaryngeal speech therapy.

Much of the early literature devoted to alaryngeal speech acquisition suggests that educational level and motivation may influence the development of alaryngeal speech production, specifically esophageal speech (Gates, Ryan, Cantu, & Hearne, 1982; Gates, Ryan, Cooper, et al., 1982; Keith, Ewert, & Flowers, 1974; King, Fowlks, & Peirson, 1968; Salmon, 1988; Volin, 1980). My personal experience, however, has not shown that educational level affects the development of verbal communication. In fact, the rehabilitation process may be expedited for those who are illiterate because the option for written communication is not available. Furthermore, I have not worked with an individual who was not motivated to communicate orally if at all possible. What motivates one individual, however, may not motivate another. Motivation seems to be a factor only in relation to the selection of the type of alaryngeal speech production. Some individuals may prefer to use the artificial larynx, whereas others may choose TE voice restoration. Still others may be interested in learning to speak using esophageal speech methods. For these reasons, I have omitted education and motivation from the list of general problems. Verbal communication remains a basic human need for the person who has spent his or her entire life communicating orally. My experience suggests that an individual, unless clinically depressed, will again seek this form of expression.

Age

Age has long been considered a factor that influences the acquisition of alaryngeal speech (Dabul & Lovestedt, 1974; Gates & Hearne, 1982; Gates, Ryan, Cantu, & Hearne, 1982; King et al., 1968; Shames, Font, & Matthews, 1963). Typically, age is a factor related to the attainment of any new skill, and alaryngeal speech production is no different. Although there are exceptions, Salmon (1988) reported that "it is generally agreed that for whatever reasons (flexibility, alertness, persistence, muscle tone, etc.), people in their mid-sixties or younger are better candidates for esophageal speech" (p. 106).

Age alone does not determine the ability to successfully use any of the alaryngeal speech alternatives. The artificial larynx offers the potential for the quickest and simplest production of speech with the fewest complications. Therefore, some patients, especially those who are older and retired from the turmoil of daily work routines and professional communications, choose the artificial larynx for its simplicity. They prefer this mode of alaryngeal speech to the lengthy period of therapy typically associated with learning esophageal speech, or the management of the voice prosthesis necessary for TE voice restoration. For others, the alternatives that offer more normal speech quality and production become the methods of choice. The use of the artificial larynx and TE speech production also require some degree of manual dexterity. With advancing age, hand–eye coordination and manual dexterity tend to decrease. These factors influence the selection of an appropriate electrolarynx and the potential use of the TE voice prosthesis and peristomal attachments. The decision as to the best alaryngeal speech alternative should be based on a thorough assessment of the individual's specific needs, personality, physical capabilities, and preference. Age alone has not been found to be significantly related to the development of alaryngeal speech and should not be considered as a single, predictive factor influencing the selection of a form of alaryngeal communication (Baugh, Lewin, & Baker, 1987; Dabul & Lovestedt, 1974; Volin, 1980; see also Chapter 3 in this text).

Radiation Therapy

Radiation therapy will affect alaryngeal speech production for both short and long terms, yet the magnitude of this effect will vary from patient to patient. Tissue that has been irradiated suffers some degree of change in elasticity, viscosity, vascularization, and healing ability. Individuals who have had preoperative radiation can experience longer postoperative healing rates and more complications, including wound breakdown and fistulization. The effects of radiation therapy tend to be greater for those who receive large doses of postoperative radiation, approximately 7,000 to 8,000 rads (70–80 Gy), generally over a course of 6 to 8 weeks (Wang, 1990). Patients will often experience erythema of the skin and related tissue edema. Late effects of radiation consist of atrophy and fibrosis of subcutaneous tissues. In severe cases, extensive fibrosis, necrosis, and poor wound healing after surgery or slight trauma may occur (see Chapters 7 and 10 in this text).

Mucous membranes react to the radiation in the form of radiation mucositis. Near the end of the second week of radiation, patients may complain of sore throat, xerostomia, and loss of taste. The mucosa will appear erythematous. Some patients with severe mucositis in the oropharynx may experience dysphagia or odynophagia. Sometimes a break in treatment may be required to lessen the symptoms. Gates and Hearne (1982) postulated that postoperative radiation therapy has a direct effect on learning esophageal speech because patients experience pharyngeal pain and dryness during the period in which they are attempting to learn esophageal speech. Therefore, postponing the start of alaryngeal speech therapy until the effects of radiation therapy have subsided may be beneficial. The patient may find communication easiest with the use of an electrolarynx during this period. Intraoral or cheek placement may be best during the immediate postoperative period, due to the acute edema and tenderness caused by the irradiation of neck tissues (see Chapter 22 in this text).

Lewin, Baugh, and Baker (1987) found that the effects of radiation-induced edema on tissue elasticity interfere with the accurate preoperative assessment and prediction of postoperative TE speech fluency. Intraesophageal pressure measurements, obtained using objective methods of esophageal insufflation testing prior to TE puncture, may be elevated in irradiated patients. One may be tempted to attribute the lack of sound to the presence of pharyngeal constrictor spasm when in fact the elevations in intraesophageal pressures and the inability to produce voice are temporarily the result of radiation-induced tissue edema. Lewin et al.'s findings suggest that preoperative insufflation testing for secondary TE punctures should be delayed until after the effects of radiation therapy have resolved (approximately 4 to 6 weeks following completion of radiation therapy).

Hamaker, Singer, Blom, and Daniels (1985) noted loss of voice in TE speakers, usually in the third or fourth week of postoperative radiation therapy. They found the effect usually transient, with the return of voice following the resolution of radiation effects. Garth, McRae, and Rhys-Evans (1991) also reported vocal deterioration and loss in prosthetic speakers as a result of the inflammation and edema of the pharynx and neck following radiation therapy.

Individuals undergoing radiation therapy may experience tenderness or pain and find it difficult to occlude, remove, clean, and replace the voice prosthesis. Removing the prosthesis and replacing it with a catheter or a "dummy" prosthesis during the course of radiation ensures patency of the fistula and prevents spontaneous closure of the TE tract. The "dummy" prosthesis is sealed on the esophageal side and, like the catheter, prevents inadvertent gastric filling when the prosthesis cannot be used for TE speech due to edema. Additionally, most patients are able to leave the "dummy" prosthesis in place without removing it through the course of radiation and often find it more comfortable than a catheter (see Chapter 19 in this text).

Following radiation therapy, some patients may experience leakage of saliva around the TE prosthesis, with salivary contamination of the trachea via aspiration. It is postulated that this happens because the TE puncture (TEP) accommodates the dilating effect of the prosthesis in irradiated patients, resulting in a circumferential enlargement of the TEP. In other words, the puncture becomes enlarged in comparison to the diameter of the prosthesis, permitting leakage around the prosthesis as a result of the effects of radiation. In most instances, the problem can be alleviated by removing the prosthesis and inserting a catheter one size smaller (French) in diameter than the prosthesis for 24 hours. In other cases, cauterization of the TEP will facilitate stenosis of the puncture back to its original size. In severe cases, intractable leakage may require surgical closure and repuncture (Silver, Gluckman, & Donegan, 1985; Singer, Blom, & Hamaker, 1981).

Additionally, irradiated patients may develop inflammatory reactions around the stoma. Singer et al. (1981) proposed use of a silicone tracheal vent tube or laryngectomy tube until the reaction subsides. Irradiation may also result in stomal stenosis. The use of a laryngectomy vent or tube, stoma button, or Barton-Mayo button (Bivona Medical Technologies, Gary, Indiana) helps dilate and prevent further stenosis of the tracheostoma.

Although the use of a vent or tube is not a problem for the artificial larynx or esophageal speaker, it is usually a problem for the TE speaker. The laryngectomy tube frequently blocks the opening of the TE puncture. Although modifications can be made, the results are often disappointing. (See the later section in this chapter titled "Stomal Stenosis and Irregularity" for further discussion.)

Finally, the literature often presents radiation therapy as a limiting factor to the success of alaryngeal speech production. It has often been cited as a contraindication to TE puncture. Although radiation therapy will, in most cases, affect the development or production of alaryngeal speech production, it is not a deterrent to the use of any of the communicative alternatives (Baugh et al., 1987; Trudeau, Schuller, & Hall, 1989; Volin, 1980). Thus, radiation treatment cannot be considered a contraindication to any method of alaryngeal speech production.

Cognitive–Mental Status

Communication is no less a basic human need for the patient who suffers from cognitive–mental limitations than for the patient who is cognitively and mentally intact. Impaired cognitive–mental functioning is limiting to the extent that lack of memory and behavior interfere with day-to-day management and carryover of learned skills to new tasks and daily routines. Simply put, if the patient cannot find his or her electrolarynx or forgets how to use it, recovery will be inhibited. The speaker who uses a TE voice prosthesis and who has impaired cognitive–mental functioning will experience similar difficulties. The esophageal speaker must understand, assimilate, and produce a complex hierarchy of new behaviors (see Chapter 16 in this text). The patient's cognitive and mental functioning will significantly influence the choice of alaryngeal speech alternative. Even with careful selection, success may be compromised. The patient may have the physical ability, but his or her mental status may prevent actualization of the skill.

Maniglia, Lundy, Casiano, and Swim (1989) suggested that proper selection of patients for TE puncture is important. Based on the requirements for daily management and use of the prosthesis, they proposed that the "informed, motivated patient with good comprehension of the mechanics of TE speech is the best candidate" (p. 490). Garth et al. (1991) found that poor intellectual capacity, although not an absolute contraindication for use of a TE speech prosthesis, was a considerable problem for 2 of 119 patients, one of whom suffered from dementia and the other from a cerebral vascular accident.

Thus, the level of the individual's cognition is important to consider when selecting an appropriate method for alaryngeal speech production. Although the individual may be highly motivated, cognitive impairment may limit his or her alaryngeal speech choices.

General Health and Medical History

Although carcinoma of the larynx is the most common upper aerodigestive tract cancer, its overall incidence is rare. Laryngeal cancer represents only 1% of all cancers, which translates into approximately 4 cases per 100,000 population (American Cancer Society, 1996). Laryngeal cancer generally strikes males with long-standing habits of cigarette smoking and alcoholism, usually in the seventh decade of life. Even though males predominate over females by a ratio of 4.6:1, the demographics of the disease are changing due to the increased frequency of smoking (Weber, 1998). As such, the patient's general health and medical history are important contributing factors to alaryngeal speech acquisition.

In general, individuals with laryngeal carcinoma are older and often have engaged in a variety of abuses, most notably alcohol and smoking. Advanced age, however, may also bring with it degenerative conditions, such as arthritis, cardiovascular and cerebrovascular disease, visual and hearing impairments, and dental problems. Each of these conditions will affect the rehabilitation of the individual who is laryngectomized. Critical evaluation of the patient's general health and abilities (e.g., manual dexterity, visual acuity) must be completed to ensure appropriate candidacy for each of the alaryngeal speech alternatives, to facilitate communicative success, and to prevent rehabilitative failure (see Chapter 3 in this text).

Pulmonary Health

Total laryngectomy permanently alters respiratory anatomy and function. Pulmonary diseases such as asthma or emphysema, commonly a result of long-term cigarette smoking, reduce lung capacity and airflow for speech and reduce the ability to clear mucous secretions from the airway. Use of an electrolarynx is not affected by limited respiratory function; however, there are implications for the esophageal and, to a greater degree, the TE speaker.

Salmon (1986) indicated that the successful esophageal speaker must be able to simultaneously coordinate and control air intake through the mouth and the lungs. For example, the inhalation method for esophageal speech production requires an ability to inhale air quickly through the stoma and into the lungs, creating an instantaneous negative pressure within the thoracic cavity and esophagus, thereby facilitating the flow of atmospheric air into the esophagus. Subsequently, the individual must expel the air from the stoma in a soft and easy manner while attempting to say "ah" using the atmospheric air within the oral cavity and esophagus. If the air passing from the stoma is audible, it may mask the esophageal sound. Consequently, an increase in the amount of air escape from the stoma during voicing may limit successful production of esophageal voice.

Control of air exchange through the stoma using either of the injection methods, tongue pumping or consonant press, is also important in preventing stomal blasting and associated noise. Although little documentation exists regarding the effect of pulmonary disease on the production of esophageal speech, logic suggests that respiratory compromise might be a limiting factor to its acquisition. Good pulmonary health is important for the production of esophageal speech, as well as for the production of TE speech. TE speech production depends primarily on pulmonary support and airflow. Pulmonary diseases such as emphysema and increased copious mucous secretions will likely affect the use of the TE voice prosthesis and the two-way tracheostoma breathing valve for hands-free speech production. The reduction in the laryngectomized individual's ability to clear secretions effectively often leads to plugging of the prosthesis with mucus. This plugging prevents airflow through the prosthesis into the pharyngoesophagus, which inhibits sound production. The patient often complains of a continual need to remove and clean the prosthesis, a frustrating, annoying, and time-consuming problem. In some instances, the use of a heat and moisture exchanger will help reduce mucous secretions (see Chapter 20 in this text).

Pulmonary disease frequently prevents the use of the tracheostoma breathing valve for hands-free TE speech. An inability to build up the necessary air pressure to automatically close the valve diaphragm prevents its successful use. Proper valve closure is necessary for automatic diversion of air into the esophagus for voice production. When pulmonary pressure is inadequate, the TE speaker must rely on digital occlusion of the stoma for speech production. A history of pulmonary disease, however, should not bias the clinician's decision to evaluate the patient for TE voice restoration, because each patient is different. Despite respiratory problems, some patients can successfully use the valve and enjoy hands-free TE speech production, and therefore should be given the opportunity to attempt to use the tracheostoma breathing valve.

Although all laryngectomized persons will experience some alteration in swallowing as a result of the removal of the larynx, swallowing problems are usually not a significant complaint following total laryngectomy. Most patients are able to swallow without difficulty; however, some may complain that eating takes longer and taste is not as distinct. This problem is exacerbated with extended laryngectomy procedures (Ward, Bishop, Frisby, & Stevens, 2002), which also have implications for speech (Deschler & Gray, 2004). The larynx is important to the opening of the pharyngoesophageal (PE) segment and the development of a negative pressure that facilitates bolus passage. Following total laryngectomy, there is an absence of negative pressure to drive bolus flow. The patient accommodates with increased propulsive pressure by the tongue. This decreased pressure gradient is reflected in delayed transit of the bolus through the passage (McConnel, Cerenko, & Mendelsohn, 1988), but again this is usually not a significant complaint. The reader is encouraged to consult the discussion provided by Lazarus (in Chapter 14 of this text) for further details related to swallowing disorders following head and neck surgery.

Gates, Ryan, Cantu, and Hearne (1982) found that difficulty swallowing after laryngectomy can occur as a result of radiation-induced mucositis, which often results in transient dysphagia. Dysphagia may also result from postoperative pain, persistent or recurrent cancer, or stricture (see Chapter 14 in this text).

Persistent or recurrent cancer and hypopharyngeal stricture can also be important causes of failure to achieve fluent esophageal or TE speech. In such instances, sustained voicing is limited by obstruction of the airflow from the pharynx and esophagus. Baugh, Lewin, and Baker (1990) indicated that dilation or surgical treatment is often necessary to relieve the obstruction to facilitate voice production and swallowing.

Sensory Changes

Hyposmia, or diminished smell, is a frequently reported problem in those who have undergone laryngectomy. This problem results from the lack of nasal airflow over the olfactory mucosa following the surgical separation of the lower from the upper airway. Although hyposmia can be considered a serious impairment, laryngectomized persons rarely complain about this problem in comparison to other changes, such as the loss of voice, presence of a stoma, respiratory problems, and psychosocial problems. Research has shown that laryngectomized patients have intact olfactory mechanisms that function normally when adequate airflow volume is provided (Tatchell, Lerman, & Watt, 1985). Interestingly, laryngectomized individuals can use successful strategies for "sniffing," including a glossopharyngeal press, a technique often used by esophageal speakers to improve smell, as well as taste. This along with other techniques may provide sufficient stimulation so that the perception of smell is acceptable to the individual (Tatchell et al., 1985; van Dam et al., 1999).

Decreased hearing and visual acuity are additional sensory sequelae of advancing age. Poor auditory sensitivity can impede the acquisition of esophageal speech. Hearing loss interferes with the laryngectomized individual's ability to hear instructions, monitor the adequacy of his or her own productions, and control the production of unwanted behaviors such as stomal blasts (Cameron, Green, & Gulliver, 2000; Diedrich & Youngstrom, 1966; Gates, Ryan, Cooper, et al., 1982; Kahane & Irwin, 1975; Martin, Hoops, & Shanks, 1974).

Although it is of little consequence to either the use of the electrolarynx or the acquisition of esophageal speech production, visual acuity should be a consideration for TE speech candidacy. Patients with decreased visual acuity often have difficulty locating the puncture site to remove and replace the prosthesis. Good visual acuity, however, is not a requirement for TE speech candidacy, as long as the care and management can be provided by a capable other person.

Poor manual dexterity may limit the use of hand-held electrolarynxes and the TE prosthesis. Special adaptations for the electrolarynx are available for laryngectomized persons with upper body disabilities. Considerable thought should be given, however, before recommending TE puncture for laryngectomized individuals with upper extremity limitations. Digital occlusion of the stoma is usually a basic prerequisite to TE speech production. If the patient is unable to cover the stoma digitally, the speech pathologist must be confident that the patient can use the tracheostoma breathing valve efficiently because the patient must rely on it solely in the absence of manual occlusion. Furthermore, a capable other person must be available to remove the prosthesis and properly adhere and remove the breathing valve.

Extent of Surgery

The majority of data regarding alaryngeal speech restoration focuses on rehabilitation following simple laryngectomy. Much less attention has been given to vocal rehabilitation of those patients undergoing the removal of the larynx, as well as significant portions of the oral cavity, oro- and hypopharynx, and cervical esophagus. The extent of surgical resection markedly influences both the choice and the quality of alaryngeal speech production (Deschler & Gray, 2004; see also Chapters 8 and 13 in this text).

Total glossectomy and laryngectomy offer a unique rehabilitative challenge to the speech pathologist. Loss of the tongue, the single most important structure for articulation and hence speech intelligibility, severely decreases successful communication, regardless of the method of alaryngeal speech production. The excessive, copious oral secretions that accompany glossectomy generally prevent the use of intraoral types of electrolarynxes. The neck- and cheek-placed devices are efficient in transmitting sound into the oral cavity, but the loss of articulatory competency severely limits verbal intelligibility, which is fair at best. The consequences of total glossectomy and laryngectomy on esophageal speech production also are profound. The patient must rely solely on methods of inhalation to draw air into the esophagus because injection methods, which rely on movement of the lingual musculature, are no longer possible. There are few reports of successful development of esophageal speech following these procedures (Anderson & Thomas, 1978).

Probably the best results for speech production following total glossectomy and laryngectomy are obtained using surgical–prosthetic alternatives, such as TE voice restoration. This may be true for two reasons. First, the sound quality more closely resembles normal laryngeal sound. Second, sound generation does not rely on the ability to learn new methods of air intake and expulsion that are frequently unsuccessful due to loss of the tongue. Therefore, the patient can concentrate strictly on compensatory strategies to enhance verbal intelligibility, and the listener is not distracted by unfamiliar methods of artificial sound generation. Nevertheless, verbal intelligibility is severely reduced and is unlikely to be improved to levels at which it is considered good.

Communicative success depends on listener familiarity and the use of contextual clues to facilitate semantic content. Frequently, the patient is forced to rely on nonoral methods of communication with unfamiliar and untrained listeners in public places. Communication in these situations is usually short, impersonal, and rushed. The outcome is usually frustrating and inefficient. The patient often is forced to depend on another person to translate his or her needs. In some cases, assistive devices such as computers with synthesized voice output may be more appropriate for communication.

Two other types of extended surgeries—the total laryngopharyngectomy and the total laryngopharyngoesophagectomy—create unique obstacles and warrant special attention to facilitate communicative restoration. Both surgeries include extirpation of the larynx and hypopharynx; the latter also includes removal of the esophagus. Reasons that lead to these radical types of surgical resection include an aggressive cancer, the extent to which the tumor has invaded other organs, and the high incidence of distant metastasis. Attention in these cases has focused on the surgical management of advanced carcinoma and more on the ideal method of reconstruction following tumor ablation than on vocal restoration. The various surgical options for reconstruction have included the use of local or regional skin flaps and visceral transposition techniques, including jejunal interposition and gastric pull-up (see Chapter 12 in this text). In some cases, a piece of the intestine, jejunum, or colon, or in the case of the gastric pull-up, the stomach, is used to reconstruct the defect. During gastric pull-up, the stomach is anastomosed to the base of the tongue and the posterior pharyngeal wall. When surgery does not involve the esophagus, the interposition of portions of the colon or free jejunal grafts in effect reconnect the base of the tongue to the remaining esophagus. The decision as to the choice of surgical procedure has focused primarily on the option with the least chance for surgical complications and the greatest chance for restoration of swallowing function. Until recently, little attention has been given to vocal rehabilitation of patients undergoing these types of surgeries (Gluckman et al., 1985; Gluckman et al., 1987; Harrison, 1969; Wenig, Keller, Levy, Mullooly, & Abramson, 1989). However, the current focus of quality-of-life issues on research investigating head and neck surgical outcomes has demonstrated the importance of speech production following cancer treatment (de Graeff et al., 1999; Deleyiannis, Weymuller, Coltrera, & Futran, 1999; Hynds Karnell, Funk, Tomblin, & Hoffman, 1999).

The few studies that have examined vocal restoration following extended surgical procedures have focused on current surgical–prosthetic methods of voice restoration. Wenig et al. (1989) reported satisfactory communication in 5 patients, 4 of whom had jejunal grafts and 1 in whom a radial forearm graft was used to replace a complete hypopharyngeal–esophageal defect. Although the investigators reported "coarse" vocal quality and lack of projection, all patients achieved fluent voice as judged by 2 voice professionals and 1 independent non-professional listener. The investigators felt that the bowel segment did not provide as good a vibratory source as the residual pharyngeal wall. Ziesmann, Boyd, Manktelow, and Rosen (1989) also reported good speech results in 2 of 3 patients who underwent neoglottic and neopharyngeal reconstruction using jejunum. Lewin and Lapine (1998) postulated that although tracheojejunal speech may be intelligible, the increased effort required to produce it may be a limiting factor to its successful use for routine communication. Maniglia, Leder, Goodwin, Sawyer, and Sasaki (1989) reported intelligible speech in 5 of 5 patients who used a Blom–Singer duckbill prosthesis following tracheogastric puncture; however, 3 of the 5 patients subsequently removed their prostheses as a result of dissatisfaction with their voices.

Based on my clinical experience, patients who receive tracheogastric puncture report marked gastric filling with air during speech attempts. Voice and speech characteristics of low pitch, decreased intensity, "wet" vocal quality, and slower rate of production, along with the air in the stomach, are most likely related to the physiologic properties of the stomach wall as a vibratory source. Specifically, the wider diameter of the pharyngogastric anastomosis is less effective as a vibratory source and permits excessive air to flow inferiorly to the stomach, resulting in gastric filling. Maniglia et al. (1989) proposed that digital pressure over the cervical stomach above the stoma can improve vocal quality. Although patients are able to produce sound, my clinical experience has not shown this to be successful for functional speech production and communication.

Successful speech restoration following radical surgical resection is often complicated. It frequently requires ingenuity, patience, and perhaps the use of some methods that seem unconventional. The previous discussion is not meant to dissuade speech pathologists from pursuing various forms of alaryngeal speech production with patients who have had extended surgical procedures. In fact, vocal restoration is especially rewarding in such patients. It is imperative, however, that other factors be considered so that successful communication is achieved. Although not always the case, in my experience, patients who are younger, who have strong motivation and commitment to success, who are independent, and who have reason to communicate, tend to demonstrate better adjustment and success.

Alaryngeal Speech Therapy

A discussion of special problems for alaryngeal speakers would not be complete without giving some attention to the availability and, more important, quality of speech therapy the patient will receive. When one considers that (a) alaryngeal speech production is basically a subspecialty within the larger class of voice disorders as a whole, (b) most academic training programs devote perhaps two or three lectures as part of a single voice disorders course to laryngectomy and alaryngeal voice production, (c) students get little if any hands-on training with laryngectomized individuals as part of their overall clinical practicum, and (d) the majority of alaryngeal speakers are usually treated in large head and neck cancer centers across the country, it is not surprising that few speech pathologists develop the skills and expertise necessary to provide good alaryngeal speech rehabilitation. I do not mean to imply that speech pathologists lack the caring or willingness to help the laryngectomized individual develop speech; however, without adequate knowledge, training, and experience, speech pathologists cannot be expected to be expert in their conduct of treatment.

Ironically, many patients treated in the large head and neck cancer centers around the country do not live close enough to return to the same institution for weekly, ongoing therapy. In fact, once most patients have healed from surgery, routine follow-up medical care is referred back to local physicians. Many laryngectomized persons choose to receive their postoperative radiation therapy at their local hospitals. Clearly, speech pathologists are faced with a dilemma. By the time a patient has healed enough to receive and benefit from therapy, he or she is ready to be discharged home to a location where services may not be available, let alone appropriate to his or her special needs (see Chapter 5 in this text). These issues need to be considered and discussed with the patient and family prior to selection of the optimal alaryngeal speech alternative.

Regardless of the extent of surgery, speech therapy usually begins postoperatively as soon as the patient has recovered sufficiently and can benefit from the intervention. Therapy generally begins while the patient is still in the hospital. During this time, various types of electrolaryngeal devices may be tried and practiced. Because neck irritation and swelling usually have not yet resolved, and the stoma remains tender, most patients begin with an intraoral device.

Although some surgeons and speech pathologists advocate fitting and placing the TE prosthesis 2 or 3 days postoperatively, most patients are not ready physically or emotionally. The stoma is sore, and sutures and staples prevent adequate digital occlusion. If the voice prosthesis is placed, it usually is not used until the patient has adequately healed and returns to the speech pathologist following hospital discharge for further treatment. During this time, the prosthesis may cause yet another worry and frustration. Therefore, based on my experience, most patients prefer to wait until they return for their first postoperative visit, approximately a week after discharge, to fit the prosthesis. Full attention can then be concentrated on TE voice production and management of the prosthesis (see Chapters 17 and 19 in this text). Although still tender, the tracheostoma and TE puncture site likely have healed sufficiently to tolerate placement and removal of the TE voice prosthesis as well as attempts at digital occlusion for voice production.

Similarly, success is limited when esophageal speech is begun prior to adequate healing. Although esophageal speech training in the immediate postoperative period should begin to focus on the various methods of air intake, inadequate healing of the neck tissue will inhibit sound production. The inability to produce sound at this time should not be interpreted as esophageal speech failure. As healing occurs, the ability to produce sound and the quality of the sound should improve. The patient's level of fatigue and emotions are high at this time. Furthermore, the patient is learning new techniques of self-care and is adjusting to a new body image. Again, esophageal speech development and progress are usually limited while the patient remains in the hospital.

Another barrier to receiving therapy while the patient remains hospitalized is the high cost of medical insurance, which has severely shortened the length of covered hospital stays. Thus, the patient is often discharged just as he or she is beginning to benefit from speech therapy. This brings us back to the first problem discussed in this section—the difficulty of accessing appropriate services from well-trained professionals following hospital discharge.

The speech pathologist should give sufficient thought to the availability of adequate therapy resources for the patient when discussing and recommending the various alaryngeal speech alternatives. A well-meaning attitude and good intentions are not sufficient. It never fails that, several weeks after a patient returns home, 250 miles from the clinic, having learned to speak and competently managing the TE voice prosthesis, an emergency room physician calls. The patient either has swallowed, has inhaled, or cannot replace the prosthesis. The TE puncture site is closing, and the doctor is not familiar with the TE puncture. What should be done? These kinds of incidents emphasize the need to be sure that the TE speaker is well informed about this alaryngeal method and understands and can demonstrate the management of the TE voice prosthesis so that the potential for problems is minimized.

Although the availability of adequate professional assistance is of concern, geographic factors have not dissuaded me from recommending surgical–prosthetic alternatives. I believe the benefits outweigh the risks, provided that the patient and significant other clearly understand early warning signs and can demonstrate techniques of management and prevention of possible problems. I have spent many hours on the telephone seeking speech pathologists who, if not already trained, are willing to work with me, via phone and mail, to ensure that the laryngectomized person develops and maintains the alaryngeal communication alternative of his or her choice. It is challenging work, but it is well worth the time and effort.

SPECIFIC PROBLEMS

Up to this point in the chapter, I have discussed problems that apply to all alaryngeal speakers regardless of the method used for speech production. The remainder of this chapter focuses on some problems faced by the laryngectomized individual as a function of the type of alaryngeal speech alternative, specifically TE voice restoration. I focus on the problems associated with the acquisition of TE speech production for three reasons. First, specific problems associated with use of the electrolarynx usually occur as a result of problems in manual dexterity or oral cavity alterations following various surgical resections, both of which have been addressed under the previous section on general problems. Second, many of the problems associated with the production of TE speech have relevance to esophageal speech production because both rely on the same structures—the pharynx and esophagus—as vibratory sources, and both depend on the resistance of airflow created by the pharynx and esophagus for sound production (see Chapter 6 in this text). Last, although TE speech restoration is not the optimal choice for all patients, it has become the preferred choice for alaryngeal speech production following total laryngectomy by a majority of patients and health care professionals as a result of limitations with both the artificial larynx and esophageal speech rehabilitation.

Specific problems associated with the production of TE speech can be subdivided into two general groups. The first group encompasses problems that occur as a result of physiological or anatomical variations in structure and function (Blom, 1986, 1988; Stafford, 2003). These problems may be directly related to the laryngectomy itself, such as pharyngeal constrictor spasm, hypopharyngeal stricture, flaccidity of the neoglottic segment, and stomal stenosis and irregularity.

Such problems also may be aggravated following laryngectomy, as is typical in patients with gastroesophageal reflux and candida colonization within the pharynx.

The second group of problems that specifically affects the production of TE speech might best be classified as mechanical. These problems are most often related to the management and use of the TE voice prosthesis (Blom, 1986). They tend to include problems experienced during sizing, fitting, removing, and replacing of the TE voice prosthesis. Although this information goes beyond the intent of the present chapter, a brief categorical summary is included in Table 24.1. A brief overview of the first group of problems—those variations in structure and function related to the laryngectomy—is provided in the subsequent section.

Pharyngeal Constrictor Hypertonicity or Spasm

Singer and Blom (1981) first used "pharyngoesophageal spasm" to refer to a lack of coordinated relaxation of the pharyngeal constrictor musculature, which results in an inferior egress of airflow to the stomach and thus prevents air escape into the pharynx for voice production. Along with resection of the larynx, the recurrent laryngeal nerve and the external and internal branches of the superior laryngeal nerve are sacrificed during total laryngectomy; however, the glossopharyngeal nerve and vagal innervation to the pharyngeal plexus should remain intact. Thus, contraction of the pharyngeal constrictor muscles may occur in response to insufflation (see Chapter 6 in this text). Figure 24.1 depicts the nerve supply following total laryngectomy. Studies have shown that in those cases in which constrictor spasm has been suspected, selective myotomy of the middle and inferior pharyngeal constrictors, including the cricopharyngeus, allows a superior egress of air for speech production (Baugh et al., 1987; Singer & Blom, 1981; Singer, Blom, & Hamaker, 1986). Singer et al. (1986) proposed that neurectomy of the pharyngeal plexus be performed at the time of laryngectomy to disrupt the pharyngeal constrictor muscle innervation, thereby preventing spasm. This procedure has the advantage of being less anatomically destructive than myotomy. It preserves the vascular integrity to the pharyngeal wall while retaining the residual resting tone of the upper esophageal segment. The residual tone has been thought to be a contributing factor to better TE voice production. Neurectomy, however, is frequently technically difficult anatomically and may not be possible in irradiated patients.

More recently the injection of botulinum neurotoxin (Botox) as a noninvasive treatment for the relief of pharyngeal constrictor spasm has been equally successful and much preferred over surgical alternatives. Botox is capable of chemically denervating focal areas of excessive muscle contraction by blocking the presynaptic release of the neurotransmitter acetylcholine at the neuromuscular junction, causing a paralysis of the involved musculature. Thus, Botox-induced paralysis alleviates muscular hypercontraction and allows the superior egress of air through the PE segment, facilitating sound and TE speech production (Blitzer,

(text continues on p. 613)

TABLE 24.1

Summary of Problems Associated with Use of the
Tracheoesophageal (TE) Puncture Voice Prosthesis and Treatment Suggestions

Indicators	Treatment
Leakage Through Prosthesis	
1. Prosthesis old and deteriorated	1. Replace prosthesis
2. Frequent need to replace prosthesis, or fungal deposits in or on valve	2. Use amphotericin B lozenges; use Nystatin oral rinse; chemically coat and disinfect prosthesis
3. Duckbill tip against posterior pharyngeal wall	3. Resize and replace with shorter prosthesis or change to low-pressure, indwelling, or ultra–low-pressure prosthesis
Leakage Around Prosthesis	
1. Prosthesis too long or pistoning in TE tract	1. Resize and replace with shorter prosthesis or place retention collar on tracheal side of prosthesis
2. Tract dilation	2. Down-stent fistula with catheters; cauterize tract; use flap reconstruction
3. Superior migration of TE tract with vertical positioning of prosthesis	3. Place catheter inferiorly or repuncture
Difficulty Inserting Prosthesis	
1. Superior migration of TE tract	1. Replace catheter inferiorly or repuncture
2. Granulation tissue	2. Remove granulation tissue; use duckbill-type prosthesis; use gel-cap insertion system; have patient in supine position; place indwelling-type prosthesis; dilate TEP (e. g., increase from 16 Fr prosthesis to 20 Fr catheter or 20 Fr prosthesis to 24 Fr catheter)
3. Tracheostomal stenosis	3. Dilate stoma with stoma button, laryngectomy tube or vent, or Barton-Mayo button; perform stomaplasty
4. Deep-set stoma	4. Use indwelling prosthesis
Gastric Filling	
1. Valve opening upon quiet respiration	1. Change to duckbill-type prosthesis or increased resistance prosthesis
2. Pharyngeal constrictor hypertonicity	2. Compromise constrictor musculature medically (Botox)
Immediate Postfitting Aphonia	
1. Overfitting/underfitting prosthesis	1. Remove prosthesis and resize
2. Prosthesis valve tip is closed	2. Remove prosthesis, inspect, and gently squeeze end to open
3. Forceful stomal occlusion	3. Apply light digital contact
4. Difficulty with intermittent voicing	4. Compare voice with and without prosthesis; compromise constrictor musculature (Botox)

(continues)

TABLE 24.1 *Continued.*

Summary of Problems Associated with Use of the
Tracheoesophageal (TE) Puncture Voice Prosthesis and Treatment Suggestions

Indicators	Treatment
Delayed Postfitting Aphonia	
1. Prosthesis valve tip is closed	1. Remove prosthesis, inspect, and gently squeeze end to open
2. TE tract stenosis/closure secondary to underfitting	2. Dilate, resize, and reinsert longer prosthesis
3. Prosthesis not fully inserted	3. Dilate and reinsert prosthesis
4. False tract formation associated with reinsertion of prosthesis	4. Replace catheter and insert prosthesis or perform radiologic study to confirm; re-puncture
Soreness or Sensitivity During Prosthetic Insertion	
1. Effects of X-ray therapy, sutures, infection, nonhealed TEP	1. Change to duckbill prosthesis; replace with TEP prosthesis with softer retention collar; use gel-cap insertion; use topical lidocaine and change to indwelling-type prosthesis; delay placement; use antibiotics if infected
Pharyngeal Constrictor Hypertonicity (spasm)	
1. Nonfluent speech	1–7. Compromise constrictor musculature tonicity (Botox)
2. Strained, tight, effortful speech	
3. Similar voice results with or without prosthesis	
4. Elevated intraesophageal pressure during objective insufflation	
5. No dysphagia or stricture	
6. Patent TE tract	
7. Voice improvement following lidocaine block	
Granulation Tissue Formation	
1. Inflammation secondary to frequent removal of prosthesis	1. Remove granulation tissue; clean prosthesis in situ; remove prosthesis due to difficulty in voicing or leakage
Soft TE Voice	
1. Prosthesis is not fully inserted	1. Dilate and resize prosthesis
2. Pharyngeal outpouching, diverticulum, or PE hypotonicity	2. Apply pressure band or anterior neck pressure; use digital occlusion instead of breathing valve
3. Radiation effects	3. Use humidification
4. Anterior protrusion of prosthesis, underfitting	4. Dilate and resize prosthesis

(continues)

TABLE 24.1 *Continued.*

Summary of Problems Associated with Use of the
Tracheoesophageal (TE) Puncture Voice Prosthesis and Treatment Suggestions

Indicators	Treatment
Elevation in Intraesophageal Pressures (>20 mm Hg) or Nonfluent TE Speech	
1. Pharyngeal constrictor hypertonicity	1. Confirm with pharyngeal plexus nerve block; compromise constrictor muscula-ture (Botox)
2. Radiation-induced edema	2. Repeat testing in 4 weeks
3. Simultaneous use of traditional methods of esophageal air injection	3. Extinguish esophageal injection behaviors
4. Gastroesophageal reflux	4. Use antireflux protocol or medication
5. Hypopharyngeal stricture	5. Perform hypopharyngeal dilatation
Small Tracheostoma or Stomal Stenosis	
1. Shortness of breath; difficulty inserting prosthesis	1. Gradually dilate stoma with stoma button, laryngectomy tube or vent, Barton-Mayo button, or modified button; perform stomaplasty
DIfficulty with Stomal Occlusion	
1. Large tracheostoma	1. Use valve housings/base plates, custom housing/button, rubber washers, suction cup, etc.
2. Irregular shape of stoma	2. Use valve housings/base plates, or custom housing/button
3. Digit obstructs airflow into the prosthesis	3. Use valve housings/base plates, custom housing/button, or suction cup; apply light digital contact
4. Forceful stomal occlusion	4. Apply light digital contact
Small Esophageal Lumen	
1. Tight, strained voice to no speech	1–3. Trim prosthestic hood; replace with InHealth InDwelling prosthesis
2. Voice better without prosthesis	
3. Dysphagia	
Separation or Edema Between Party Wall	
1. Weaker voice with prosthesis in place	1–4. Insert measuring tool fully so it is flush against puncture site; confirm radiographi-cally; replace catheter to dilate, align tract, and heal; repuncture if needed
2. Catheter passes only part way, resistance (puncture misaligned)	
3. Difficulty fully inserting measuring tool	
4. Progressive deterioration in voice	
Poor Tracheostoma Valve Adherence	
1. Skin irritation, peristomal erythema, soreness	1. Use protective barrier wipes; use DuoDerm adhesive patch; use Optiderm housing; use hydrocolloid base plates; use Montgomery straps; use benzoine tincture; properly clean skin; change liquid adhesive brand

(continues)

TABLE 24.1 *Continued.*

Summary of Problems Associated with Use of the
Tracheoesophageal (TE) Puncture Voice Prosthesis and Treatment Suggestions

Indicators	Treatment
Poor Tracheostoma Valve Adherence (*continued*)	
2. Excessive mucous secretions	2. Use heat and moisture exchangers; remove valve from housing prior to coughing; position housing correctly; use mucolytics
3. Increased back pressure	3. Speak softer; increase diameter of prosthesis to 20 Fr; use low-resistance prosthesis; use Barton-Mayo button or custom button; put tape over housing; inject Botox for hypertonicity
4. Irregular stoma or peristomal topography	4. Use custom housing or flexiderm housing; put tape over housing; perform stomaplasty
Difficulty with Tracheostoma Valve Closure	
1. Difficulty closing valve or diaphragm for speech	1. Adjust diaphragm position; use spring-loaded valve device
2. Difficulty breathing through valve	2. Adjust position of diaphragm
3. Emphysema or asthma	3. Manage medically; use digital occlusion
Aspiration of Voice Prosthesis	
1. Tracheal aspiration upon insertion or removal of prosthesis	1–2. Attach button larger than stoma to strap; change to a prosthesis with a thicker retention collar; thread string through strap around neck
2. Excessive coughing	
Stenosis or Closure of the Fistula or Puncture	
1. Anterior protrusion of prosthesis	1. Dilate, resize, refit prosthesis
2. Unable to pass catheter	2. Insert smaller catheters (8, 10, 12, 14 Fr) and dilate TE tract
3. No liquid noted through TEP upon swallowing	3. Dilate; repuncture
4. Granulation tissue	4. Remove granulation tissue; reduce frequency of prosthetic removal
Radiation-Induced Edema	
1. Minimal to no sound, but easy catheter insertion	1. Delay prosthetic placement; replace with catheter or dummy prosthesis for longer durations
2. Tenderness, soreness with prosthetic insertion	2. Use topical lidocaine prior to insertion; use gel-cap insertion; change to prosthesis with duckbill or soft retention collar
3. Increased intraesophageal pressures or nonfluent speech	3. Maintain prosthesis; retest 4 to 6 weeks postradiation

Note. PE = pharyngoesophageal; TEP = tracheoesophageal puncture.
Sources for this table are Baugh, Lewin, and Baker (1990); Biota (1986, 1988); Garth, McRae, and Rhys-Evans (1991); Johnson, Beery, Aramany, and Sigler (1986); and Mahieu, van Saene, Rosingh, and Schutte (1986).

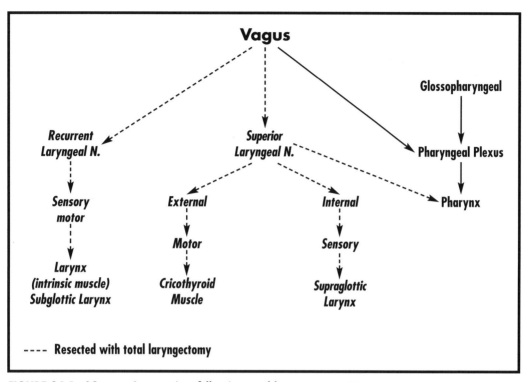

FIGURE 24.1. Nervous innervation following total laryngectomy. N. = nerve.

Komisar, Baredes, Brin, & Stewart, 1995; Hamaker & Blom, 2003; Ramachandran, Arunachalam, Hurren, Marsh, & Samuel, 2003; Terrell, Lewin, & Esclamado, 1995). Usually, a single injection is sufficient; however, some patients may need a subsequent injection to achieve fluent speech production should the initial injection fail to completely relax the musculature. Although the effect of Botox may be temporary, necessitating reinjection as the effect wears off, a majority of patients obtain long-term results without need for reinjection.

Researchers have also described and recommended various methods of preoperative esophageal insufflation to identify patients with spasm who were candidates for myotomy at the time of TE puncture, thereby avoiding additional surgery and further postpuncture speech delay (Blom, Singer, & Hamaker, 1985; Lewin et al., 1987; Schuller, Jarrow, Kelly, & Miglets, 1983). Figure 24.2 shows the testing apparatus used to perform objective intraesophageal insufflation as proposed by Lewin et al. (1987). The results of the study demonstrated a direct relationship between intraesophageal pressures and TE speech production. As intraesophageal pressure measurements increased, TE speech fluency decreased. Elevations in intraesophageal pressure measurements above 20 mm Hg during preoperative esophageal insufflation were associated with nonfluent TE speech production post–TE puncture. This method provided objective indication for myotomy at the time of TE puncture, rather than as a postoperative procedure. Currently, this method and the self-insufflation method proposed by Blom et al.

FIGURE 24.2 Testing apparatus for objective intraesophageal air insufflation demonstrating catheter placement and attachment to pressure recorder, and insufflation source. From "An Objective Method for Prediction of Tracheoesophageal Speech Production" by J. S. Lewin, R. F. Baugh, and S. R. Baker, 1987, *Journal of Speech and Hearing Disorders, 55,* 212–217. Copyright 1987 by the American Speech-Language-Hearing Association. Reprinted with permission.

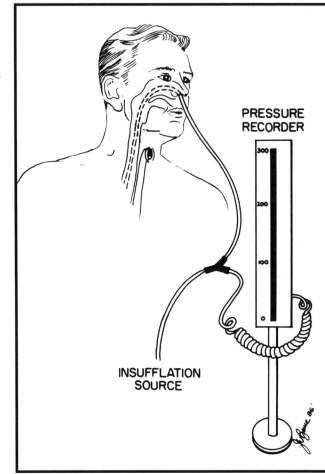

(1985) continue to be useful tools for identifying patients who may benefit from Botox injection prior to TE puncture and, at the same time, allow the patient to hear his or her "new" voice preoperatively. Preoperative insufflation may not be as critical as it once was, however, given the simple procedure of Botox injection should the patient fail to achieve fluent TE speech production postoperatively. A protocol for objective air insufflation testing is presented in Figure 24.3.

Hypopharyngeal Stricture

Constrictions of the hypopharynx can be an important cause of failure to achieve fluent TE speech. They are best classified as structural or anatomical abnormalities that hinder TE speech ability by impeding airflow from the pharynx and esophagus, thereby limiting sound production. Simpson, Smith, and Gordon (1972) referred to one type of permanent, organic stricture above the pharyngoesophageal junction as a constant area of narrowing that does not distend even during swallowing. This type of stricture is most likely related to loss of mucosa due to excision and related fibrosis and/or scarring secondary to delayed healing. Management usually entails medical or surgical treatment, including repeated dilatation or surgical reconstruction of the stenotic area. Strictures do not improve with relaxation or voice therapy.

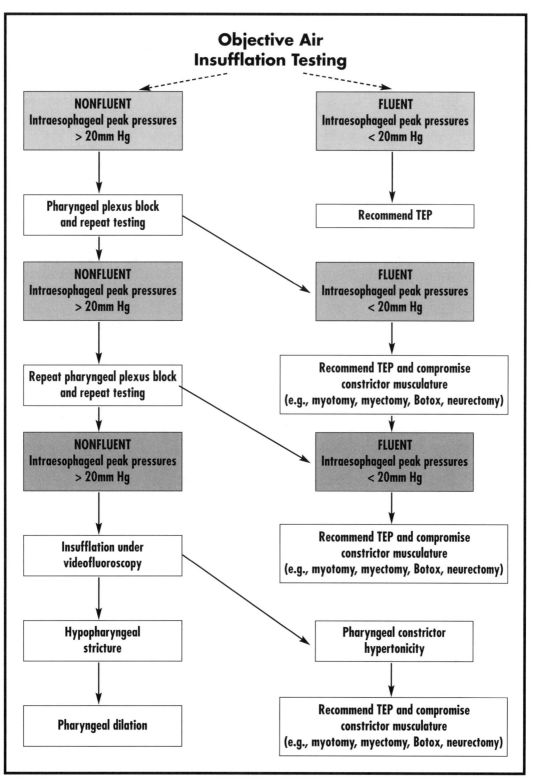

FIGURE 24.3. Assessment protocol for fluent TE speech.

Baugh et al. (1990) proposed the use of objective air insufflation testing to substantiate a need for further testing when hypopharyngeal stricture is suspected. During preoperative insufflation, absence of reduced intraesophageal pressures, along with a lack of improvement in TE speech production following relaxation of the musculature with pharyngeal plexus nerve block, may suggest hypopharyngeal stricture. Frequently, the patient will also report difficulty swallowing. Given these indications, videofluoroscopic recording of swallowing will usually confirm a diagnosis of hypopharyngeal stricture.

Neoglottic Tonicity

Much has been written regarding the proper tonicity of the neoglottic segment following total laryngectomy for both esophageal and TE speech production. Proper tonicity of the neoglottic segment is critical to phonatory success. A vibratory segment that is too loose or flaccid is as great a problem as one that is too tight and unyielding. Previous discussions within this chapter centered around management of the PE sphincter that is too tight. The flaccid segment is frequently helped with the use of external digital pressure, neck bands, and other prosthetic devices. Although Montgomery and Lavelle (1974) reported a surgical procedure called a sternomastoid muscle swing to provide extrinsic compression to the anterior wall of the pharynx using the added bulk provided by repositioning the sternomastoid muscle anteriorly, my experience has not shown surgical correction to be a common method of choice for relief of the flaccid neoglottic segment.

Stomal Stenosis and Irregularity

Stenosis of the tracheostoma is not an infrequent complication following total laryngectomy (Montgomery, 1973). It may occur immediately following surgery or years later. The most common causes of stenosis are (a) excessive scar tissue formation, usually resulting from postoperative infection or fistulization; (b) fibrosis; (c) excessive fat surrounding the stoma; (d) defective or absent tracheal rings; and (e) tumor recurrence. Frequently, a laryngectomy tube or stoma button may be used to dilate the stoma and maintain an adequate airway. The use of these devices usually interferes with TE speech production by occluding the TE puncture and prosthesis, which prevents airflow into the pharynx for voice production. Shapiro and Ramanathan (1982) combined both the voice prosthesis and the stoma button into one unit to compensate for this problem; however, their prosthesis was often difficult to place and not always effective in accomplishing voice production while maintaining stomal patency. For these reasons, this type of prosthesis is neither readily available nor frequently used.

Some patients are able to maintain an adequate airway by wearing a stoma button or laryngectomy tube while sleeping and removing it during the day for speech purposes. When necessary, the laryngectomy tube or vent may be fenestrated to accommodate the prosthetic inlet for airflow and speech production. Granulation tissue may develop, however, within the fenestrated area as a result of the mucosal irritation from long-term placement in the trachea. Also, the rotational movement of the vent may cause misalignment of the TE puncture and the fenestration, which is often a frustrating problem for some patients (Lewin, 1998). Alternatively, the use of the standard or customized Barton-Mayo button may provide the same benefit as a laryngectomy tube or vent, while at the same time permitting the attachment of a tracheostoma breathing valve for hands-free TE speech. The size of the stoma facilitates snug retention of the button while maintaining the patency of the stoma (Lewin et al., 2000).

When tracheostomal stenosis persists despite prosthetic attempts to maintain an adequate airway, surgical procedures may be used to revise the tracheostoma (Ogura & Thawley, 1979). Unfortunately, the resulting stomal configuration may be irregular and, therefore, difficult to manually occlude for TE voice production. One of the most common problems that those with irregular stomal configurations experience is difficulty with adherence of the tracheostoma breathing valve to the neck. Sometimes, prosthetic insertion may also be difficult when the stoma and, hence, the TE puncture are deeply recessed into the neck. Patients with irregular stomal configurations most often rely solely on digital occlusion of the tracheostoma for voice purposes. Stomal plugs and rubber washers have been used to help patients occlude a large irregular stoma when digital occlusion is difficult (Garth, Fenton, Pearson, Riden, & Thomas, 1993; Johnson, Beery, Aramany, & Sigler, 1986; Lewin, 2004). Additionally, modification of standard tracheostoma valves has been shown to be successful (Cantu, Shagets, Fifer, Andres, & Newton, 1986; Doyle, Grantmyre, & Myers, 1989). Successful TE speech production often depends on designing and using custom-made devices. The maxillofacial prosthodontist can often help facilitate the patient's success by custom-molding peristomal or intraluminal devices that will improve digital occlusion or permit attachment of a tracheostoma breathing valve for hands-free speech production.

Gastroesophageal Reflux

TE speakers who suffer from gastroesophageal reflux—that is, spontaneous flowing of stomach contents back into the esophagus—experience specific problems related to speech production. The literature is replete with documentation as to the necessity for a competent distal esophageal sphincter for the development of esophageal speech. The distal esophageal sphincter separates the esophageal and gastric (stomach) lumens. When this sphincter fails to remain closed, the result may be the reflux of gastric contents into the throat. The development of a hiatal hernia is commonly seen in patients with gastroesophageal reflux. Wolfe, Olson, and Goldenberg (1971) reported failure to acquire esophageal speech in patients who demonstrated gastroesophageal reflux, hiatal hernia, and varying degrees of esophagitis. These investigators also suspected that, in many of the patients, the hiatal hernia and reflux were most likely present prior to the laryngectomy. It also has been suggested that the air charging associated with esophageal speech production may aggravate this gastric problem (Lewin et al., 2000).

The pharynx is normally guarded by the upper esophageal sphincter. The cricopharyngeus muscle arising from the cricoid cartilage provides the sphincteric action at this part of the gastrointestinal tract. It has a constant resting tone and relaxes and contracts in response to distension. This segment has been referred to as the PE sphincter (Henderson, 1986). As far back as 1957, Creamer and Schlegel found that pressure at the PE sphincter increased immediately following esophageal distension, with an 80% response rate. The muscle contraction at the PE sphincter occurred without relaxation, followed by initiation of a peristaltic wave and relaxation of the gastroesophageal sphincter. The authors speculated that the entire response prevented the spontaneous return of gastric contents into the pharynx, while propelling the contents into the stomach. Other authors have substantiated this finding and have found that acid stimuli, along with intraluminal distension of the esophagus, strongly initiate the physiologic response of this reflex contraction (Enzman, Harell, & Zboralske, 1977; Gerhardt, Shuck, Bordeaux, & Winship, 1978).

Laryngectomized individuals with a known history of gastroesophageal reflux may be at a higher risk for the occurrence of pharyngeal constrictor spasm, reducing TE speech abilities. Disruption of the upper esophageal sphincter following pharyngeal constrictor myotomy or Botox injection may improve speech fluency, but at the same time destroy the pharyngeal barrier to esophageal reflux. Thus, patients may complain of increased regurgitation into the oropharynx and oral cavity, especially after meals and when stooping or bending over. The resulting voice often has a liquid vocal quality that is unappealing to many TE speakers.

Many patients are able to control or avoid reflux occurrences once they are aware of the postural and dietary irritants. In some cases, anti–gastroesophageal reflux medications may be recommended by the physician to reduce the symptoms and occurrences.

Candida

Although all TE voice prostheses require replacement as a result of natural wear and tear, the duration of wear time will vary from patient to patient. The need to replace the prosthesis is usually indicated by leakage through the prosthesis, tracheal aspiration, or progressive changes in airflow resistance. Most patients report the average life of a TE voice prosthesis to be between 3 and 5 months, although durations of up to 14 months have been reported by various investigators (Hilgers & Schouwenburg, 1990).

The most common cause of prosthetic deterioration is the formation of yeasts on the valved side of the prosthesis, which tend to colonize and eventually cause prosthetic malfunction. Proper valve closing is impeded due to this colonization, and the prosthesis begins to leak. If the prosthesis is not removed, leakage progressively worsens as colonization continues. Additionally, airflow resistance increases and the patient may experience greater effort speaking. Because the tongue is the main source of yeasts in the oral cavity, it is not surprising to find that the voice prosthesis sitting in the pharyngoesophagus is severely susceptible to the formation of these yeast strains, with *Candida albicans* being the most commonly isolated strain (Busscher & van der Mei, 1998).

Attempts to control the formation of yeasts on voice prostheses have relied primarily on the application of antimycotics. In some studies, applying antimycotics has effectively reduced the candida formation and increased prosthesis lifetime. Unfortunately, the use of antimycotics, such as amphotericin B lozenges (Mahieu, van Saene, den Besten, & van Saene, 1986; van Lith-Bijl, Mahieu, Patel, & Zijlstra, 1992), and rinsing the mouth twice a day with nystatin (Blom & Hamaker, 1996) do not completely eliminate yeast formation on the prosthesis. Furthermore, the long-term use of antimycotics may actually stimulate the development of resistant strains. Alternatively, studies have shown that the consumption of dairy products containing active probiotic bacteria, such as buttermilk and yogurt, may prohibit yeast formation on silicone rubber voice prostheses (Bos, Busscher, Geertsema-Doornbusch, & van der Mei, 1997; Busscher, et al., 1998). Investigations are ongoing to develop prostheses that are inherently resistant to candida colonization.

SUMMARY

This chapter has sought to familiarize the reader with special problems faced by individuals who have undergone laryngectomy as they attempt to acquire and further develop alaryngeal speech. Speech pathologists must understand and consider both the general and the specific problems each laryngectomized individual faces as he or she adjusts to the changes that affect the daily routines and communication that most people take for granted. Speech pathologists must be adequately informed and trained so that they can provide appropriate counseling and treatment to help the laryngectomized person attain the type of alaryngeal speech alternative of his or her choice. Although this work is often challenging, the results are well worth the time and effort and increase each patient's chance of optimizing alaryngeal communication.

REFERENCES

American Cancer Society. (1996). *Cancer facts and figures.* New York: Author.

Anderson, J. D., & Thomas, S. (1978). Speech rehabilitation of a laryngectomized–glossectomized patient. *Laryngoscope, 88,* 1666–1670.

Baugh, R. F., Lewin, J. S., & Baker, S. R. (1987). Preoperative assessment of tracheoesophageal speech. *Laryngoscope, 97,* 461–466.

Baugh, R.F., Lewin, J.S., & Baker, S.R. (1990). Vocal rehabilitation of tracheoesophageal speech failures. *Head & Neck, 12,* 69–73.

Biota, E. D. (1986, November). *Tracheoesophageal puncture: Problems and solutions.* Paper presented at the annual meeting of the American Speech-Language-Hearing Association, Detroit.

Biota, E. D. (1988). Tracheoesophageal valves: Problems, solutions, and directions for the future. *Head and Neck Surgery, 10*(Suppl. 2), 142–145.

Blitzer, A., Komisar, A., Baredes, S., Brin, M. F, & Stewart, C. (1995). Voice failure after tracheo-esophageal puncture: Management with botulinum toxin. *Otolaryngology—Head & Neck Surgery, 113,* 668–670.

Blom, E. D. (1986, November). *Tracheoesophageal puncture: Problems and solutions.* Paper presented at the annual meeting of the American Speech-Language-Hearing Association, Detroit, MI.

Blom, E. D. (1988). Tracheoesophageal valves: Problems, solutions, and directions for the future. *Head & Neck Surgery, 10*(Suppl. 2), 142–145.

Blom, E. D., & Hamaker, R. C. (1996). Tracheoesophageal voice restoration following total laryngectomy. In E. N. Myers & J. Suen (Eds.), *Cancer of the head and neck* (pp. 839–852). Philadelphia: Saunders.

Blom, E. D., Singer, M. I., & Hamaker, R. C. (1985). An improved esophageal insufflation test. *Archives of Otolaryngology, 111,* 211–212.

Bos, R., Busscher, H. J., Geertsema-Doornbusch, G. I., & van der Mei, H. C. (1997). Adhesions competition between Streptococcus thermophilus and Candida species. In J. Wimpenny, P. Hadley, P. Gilbert, & H. Lappin-Scott (Eds.), *Biofilm: community interaction and control* (pp. 113–117). Chippenham, UK: BioLine-Antony Rose.

Busscher, H. J., Bruinsma, G., van Weissenbruch, R., Leunisse, C., van der Mei, H. C., Dijk, F., & Albers, F. W. (1998). The effect of buttermilk consumption on biofilm formation on silicone rubber voice prostheses in an artificial throat. *European Archives of Oto-Rhino-Laryngology, 255,* 410–413.

Busscher, H. J., & van der Mei, H.C. (1998). Biofilm formation and its prevention on silicone rubber voice prostheses. In E. D. Blom, M. I. Singer, & R. C. Hamaker (Eds.), *Tracheoesophageal voice restoration following total laryngectomy* (pp. 89–102). San Diego, CA: Singular.

Cameron, P., Green, W. B., & Gulliver, M. (2000). *Journal of Speech–Language Pathology and Audiology, 24,* 122–126.

Cantu, E., Shagets, F. W., Fifer, R. C., Andres, C. J., & Newton, A. D. (1986). Customized valve housing. *Laryngoscope, 96,* 1159–1163.

Creamer, B., & Schlegel, J. (1957). Motor responses of the esophagus to distention. *Journal of Applied Physiology, 10,* 498–504.

Dabul, B., & Lovestedt, I. (1974). Prognostic indicators of esophageal speech. *Journal of Surgical Ontology, 6,* 461–469.

de Graeff, A., de Leeuw, R. J., Ros, W. J. G., Hordijk, G., Battermann, J. J., Blijham, G. H., Winnubst, J. A. M. (1999). A prospective study on quality of life of laryngeal cancer patients treated with radiotherapy. *Head & Neck, 21,* 291–296.

Deleyiannis, F. W.-B., Weymuller, E. A., Coltrera, M. D., & Futran, N. (1999). Quality of life after laryngectomy: Are functional disabilities important? *Head & Neck, 21,* 319–324.

Deschler, D. G., & Gray, S. T. (2004). Tracheoesophageal speech following laryngopharyngectomy and pharyngeal reconstruction. *Otolaryngologic Clinics of North America, 37*(3), 567–583.

Diedrich, W. M., & Youngstrom, K. A. (1966). *Alaryngeal speech.* Springfield, IL: Thomas.

Doyle, P. C., Grantmyre, A., & Myers, C. (1989). Clinical modifications of the tracheostoma breathing valve for voice restoration. *Journal of Speech and Hearing Disorders, 54,* 189–192.

Enzman, D. R., Harell, G. S., & Zboralske, F. F. (1977). Upper esophageal responses to intraluminal distension in man. *Gastroenterology, 72,* 1292–1298.

Garth, R. J., Fenton, C. J., Pearson, C. R., Riden, K., & Thomas, M. R. (1993). The tracheostomal washer: A simple aid for tracheo-oesophageal speakers with a large tracheostome. *Journal of Laryngology and Otology, 107,* 824–825.

Garth, R. J. N., McRae, A., & Rhys-Evans, P. H. (1991). Tracheo-esophageal puncture: A review of problems and complications. *Journal of Laryngology and Otology, 105,* 750–754.

Gates, G. A., & Hearne, E. M. (1982). Predicting esophageal speech. *Annals of Otology, Rhinology and Laryngology, 91,* 454–457.

Gates, G. A., Ryan, W., Cantu E., & Hearne, E. (1982). Current status of laryngectomee rehabilitation: II. Causes of failure. *American Journal of Otolaryngology, 3,* 8–14.

Gates, G. A., Ryan, W., Cooper, J. C., Lawlis, G. F., Cantu, E., Hayashi, T., Lauder, E., Welch, R. W., & Hearne, E. (1982). Current status of laryngectomee rehabilitation: I. Results of therapy. *American Journal of Otolaryngology, 3,* 1–7.

Gerhardt, D. C., Shuck, T. J., Bordeaux, R. A., & Winship, D. H. (1978). Human upper esophageal sphincter: Response to volume, osmotic, and acid stimuli. *Gastroenterology, 75,* 268–274.

Gluckman, J. L., McDonough, J. J., McCafferty, G. J., Black, R. J., Coman, W. B., Cooney, T., Bird, R. J., & Robinson, D. W. (1985). Complications associated with free jejunal graft reconstruction of the pharyngoesophagus: A multi-institutional experience with 52 cases. *Head and Neck Surgery, 7,* 200–205.

Gluckman, J. I., Weissler, M. C., McCafferty, G., Black, R. J., Coman, W. W., Cooney, T., & Bird, R. J. (1987). Partial vs. total esophagectomy for advanced carcinoma of the hypopharynx. *Archives of Otolaryngology—Head and Neck Surgery, 113,* 69–72.

Gress, C. D., (2004). Preoperative evaluation for tracheoesophageal voice restoration. *Otolaryngology Clinics of North America, 37*(3), 519–530.

Hamaker, R. C., & Blom, E. D. (2003). Botulinum neurotoxin for pharyngeal constrictor muscle spasm in tracheoesophageal voice restoration. *Laryngoscope, 113,* 1479–1482.

Hamaker, R. C., Singer, M. I., Blom, E. D., & Daniels, H. A. (1985). Primary voice restoration at laryngectomy. *Archives of Otolaryngology, 111,* 182–186.

Harrison, D. F. N. (1969). Surgical management of cancer of the hypopharynx and cervical esophagus. *British Journal of Surgery, 56,* 95–103.

Henderson, R. D. (1986). Gastroesophageal reflux. In C. W. Cummings & J. M. Fredrickson (Eds.), *Otolaryngology—Head and neck surgery: Vol. 3. Larynx/hypopharynx, trachea/esophagus, thyroid/parathyroid* (pp. 2377–2400). St. Louis, MO: Mosby.

Hilgers, F. J. M., & Schouwenburg, P. F. (1990). A new low-resistance, self-retaining prosthesis (Provox) for voice rehabilitation after total laryngectomy. *Laryngoscope, 100,* 1202–1207.

Hynds Karnell, L., Funk, G. F., Tomblin, J. B., & Hoffman, H. T. (1999). Quality of life measurements of speech in the head and neck cancer patient population. *Head & Neck, 21,* 229–238.

Johnson, J. T., Beery, Q. C., Aramany, M. A., & Sigler, B. (1986). Vocal restoration and the large irregular tracheostoma. *Laryngoscope, 96,* 214–215.

Kahane, J. C., & Irwin, J. A. (1975, November). *Comparison of hearing sensitivity and stoma noise in 90 esophageal speakers.* Paper presented at the annual convention of the American Speech and Hearing Association, Washington, DC.

Keith, R. L., Ewert, J. C., & Flowers, C. R. (1974). Factors influencing the learning of esophageal speech. *British Journal of Disorders in Communication, 9,* 110–116.

King, P. S., Fowlks, E. W., & Peirson, G. A. (1968). Rehabilitation and adaptation of laryngectomy patients. *American Journal of Physical Medicine, 47,* 192–203.

Lewin, J. S. (1998). Maximizing tracheoesophageal voice and speech. In E. D. Blom, M. I. Singer, & R. C. Hamaker (Eds.), *Tracheoesophageal voice restoration following total laryngectomy* (pp. 67–72). San Diego, CA: Singular.

Lewin, J. S. (2004). Nonsurgical management of the stoma to maximize tracheoesophageal speech. *Otolaryngology Clinics of North America, 37*(3), 585–596.

Lewin, J. S., Baugh, R. F., & Baker, S. R. (1987). An objective method for prediction of tracheoesophageal speech production. *Journal of Speech and Hearing Disorders, 52,* 212–217.

Lewin, J. S., & Lapine, P. R. (1998). Intraluminal pressure evaluation during vowel and word production in patients with TE and TJ puncture. *Journal of Medical Speech Pathology, 6*(1), 27–37.

Lewin, J. S., Lemon, J., Bishop-Leone, J. K., Leyk, S., Martin, J. W., & Gillenwater, A. M. (2000). Experience with Barton button and peristomal breathing valve attachments for hands-free tracheoesophageal speech. *Head & Neck, 22,* 142–148.

Mahieu, H. F., van Saene, H. K., Rosingh, H. J., & Schutte, H. K. (1986). Candida vegetations on silicone voice prostheses. *Archives of Otolaryngology—Head and Neck Surgery, 112*(3), 321–325.

Mahieu, H. F., van Saene, J. J. M., den Besten, J., & van Saene, H. K. F. (1986). Oropharynx decontamination preventing candida vegetation on voice prostheses. *Archives of Otolaryngology—Head and Neck Surgery, 112,* 1090–1092.

Maniglia, A. F., Leder, S. B., Goodwin, W. J., Jr., Sawyer, R., & Sasaki, C. T. (1989). Tracheogastric puncture for vocal rehabilitation following total pharyngolaryngoesophagectomy. *Head and Neck Surgery, 11,* 524–527.

Maniglia, A. J., Lundy, D. S., Casiano, R. C., & Swim, S. C. (1989). Speech restoration and complications of primary versus secondary tracheoesophageal puncture following total laryngectomy. *Laryngoscope, 99,* 489–491.

Martin, D. E., Hoops, H. R., & Shanks, J. C. (1974). The relationship between esophageal speech proficiency and selected measures of auditory function. *Journal of Speech and Hearing Research, 74,* 80–85.

McConnel, F. M., Cerenko, D., & Mendelsohn, M. S. (1988). Dysphagia after total laryngectomy. *Otolaryngologic Clinics of North America, 21,* 721–726.

Montgomery, W. W. (1973). *Surgery of the upper respiratory system.* Philadelphia: Lea & Febiger.

Montgomery, W. W., & Lavelle, W. G. (1974). A technique for improving esophageal and tracheopharyngeal speech. *Annals of Otology, Rhinology and Laryngology, 83,* 452–461.

Ogura, J. H., & Thawley, S. E. (1979). Complications of alaryngeal surgery. In J. J. Conley (Ed.), *Complications of head and neck surgery* (pp. 246–273). Philadelphia: Saunders.

Ramachandran, K., Arunachalam, P. S., Hurren, A., Marsh, R. L., & Samuel, P. R. (2003). Botulinum toxin injection for failed tracheo-oesophageal voice in laryngectomees: The Sunderland experience. *Journal of Laryngology & Otology 117,* 544–548.

Salmon, S. J. (1986). Methods of air intake for esophageal speech and their associated problems. In R. L. Keith & F. L. Darley (Eds.), *Laryngectomee rehabilitation* (pp. 55–69). Austin, TX: PRO-ED.

Salmon, S. J. (1988). Factors predictive of success or failure in acquisition of esophageal speech. *Head and Neck Surgery, 10*(Suppl. 11), 105–109.

Schuller, D. E., Jarrow, J. E., Kelly, D. R., & Miglets, A. W. (1983). Prognostic factors affecting the success of duckbill vocal restoration. *Otolaryngology—Head and Neck Surgery, 91,* 396–398.

Shames, G. H., Font, J., & Matthews, J. (1963). Factors related to speech proficiency of the laryngectomized. *Journal of Speech and Hearing Disorders, 28,* 273–287.

Shapiro, M. J., & Ramanathan, V. R. (1982). Trachea stoma vent voice prosthesis. *Laryngoscope, 92,* 1126–1129.

Silver, F. M., Gluckman, J. L., & Donegan, J. O. (1985). Operative complications of tracheoesophageal puncture. *Laryngoscope, 95,* 1360–1362.

Simpson, I. C., Smith, J. C., & Gordon, M. T. (1972). Laryngectomy: The influence of muscle reconstruction on the mechanism of oesophageal voice production. *Journal of Laryngology and Otology, 86,* 961—990.

Singer, M. I., & Blom, E. D. (1981). Selective myotomy for voice restoration after total laryngectomy. *Archives of Otolaryngology, 107,* 670–673.

Singer, M. I., Blom, E. D., & Hamaker, R. C. (1981). Further experience with voice restoration after total laryngectomy. *Annals of Otology, Rhinology and Laryngology, 90,* 498–502.

Singer, M. I., Blom, E. D., & Hamaker, R. C. (1986). Pharyngeal plexus neurectomy for alaryngeal speech rehabilitation. *Laryngoscope, 96,* 50–53.

Stafford, F. W. (2003). Current indications and complications of tracheoesophageal puncture for voice restoration after laryngectomy. *Current Opinion in Otolaryngology—Head and Neck Surgery, 11,* 89–95.

Tatchell, R. H., Lerman, J. W., & Watt, J. (1985). Olfactory ability as a function of nasal air flow volume in laryngectomees. *American Journal of Otolaryngology, 6,* 426–432.

Terrell, J. E., Lewin, J. S., & Esclamado, R. (1995). Botulinum toxin injection for post-laryngectomy TE speech failure. *Journal of the American Academy of Otolaryngology—Head and Neck Surgery, 113,* 788–791.

Trudeau, M. D., Schuller, D. E., & Hall, D. A. (1989). The effects of radiation on tracheoesophageal puncture. *Archives of Otolaryngology—Head and Neck Surgery, 115,* 1116–1117.

van Dam, F. S. A. M., Hilgers, F. J. M., Emsbroek, G., Touw, F. I., van As, C. J., & de Jong, N. (1999). Deterioration of olfaction and gustation as a consequence of total laryngectomy. *Laryngoscope, 109,* 1150–1155.

van Lith-Bijl, J. T., Mahieu, H. F., Patel, P., & Zijlstra, R. J. (1992). Clinical experience with the low-resistance Groningen button. *European Archives of Oto-Rhino-Laryngology, 249,* 354–357.

Volin, R. A. (1980). Predicting failure to speak after laryngectomy. *Laryngoscope, 90,* 1–10.

Wang, C. C. (1990). *Radiation therapy for head and neck neoplasms: Indications, techniques, and results.* Chicago: Year Book Medical Publishers.

Ward, E. C., Bishop, B., Frisby, J., & Stevens, M. (2002). Swallowing outcomes following laryngectomy and pharyngolaryngectomy. *Archives of Otolaryngology—Head and Neck Surgery, 128,* 181–186.

Weber, R. S. (1998). Advanced laryngeal cancer: Defining the issues. In K. T. Robbins & T. Murry (Eds.), *Head & neck cancer* (pp. 33–36). San Diego, CA: Singular.

Wenig, B. L., Keller, A. J., Levy, J., Mullooly, V., & Abramson, A. L. (1989). Voice restoration after laryngopharyngoesophagectomy. *Otolaryngology—Head and Neck Surgery, 101,* 11–13.

Wolfe, R. B., Olson, J. E., & Goldenberg, D. D. (1971). Rehabilitation of the laryngectomee: The role of the distal esophageal sphincter. *Laryngoscope, 81,* 1971–1978.

Ziesmann, M., Boyd, B., Manktelow, R. T., & Rosen, I. B. (1989). Speaking jejunum after laryngopharyngectomy and neoglottic and neopharyngeal reconstruction. *American Journal of Surgery, 158,* 321–323.

Chapter 25

Peer Group Support in Laryngectomy Rehabilitation

Leslie E. Glaze

Successful alaryngeal speech rehabilitation relies on many factors, including the individual's potential for and dedication to recovery, the availability of competent professional services, and support from family members, friends, and coworkers. This chapter identifies another prime source of support to laryngectomized individuals, that of a group approach to alaryngeal speech treatment and sociocommunicative rehabilitation. Laryngectomy rehabilitation is primarily an individual journey for each patient. Nonetheless, the collective emotional support from a laryngectomized individual's peer group of other, more advanced alaryngeal speakers may provide an invaluable resource throughout the rehabilitation period. These individuals have obtained relevant experience and wisdom, simply by having "been there." Patients often respond profoundly and positively to these role models as they connect to the credibility, compassion, and personal disclosure offered by peers in a group setting. The group treatment situation also provides an ecologically valid communication interaction that cannot be duplicated by any other health professional or support personnel. Thus, the use of peer group treatment in the form of direct alaryngeal speech therapy groups or social laryngectomy clubs has become a time-honored and valued source of teaching, learning, and communication exchange (Lerman, 1999; Salmon & Mount, 1991).

Patients recovering from laryngectomy surgery seem to experience both social and communicative benefits from peer group interactions (see Chapter 26 in this text). They make new friends, observe role models, and achieve speech goals. Patients can also discuss the adjustments to total laryngectomy with other group members, while observing the leadership skills exhibited by some who have experienced positive rehabilitation outcomes. This chapter will explore some of the clinical advantages of different forms of group therapy for laryngectomized individuals and provide suggestions for involving patients, spouses, and other close family members throughout the rehabilitation process.

EVIDENCE OF BENEFICIAL PEER MODELS AND SUPPORT

The potential benefits of peer interactions on recovery following laryngectomy are difficult to measure empirically because their impact is not easily separated from individual progress in rehabilitation. Furthermore, the effects of group therapy probably vary from individual to individual. Clinical experience, however, has provided many examples of the positive utility of peer support in all kinds of rehabilitation. In the cancer rehabilitation literature, studies conducted in the last decade underscore the clinical effectiveness of supportive group models for patients who are recovering from various forms of cancer. Evans and Connis (1995) conducted a controlled study of depression in patients undergoing radiation treatments for a variety of cancers. Subjects were assigned randomly to three study groups. The first group received adjunctive cognitive-behavioral group therapy, the second received social support group therapy, and the third received no group therapy. Psychological profiles for subjects who participated in either of the group therapies revealed fewer symptoms of depression and anxiety than the control subjects who received no group treatment. Subjects who participated in the social support group therapy were the most resistant to other symptoms of psychiatric distress, including depression, hostility, anxiety, and breakdowns in interpersonal relationships (Doyle 1999a, 1999b; Ramirez et al., 2003; see also Chapter 26 in this text). Therefore, the authors concluded that the strongest positive benefits were displayed following social support group therapy. These subjects even demonstrated positive benefits in psychological assessment probes conducted 6 months following the completion of their radiation treatment. Evans and Connis (1995) demonstrated the clinical value of both cognitive-behavioral and social support group therapies, but suggested that the social support format yielded the most robust effects for these individuals.

Other studies in the breast cancer treatment literature describe the positive impact of various group therapy approaches, including both cognitive-behavioral and social support groups. Gray, Fitch, Davis, and Phillips (1997) conducted interviews with 24 women who were undergoing treatment for breast cancer. These subjects participated in four different group therapy settings where they were able to meet other breast cancer survivors to receive practical information, advocacy tips, and emotional support. Regardless of the type of setting, patients described overwhelmingly positive response and appreciation for the group therapy experience, especially for answering questions and learning about self-advocacy. These findings confirm the long-standing clinical belief that the impact of group support is a strong adjunct to the information given by individual health care providers. Similarly, Coward (1998) documented statistically significant improvements in ratings of functional performance status, mood state, and satisfaction with life in subjects with breast cancer who underwent a group treatment course focusing on emotional and physical well-being. Samarel et al. (1998) chronicled telephone interviews of 70 women who had participated in structured group therapy as an adjunct to treatment for breast cancer. All subjects found the experience beneficial, and the majority credited the group experience with providing benefits of emotional support, improved physiological adaptation, and an improved attitude toward breast cancer overall.

The impact of group support has also been studied in two nontraditional, innovative models designed to accommodate individuals who cannot participate in live, face-to-face meetings. The reports describe the effectiveness of group support using telephone conferencing and computer-based bulletin boards. Colon (1996) reported that a weekly telephone conference call was a viable alternative to face-to-face group meetings for individuals recovering from cancer but who were homebound or otherwise unable to travel to conventional (live) support groups. Weinberg, Schmale, Uken, and Wessel (1996) presented perhaps the most forward-thinking model for group interactions: a computer-mediated support group accessed via home computers for 6 patients recovering from breast cancer. Despite the distance approach to group interactions, patients in both of these studies perceived and reported benefits of mutual support, empathy, advocacy, and mentorship similar to those noted for other traditional face-to-face group situations. All of these findings illustrate the important contribution of group cohesion that evolves when participants feel a shared emotional connection to support each other through the process of cancer rehabilitation by communicating openly and with mutual respect and positive regard for each other. Remarkably, this hallmark feature of successful group therapy emerged even in the nontraditional and asynchronous exchanges allowed by a "virtual" support group, conducted without face-to-face interactions and across a time series of computer bulletin postings.

THE MECHANICS OF PEER GROUP SUPPORT AND THERAPY

Group interactions in communication disorders are a logical and natural extension of the individual treatment process. For some individuals, the subtle hierarchy of the patient-to-professional communication will limit the patient's willingness to express all of his or her feelings and concerns. The group setting provides an environment where individuals and their families can share common experiences in a peer relationship that is supported but not directed by professionals. Newer speech–language pathologists may be surprised to hear the number of questions and topics of discussion that unfold between newer and more senior group members. These topics range from conventional communication dilemmas to more intimate details of personal self-care; changes in relationships with family members, friends, and coworkers; feelings about the cancer diagnosis and its potential recurrence; and their self-confidence and self-esteem as alaryngeal speakers (see Chapters 26 and 28 in this text).

As a new clinician, I recall observing this virtual explosion of questions, discussion, and disclosure at my patient's first visit to an alaryngeal speech group. At the time, I wondered whether this intense interest in peer exploration reflected a failing on my part. Had I not offered enough information to the patient in individual sessions? Had I neglected to establish comfortable rapport to allow the patient to ask any of these questions? Had I not already described with the patient the same questions I heard repeated to other group members? With time and experience, I learned that the success of the group interaction is not always a reflection of the speech–language pathologist's (or other health care professional's) deficiencies as an information source. Rather, this positive group exchange is a healthy response of individuals who are willing to share with and care for each other, based on a common experience as a laryngectomized individual. Indeed, Salmon and Mount (1991) may have stated it best: "We are convinced that patients and spouses are the best teachers" (p. 94).

The group setting differs from the patient–professional relationship in other ways. Group discussion supplies a functional alternative to the clinician–client dyad, and redirects conversation from the limits of a two-person exchange to a more natural and spontaneous conversation with more than one communication partner. Because of the heterogeneous backgrounds of various group participants, every member of the group has the potential to be both a teacher–mentor and a learner. To foster this evolution of skills and mentorship, the speech–language pathologist must be prepared to relinquish some control and commit to a role as discussion facilitator, without overmanaging the group flow of topics or information. In healthy and productive group interactions, all members and all contributions are valued. Thus, leadership shifts subtly but importantly from the clinician to the members of the group, who share control of the group's goals, plans, functions, and activities.

This transfer of "control" from the professional to the patient and his or her peers is in itself especially empowering for newly laryngectomized individuals who, in the early stages of cancer diagnosis, surgery, and inpatient recovery, typically had very little control over any aspect of their care. In the immediate post-operative outpatient period, they have regained some autonomy over self-care routines, but often still rely on the speech–language pathologist and close family members to assist with and interpret their communications. In the group setting, new patients see for themselves the functional outcomes of well-rehabilitated laryngectomized speakers who have recovered and once again established independent and communicatively competent lifestyles (Eadie & Doyle, 2004). Because of this shared history, there emerges a mutual trust and a camaraderie among laryngeal cancer survivors, marked by elements of credibility, compassion, and benevolence. The most important role of clinicians in the group setting is to ensure that

- all participants and contributions are valued
- honest, yet mutually respectful comments and opinions prevail
- individuals are able to cross-mentor and learn from each other in an environment of free-flowing conversation

When this balance of shared disclosure and learning is achieved, a supportive group environment becomes an essentially self-sustaining source of personal discovery and learning for alaryngeal speakers and other participants.

Luterman (1996) expanded on the emotional vitality and interpersonal connection that is central to well-functioning group therapy. He cited work by Yalom (1975), who described many potential curative benefits of group therapy in psychiatric treatment. Three of these benefits are intrinsic to the success of alaryngeal speech groups and laryngectomy clubs. The first benefit is *universality*, a concept that helps patients to understand that they are not alone in the process of recovery and rehabilitation from head and neck cancer. Nearly every patient feels alone at some point in the process from diagnosis to rehabilitation. Group treatment settings help patients to recognize that many others have gone before and will follow their experience of receiving the diagnosis of cancer and living life with a total laryngectomy.

The second benefit is *altruism,* which arises when patients are able to empathize with and support each other emotionally. Altruism broadens the patient's egocentric view of the disorder ("Why me?") and allows him or her to take the perspective of another individual. In alaryngeal speech groups, I have observed the rapid blossom of friendships and the appropriate gestures of mutual respect based on the common knowledge of a shared history with head and neck cancer. These connections cross differences in ethnicity, socioeconomic status, home culture, and other societal divisions.

The third curative factor that applies to alaryngeal group members is their ability to develop into reliable *teachers and mentors.* The predominance of information shared between patients is a candid disclosure of personal experiences and anecdotes. In a tradition similar to oral history, this exchange between participants becomes the essential component that establishes the core connection leading to group cohesiveness, bolstering the esteem of participants individually and collectively. A group environment of friendship and cooperative learning emerges and evolves because individuals have the opportunity to gain the confidence and the willingness to mentor others.

ROLE OF THE FACILITATOR IN GROUP SPEECH THERAPY

Successful group therapy requires the skills of a sensitive and diplomatic facilitator who is charged with several responsibilities. First, the group facilitator must identify an appropriate referral base of alaryngeal speakers to participate in group therapy and, if possible, include participants with a range of communicative experience. To encourage regular attendance, the meetings should be held at a consistent place and at a regular time. Attendance at meetings should be an individual choice, and not every patient who is referred may wish to participate; however, the consistent presence of the group may foster a longer term commitment to periodic attendance, especially for older members who may return only occasionally. In this regard, it is often beneficial for newer patients and family members to attend groups soon after their release from the hospital, well before alaryngeal speech skills are mastered. Encouraging such early participation may facilitate continued patient involvement, with added benefit to long-term outcomes. This early experience in a group setting allows patients to listen to and observe the communication methods and skills of other alaryngeal speakers. Advanced speakers provide outstanding speech role models for new patients; similarly, less successful speakers may motivate and compel the new patient to develop his or her own standards of acceptable speech criteria. Occasionally, these models help new patients to elect their own preferred method of alaryngeal speech.

The second role of the facilitator is to devise a series of flexible lesson plans for group therapy sessions. These plans provide the group with some direction for making progress in speech skills, while varying topics to maintain interest. Session plans must allow the facilitator to spontaneously modify approaches based on individual and collective needs and interests. In some settings, it may be possible to pair newer patients with advanced speakers for more focused peer interaction and mentorship. Thus, the skilled group leader will plan lessons that address a sufficiently broad range of speech practice targets from which both novices and advanced speakers can benefit. In most groups, attendance is variable and unpredictable, both in the number of participants and in the skill levels available. Thus, the group leader must devise session plans that remain sufficiently flexible to modify tasks and targets as needed to accommodate the interests and communication skills of the members in attendance.

The third role of the group facilitator is to model and promote a group attitude and philosophy that is consistently inclusive and respectful of all levels of ability and all individual personalities. Successful group interactions are sustained when members receive satisfaction from their participation in group interactions and from their emotional connection to the other members. Indeed, group interactions are most productive and successful when every member feels that he or she has a functional role in the group, whether it be as mentor to new visitors, leader for speech activities, helper in the kitchen, or greeter at the door. Thus, the professional is responsible for monitoring and guiding the welcoming and supportive nature of group interactions, including universal positive regard, mutual respect, and positive and constructive feedback for all participants at all times.

In fostering and mentoring this attitude of group collegiality, the professional must be prepared to relinquish some control of the group direction over time. If the clinician can withdraw from actively managing the group dynamics, he or she can impart to the participants a confirmed belief in the power of the group's self-sufficiency and competence as a support team. The clinician, however, still has the responsibility to monitor the progress and direction of group themes and conversation, assess group treatment outcomes, and troubleshoot any stalling points in the lessons. By doing so, essential communication goals are met, while the growing self-sufficiency of the group as a whole and its individual members is facilitated and maintained.

SPEECH THERAPY GROUPS

Two complementary but different approaches to group therapy are common in alaryngeal speech rehabilitation: the speech treatment group and the social laryngectomy club. The *speech treatment group* exists expressly for laryngectomized patients to work together on alaryngeal speech and communication targets, under the direction of a speech–language pathologist. These group lessons are organized to provide general alaryngeal voice and speech therapy to all members. Often, group participants will exhibit heterogeneous methods of alaryngeal speech and skill levels. This requires the clinician to create speech lessons that will benefit a broad range of alaryngeal speech competencies and methods (see Chapter 3 in this text). For example, a target goal might address speech intelligibility using increased articulatory loudness and precision, appropriate for various skill levels and any of the alaryngeal speech methods. Typical sessions will include several components:

- Introductions (as needed) and a warm-up icebreaker
- Specific focus or goal for the session
- Planned speech activity that targets the goal in structured or natural contexts
- Closing evaluative period to reflect on what has been learned
- Summary of important take-home practice routines

The overall purpose for using an alaryngeal speech group therapy approach is to improve the communication effectiveness of all the group participants, regardless of their skill level or time postsurgery (see Chapters 16 and 27 in this text). Ideally, the format will include group speech practice regimens that give patients the opportunity to communicate in natural conversation and with different communication partners. Because of the potential for different skill levels, however, all patients must be encouraged to demonstrate patience and tolerance for each other's alaryngeal speech ability and performance. The notions of continuing practice, refining skills, and lifelong learning apply to all. When a high level of trust and support is achieved in the group, the group becomes an emotionally safe place for new patients to receive critical feedback on speech production, express their frustrations, discuss the limits of alaryngeal speech, and troubleshoot periodic plateaus in speech progress with more advanced speakers. Thus, even though speech skills remain central to the purpose for alaryngeal speech group therapy, broader socialization skills and communicative benefits arise through the experience.

In contrast, the *social laryngectomy club* serves as another approach to group therapy. The express purpose of the social laryngectomy group is to develop friendships and offer social support to patients and family members who live with total laryngectomy. The names of these clubs (e.g., Lost Chord Club, New Voice Club) reflect the identity of the common experience of its members. These groups meet periodically and can involve a broader circle of participants in the life of the laryngectomized individual, including spouses, significant others, and extended family members. Social clubs try to identify and meet the needs of patients, spouses, significant others, and extended family members. It is common to see children, in-laws, grandchildren, friends, and other close support persons attending and enjoying the club meetings or the social gatherings.

Social clubs are organized and directed by patients, with help from club sponsors, such as the American or Canadian Cancer Society, the International Association of Laryngectomees (IAL), local hospital auxiliaries, and others. These clubs typically elect officers, collect modest dues, take minutes, and produce a mailing list or newsletter. Laryngectomy club officers and regularly attending members can establish their niche in the group dynamic by serving as positive role models for new members. Spouses can also become involved by volunteering to arrange for guest speakers, planning an activity or special outing, or arranging for refreshments.

A socially oriented laryngectomy club reinforces the need for social rehabilitative support to laryngectomized individuals and their families, by introducing and greeting new members, maintaining contact with current members, supporting relationships with spouses, and exploring challenges beyond the goals of alaryngeal speech acquisition. Although these clubs may dedicate a portion of the meeting time to a formal group speech therapy lesson, the emphasis is lessened in comparison to a stand-alone speech treatment group. The speech–language pathologist often serves as a consultant to the group, charged with the responsibility for planning and directing the speech treatment portion of the meeting; however, speech therapy is only one among a number of different agenda items that form the "business" of a social laryngectomy club. At least three different purposes and goals are common to social laryngectomy clubs:

1. Interpersonal support and friendship for patients and family members
2. Organized service mission or advocacy projects
3. Planning special social events

As an added dimension, many clubs have members who are committed to staying in contact with elderly members through phone calls, visits, and cards. Members keep each other apprised of each other's health and medical status, especially for patients who have become ill or experienced a recurrence of cancer (Blanchard, Albrecht, Rucksdeschel, Grant, & Hammick, 1995; see also Chapter 26 in this text).

Laryngectomy clubs often adopt and work toward service missions of their sponsoring organizations, such as the IAL and the American or Canadian Cancer Societies, or other cancer or antitobacco support groups. For example, a guest speaker may be invited to present information about research or specially funded projects in these organizations. Some group members and spouses elect to attend sponsored training to qualify as a laryngectomized hospital visitor for new inpatients. Other members demonstrate tireless advocacy efforts by conducting organized lobbying to support relevant causes such as antitobacco legislation or health care access for other individuals. Still other experienced members have provided inservice visits to local emergency and paramedic personnel, to inform them of the specialized needs of a "neck breather." All of these examples illustrate the strong positive effects of increased awareness, group cohesiveness, and confidence stimulated by group interactions.

The Lost Chord Club of St. Paul, Minnesota, like many other clubs, promotes awareness of alaryngeal speech and the threat of laryngeal cancer. Consequently, this club has been featured in local newspapers, on television broadcasts, and in community newsletters. Other members join organized local and statewide speaker bureaus to present antismoking information to schools and community groups. Every few years, all of the Minnesota State clubs work together to plan and execute a professional workshop to educate patients, family members, allied professionals, and students about laryngectomy rehabilitation.

Finally, no social club would be complete without the special gatherings planned to celebrate seasonal holidays, host a summertime picnic, reconnect at conventions, share a potluck dinner, and join a sing-along. Some clubs organize community appreciation receptions, at which speech–language pathologists, head and neck surgeons, oncology nurses, and other professionals are recognized for their contributions to laryngectomy rehabilitation. These events vary from group to group, but all combine to strengthen the cohesiveness and the heritage of social laryngectomy clubs. Volunteering to help with these special social events offers the new patient or spouse a chance to give to others and experience a renewed sense of autonomy, self-sufficiency, and perhaps even a potential for leadership within the alaryngeal speech community or club. Groups that are organized and run by rehabilitated laryngectomized individuals provide enormously positive role models for the new patient and members of his or her family, who can observe directly how others have survived and continued to participate in life.

GROUP THERAPY TOPICS AND LESSONS

Alaryngeal Speech Activities

The clinician who plans group speech therapy must acknowledge from the outset that successful group therapy requires significant planning, as well as the flexibility and willingness to spontaneously alter treatment targets or lessons based on group needs and the individual competencies of participants in a given session. To that end, session activities should benefit alaryngeal speakers at all levels, from the novice to the experienced communicator. For example, activities should be sufficiently challenging but noncompetitive, thus allowing each individual to receive praise and suggestions from his or her peers.

Because alaryngeal speech intelligibility is at the core of most target goals, group therapy allows a useful opportunity to break the speech signal into various relevant segments and topics, each of which could serve as a viable lesson. For example, to maximize the potential for relevant speech practice in the context of natural conversation, it is possible to embed targets in real-world stimulus materials, such as readings, question-and-answer formats, newspaper clippings, jokes and anecdotes, headlines and advertising slogans, famous quotations and quotables, and even song lyrics. Practice items can also be adapted into role plays using supportive props, such as telephone books, mail-order catalogs, restaurant menus, and direct-mail advertisement circulars. These practice items seem to stimulate greater interest and expanded conversation than do contrived practice sentences. Using these materials, various sessions can focus on traditional speech therapy targets, including the following:

- Precise and exaggerated articulation, including increased loudness and length of sound production
- Natural and pleasant intonation, using contrastive stress and rising and falling suprasegmental patterns
- Increased and decreased speech rate and speech loudness, to alter emotional content or meet other contextual needs
- Achieving optimal sound naturalness, by monitoring phrasing, duration, and timing

Metacommunication Skills

Another useful focus for alaryngeal speech therapy groups is to address larger communication issues in alaryngeal speech (see Chapters 3, 5, and 24 in this text), through practice and discussion. Special challenges unique to alaryngeal speech can be described (e.g., speaking in background noise); then group participants are asked to troubleshoot appropriate and creative compensations for the communication challenge. These speech dilemmas and accommodations can be explored via role playing, barrier games, and partner dyads. The entire group then returns to discuss and propose solutions or alternatives to the problems observed. Many times, experienced alaryngeal speakers will be able to share specific anecdotes from their own experiences to highlight these challenges and how they were resolved, if at all. Some possible examples include speaking

- with and without visual (lip) cues
- in background noise
- on the telephone
- when a whisper is desired
- with increased time pressure demands
- in the workplace or at social gatherings
- from distances or outside
- with unfamiliar, impatient, or reluctant listeners
- using an augmentative voice amplifier

Special Abilities and Special Problems

The speech–language pathologist, in planning alaryngeal group therapy lessons, should consider the many physiological adaptations that alaryngeal speakers are required to make to regain abilities to smell, spit, blow, cough, sneeze, drink from a fountain, suck on a straw, gargle, whistle, and blow one's nose. Often, laryngectomized individuals have been told that these abilities will be lost forever after the surgery. On the contrary, most experienced alaryngeal speakers can demonstrate remarkable compensations and help newer patients learn to develop these special adaptations. Sometimes special equipment or devices are useful to introduce workable compensations to allow laryngectomized individuals to perform these skills. A fun and revealing session can be planned with rotating "stations" where individuals try their skills at these so-called impossible tasks, such as using a straw, bean spitting, whistling, blowing bubbles, and using the smelling tube (nipple coupled to a flexible tube), as reported by Bosone (1984). Using the smelling tube, patients try to detect various scents (e.g., coffee, peppermint, citrus, cinnamon) while blindfolded. Another session is planned to view and learn about the LARKEL laryngectomy snorkel device (Andreas Fahl Medizintechnik-Vertrieb, Koln, Germany), which allows individuals who have been larygectomized to participate in swimming activities. These individuals must receive specialized training to fully understand the design and application of the device. Finally, other sessions review challenges in returning to preferred hobbies and recreational activities after total laryngectomy. These topics include safety tips while on or near the water, as well as effective ways to continue active sports, gardening, cooking, woodworking, and other skilled avocations that may be altered by the presence of a stoma or by the need to use alaryngeal speech. Again, the source of an alaryngeal group's benefits is founded in the members' own direct experience, creativity, empathy, and friendship toward each other.

Counseling

Regardless of the lesson plan, a consistent and essential element that infuses all successful group therapy is the ability for group members to share, disclose, and counsel each other. Consider several classic and familiar images of a support group scene: a new patient and spouse being introduced to the club, seasoned members mentoring newly laryngectomized individuals, and speech–language pathology students learning from candid discussions with well-rehabilitated laryngectomized speakers. Groups that are organized and run by individuals who have undergone laryngectomy provide enormously positive role models for the new patient and his or her family and are hallmarks of effective group interactions. These positive exchanges establish the basis for the peer support and friendship that pass from one individual to another, across months, years, and decades. Many alaryngeal speech groups have been in existence nearly 50 years, and old-timers can recall the welcome and guidance that they received, even as they advance to senior positions as "elder statesmen" within the group. This willingness to support each other lies at the very core of the psychosocial rehabilitation achieved in group therapy. I am reminded of the Laryngectomy Oath, taken at the start of every meeting of a Lost Chord Club I attended regularly in Minneapolis:"I will use every available means to perfect my speech and affect my rehabilitation, and I pledge all my efforts to assist fellow [laryngectomees] in achieving these goals." Additionally, the charter mission for this club states that its purpose is to do "all things possible to bring about the total rehabilitation of all laryngectomees who sincerely desire it." This commitment to each other and to the advancement of quality of life (Doyle, 1994; see also Chapter 28 in this text) in laryngectomized individuals and their family members represents the essential power of group therapy: to promote the best possible outcomes by learning, teaching, and passing on a spirit of friendship, wellness, and group support.

SUMMARY

Group therapy is a productive, supportive, and enjoyable form of adjunctive treatment for laryngectomized individuals. Group therapy formats may serve several purposes including speech rehabilitation for laryngectomized individuals, social interaction for patients and families, or both. Regardless, the group therapy experience provides many distinct advantages that cannot be achieved exclusively through patient–professional relationships. These opportunities range from forming new friendships with other laryngectomized individuals, learning from different alaryngeal speaker models, providing a supportive network of spouses and extended family members, and creating a community of mutually respectful, credible, and compassionate group support. Within the group setting, laryngectomized individuals develop leadership skills as peer mentors and often regain a sense of communicative self-confidence that may not be readily recaptured in external environments (Eadie, 2003). The role of the speech–language pathologist in group therapy models is strictly as a facilitator, with sufficient flexibility to

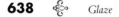

foster group direction and goals that evolve according to the needs of individual members. By promoting group dynamics that emphasize a philosophy of support, mutual respect, and cohesiveness, the speech–language pathologist contributes greatly to the success of the group therapy approach.

REFERENCES

Blanchard, C. G., Albrecht, T., Rucksdeschel, J., Grant, D., & Hammick, R. (1995). The role of social support in adaptation to cancer and to survival. *Journal of Psychosocial Oncology, 13,* 75–95.

Bosone, Z. (1984). The nipple tube: A simple device for olfaction and nose blowing after laryngectomy. *Journal of Speech and Hearing Disorders, 49,* 106–107.

Colon, Y. (1996). Telephone support groups: A nontraditional approach to reaching underserved cancer patients. *Cancer Practice, 4*(3), 156–159.

Coward, D. D. (1998). Facilitation of self-transcendence in a breast cancer support group. *Oncology Nursing Forum, 25*(1), 75–84.

Doyle, P. C. (1994). *Foundations of voice and speech rehabilitation following laryngeal cancer.* San Diego, CA: Singular.

Doyle, P. C. (1999a). Laryngectomy rehabilitation: Past, present, and future. *Journal of Speech–Language Pathology and Audiology, 23,* 50.

Doyle, P. C. (1999b). Postlaryngectomy speech rehabilitation: Contemporary considerations in clinical care. *Journal of Speech–Language Pathology and Audiology, 23,* 109–116.

Eadie, T. L. (2003). The ICF: A proposed framework for comprehensive rehabilitation of individuals who use alaryngeal speech. *American Journal of Speech–Language Pathology, 12,* 189–197.

Eadie, T. L., & Doyle, P. C. (2004). Auditory–perceptual scaling and quality of life in tracheoesophageal speakers. *Laryngoscope, 114,* 753–759.

Evans, R. L., & Connis, R. T. (1995). Comparison of brief group therapies for depressed cancer patients receiving radiation treatment. *Public Health Reports, 110,* 306–311.

Gray, R., Fitch, M., Davis, C., & Phillips, C. (1997). A qualitative study of breast cancer self-help groups. *Psychooncology, 6,* 279–289.

Lerman, J. W. (1999). Group therapy for laryngectomees. In S. Salmon (Ed.), *Alaryngeal speech rehabilitation: For clinicians by clinicians* (2nd ed., pp. 269–284). Austin, TX: PRO-ED.

Luterman, D. M. (1996). *The group process in counseling persons with communication disorders and their families* (3rd ed.). Austin, TX: PRO-ED.

Ramirez, M. J., Ferriol, E. E., Domenech, F. G., Llatas, M. C., Suarez-Varela, M. M., & Martinez, R. L. (2003). Psychosocial adjustment in patients surgically treated for laryngeal cancer. *Otolaryngology—Head and Neck Surgery, 129,* 92–97.

Salmon, S. J., & Mount, K. H. (1991). Group therapy. In S. J. Salmon & K. H. Mount (Eds.), *Alaryngeal speech rehabilitation: For clinicians by clinicians* (pp. 93–105). Austin, TX: PRO-ED.

Samarel, N., Fawcett, J., Krippendorf, K., Piacentino, J. C., Eliasof, B., Hughes, P., Kowitski, C., & Ziegler, E. (1998). Women's perceptions of group support and adaptation to breast cancer. *Journal of Advanced Nursing, 28,* 1259–1268.

Weinberg, N., Schmale, J., Uken, J., & Wessel, K. (1996). Online help: Cancer patients participate in a computer-mediated support group. *Health and Social Work, 21,* 24–29.

Yalom, I. (1975). *The theory and practice of group psychotherapy.* New York: Basic Books.

Chapter 26

Group Treatment Models for Head and Neck Cancer

Candace Myers

Social support has long been recognized as a significant contributor to the recovery and adjustment of individuals living with cancer. Because those dealing with head and neck cancer also experience the devastating loss of their traditional means and ease of communication and social interaction with others, social support is especially beneficial. Social support may include spouses and partners, other family members, health care professionals, special support groups, and one-to-one peer visits (Blanchard, Albrecht, Rucksdeschel, Grant, & Hemmick, 1995; Mathieson, Logan-Smith, Phillips, MacPhee, & Attia, 1996). This chapter reviews the literature pertaining to social and peer support for those with cancer in general, and head and neck cancer patients specifically; presents a rationale for and the benefits associated with support programs; discusses similarities and differences between group treatment approaches; and offers practical suggestions for organizing and conducting support programs.

REVIEW OF THE LITERATURE

At all stages between diagnosis and recovery, people diagnosed with and treated for head and neck cancer suffer a multitude of psychosocial concerns, including depression, anxiety, anger, psychological distress, and loss of self-esteem (Baile, Gibertini, Scott, & Endicott, 1992; Breitbart & Holland, 1988; Gibson & McCombe, 1999; McQuellon & Hurt, 1997; Morton, Davies, Baker, Baker, & Stell, 1984; Olson & Shedd, 1978; Pruyn et al., 1986; Rapoport, Kreitle, Chaitchik, Algor, & Weissler, 1993; Stam, Koopmans, & Mathieson, 1991; Strauss, 1989; Watt-Watson & Graydon, 1995). Individuals who have undergone treatment for head and neck cancer also experience social isolation, stigmatization, and relationship difficulties (de Boer et al., 1995; Harwood & Rawlinson, 1983; Mathieson, Stam, & Scott, 1991; McDonough et al., 1996). These difficulties are experienced not only by newly diagnosed patients, but also by those who have completed treatment and may be considered "cured." Recent studies on cancer survivors demonstrate that cancer patients in general suffer high levels of disease- and treatment-related symptoms, quality-of-life (QOL) impairment, and psychosocial concerns for many years after treatment (Ferrell, Hassey Dow, Leigh, Ly, & Gulasekaram, 1995; Gallo, Sarno, Baroncelli, Bruschini, & Boddi, 2003; Loescher, Clark, Atwood, Leigh, & Lamb, 1990). These areas of concern appear to be of greater significance for head and neck cancer patients in particular (Bjordal, Kassa, & Mastekaasa, 1994; de Boer et al., 1995; Rapoport et al., 1993). Loescher et al. (1990) noted that cancer survivors have ongoing needs for information (e.g., why the cancer occurred; how to monitor changes in their health, such as new symptoms or signs of recurrence), support from peers and health care professionals, access to rehabilitation strategies and services, reassurance, and control of their ongoing health care (e.g., choice of health care provider, ways to minimize the effects of cancer-related physical and emotional stresses). There is clearly an identified and ongoing need for the provision of information and support throughout the course of treatment and rehabilitation, and continuing long after formal follow-up has ended (Doyle, 1999). When such information and support is provided, patients may cope better throughout the course of their illness, and beyond.

Researchers have found that social support can have many benefits for cancer patients in general. In a review of the effectiveness of cancer support programs, Fobair (1997a) discussed five types of support groups: (a) open-ended support, (b) educational–cognitive, (c) self-help, (d) mutual aid, and (e) supportive–expressive. Two of the most widely used types of group programs in health care settings are educational–cognitive and supportive–expressive. Educational–cognitive groups, which focus on learning about and coping with the illness, were thought to increase one's sense of meaning of life, and ultimately enhance quality of life. Supportive–expressive groups are structured to build social support and help members express their emotions and feelings of vulnerability, thus helping them come to terms with myriad treatment-related concerns and the impact of illness on their family. This social support process takes place in an atmosphere of empathy and unconditional, positive regard through the facilitation of a professional group leader. Programs based on education and support, mutual aid (i.e., peer support), cohesiveness, and acceptance were found to reduce members' uncertainty, anxiety, and levels of distress. Additional benefits included increased psychosocial adjustment, improved coping and communication skills, improved mood, and reduction of confusion and fatigue. Participants in such groups demonstrated increased knowledge about disease and treatment, greater use of active coping skills, greater use of health-enhancing behaviors, less tension and more vigor, healthier immune systems, fewer recurrences of disease, and lower rates of death (see Fobair, 1997a). Fobair concluded that group interventions demonstrated substantial patient benefit across the board, whether the group is educational–cognitive, self-help, or supportive–expressive, and that although all groups demonstrate positive impact on quality of life, supportive–expressive interventions appear to be the most effective (Fobair, 1997a).

The absence of social support in those treated for cancer can lead to a deterioration in psychosocial status. Bottomley, Hunton, Roberts, Jones, and Bradley (1996) compared group cognitive-behavior therapy for psychologically distressed cancer patients with a social support group and a standard-care nonintervention group. Their results suggested that both types of intervention groups (i.e., cognitive-behavior and social support) may help to "buffer" the patient against psychological distress. Furthermore, those who do not receive such services "may be prone to a deterioration in psychological well-being" (Bottomley et al., 1996, p. 80). Interestingly, the social support group evaluated in this study had no specific psychotherapeutic intervention strategies other than to facilitate group discussion. The role of the therapist was "to intervene at times when group discussions became fragmented or when the group members required assistance or guidance" (p. 72). The results indicate that even minimal peer support and guided discussion by a health care professional can have significant benefits for cancer patients.

The impact of psychosocial support on survival has also been addressed in the literature. In a review of published articles that focused on psychosocial interventions and survival, Cwikel, Behar, and Zabora (1997) noted that the strongest predictors of survival are biological (i.e., tumor status) and that the effects of psychosocial factors are inconsistent in early-stage disease, and insignificant in cases of metastatic cancer. Involvement in social networks, however, is positively correlated with survival, and psychosocial interventions are most effective at early stages of disease and in younger patients (under 55 years). Furthermore, the benefits of social support on reducing psychological distress, improving coping, and enhancing QOL are well documented. The authors also stressed the importance of reaching out to "at-risk" groups, including those who are poor, are unmarried, have few social supports, live in disadvantaged neighborhoods, are non–English-speaking, and are nonwhite. These groups traditionally have difficulty accessing adequate health care services, let alone psychosocial support.

Many studies have demonstrated the benefits of group support, peer support, and early socialization for head and neck cancer patients (de Boer et al., 1995; see also Chapter 25 in this text). The impact on the psychosocial dimension is particularly important, given the high rate of psychosocial distress among these patients. Baker (1992) surveyed 52 patients with head and neck cancer and found that social interaction, communication, emotional behavior, and alertness were positively correlated with perceived social support. Hammerlid, Persson, Sullivan, and Westin (1999) compared two types of psychosocial intervention for head and neck cancer patients, a long-term group psychological therapy program for newly diagnosed patients, and a short-term psychoeducational program 1 year after treatment. QOL measures indicated benefits in the areas of social and emotional functioning and global QOL, as well as reduction in psychiatric morbidity (Hammerlid et al., 1999). Stam et al. (1991) and Mathieson et al. (1996) found that satisfaction with social support from family, friends, and acquaintances had a significant effect on both psychological distress and QOL for individuals who had undergone laryngectomy. In addition, adjustment postlaryngectomy is positively influenced by social support. This may be particularly true among patients with newly (i.e., within the first 6-month period) diagnosed cancer (Rustoen, Moum, Wiklund, & Hanestad, 1999). Zabora (1999) suggested that educational programs may be beneficial for patients with lower levels of psychological distress, whereas support groups might be best suited for those with moderate levels of distress and fewer existing social supports. Among head and neck cancer patients, psychological distress levels are frequently at least moderate, suggesting that the social support program might be the preferred model of intervention with this population.

In addition to reducing distress, social support may also provide an atmosphere in which hope can develop among patients with head and neck cancers. The role of hope in improving effectiveness of treatment interventions and enhancing well-being is well supported (McGee, 1984; Menninger, 1959). Bunston, Mings, Mackie, and Jones (1995) proposed an empirical model of the determinants of hope, based on a cross-sectional survey of 194 outpatients (96 with ocular melanoma and 98 with head and neck cancer). These authors expressed particular concern about the impact of continued alcohol consumption among many of these patients, which can affect the severity of illness, emotional and physical functioning, and coping ability (Bunston et al., 1995). These authors unexpectedly found that social support itself had no influence, either direct or indirect, on hope; however, they emphasized the importance of locus of control, or personal sense of control over one's life, as either a direct determinant of hope or as a factor that buffers distress and promotes coping. Furthermore, the authors' findings "emphasize the importance of helping patients lessen the twin burdens of physical and emotional distress, thus creating an environment in which hopefulness can flower" (Bunston et al., 1995, p. 99). Thus, while not directly impacting hope, social support may indirectly promote its development, through both the provision of information, which may foster increased locus of control, and the reduction of emotional distress through psychosocial support in peer group programs.

The impact of support on psychosocial adjustment and speech recovery has been widely reported in the literature as well. Breitbart and Holland (1988) noted that support from other well-rehabilitated individuals who had undergone laryngectomy can assist patients and families with practical problems of adaptation. Harris, Vogtsberger, and Mattox (1985) noted that attendance at weekly support group meetings for those who have been laryngectomized resulted in improved patient morale, patient compliance, support between patients, and fewer patients discharged against medical advice. Martin (1963) demonstrated that peer support groups provided strong motivation to rehabilitation and acted as a buffer against the trauma of the loss of speech. Similarly, Pruyn et al. (1986) noted the importance of social support in speech rehabilitation outcomes, social functioning, and reduction of anxiety and depression. Thus, peer support has a wide range of potential benefits for the person who has undergone treatment for head and neck cancer.

Social isolation is not uncommon following treatment for head and neck cancer, and support from well-rehabilitated peers can contribute greatly to the reintegration of these patients into society (Salmon, 1986). Doyle (1994) described the subtle yet significant ways in which a person who is laryngectomized may be socially penalized by the multiple stigma of altered physical appearance, communication differences and limitations (alaryngeal speech), and the diagnosis of cancer. He further described the benefits of peer support as the "potential to offer patients and members of their family excellent access to information" from a patient's perspective (p. 250). Because survivors of head and neck cancer who have regained functional communication know the challenges of learning to speak again, they may be more likely to show patience, acceptance, and tolerance as new patients struggle with speech initiation, fluency, acceptability, and intelligibility. Darvill (1983) noted that "the positive and encouraging atmosphere of a [laryngectomy] club can act as a valuable bridge between therapy and the return to an active social life" and "many helpful and practical hints are handed on and firm friendships made" (p. 213). McQuellon and Hurt (1997) reviewed the psychosocial impact of laryngeal cancer and noted the importance of having support group meetings and ongoing contact with well-rehabilitated laryngectomy patients. McDonough et al. (1996) also noted the importance of social support, particularly at difficult times during the rehabilitation process (e.g., following surgery and during radiotherapy), to reduce levels of social avoidance and alleviate distress.

Support group programs can have particular benefits in terms of postlaryngectomy speech and communication development. Richardson and Bourque (1985) identified variables that were related to methods of communication after laryngectomy. Data were collected from persons who were laryngectomized regarding support received from family, friends, and other persons who were laryngectomized, as well as characteristics of voice therapy experiences, the extent of surgery, and demographic characteristics. Persons who were laryngectomized were divided into three groups based on mode of communication: esophageal speakers, electrolarynx users, and nonverbal communicators. The authors found that the higher the level of association and interaction with other persons who were laryngectomized, the greater the likelihood that the individual would learn esophageal speech. Successful speech rehabilitation was strongly affected by social support.

Blood et al. (1994) studied the needs and perceived social support among persons who were laryngectomized in an attempt to define the role of the speech–language pathologist in facilitating mutual support and self-help groups. These authors found that individuals who were laryngectomized who were "good copers" and had adapted well to their laryngectomy perceived themselves as having better quality social networks and more functional support. Functional support included such characteristics as chances to talk to someone, invitations to go out, and having the perception that someone cares about them. Those individuals who coped well had a more favorable perception of their own voice quality; it is possible that these individuals received encouragement specifically related to speech and voice from peers and health care professionals. Furthermore, good copers reported a higher likelihood of helping others. This suggests that once persons who have been laryngectomized are able to turn their attention to assisting new patients in their adjustment to the laryngectomy, the well-rehabilitated individual may continue to benefit from such involvement with others. Blood et al. suggested that rehabilitation of laryngectomees should include more direct nurturing through professional support, counseling, or attendance in self-help programs.

Based on the literature, there are many and varied benefits of social support in general and support group programs in particular for those who are laryngectomized. For the individual with few social supports, it may be even more important to provide support in a more formal manner (i.e., through structured group programs). Furthermore, psychosocial interventions such as group support may result in broader benefits in addition to improved individual quality of life and patient satisfaction. By alleviating patients' symptoms of distress and anxiety, health outcomes may improve. Also, support group programs may subsequently lead to fewer clinic visits and reduced health care costs (Fobair, 1997b; Zabora, 1999). Such considerations have clear and direct impact in the ever-changing health care environment.

GROUP SUPPORT MODELS: COMMON FEATURES

In the next section of this chapter, I review three types of support group programs for individuals living with head and neck cancer. Two groups are specifically designed for individuals who have undergone laryngectomy; one is hospital based and professionally led, whereas the other is a community-based, self-help group. These are typically referred to as "New Voice" groups, although community groups may have participants who are long-term survivors. The third group is for head and neck cancer patients who have not undergone laryngectomy. All were established through informal identification of patient need and desire for peer support. I have participated in the establishment and ongoing facilitation of all three types of programs since 1990.

Objectives

The goal of support groups is to meet the following objectives:

1. To provide the opportunity to meet with others who have experienced a diagnosis of head and neck cancer. Networks are formed among participants, and social isolation is reduced.

2. To offer education on the topics of cancer diagnosis, treatment, and sequelae (e.g., functional limitations; changes in eating, swallowing, speech/voice/communication, senses of taste and smell, disfigurement and body image, and social and vocational roles; pain; adjustment to change and loss), all of which are QOL issues. With the trend toward shorter hospital stays, patients are often discharged with acute concerns addressed, but little time to learn and absorb knowledge about the disease and the implications of treatment. Patient education can be reinforced in professionally facilitated group support settings. The education–discussion approach conveys respect for the patient's ability to assume responsibility for his or her own care (Fobair, 1997b). Receiving adequate information related to the disease and its consequences also reduces anxiety and lessens psychosocial distress (Lonergan, 1985), reduces uncertainty and increases a sense of personal control (Albrecht & Adelman, 1987), and is a predictor of positive rehabilitation outcomes (de Boer et al., 1995).

3. To provide emotional and practical support to enhance coping and adjustment to the diagnosis of cancer, treatment and its side effects, and fears of recurrence.

4. To provide an accepting, patient, encouraging, and tolerant setting in which a newly laryngectomized individual or person with head and neck cancer can communicate freely with others while struggling to learn to speak again. One can witness great sensitivity and support from other patients to the new member practicing his or her new and altered form of speech. This support fosters confidence in communication by providing opportunities for successful and supported communication with people other than the speech–language pathologist. The person with head and neck cancer can practice enhancing his or her intelligibility, managing communication in noise, or communicating with listeners with hearing impairments. This interaction promotes independence and reduces social isolation.

5. To develop a compendium of resources available to both patients and members of their families.

6. To educate health care professionals and the general public about issues pertinent to the population of laryngectomized individuals and persons with head and neck cancer. Initiatives taken include school presentations on the dangers of smoking; talks to medical, dental, and nursing students; education of dentists through the dental association;

educational sessions for Emergency Medical System (EMS) responders on aspects of artificial resuscitation for neck breathers; and so on.

7. To advocate for better services at various levels—individual, program, health care system, and community agencies.

Format and Content of Group Programs

The group format is open ended, which means that members can attend for as few or as many sessions as they choose; intake into the group is continuous as new patients appear. The continuity of the group, therefore, is not dependent on new members for a commitment to attend a set number of sessions or weeks. This format is appropriate for small, specialized patient populations and allows easy, immediate access for new patients or for patients on an as-needed basis. It also permits the ongoing attendance of "senior" members, who assist with information provision and guidance. Sessions may be informal and flexible depending on the immediate needs of members. Meetings generally begin with a welcome to new members and individual introductions. Assistance from facilitators or group leaders is offered to those who have difficulty with speech intelligibility. Formal presentations from invited speakers (usually health care professionals) may alternate with informal discussion sessions guided by the facilitator(s). A list of suggested presentation topics is presented in Table 26.1. Meetings allow for refreshments and mingling, either before, during, or after the sessions.

Recruitment of Members

Clinic staff (nursing, physicians) are encouraged to refer patients and families to the support groups. Handouts and pamphlets with dates, times, locations, and the program of meetings are made available. Due to disfigurement and communication problems, many patients tend to isolate themselves initially. Therefore, it is often helpful to first establish a connection with a health care professional associated with the group or a trained visitor who understands patients' fears and concerns. This can facilitate entry to the group for new members. Potential members need to be informed that some group members may be experiencing trying times and their stories might be overwhelming. They also need to know that although many patients find the group helpful, others prefer to use other types of resources such as one-to-one counseling or individual peer support.

Attendance

Members may choose to attend regularly early on, then withdraw for various reasons, such as adjustment problems, return to work, illness during treatment, or recurrence. Some individuals attend specifically for formal educational sessions and do not attend the more informal sharing, mutual-support sessions. In

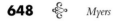

TABLE 26.1

Suggested Topics for Group Sessions

Communication options and practice

Assistive devices

Tracheoesophageal management and new products

Voice and hearing management in noisy conditions or with people who have hearing
   impairments

Radiotherapy

Medical and surgical options and innovations (e.g., laryngeal transplant, reconstructive
   techniques)

Prevention of recurrence

Pain management

Unconventional and alternative treatments

Eating and swallowing

Diet and nutrition

Dental and oral care

Relaxation and stress management

Yoga and mind–body techniques

Coping with loss and change

Bereavement and grieving

Quality-of-life issues

Cancer resources

Visitor guidelines

Improving communication with medical staff

Return-to-work issues

Financial and income tax implications

---

contrast, some individuals attend the support group for long periods of time, even after treatments have ended. This is not surprising, given evidence that head and neck cancer patients experience QOL impairment for many years after the event (Bjordal et al., 1994; Ferrell et al., 1995) and that social isolation and loss of social contacts are not uncommon in this population (Pruyn et al., 1986). Family members also frequently attend; de Boer et al. (1995) stressed the importance of including the spouse or partner and other family members in rehabilitation and support programs. Health care professionals and students or interns are welcome and encouraged to attend.

Individuals with head and neck cancer attend support group programs for a variety of reasons. Bauman, Gervey, and Siegel (1992) found that patients who feel that their social support network is inadequate are most likely to participate in a support group. Bauman and colleagues also found that major motivations to attend a support group were to compare one's physical progress and emotional status with that of others, to learn more about one's illness, and to share concerns with others. Fobair (1989) suggested that although women may be more likely to join a group, men will do so if they feel they need more information, feel misunderstood at home, or experience a loss of control. Sutherland and Goldstein

(1992) found that patients who chose not to participate in group activities felt unable to relate to others, felt that being with others was frightening or depressing, believed they were better off than others, or wanted to put the cancer behind them. Blanchard et al. (1995) suggested that some patients may not attend because of embarrassment; fear of appearing weak or less competent; concerns about imposing on others, becoming overly dependent, or being obligated; or anxiety over potential rejection by other group members.

Common Themes in Groups for Persons With Head and Neck Cancer[1]

Emotional Impact of the Illness

Patients who have been diagnosed and treated for head and neck cancer report feeling overwhelmed and anxious, and generally describe their experience with cancer as the harshest and most difficult life event. In hospital-based programs with new patients, the value and importance of cofacilitation with a psychosocial oncology specialist (e.g., social worker) cannot be overstated. Members frequently exhibit signs of various stages of grief and adjustment; feelings of bereavement and loss, anger, self-recrimination, guilt, and regret; and fears of recurrence and death. Expert guidance on an emotional level is crucial when these issues arise. It is important not only to support the patient who expresses these feelings, but also to provide hope and encouragement to other patients attending the group, lest they themselves become overwhelmed and discouraged. Some members need to repeat their stories over and over again (e.g., the consequences of a late diagnosis or the extent of their surgery or treatment). It appears necessary for these individuals to reiterate their experience until they are personally ready to move on. Confidentiality is stressed, and members must be directly and regularly advised of the importance of protecting the privacy of others.

Coping with Disease and Treatment-Related Changes

As a result of the disease and its treatments, patients with head and neck cancer experience significant physical, psychological, and social changes. These include changes in eating and swallowing; sense of taste and smell; voice, speech, and communication; stoma care and hygiene; management of tracheoesophageal puncture (TEP); loss of energy; concentration problems; anxiety; depression; disfigurement; body image; loss of self-esteem; roles and relationships; sense of isolation; stigma; and cancer-specific concerns, such as fears of recurrence (Eadie, 2003; see also Chapters 1 and 28 in this text). These individuals require accurate information and practical strategies to cope with and adjust to changes. They also seek validation of their unique experience of cancer and the recognition of the impact of many individual changes and losses.

---

[1]This section is adapted from Bisson (1995).

Negotiating the Health Care System

Patients may feel overwhelmed by the many appointments, the costs, and the impact on their time and resources. They may express concerns that early symptoms
were reported to but were not addressed by health care professionals. In my clinical experience, this seems to be a particularly common theme among members
of the nonlaryngectomy support group for persons with head and neck cancer.
Sometimes these individuals express frustration about getting professionals to
take their concerns seriously.

Practical suggestions about managing health care are beneficial. For example,
the facilitators should support and encourage the patient to seek follow-up for
troubling symptoms, to communicate concerns to health care professionals in a
more clear or effective way, or to continue with health habits or lifestyle changes
that appear to have a positive impact on their QOL.

Sense of Vulnerability

Feelings of "chaos"—that is, a lack of control, fear of the unknown, and uncertainty—are frequently expressed by head and neck cancer patients. The nature
and level of fear may vary within the individual during the various stages of recovery: at the time of diagnosis, during treatment, after treatment, with recurrence, around the time of routine follow-up visits, and with significant life events,
such as a return to work. Patients may experience heightened distress when dealing with a cancer recurrence or the death of another member of the group; these
individuals require an opportunity to confront and work through fears in an atmosphere of understanding, acceptance, and support. Again, it is invaluable to
have the guidance of a professional in the area of psychosocial oncology to facilitate such discussions.

Quality of Life

Among people living with head and neck cancers, QOL is assessed from a unique
and personal perspective and changes over time in response to the disease and
its treatments (Schipper, 1990). Among members of a peer support group, there
is frequently wide variation in the experience of handicap versus disability, even
given similar degrees of impairment (World Health Organization, 1993). For
further discussion on these issues, see Eadie (2001) and Chapter 28 in this text.

Clinical Issues[2]

A strength of hospital-based programs is the opportunity for interdisciplinary
collaboration and support, which ensures accurate and appropriate management
of the varied and changing needs of group attendees. Because new group mem-

---

[2]This section is adapted from Bisson (1995).

bers in particular often feel overwhelmed with others' stories and fear they may experience similar outcomes, facilitators need to validate the member's feelings and provide encouragement. It is important to highlight the patient's strengths and coping ability to date, without minimizing his or her experience. There is a frequent need to emphasize that no two people are the same, and therefore their experiences will be different.

In some cases, family members attend group meetings when the individual experiencing cancer feels too fatigued or ill to attend. Educational sessions and support are often beneficial for the family member, who can convey information to the patient. In some instances, a spouse may continue to attend meetings after the husband or wife has passed away from recurrent cancer. The need for support in the bereavement process is obvious. The family member should be encouraged to attend individual sessions with the social worker and bereavement support services as needed.

Patients dealing with recurrent cancer continue to be welcome at support group meetings. Discussion often centers around the importance of continuous monitoring, early detection, and the nature of additional curative and palliative treatments, as well as "unconventional treatments" (i.e., alternative or complementary therapies). Knowledge of a member's recurrent disease, however, can provoke anxiety or distress in other members. The skilled guidance of a psychosocial support professional can promote valuable discussion. This provides a direct opportunity for members to face their own fears associated with recurrence. It is not unusual to have group members who have survived a second and even third recurrence or unrelated cancers, or a subsequent illness such as cardiac disease. The member's subsequent recovery and survival provides hope in the face of reality for many patients.

Hospital-based programs are generally supported through the allocation of clinical time devoted to the groups. Funding obtained through organizations such as the local cancer society may permit publication and distribution of a regular newsletter. The newsletter provides educational information, meeting times and locations, and contact persons. Patients who live far away from the facilities where group meetings are held often appreciate a newsletter.

DIFFERENT GROUP TREATMENT MODELS

New Voice Clubs

The International Association of Laryngectomees (IAL) is a self-help organization founded by the American Cancer Society (ACS) in 1952. It presently has over 250 member clubs throughout North America and the world, and distributes a newsletter to over 30 foreign countries. The ACS and the Canadian Cancer Society (CCS) often provide financial support and meeting facilities for member groups. IAL clubs are led by well-rehabilitated individuals who have been laryngectomized and are often called the "New Voice Club" or the "Lost

Chord Club." Members are outpatients. Professional assistance, such as organizational support or provision of educational sessions, is provided on request. Health care professionals may serve as invited consultants (vs. facilitators who attend on a regular basis and lead the group). IAL chapters are seen as a complement to hospital-based support groups and one-to-one professional psychosocial support. IAL group leaders frequently visit new patients pre- or postoperatively, and may also attend the hospital-based group on occasion.

Self-help groups have multiple benefits, as listed in Table 26.2. Fobair (1997b) noted that self-help groups "create a support system through the structure of their membership, group commitment to goals, and members' identification with the group" (p. 129). Furthermore, Fobair noted that such groups "remove the stigma of the patient role, reduce social isolation, and provide social and emotional support" (Fobair, 1997b, p. 129).

Hospital-Based Laryngectomy Support Group

The hospital-based laryngectomy support group is formed in an effort to bring together people who have had similar experiences at early stages in their adjustment to laryngectomy. Given that laryngectomy results in a significant change in communicative ability, it may be difficult for a person to attend a group with strangers when just learning to speak again. Meetings are typically held weekly during the day to facilitate the attendance of (a) inpatients, (b) members who are retired or not working and prefer not to attend evening meetings, and (c) rural or out-of-town patients, who are often unable to attend evening meetings of the local IAL chapter. A nucleus of people attend regularly; others attend intermittently or only once or twice. Members vary from having been recently diagnosed (prior to the start of treatment) to being long-term cancer survivors. In general, however, this group includes more recently diagnosed patients who are undergoing radiotherapy. Hospital-based groups are particularly suited to open formats; because membership changes, the needs vary according to who attends. New inpatients struggling with communication and lifestyle adjustment can benefit from the ongoing presence and expertise of outpatients and senior members of the group. Attendees who have adjusted to living with the loss of their larynx seem to benefit from assisting new patients. Senior members appreciate being able to support and educate new patients, and this contact reminds them how much progress they themselves have made.

Although professional facilitation provides multiple benefits for the hospital-based groups serving those with head and neck cancer, less formal participation by a professional also may be beneficial in such support groups. A speech–language pathologist or social worker can provide practical, logistical support in the form of booking rooms and facilitating attendance of new patients, and establishing contacts between participants. Other functions of the speech–language pathologist include consultation and direct intervention; provision of referrals to other professionals; and providing data, contacts, and consultation for public education, political action, and advocacy (Wax, 1985, p. 3). Open-ended groups may

Table 26.2
Benefits of Self-Help Groups

Self-help groups do the following:

1. Transform adversity into bonding: "Intense attachments are formed with people who are there with you, are there for you, and are like you because of the power of the life experience you share" (p. 2). Group members form ties stronger than those dictated by economics or ethnicity.

2. Transform stigma into honor: "The gradual desensitization and destigmatization make a badge of honor out of what had been a curse" (p. 2).

3. Offer role transformation: "Helpees to helpers, students to teachers, patients to staff members, dependent individuals to masterful ones, consumers of services to producers of services" (p. 2).

4. Provide a transformed environment: Status is based on mastery of adversity and ability to help others, rather than on factors relating to economics, age, or occupation. The environment is egalitarian, rather than stratified by religious, political, or economic issues.

5. Help to transform deviant behavior into normative behavior. For example, all laryngectomees share features and behaviors that would stand out as different in society as a whole (e.g., the diagnosis of cancer, fears of recurrence, status as a neck-breather, unusual speech and voice patterns, a noticeable cough).

6. Transform experiential or folk knowledge into wisdom (p. 3). Certain information is owned, trusted, and shared among the members. Practical knowledge is freely exchanged and sometimes contrasts with that provided by health-care professionals, which is sometimes viewed as insensitive to patient realities.

7. Allow powerful emotions to be expressed and legitimized. Strong helping commitments are formed, and members are free to explore the stages of grief with acceptance and support.

8. Encourage active involvement in politics by transforming personal experiences into opportunities for public service, increased public education and awareness, and advocacy for better services.

Note. Adapted from "Self-Help Groups," by J. Wax, 1985, *Journal of Psychosocial Oncology, 3*(3), pp. 1–4.

lack focus and cohesiveness due to continuous and changing membership intake or small patient populations with short hospital stays. Facilitators can provide structure and facilitate cohesiveness through introductions and establishing group focus and purpose.

Professional input is often helpful in clarifying misconceptions and inaccuracies that may arise as participants share information. Content is a combination of education–discussion and counseling–support (see Fobair, 1997b). Specialized expertise enables the speech–language pathologist and the social worker to fill both these roles. In open-ended groups, there are often new members who are struggling with a multitude of issues, including the ability to communicate readily and intelligibly, as well as the newness of participating in a group setting. The speech–language pathologist can assist the new members with communication efforts and support participation of all members, as well as offer education about communication options and the lifestyle consequences of laryngectomy. The facilitator must be especially sensitive to the possibility of some members monopolizing discussion or providing inaccurate information, because newer communicators have less ease and confidence in speaking.

The social worker is invaluable in terms of managing group processes and handling negative group processes. In contrast to organized psychotherapy group formats, there is less stigma attached to the head and neck cancer group program content. Although issues related to dealing with the emotional impact of the disease and consequences arise and are addressed, they are not the primary focus of the group. Members view the group as primarily providing information, education, and support. The social worker can provide guidance with negative discussion, such as dwelling on discouraging news, and can balance realities with accuracy of information presented. Maintaining a realistic yet positive focus can be problematic when issues arise related to recurrence or death of a member. This information can be particularly discouraging for new members. The facilitator can balance the discussion by addressing these concerns directly, acknowledging the reality of one's fear of recurrence and death, and guiding discussion toward providing strategies for coping with these fears and uncertainties. Feelings are legitimized and normalized; that is, one learns that one's thoughts and emotions are valid and normal, and are frequently experienced by others with a similar diagnosis. Active coping techniques for group members are discussed. These techniques may include "giving themselves permission ... to feel, identifying and naming their feelings, accepting situations that are beyond their control, and using constructive thinking and problem-solving to change what can be changed" (Fobair, 1997b, p. 128).

The benefits of support from members of the health care team are well recognized. Slevin et al. (1996) evaluated patients' attitudes to different sources of support, including that of individuals, support groups, and information sources. The authors found that the three most important sources of emotional support were senior registrars (i.e., patients who were further along in their recovery and in the adjustment process), followed by family and consultants, and that patients preferred doctor- or nurse-led support groups to patient-led groups. Dunkel-Schetter (1984) found that health care providers were considered a particularly important source of social support for cancer patients and that patients viewed medical care as unhelpful if the professionals did not provide sufficient emotional support. Facilitators are effective when respectful, attentive, warm, and willing to talk about themselves (Yalom, 1975).

Hospital-based groups in which new patients are encouraged to attend by the health care professional may be a way to demonstrate the benefits of peer support at an early and critical stage and, therefore, promote continued later attendance in groups. Inpatients invariably report that their attendance at the hospital-based group is a positive experience.

Members are sometimes divided into discussion groups according to patient demographics, circumstances, or specific concerns. Groups might be based on younger versus older patients, speech and swallowing difficulties, adjustment issues, patient versus spouse and family member concerns, return-to-work issues, or female versus male patients. Each group may include a facilitator, either a health care professional or a trained volunteer. The creation of subgroups within a larger meeting can allow specific focus on identified needs. The larger group is brought together to share information that can be of benefit to all and to explore common concerns (e.g., negotiating the health care system, communicating with physicians, coping with the effects of radiotherapy, communicating with family and friends).

Additional considerations for facilitator-led groups include maintenance of records, evaluations (e.g., patient satisfaction surveys), scheduling or rotation of leaders to ensure coverage and prevent burnout, and potential publications (Heiney & Wells, 1989).

Head and Neck Cancer Support Groups (Not Including Laryngectomees)

People who have had cancers of the head and neck and are not laryngectomized may find that their unique needs are not met within a support group for those who have undergone laryngectomy. In my experience, when these patients are invited to attend a laryngectomy support group, they may express that they have "nothing in common" with laryngectomized individuals, despite a similar diagnosis of cancer, fears of recurrence, and physical and functional changes in appearance, eating, and swallowing. Additionally, they may feel that talking to another cancer survivor with a different type of cancer (e.g., breast, colon) is not helpful. Furthermore, in my experience, the demographics of the nonlaryngeal head and neck cancer population appear to be different, with a younger average age and dissimilar lifestyle factors (better overall health, a lesser or nonexistent smoking and drinking history). Because of the absence of typical risk factors or the presence of unusual or rare tumors, nonlaryngeal cancers may be diagnosed when the cancer is more advanced, with resulting devastating consequences requiring extensive surgery, aggressive treatment, or both. These individuals may have major functional limitations affecting their physical and psychosocial well-being (see Chapter 28 in this text).

Groups for nonlaryngectomized head and neck cancer patients are uncommon. In 1993, contact with the ACS revealed that of more than 1,000 support groups affiliated with the ACS, none existed specifically for this population, but over 250 support groups existed for the laryngectomized. Support for People with Oral and Head and Neck Cancer and Let's Face It: A Network for People with a Facial Difference are support programs that can offer much to individuals with head and neck cancers (see contact information in Appendix 26.A).

The target population for the head and neck cancer group is people with a diagnosis of cancer in the head and neck area; those with brain tumors and laryngectomies are generally excluded because groups typically exist for these people. This unique population requires skilled multidisciplinary professional support (e.g., dietetics, physiotherapy, psychosocial support, speech–language pathology, dentistry, prosthodontics). Family members and significant others are included in meetings. Handouts or newsletters are provided with dates, location, planned sessions, and contact persons. Due to communication impairments and disfigurement, many patients tend to isolate themselves initially. Connecting first with a health care professional (speech–language pathologist, social worker, dentist, or nurse) or a veteran patient who understands their fears and concerns often facilitates entry to the group. Potential members need to be made aware that some members are going through very trying times and their stories might be overwhelming. They also need to know that although many people find the group helpful, some prefer one-to-one support by peers or professionals.

Meetings at St. Boniface Hospital in Winnipeg, Manitoba are usually held monthly and during the evenings to facilitate attendance of persons who have returned to work. Out-of-town patients arrange clinical follow-up on meetings days. Meetings are held in a parlor room at the hospital—a warm and inviting atmosphere away from the clinic and treatment areas, conducive to sharing and support. The format is open with no registration required. Demographics reflect population trends; most members are younger, urban, and in the workforce. A nucleus of people attend regularly, whereas others attend once or twice for specific educational sessions.

Women-Only Group

It has been beneficial to bring together women who have experienced laryngectomy, either one to one or in a small group setting. Brown and Doyle (1999) described some of the unique concerns of women who are laryngectomized, including perceptions of femininity, disfigurement and body image, stigma associated with altered communication and diagnosis of cancer, intimacy, independence, and the ability to perform daily tasks. In addition, some laryngectomized females express special needs related to stoma protection and safety (many female patients live alone and have expressed concern about security and harassing phone calls).

One-to-One Peer Support

Finally, it is important not to discount the value of one-to-one support for some patients. To quote Betsy Wilson, founder and coordinator of Let's Face It: "Don't be burdened by the word 'group.' One person is enough. The last thing some of us want is to be part of a group" (personal communication, 1995).

PRACTICAL STRATEGIES FOR ORGANIZING AND RUNNING GROUPS

The following suggestions are provided as a guide for organizing and conducting support group programs for people with head and neck cancer.

First Steps
- Begin with a small group of interested patients.
- Collaborate with other interested health care professionals and trained cancer patients. The workload can be shared, and the wider professional perspective enhances patient care.

Support
- Link with a sponsoring agency, such as the Canadian or American Cancer Society, to assist with practical support such as funding, educational materials, meeting rooms, and newsletter costs and distribution.
- Seek the active support and endorsement of program managers, as well as physicians (oncologists, surgeons) and nurses. Doing so helps to ensure consistent referrals. Invite these individuals to attend a meeting or present an educational session so they can see firsthand the benefits of the program.

Logistics
- Organize regular meetings in conjunction with clinic days to facilitate the attendance of out-of-town patients. Try to accommodate the needs of rural patients for whom contact with others who share the same experience is a lifeline.
- Ensure consistency in meeting days and times, an easily accessible location, and contact persons. This facilitates the attendance of members who are unable to attend regularly. Ensure accuracy of pamphlets and newsletters; out-of-date materials do circulate.
- Find volunteers to produce a newsletter; supply them with accurate educational articles and offer to proofread the newsletter. Citing sources is important.
- Encourage members to avail themselves of opportunities to become trained laryngectomee or cancer-survivor visitors. The Canadian Cancer Society offers an excellent program for cancer survivors, who can then become one-to-one visitors or participate in or lead a group program.

Format
- Encourage patient-run groups with professional support wherever possible.
- Begin by having members introduce themselves (including name, diagnosis and update since last meeting, and surgery date and type). Reiterate the names if poor speech intelligibility or hearing loss is an issue.
- Have a format that is informal and flexible, especially for groups where membership is fluid and new patients are dealing with a multitude of changing issues. The group can then meet needs as they arise.
- Establish a "back-up" educational plan to help provide structure as the facilitator gets used to running a group.
- Honor "senior" members (i.e., well-rehabilitated patients). They are the backbone of the group and can provide invaluable assistance in terms of

practical and direct patient support. Regularly encourage their sharing of experiences and input on issues. They are the true experts on living with the effects of head and neck cancers, coping, and adjustment. Acknowledge their contribution at the end of each meeting. Acknowledge their support annually through a thank-you note, a small token of appreciation, or a nomination for a volunteer award. Frequent acknowledgment and recognition will ensure their continued attendance.

- Encourage attendees to bring in samples and share information on new products. Sometimes patients are the first to be informed of new technological developments and products.
- Facilitate involvement of all members at meetings. Some may be dominant, and new patients may have a communication deficit that interferes with easy involvement in the group.
- Bring new patients to meetings, or have a well-rehabilitated "friendly visitor" bring them. It can be difficult enough to attend a meeting of strangers, let alone when a communication impairment is present. Early attendance and connection with other laryngectomees can promote continued participation.

Refreshments

- Consider the limitations of your patient group in choosing refreshments. Provide noncaffeinated, nonacidic beverages; easy to eat and swallow foods; and water.

Finally, the facilitator should not be discouraged by lack of interest in attendance by some patients. The value of one-to-one peer support cannot be underestimated for some patients.

For further information on group organization and maintenance strategies, the reader is encouraged to refer to Cella and Yellen (1993), Fobair (1997b), and Wax (1985). Fobair (1997a, 1997b) provides further discussion of group treatment models. Heiney and Wells (1989) provide a comprehensive overview of the philosophical and practical considerations for patient support groups, including an excellent timeline for establishing a group "from scratch," and suggestions for managing group processes.

SUMMARY

The effects of cancer on the individual and the family are well documented. Studies indicate that people who attend psychosocial–educational support programs report a reduction in anxiety and depression, and improved QOL. However, the impact of participation in such groups in terms of survival rates is still unknown. Programs such as those described must be examined in the context of evaluative research. Specifically, the following questions merit further attention: Are different formats better suited to individuals at different stages of recovery (e.g., are professionally facilitated groups more beneficial for patients at early stages of treatment and recovery, and peer-conducted groups more valued at later stages of recovery)? How does participation in support group programs affect QOL among individuals with head and neck cancer? What type of content and frequency of meeting is most beneficial, and at what stages? Do educational sessions lead to behavioral changes (e.g., tobacco reduction, change in diet or oral care, better stress management) among those individuals with head and neck cancer? Do educational sessions lead to improved outcomes (e.g., improved health status, fewer medical visits)? Is there a role for technology (e.g., e-mail, Internet) in psychosocial or peer support for those individuals who are in remote locations or are unable to attend support group programs? Documented efficacy studies may substantiate the clinically observed benefits of support group programs and ensure the survival of such programs in times of health care reform. Finally, as Fobair (1997b) stated,

> The personal benefits of being a group leader become clear when group members let us know that we have had a significant impact on their lives. As group leaders, we enjoy the opportunity to be transformed by special moments in our groups and experience for ourselves how we are all connected. (p. 143)

ACKNOWLEDGMENTS

The author is particularly grateful to Agathe Bisson, social worker at St. Boniface General Hospital, Winnipeg, Manitoba, and to the members of the Psychosocial Oncology Department at CancerCare Manitoba, who have so willingly shared their expertise in the psychosocial aspects of client care among cancer patients, and to the members of the support group programs in which I have been involved, and who continue to be an inspiration.

Financial and practical support, such as provision of written educational materials, has been provided for the St. Boniface meetings by the pharmaceutical company, Pharmacia and Upjohn, which produces the xerostomia remedy, pilocarpine (Salagan). The CCS has provided financial support for a newsletter, which is an important source of information and support for patients unable to attend due to illness, treatment, or distance. Let's Face It, an organization for people with a facial difference, also has provided valuable information and resources.

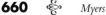

Appendix 26.A

Resources

American Cancer Society
(phone for nearest regional office)
Phone: 800/ACS/2345
www.cancer.org

Canadian Cancer Society
National Office
10 Alcorn Avenue, Suite 200
Toronto, ON M4V 3B1 Canada
Phone: 416/961-7223
www.cancer.ca
E-mail: ccs@cancer.ca

International Association of Laryngectomees
7822 Ivymount Terrace
Potomac, MD 20854
Phone: 301/983-9323
Fax: 301/983-4397
www.larynxlink.com
E-mail: ialwebmaster@larynxlink.com

Let's Face It: A Network for People with a Facial Difference
P.O. Box 29972
Bellingham, WA 98228-1972
Phone: 306/676-7325
www.faceit.org
E-mail: letsfaceit@faceit.org

SPOHNC: Support for People with Oral and Head and Neck Cancer
P.O. Box 53
Locust Valley, NY 11560-0053
Phone: 800/377-0928
www.spohnc.org
E-mail: webmaster@spohnc.org

REFERENCES

Albrecht, T. L. & Adelman, M. B. (1987). *Communicating social support*. Newbury Park, CA: Sage.

Baile, W. F., Gibertini, M., Scott, L., & Endicott, J. (1992). Depression and tumor stage in cancer of the head and neck. *Psycho-oncology, 1,* 15–24.

Baker, C. A. (1992). Factors associated with rehabilitation in head and neck cancer. *Cancer Nursing, 15,* 395–400.

Bauman, L. J., Gervey, R., & Siegel, K. (1992). Factors associated with cancer patients' participation in support groups. *Journal of Psychosocial Oncology, 10*(3), 1–20.

Bisson, A. (1995, May). *Laryngectomee support group: Six years experience.* Paper presented at Canadian Association for Psychosocial Oncology Annual Conference, Saskatoon, Saskatchewan, Canada.

Bjordal, K., Kaasa, S., & Mastekaasa, A. (1994). Quality of life in patients treated for head and neck cancer: A follow-up study 7 to 11 years after radiotherapy. *International Journal of Radiation Oncology, Biology, Physics, 28*(4), 847–856.

Blanchard, C. G., Albrecht, T. L., Ruckdeschel, J. C., Grant, C. H., & Hemmick, R. M. (1995). The role of social support in adaptation to cancer and to survival. *Journal of Psychosocial Oncology, 13*(1/2), 75–95.

Blood, G. W., Simpson, K. C., Raimondi, S. C., Dineen, M., Kauffman, S. M., & Stagaard, K. A. (1994). Social support in laryngeal cancer survivors: Voice and adjustment issues. *American Journal of Speech–Language Pathology, 1,* 37–44.

Bottomley, A., Hunton, S., Roberts, G., Jones, L., & Bradley, C. (1996). A pilot study of cognitive behavioral therapy and social support group interventions with newly diagnosed cancer patients. *Journal of Psychosocial Oncology, 14*(4), 65–83.

Breitbart, W., & Holland, J. (1988). Psychosocial aspects of head and neck cancer. *Seminars in Oncology, 15*(1), 61–69.

Brown, S. I., & Doyle, P. C. (1999). The woman who is laryngectomized: Parallels, perspectives, and reevaluation of practice. *Journal of Speech–Language Pathology and Audiology, 23*(2), 54–60.

Bunston, T., Mings, D., Mackie, A., & Jones, D. (1995). Facilitating hopefulness: The determinants of hope. *Journal of Psychosocial Oncology, 13*(4), 79–103.

Cella, D. F., & Yellen, S. B. (1993). Cancer support groups: The state of the art. *Cancer Care, 1*(1), 56–61.

Cwikel, J. G., Behar, L. C., & Zabora, K. R. (1997). Psychosocial factors that affect the survival of adult cancer patients: A review of the literature. *Journal of Psychosocial Oncology, 15*(3/4), 1–34.

Darvill, G. (1983). Rehabilitation—Not just voice. In Y. Edels (Ed.), *Laryngectomy: Diagnosis to rehabilitation* (pp. 192–217). Rockville, MD: Aspen.

de Boer, M. F., Pruyn, J. F., van den Borne, B., Knegt, P. P., Ryckman, R. M., & Verwoerd, C. D. (1995). Rehabilitation outcomes of long-term survivors treated for head and neck cancer. *Head & Neck, 17,* 503–515.

Doyle, P. C. (1994). *Foundation of voice and speech rehabilitation following laryngeal cancer.* San Diego: Singular.

Doyle, P. C. (1999). Postlaryngectomy speech rehabilitation: Contemporary considerations in clinical care. *Journal of Speech–Language Pathology and Audiology, 23,* 109–116.

Dunkel-Schetter, C. (1984). Social support and cancer: Findings based on patient interviews and their implications. *Journal of Social Issues, 40,* 77–98.

Eadie, T. L. (2001). The ICIDH–2: Theoretical and clinical implications for speech–language pathology. *Journal of Speech–Language Pathology and Audiology, 25,* 181–200.

Eadie, T. L. (2003). The ICF: A proposed framework for comprehensive rehabilitation of individuals who use alaryngeal speech. *American Journal of Speech–Language Pathology, 12,* 189–197.

Ferrell, B. R., Hassey Dow, K., Leigh, S., Ly, J., & Gulasekaram, P. (1995). Quality of life in long-term cancer survivors. *Oncology Nursing Forum, 22*(6), 915–922.

Fobair, P. (1989, November). *Twelve clinical indicators of the level of distress among cancer patient survivors.* Paper presented at the 35th Annual Meeting of the National Association of Social Workers, Health and Mental Health Section, San Francisco.

Fobair, P. (1997a). Cancer support groups and group therapies: Part I. Historical and theoretical background and research on effectiveness. *Journal of Psychosocial Oncology, 15*(1), 63–81.

Fobair, P. (1997b). Cancer support groups and group therapies: Part II. Process, organizational, leadership, and patient issues. *Journal of Psychosocial Oncology, 15*(3/4), 123–147.

Gallo, O., Sarno, A., Baroncelli, R., Bruschini, L., & Boddi, V. (2003). Multivariate analysis of prognostic factors in T3 N0 laryngeal carcinoma treated with total laryngectomy. *Otolaryngology—Head and Neck Surgery, 128,* 654–662.

Gibson, A. R., & McCombe, M. D. (1999). Psychological morbidity following laryngectomy: A pilot study. *The Journal of Laryngology and Otology, 113,* 349–352.

Hammerlid, E., Persson, L.-O., Sullivan, M., & Westin, T. (1999). Quality-of-life effects of psychosocial intervention in patients with head and neck cancer. *Otolaryngology—Head and Neck Surgery, 120,* 507–516.

Harris, L. L., Vogtsberger, K. N., & Mattox, D. E. (1985). Group psychotherapy for head and neck patients. *Laryngoscope, 95,* 585–587.

Harwood, A. R., & Rawlinson, E. (1983). The quality of life of patients following treatment for laryngeal cancer. *International Journal of Radiation Oncology, Biology, Physics, 9,* 335–338.

Heiney, S. P., & Wells, L. M. (1989). Strategies for organizing and maintaining successful support groups. *Oncology Nursing Forum, 16*(6), 803–809.

Loescher, L. J., Clark, L., Atwood, J. R., Leigh, S., & Lamb, G. (1990). The impact of the cancer experience on long-term survivors. *Oncology Nursing Forum, 17*(2), 223–229.

Lonergan, E. C. (1985). Mobilizing group members' coping devices. In *Group intervention: How to begin and maintain groups in medical and psychiatric settings* (pp. 171–210). New York: Aronson.

Martin, H. (1963). Rehabilitation of the laryngectomee. *Cancer, 16*(7), 823–841.

Mathieson, C. M., Logan-Smith, L. L., Phillips, J., MacPhee, M., & Attia, E. L. (1996). Caring for head and neck oncology patients: Does social support lead to better quality of life? *Canadian Family Physician, 42,* 1712–1720.

Mathieson, C. M., Stam, H. J., & Scott, J. P. (1991). The impact of laryngectomy on the spouse: Who is better off? *Psychology and Health, 5,* 153–163.

McDonough, E. M., Varvares, M. A., Dunphy, F. R., Dunleavy, T., Dunphy, C. H., & Boyd, J. H. (1996). Changes in quality-of-life scores in a population of patients treated for squamous cell carcinoma of the head and neck. *Head & Neck, 18,* 487–493.

McGee, R. (1984). Hope: A factor influencing crisis resolution. *Advances in Nursing Science, 6*(4), 34–44.

McQuellon, R. P., & Hurt, G. J. (1997). The psychosocial impact of the diagnosis and treatment of laryngeal cancer. *Otolaryngology Clinics of North America, 30,* 213–241.

Menninger, K. (1959). Hope. *American Journal of Psychiatry, 116,* 481–491.

Morton, R. P., Davies, A. D. M., Baker, J., Baker, G. A., & Stell, P. M. (1984). Quality of life in treated head and neck cancer patients: A preliminary report. *Clinics in Otolaryngology, 9,* 181–185.

Olson, M. L., & Shedd, D. P. (1978). Disability and rehabilitation in head and neck cancer patients after treatment. *Head and Neck Surgery, 1,* 52–58.

Pruyn, J. F., de Jong, P. C., Bosman, L. J., van Poppel, J. W., van den Borne, H. W., Ryckman, R. M., & de Meij, K. (1986). Psychosocial aspects of head and neck cancer: A review of the literature. *Clinics in Otolaryngology, 11,* 469–474.

Rapoport, Y., Kreitle, S., Chaitchik, S., Algor, R., & Weissler, K. (1993). Psychosocial problems in head-and-neck cancer patients and their change with time since diagnosis. *Annals of Oncology, 4,* 69–73.

Richardson, J. L., & Bourque, L. B. (1985). Communication after laryngectomy. *Journal of Psychosocial Oncology, 3*(3), 85–97.

Rustoen, T., Moum, T., Wiklund, I., & Hanestad, B. R. (1999). Quality of life in newly diagnosed cancer patients. *Journal of Advanced Nursing, 29*(2), 490–498.

Salmon, S. J. (1986). Laryngectomee visitations. In R. L. Keith & F. L. Darley (Eds.), *Laryngectomy rehabilitation* (pp. 351–369). San Diego: College-Hill Press.

Schipper, H. (1990). Quality of life: Principles of the clinical paradigm. *Journal of Psychosocial Oncology, 8*(2/3), 171–185.

Slevin, M. L., Nichols, S. E., Downer, S. M., Wilson, P., Lister, T. A., Arnott, S., Maher, J., Souhami, R. L., Tobias, J. S., Goldstone, A. H., & Cody, M. (1996). Emotional support for cancer patients: What do patients really want? *British Journal of Cancer, 74,* 1275–1279.

Stam, H. J., Koopmans, J. P., & Mathieson, C. M. (1991). The psychosocial impact of a laryngectomy: A comprehensive assessment. *Journal of Psychosocial Oncology, 9*(3), 37–58.

Strauss, R. P. (1989). Psychosocial responses to oral and maxillofacial surgery for head and neck cancer. *Journal of Oral Maxillofacial Surgery, 47,* 343–348.

Sutherland, C. E., & Goldstein, M. S. (1992). Joining a healing community for cancer: Who and why? *Social Science and Medicine, 35,* 323–333.

Watt-Watson, J., & Graydon, J. (1995). Impact of surgery on head and neck cancer patients and their caregivers. *Nursing Clinics of North America, 30,* 659–671.

Wax, J. (1985). Self-help groups. *Journal of Psychosocial Oncology, 3*(3), 1–4.

World Health Organization. (1993). *International classification of impairments, disabilities, and handicaps: A manual of classification relating to the consequences of disease.* Geneva, Switzerland: World Health Organization.

Yalom, I. D. (1975). *The theory and practice of group psychotherapy.* New York: Basic Books.

Zabora, J. (1999). Screening procedures for psychological distress. In J. Holland (Ed.), *Psychooncology* (pp. 653–661). New York: Oxford University Press.

Chapter 27

Accountability in Alaryngeal Speech Rehabilitation

Minnie S. Graham

To be proficient clinicians, we bear the responsibility of being knowledgeable of alaryngeal speech rehabilitation, determined in our efforts, deeply caring in our relationships, and constant in our desire to help the laryngectomee and the family. To the laryngectomee and family, to our profession, and to ourselves, we owe nothing less. (Graham, 1997, p. 182)

The impetus in today's professional health care arena is for streamlined, efficient, and low-cost patient management. In response to the rising costs of hospitalization, medical treatment, and rehabilitative services, the payers for these services—Medicare, Medicaid, insurance companies, and individuals—are demanding justification for each and every procedure. Professionals are being charged with the responsibility to support their recommendations and methods of treatment using outcome data. In recent years, the American Speech-Language-Hearing Association (ASHA) has actively engaged its membership in the collection and publication of outcome data for the treatment and management of a variety of communicative disorders (for outcomes and clinical trial initiatives and other projects, see ASHA, 1995; Baum, 1998; Gallagher, 1998; Johnston & Granger, 1994; Pietranton & Baum, 1995). Using the available data, ASHA staff are lobbying actively for health care reform that is directly beneficial to rehabilitation efforts. Within the clinical setting, speech–language pathologists are advocating for professional services on behalf of those individuals with communicative disorders. In the process, clients are becoming the recipients of intervention methods that are based on collective research and clinical experiences that have undergone professional scrutiny.

In alaryngeal speech rehabilitation, regardless of the selected communication method—artificial larynx, esophageal speech, or tracheoesophageal (TE) speech—periodic evaluation and reevaluation are required. The rationale behind evaluation that is often foremost in the clinician's mind is the need to establish baselines that give direction for therapy and to provide an index for progress. The clinician is committed ethically to identifying and adapting training methods for each client so that the desired outcome is achieved with an economy of time, expense, and effort. Given the current and ever-changing economic climate, the speech–language pathologist is obligated to provide (a) a strong supporting basis for the initiation of therapy, (b) ongoing data that reflect whether or not progress is occurring during therapeutic intervention, and (c) data-based summary reports that advocate the continuation or termination of therapy. The purpose of this chapter is to review the procedures for alaryngeal speech rehabilitation from an accountability perspective. Terms that define and describe the methods of alaryngeal speech production are introduced as the basis for goal and subgoal selection for use of the artificial larynx, esophageal speech, and TE speech. Next, the components of lesson planning, including establishing baselines and the selection of stimuli, are presented. Components of clinical training that are supported by the literature—that is, instruction and feedback, consistent and variable practice, speed versus accuracy, frequency of sessions, the task hierarchy, client performance levels, and group therapy—are outlined. A rationale for the maintenance of written records (e.g., therapy logs and report writing) is given. Finally, issues surrounding the termination of therapy are addressed.

PARAMETERS OF ALARYNGEAL SPEECH PRODUCTION

The ultimate goal of alaryngeal speech rehabilitation is functional communication. Basic to the process of goal selection is discovering how to maximize the effectiveness, efficiency, and naturalness of the individual's communication. A number of communication options are available to the client. The primary methods used are the artificial larynx, esophageal speech, and TE speech. Some individuals choose one of these as their primary method of communication; others select and use a variety of alaryngeal communication methods based on need and environmental factors (Berry, 1978; Carpenter, 1999; Doyle, 1994; Duguay, 1978, 1983; Palmer & Graham, 2004). The choice of communication option(s) should be made by the individual based on a complex interplay of physical and cognitive considerations postoperatively, environmental and occupational factors, recommendations made by the physician and speech–language pathologist, information about the advantages and disadvantages of each of the alaryngeal speech methods, and personal preference (Carpenter, 1999; Doyle, 1994; Graham, 1997). Once the method of alaryngeal speech communication has been determined, the clinician's attention turns to the appropriate procedures for assessment and intervention as supported by the literature. This concern is influenced by changes in an ever-shrinking world (Fagan, Lentin, Oyarzabal, Isaacs, & Sellars, 2002).

Frequency, intensity, quality of voicing, rate and *phrasing,* and *intelligibility* are terms commonly used in the literature to define and describe alaryngeal speech production. More often than not, measures of these parameters are used in studies comparing speech production by alaryngeal speakers to that of laryngeal speakers (e.g., Hyman, 1955; Robbins, 1984; Robbins, Fisher, Blom, & Singer, 1984; Snidecor & Curry, 1959; Tikofsky, 1965). A review of the literature, however, raises concern that a standard set of criteria is not used across studies of alaryngeal speech abilities. Although there have been efforts to establish guidelines for specific modes of alaryngeal speech—specifically artificial laryngeal speech (Hyman, 1955; Rothman, 1978; Salmon, 1994a, 1999; Weiss & Basili, 1985; see also Chapter 22 in this text), esophageal speech (Barton & Hejna, 1963; Berlin, 1963, 1965; Filter & Hyman, 1975; Hoops & Guzek, 1974; Hoops & Noll, 1969; Robe, Moore, Andrews, & Holinger, 1956; Shipp, 1967; Wepman, MacGahan, Rickard, & Shelton, 1953), and TE speech (Lewin, 1999; Schultz & Harrison, 1992; Tardy-Mitzell, Andrews, & Bowman, 1985; Trudeau, 1994; Williams, Scanio, & Ritterman, 1989)—even within specific groups of alaryngeal speakers, there is a broad range of what is considered acceptable performance.

According to Doyle (1994), a substantial diversity of performance is to be expected both within and across alaryngeal speech modes. On the other hand, based on listener ratings and instrumental measures, there is a clear distinction among poor, average, and superior alaryngeal speakers regardless of the speaking mode. Using these studies (and others), the speech–language pathologist has access to a variety of guidelines by which to make judgments about (a) the effectiveness of alaryngeal speech training and (b) the proficiency of production in individual clients.

To date, there is little standardization across the literature for assessment and reevaluation of alaryngeal speech methods (Carpenter, 1999). Graham (1997) constructed hierarchies for the evaluation of artificial larynx use, for various methods of air intake for esophageal speech, and for TE speech (see summary sheets for the evaluation of alaryngeal speech methods, presented later in this chapter as Figures 27.2 through 27.6). The characteristics specific to each of the alaryngeal speech methods are assessed systematically. For example, the clinician makes judgments about each of the components necessary for optimal use of the artificial larynx—placement, on–off control, articulation, rate, and phrasing. During testing, 10 stimuli are presented orally or in writing. Each of the client's productions is rated by the clinician using a binary scoring system (e.g., correct or incorrect; present or absent; acceptable or not acceptable). At the clinician's discretion, a more sophisticated method of scoring may be devised (e.g., a 5-point rating scale, with 1 = excellent, 2 = above average, 3 = average, 4 = below average, 5 = poor). The clinician makes a judgment about each performance aspect for that alaryngeal speech mode (e.g., for the artificial larynx, the ratings for a single production might read "appropriate placement, delayed on–off control, average articulation, slow rate, no phrasing"). The client might be asked to repeat each of the test stimuli twice to allow the clinician time to hear, observe, and assess the various components of the production. The clinician totals the client's performance for each parameter across the 10 stimulus items and calculates the percentages. If the client achieves an overall accuracy of performance of 70% or higher (e.g., placement of the artificial larynx was appropriate during 7 of the 10 stimuli), testing continues at the next level of production (longer utterances). Testing is discontinued at the level of production at which the client's performance falls below a mean of 60% accuracy across the parameters. Hence, performance of 60% accuracy or less across the parameters indicates the level of production to begin therapeutic intervention.

The benefits of the evaluation are twofold: (a) the client's current level of production (baseline of performance) is established, and (b) an indication of the behaviors to be targeted in therapy is provided. In other words, the clinician has a supporting basis for the initiation of therapy and the direction in which therapy should go (see Chapter 5 in this text). In addition, the stimuli used in the original assessment can be readministered in subsequent progress assessments, allowing the speech–language pathologist to compare and contrast previous (baseline) performance with current performance. Such an analysis presents the opportunity to support or challenge the clinician's choice of goals for the client and the effectiveness of the therapy.

GETTING STARTED: GOAL SELECTION

At the intervention stage of the rehabilitation process, the client's performance, based on the characteristics of the chosen method of alaryngeal speech production, has been documented through assessment. A series of subgoals, based on the parameters that support the terminal goal of functional communication, is identified. According to Carpenter (1999), subgoals related to alaryngeal voice production (i.e., consistency, control, and characteristics of quality, loudness, and pitch) are common to all methods of alaryngeal speech; however, their descriptions differ based on the mode of communication (see Figure 27.1). For example, consistency of voicing for artificial laryngeal speech is based on appropriate placement of the instrument and maintaining a good seal against the neck or cheek (Diedrich & Youngstrom, 1966; Duguay, 1983; Salmon, 1999; Snidecor, 1978a). Consistency of voicing for esophageal speech refers to the client's ability to move air into the upper esophagus and return it to the oral cavity (Diedrich & Youngstrom, 1966; Duguay, 1999; W. N. Gardner, 1971; Snidecor, 1978b). Consistency of voicing for TE speech is determined by the individual's level of respiratory support and ability to maintain a stoma seal and adequate respiratory pressure during speech production (Bosone, 1994, 1999; Casper & Colton, 1998; see also Chapters 17, 18, and 24 in this text).

Articulation, timing, and prosody are the subskills that relate to alaryngeal speech production. Regardless of the method of alaryngeal speech, the ability to achieve oral pressure and to make voicing contrasts are important to articulatory proficiency (Connor, Hamlet, & Joyce, 1985; Diedrich & Youngstrom, 1966; Doyle, Danhauer, & Reed, 1988; Doyle & Haaf, 1989; Robbins, Christensen, & Kempster, 1986; Snidecor, 1978b). Rate of speech and pause time affect the listener's judgment of "acceptability" (Bennett & Weinberg, 1973; Diedrich & Youngstrom, 1966; Filter & Hyman, 1975; Hoops & Guzek, 1974; Hoops & Noll, 1969; Shipp, 1967; see also Chapter 6 in this text). Prosody is reflected in the client's use of phrasing and inflection (Gandour & Weinberg, 1983). Finally, audible and visible distractions (e.g., stoma noise, klunking, loss of eye contact, double injections, facial grimacing) can interfere with successful delivery of the intended message (Diedrich & Youngstrom, 1966; Duguay, 1999; Lerman, 1999; Salmon, 1999; Sedory, Hamlet, & O'Connor, 1989; see also Chapter 3 in this text).

Baseline performances recorded during the assessment are matched to the selected subgoals for the particular mode of alaryngeal speech. Of particular interest are the subgoals that are to be targeted early in therapy. The baseline data become the standard by which the speech–language pathologist measures change, evaluates the effectiveness of therapy, and determines the need to continue, alter, or terminate treatment. Other factors that are not so easily measured but have the power to influence the speech rehabilitation process include any motor, sensory, or cognitive deficits; the level of motivation; the environmental demands; daily communication needs; and previously established communication strategies (Gilmore, 1994, 1999; Salmon, 1994c; see also Chapters 3, 4, 5, 16, 22, 25, and 26 in this text).

ALARYNGEAL SPEECH SUBSKILLS

Client _____ Date _____

Write in the scale value that best represents the client's performance per speech type: AL = artificial larynx; ES = esophageal speech; TES = tracheoesophageal speech

Scale: 1 = Very Good; 2 = Good; 3 = Average; 4 = Poor; 5 = Very Poor

	AL	ES	TES
Voice Production			
Consistency	____ Placement	____ Intake Pattern	____ Respiratory Support
	____ Tissue Seal	____ Return Pattern	____ Stoma Seal/Pressure
Control	____ On–Off	____ Duration	____ Duration
Characteristics	____ Quality	____ Quality	____ Quality
	____ Loudness	____ Loudness	____ Loudness
	____ Pitch	____ Pitch	____ Pitch
Speech Production			
Articulation	____ Oral Pressure	____ Oral Pressure	____ Oral Pressure
	____ Voicing Contrasts	____ Voicing Contrasts	____ Voicing Contrasts
Timing	____ Syllable Rate	____ Syllable Rate	____ Syllable Rate
	____ Pause Time	____ Pause Time	____ Pause Time
Prosody	____ Phrasing	____ Phrasing	____ Phrasing
	____ Inflection	____ Inflection	____ Inflection
Distracters (Describe)			
Audible	_____	_____	_____
	_____	_____	_____
Visible	_____	_____	_____
	_____	_____	_____

FIGURE 27.1. Form for assessing subskills of alaryngeal speech types. From "Treatment Decisions in Alaryngeal Speech," by M. A. Carpenter, in *Alaryngeal Speech Rehabilitation* (p. 68), by S. J. Salmon (Ed.), 1999, Austin, TX: PRO-ED. Copyright 1999 by PRO-ED. Reprinted with permission.

As previously discussed, evaluation of alaryngeal speech methods provides the clinician with the information to select subgoals specific to the individual's needs. Although subgoals may be similar across all alaryngeal speech modes, the tasks and stimuli for the specific methods are different. Stimuli used for instruction of artificial larynx use differ from those used to teach beginning esophageal speech. In Chapter 16 in this text, goals and instruction for various alaryngeal speech methods are explained, along with suggestions for problem solving. The purpose of this chapter is to assist the speech–language pathologist in determining subgoals from a technical and accountability perspective.

Subgoals should be written using a behavioral format. Being able to describe a target behavior at certain levels of the hierarchy in terms of a percentage or ratio facilitates the determination of progress or lack of progress. There are three components of a subgoal that is written in behavioral terms. The client must (a) do something, (b) do so under certain conditions, and (c) do something at a predetermined level of accuracy. For example, a behaviorally written subgoal for TE speech might read, "The client will use appropriate valving during two-syllable phrases with 80% accuracy." The *do* portion of the subgoal defines the behavior (e.g., the client will cover the stoma sufficiently so that there is minimal to no air leakage). The *conditions* under which the behavior is to be performed are given (e.g., during two-syllable phrases such as "this time" or "watch out"). Third, the *level of accuracy* predicts the minimum performance expected (e.g., at least 80% of the behaviors will be considered correct).

Behavioral goals may be developed in short- or long-term form. The short-term goals, or subgoals, are used on a session-by-session basis to outline the sequential steps of behaviors that will lead to the long-term goals. An example of a short-term goal appears in the previous paragraph regarding the individual learning to use TE speech: "The client will use appropriate valving during two-syllable phrases with 80% accuracy." The results of the daily activities are recorded in daily therapy logs (see section on therapy logs later in this chapter). Accomplishing a sequence of short-term goals will lead to the long-term or terminal goal for the particular method of communication. Most frequently, long-term goals are written in the evaluation report to describe the anticipated outcome of therapy. An example of a long-term goal for TE speech might read, "The client will develop proficiency of TE speech for a variety of conversational interactions as demonstrated by appropriate valving, articulation, rate, and phrasing."

Thus, through evaluation and periodic reevaluation, a series of short-term goals or subgoals is identified that will systematically guide clinician and client toward the desired goal of "proficiency of speech." Because these subgoals differ in their definition and description based on the method of alaryngeal speech being used, I address short- and long-term goals of the methods individually.

The Artificial Larynx

Functional use of the artificial larynx is defined as the ability to reliably communicate information, needs, and opinions. Proficient use of the artificial larynx encompasses optimal placement of the artificial larynx, coordination of the on–off control with speaking, articulatory precision, natural rate and phrasing, and absence of distractive behaviors (e.g., klunking, stoma noise, facial grimacing) (Diedrich & Youngstrom, 1966; Doyle, 1994; Duguay, 1983; Graham, 1997;

Lerman, 1991; Salmon, 1994a, 1999; Snidecor, 1978a; see also Chapter 22 in this text). For the client who has never tried the artificial larynx, the assumed baseline for these six parameters is zero. For the client who has been introduced to the artificial larynx and has undergone formal, informal, or self-instruction previously, an evaluation to obtain baseline behaviors is advised.

A sample format for recording the client's proficiency with the artificial larynx is provided in Figure 27.2. The type and placement of the artificial larynx and the percentage of time the artificial larynx is used for communication are recorded. Six levels of production based on length of utterance are listed. The components leading to proficient use of the artificial larynx (i.e., placement, "on" control, articulation, phrasing, rate, and distracting nonverbal behaviors) are assessed beginning at two- to four-syllable phrases and sentences (Level I). Ten stimuli are presented at each level of production. If the client achieves 90% or higher accuracy for each parameter at Level I, testing progresses to Level II, and so on. If the client's performance falls below 90% accuracy for any of the six parameters at a certain level of production, testing stops. Those aspects of artificial larynx use that are performed with less than 90% accuracy become the target behaviors (subgoals) for therapy. The length of stimuli used in the therapy environment is determined by the level of production at which testing was terminated.

Esophageal Speech

The terminal goal for the esophageal speaker is to be able to produce any utterance, regardless of phonetic context or syllable length, with minimal effort and maximal intelligibility. There is considerable discussion in the literature concerning the parameters that define proficient esophageal speech (Carpenter, 1999; Doyle, 1994; Haroldson, 1999; D. E. Martin, 1994; Weinberg, 1983). Weinberg (1983) associated refined esophageal speech with the client's ability to produce longer utterances using normal rate and phrasing while maintaining a high level of intelligibility in the absence of distracting behaviors. Using the terms *intelligibility* and *proficiency,* Carpenter (1999) confirmed the need for the clinician to assess the ultimate skill level of the esophageal speaker. She considered two additional components, however, when establishing outcome measures: (a) the number and variety of contexts (e.g., home, work, church, stores) and the specific activities (e.g., one-on-one, telephone, small group, public speaking) in which esophageal speech is used and (b) the client's expressed level of satisfaction with his or her speaking skills, which either supports or challenges the clinician's assessment. If the clinician's and client's opinions do not correspond, counseling by an independent third party may be helpful.

Across the literature, the goals for teaching esophageal speech tend to fall into one of two major categories: voicing or intelligibility (Graham, 1997). Subgoals for voicing include *consistency of voicing* (air from the oral cavity must be moved into the upper esophagus and returned reliably), *esophageal quality* (the returning air vibrates the pharyngeoesophageal segment to create a full, resonant sound), and *latency* (quick and efficient intake and return of the air for speech,

SUMMARY SHEET FOR THE EVALUATION OF THE ARTIFICIAL LARYNX

Client Name _____

Clinician Name _____

Type of artificial larynx used _____

Percent of time used _____   Situations used _____

Placement: ☐ Neck   ☐ Cheek   ☐ Intraoral   ☐ Stoma

Date _____

Level of Production	Parameters					
	Placement	"On" Control	Articulation	Phrasing	Rate	Distractions
I. two- to four-syllable phrases and sentences	%	%	%	%	%	%
II. five- to seven-syllable phrases and sentences	%	%	%	%	%	%
III. eight-syllable (or more) phrases and sentences	%	%	%	%	%	%
IV. Oral reading of paragraphs	%	%	%	%	%	%
V. Structured conversation	%	%	%	%	%	%
VI. Spontaneous and extended conversation	%	%	%	%	%	%

Description of error behaviors _____

_____

_____

FIGURE 27.2. Example of summary sheet for the evaluation of the artificial larynx. From *The Clinician's Guide to Alaryngeal Speech Therapy* (p. 164), by M. S. Graham, 1997, Boston: Butterworth–Heinemann. Copyright 1997 by Butterworth–Heinemann. Reprinted with permission.

as well as duration of phonation for vowels) (Diedrich & Youngstrom, 1966; Duguay, 1999; Hyman, 1994; D. E. Martin, 1994; Shanks, 1994). The subgoals for intelligibility of speech include *articulation* (crisp articulatory contacts and the ability to make voicing contrasts), natural *rate and phrasing,* use of *intonation and stress,* appropriate *loudness,* elimination of *distractive behaviors* (e.g., stoma noise, klunking, and facial grimacing), and an increase in *desirable behaviors* (e.g., eye contact, gestures, facial expression) (Diedrich & Youngstrom, 1966; Doyle, 1994; Duguay, 1999; Hyman, 1994; D. E. Martin, 1994; Shanks, 1994).

Esophageal speech training involves the teaching of one or more methods of air intake: the injection method for obstruents (IMO), the injection method of sonorants and vowels (IMSV), and the inhalation method (IM) (see Chapter 16 in this volume for a description and discussion of these methods). All of these methods of air intake share the same subgoals for voicing and intelligibility that provide the foundation for achieving proficient esophageal speech. Examples of forms for recording the client's performance for these esophageal methods are shown in Figures 27.3 through 27.5.

In the initial stages of esophageal speech training, the methods of air intake are divided into separate activities. In Figure 27.3, an example of a summary sheet for the evaluation of the IMO, six parameters are assessed at each of 10 levels of production based on length of utterance and phonetic context. The levels of production are based on phonetic theory and research in the area of alaryngeal speech that supports a therapeutic hierarchy (Diedrich & Youngstrom, 1966; Duguay, 1999; W. N. Gardner, 1971; Hyman, 1994; Salmon, 1994b; Snidecor, 1978b; see also Chapters 16 and 22 in this text). Testing starts at the one-syllable word level using 10 stimuli that begin with unvoiced obstruents paired with mid and low vowels (e.g., /tɑp/). The criterion to move to the next level of production is set at 90% or higher accuracy of performance across six aspects of esophageal speech. Failure to achieve 90% accuracy for any parameter at that level of performance indicates the starting point for therapeutic intervention.

IMSV and IM share the same seven levels of production and phonetic context hierarchy (see discussion of methods of air intake in Chapter 16). Evaluation of these methods of air intake starts with 10 one-syllable words beginning with mid or low vowels (e.g., /əp/). The criterion to proceed to the next level on the hierarchy is set at 90% or higher accuracy for each of the features of esophageal speech (see Figure 27.4).

To facilitate client awareness and mastery of the various methods of air intake, therapy activities using IMO, IMSV, and IM are kept separate up to and including the five- to six-syllable phrase and sentence levels of production. Within each activity, 10 stimuli that highlight the appropriate phonetic context for the specific method of air intake are used. The criterion to move to the next level of the hierarchy (same subgoals but in longer utterances) is 90% accuracy across all subgoals for that level. (As an example, assume the client is learning to use IMSV and has progressed to Level IV, single-syllable words beginning with sonorants and other vowels. To advance to Level V, two-syllable words and phrases beginning with sonorants and vowels, the client must first produce at least 10 stimuli at

(*text continues on p. 679*)

SUMMARY SHEET FOR THE EVALUATION
OF THE INJECTION METHOD FOR OBSTRUENTS

Client Name _____

Clinician Name _____ Date _____

Level of Production	Parameters of Voicing			Parameters of Intelligibility		
	Consistency of Voicing	Esophageal Quality	Latency	Articulation	Rate	Distractions
Single-syllable words beginning with						
I. unvoiced obstruents + mid–low vowels	%	%	%	%	%	%
II. unvoiced obstruents + other vowels	%	%	%	%	%	%
III. voiced obstruents + mid–low vowels	%	%	%	%	%	%
IV. voiced obstruents + other vowels	%	%	%	%	%	%
V. unvoiced and voiced obstruent blends	%	%	%	%	%	%
Two-syllable words and phrases						
VI. unvoiced obstruents	%	%	%	%	%	%
VII. unvoiced and voiced obstruents	%	%	%	%	%	%
VIII. voiced obstruents	%	%	%	%	%	%
Three- to four-syllable phrases and sentences						
IX. unvoiced and voiced obstruents	%	%	%	%	%	%
Five- to six-syllable phrases and sentences						
X. unvoiced and voiced obstruents	%	%	%	%	%	%

Description of error behaviors _____

FIGURE 27.3. Example of summary sheet for the evaluation of the injection method for obstruents. From *The Clinician's Guide to Alaryngeal Speech Therapy* (p. 165), by M. S. Graham, 1997, Boston: Butterworth–Heinemann. Copyright 1997 by Butterworth–Heinemann. Reprinted with permission.

SUMMARY SHEET FOR THE EVALUATION OF THE INJECTION METHOD FOR SONORANTS AND VOWELS AND FOR THE EVALUATION OF THE INHALATION METHOD

Client Name _____

Clinician Name _____   Date _____

Level of Production	Parameters of Voicing			Parameters of Intelligibility		
	Consistency of Voicing	Esophageal Quality	Latency	Articulation	Rate	Distractions
Single-syllable words beginning with						
I. mid and low vowels	%	%	%	%	%	%
II. other vowels	%	%	%	%	%	%
III. sonorants + mid–low vowels	%	%	%	%	%	%
IV. sonorants + other vowels	%	%	%	%	%	%
Two-syllable words and phrases						
V. sonorants and vowels	%	%	%	%	%	%
Three- to four-syllable phrases and sentences						
VI. sonorants and vowels	%	%	%	%	%	%
Five- to six-syllable phrases and sentences						
VII. sonorants and vowels	%	%	%	%	%	%

Description of error behaviors _____

FIGURE 27.4. Example of summary sheet for the evaluation of the injection method for sonorants and vowels and for the evaluation of the inhalation method. From *The Clinician's Guide to Alaryngeal Speech Therapy* (p. 166), by M. S. Graham, 1997, Boston: Butterworth–Heinemann. Copyright 1997 by Butterworth–Heinemann. Reprinted with permission.

SUMMARY SHEET FOR THE EVALUATION
OF COMBINED METHODS OF ESOPHAGEAL SPEECH

Client Name _____

Clinician Name _____ Date _____

Level of Production	Articulation	Rate	Phrasing	Intonation	Loudness	Distractions
I. two- to four-syllable phrases and sentences	%	%	%	%	%	%
II. five- to seven-syllable phrases and sentences	%	%	%	%	%	%
III. eight-syllable (or more) phrases and sentences	%	%	%	%	%	%
IV. oral reading of paragraphs	%	%	%	%	%	%
V. structured conversation	%	%	%	%	%	%
VI. spontaneous and extended conversation	%	%	%	%	%	%

Description of error behaviors _____

_____

_____

FIGURE 27.5. Example of summary sheet for the evaluation of combined methods of esophageal speech. From *The Clinician's Guide to Alaryngeal Speech Therapy* (p. 167), by M. S. Graham, 1997, Boston: Butterworth–Heinemann. Copyright 1997 by Butterworth–Heinemann. Reprinted with permission.

Level IV with 90% accuracy for consistency of voicing, esophageal quality, latency, articulation, rate, and absence of distracting behaviors.) The client may experience differing levels of success among the esophageal speech methods and may advance more quickly along the therapy hierarchy for one method than another. To advance, however, to combining the methods of air intake for esophageal speech, the client must be able to perform at 90% or higher accuracy for all the parameters at the five- to six-syllable phrase and sentence level of production using (a) the injection method for obstruents, *and* (b) the injection method for sonorants and vowels *or* the inhalation method. The use of combined methods of air intake provides the esophageal speaker with the ability to produce a variety of utterances without regard to phonetic context (as occurs in normal conversational speech).

In the advanced stages of esophageal speech training, the opportunity to select and combine the various methods of air intake is presented within each therapy activity so that the individual is producing utterances that include all phonetic contexts (see Figure 27.5). Articulatory precision, natural rate, phrasing, and intonation, situation-appropriate loudness, and attention to distractive behaviors are the subgoals of advanced esophageal speech training. There are six levels of production based on length of utterance; all stimuli are composed of unrestricted phonetic context. The prerequisite behavior to advance to the next level of the hierarchy (same subgoals but in longer utterances) is 90% accuracy across all subgoals at the current level of production.

The temptation to move prematurely up the hierarchy toward longer and more complex utterances is offset by the adherence to the hierarchy and requisite performance standards. Throughout esophageal speech training, periodic reevaluation allows the speech–language pathologist to reassess the client's performance and gives direction to modifications of future therapy. The results of the reassessments are shared with the individual, the family, and other rehabilitative personnel. Respect for and observance of a sequential approach to esophageal speech training has the potential to build a strong foundation for proficient esophageal speech. Following such a regimen may reduce the extraordinary failure rate reported in the literature for esophageal speech (W. N. Gardner & Harris, 1961; Gates et al., 1982; Gilmore, 1999; King, Fowlks, & Pierson, 1968; H. Martin, 1963; Putney, 1958; Salmon, 1983; Schaefer & Johns, 1982).

Tracheoesophageal Speech

TE speech is unique to the other alaryngeal speech methods in that surgical intervention has allowed the individual to access lung air again for speech production. Voicing is achieved via the passage of air through the TE puncture (TEP) voice prosthesis into the upper esophagus, where vibration of the pharyngoesophageal (PE) segment occurs. Assuming that selection and placement of the TEP voice prosthesis have been accomplished, there are five target behaviors basic to achieving proficient TE communication: valving, articulation, rate, phrasing, and attention to nonverbal behaviors (Amster & Amster, 1994; Bosone,

1999; Doyle, 1994; Graham, 1997; Lewin, 1999; see also Chapters 17 and 18 in this text).

Six levels of production, based on the length of utterance, are evaluated using the five features for intelligibility of TE speech (see Figure 27.6). *Valving* is achieved by finger occlusion or use of a tracheostoma valve; important to either method is the ability to completely occlude the stoma so that lung air is directed through the TE voice prosthesis and into the upper esophagus. An important component of intelligibility is *articulatory precision* (particularly for plosives, fricatives, and affricates). Of interest, however, is the finding that voicing errors are the primary reason for the loss of intelligibility in TE speakers (Doyle et al., 1988; Dudley, Robbins, Singer, Blom, & Fisher, 1981). Without the selective vibratory action of the vocal folds, the TE speaker is most likely to "voice" all consonants, regardless of the intended target phoneme. *Phrasing* and *rate* are interactive in that the objective for the TE speaker is to achieve as normal a speaking rate as possible while observing natural pauses during discourse. As with the other methods of alaryngeal speech, *distractive behaviors* (e.g., stoma noise, facial grimacing, excessive bodily tension) must be reduced or eliminated. Mannerisms that accompany and enhance natural speaking, such as eye contact, pausing for emphasis, and congruent gestures and facial expressions, are encouraged.

The five parameters for TE speech are evaluated beginning with 10 two- to four-syllable phrases and sentences (Level I). A 90% or higher level of accuracy for each of the five attributes indicates the need to assess at the next level, five- to seven-syllable phrases and sentences. The client's failure to achieve competency for one or more of the parameters at a particular level assists the clinician in identifying and selecting appropriate therapy tasks.

LESSON PLANNING AND THERAPY CONSIDERATIONS

The speech–language pathologist uses the client's performance during the assessment to identify the appropriate level of production to begin alaryngeal speech training. Target behaviors are selected from the level of production at which the client failed to achieve 90% or higher accuracy (given 10 stimuli) across all of the parameters for that method of alaryngeal speech. Those parameters with accuracy ratings below 90% become the target behaviors (subgoals) within the therapy activities.

For each therapy activity within the session, the specific subgoal, the baseline performance, and the procedures to implement each activity are outlined (see examples in Tables 27.1 to 27.3). As previously discussed, the subgoal is written behaviorally: "The client will do something under certain conditions with a predetermined level of accuracy." The level of accuracy during the therapy activity is expected to be higher than the baseline performance recorded during assessment.

SUMMARY SHEET FOR THE EVALUATION OF TRACHEOESOPHAGEAL SPEECH

Client Name _____

Clinician Name _____   Date _____

Level of Production	Parameters				
	Valving	Articulation	Phrasing	Rate	Distractions
I. two- to four-syllable phrases and sentences	%	%	%	%	%
II. five- to seven-syllable phrases and sentences	%	%	%	%	%
III. eight-syllable (or more) phrases and sentences	%	%	%	%	%
IV. oral reading of paragraphs	%	%	%	%	%
V. structured conversation	%	%	%	%	%
VI. spontaneous and extended conversation	%	%	%	%	%

Description of error behaviors _____

_____

_____

FIGURE 27.6. Example of summary sheet for the evaluation of tracheoesophageal speech. From *The Clinician's Guide to Alaryngeal Speech Therapy* (p. 167), by M. S. Graham, 1997, Boston: Butterworth–Heinemann. Copyright 1997 by Butterworth–Heinemann. Reprinted with permission.

TABLE 27.1

Example of a Lesson Plan for Teaching Use of the Artificial Larynx

The subgoals (or short-term goals) for this session are placement, on–off control, and articulation. (Note that each goal is addressed in separate activities.)

Subgoal 1: Using the artificial larynx, Mr. B will use appropriate placement during two- to four-syllable phrases and sentences 80% of the time.

Rationale: Appropriate placement reduces extraneous buzzing and enhances transmission of sound, thus increasing intelligibility of speech.

Baseline: 60% appropriate placement

Procedure: The clinician will model each of 10 two- to four-syllable phrases and sentences (e.g., "That's my boy," "fifteen minutes," "Pass the salt"). Mr. B will place the artificial larynx against his neck, say the stimulus phrase, and then remove the artificial larynx from his neck. The clinician will provide feedback after each production.

Performance Summary: 80% appropriate placement with clinician assistance (guidance to the correct spot on the neck)

Subgoal 2: Using the artificial larynx, Mr. B will use appropriate on–off control during two- to four-syllable phrases and sentences 80% of the time.

Rationale: Intelligibility is increased when the on–off control is coordinated with speech so that voiced and unvoiced consonants are perceived correctly by the listener. Unnecessary buzzing is eliminated.

Baseline: 50% appropriate use of the on–off control

Procedure: The clinician will model each of 10 two- to four-syllable phrases and sentences (e.g., "Come back again," "That's my cat," "Missed my train"). Mr. B will press the "on" control as he begins the phrase and release the control at the close of the phrase. If the final sound in the phrase is unvoiced, he will release the control and mouth the final silent consonant.

Performance Summary: 80% appropriate on–off control with clinician-generated cues (e.g., "Remember to turn the artificial larynx off as you say the final /t/ in the word 'cat.'")

Subgoal 3: Using the artificial larynx, Mr. B will use articulatory precision during two- to four-syllable phrases and sentences 80% of the time.

Rationale: Clear, well-articulated sounds increase the intelligibility of speech.

Baseline: 70% articulatory precision

Procedure: The clinician will model each of 10 two- to four-syllable phrases and sentences (e.g., "Before she left," "kings and queens," "mix and match"). Mr. B will first mouth the phrase, then use the artificial larynx to add sound.

Performance Summary: 80% articulatory precision when preceded by mouthing the sounds and then adding the vibration of the artificial larynx

Baseline

The baseline represents the client's performance during the most recent evaluation or during a previous therapy session. The baseline measure serves as a reference point by which to compare the client's performance in the upcoming session(s). Increased accuracy of performance may indeed confirm the appropriateness of the therapeutic intervention. No change in behavior may signal the need to alter the treatment strategy.

TABLE 27.2

Example of a Lesson Plan for Teaching Esophageal Speech

The individual is learning (a) the injection method for obstruents (IMO) and (b) the injection method for sonorants and vowels (IMSV). Subgoals for esophageal speech training include consistency of voicing, quality of voicing, latency, articulation, rate, and nonverbal behaviors. Note that at the lower levels of the hierarchy, the two methods of air intake are addressed in separate activities.

Subgoal 1: Using the IMO, Mrs. K will achieve consistency of voicing during one-syllable words beginning with voiced obstruents plus mid and low vowels 80% of the time.

Rationale: Pairing mid and low vowels with voiced obstruents facilitates production.

Baseline: 70% consistency of voicing

Procedure: The clinician will model each of 10 one-syllable words beginning with voiced obstruents plus mid and low vowels (e.g., "vote," "board," "dark"). Mrs. K will repeat each word.

Performance Summary: 80% consistency of voicing when reminded to "say the word vigorously" so as to move the air posteriorly

Subgoal 2: Using the IMSV, Mrs. K will demonstrate appropriate latency during the production of one-syllable words beginning with sonorants plus mid and low vowels 80% of the time.

Rationale: The ability to inject air and then retrieve the air from the upper esophagus in a timely manner is key to the efficiency of esophageal speech production.

Baseline: 70% appropriate latency

Procedure: The clinician will model each of 10 one-syllable words beginning with sonorants plus mid and low vowels (e.g., "more," "lunch," "rough"). Mrs. K will repeat each word.

Performance Summary: 90% appropriate latency. Mrs. K. will repeat this activity next week. If she achieves 90% appropriate latency again, she is ready to move to the next level of stimuli.

Subgoal 3: Using the IMSV, Mrs. K will reduce stoma noise during the production of one-syllable words beginning with sonorants plus mid and low vowels to 20% of the time.

Rationale: Stoma noise represents forceful exhalation, is distracting to the listener, interferes with intelligibility, and fatigues the alaryngeal speaker.

Baseline: 80% occurrence of stoma noise

Procedure: The clinician will model each of 10 one-syllable words beginning with sonorants plus mid and low vowels (e.g., "young," "wash," "name"). Mrs. K will repeat each word.

Performance Summary: 30% occurrence of stoma noise. Mrs. K responded to the clinician's suggestion to "tighten your abdomen, but do not push" during speech production.

For example, as reflected in the lesson plan in Table 27.1, during testing for use of the artificial larynx, Mr. B achieved 60% accuracy for placement of the artificial larynx at Level I (two- to four-syllable phrases and sentences). The first therapy activity will target appropriate placement using stimuli composed of two- to four-syllable phrases and sentences. The baseline for the activity is 60%

TABLE 27.3

Example of a Lesson Plan for Teaching Tracheoesophageal (TE) Speech

---

The subgoals (or short-term goals) for this session are valving, articulation, rate, phrasing, and nonverbal behaviors. (Note that each of the subgoals is addressed in separate activities.)

Goal 1: Using TE speech, Mr. W will use appropriate valving during five- to seven-syllable phrases and sentences 80% of the time.

Rationale: An airtight seal at the stoma redirects lung air through the prosthesis and into the esophagus for TE speech. Air leakage at the stoma results in stoma noise.

Baseline: 70% appropriate valving

Procedure: The clinician will model 10 five- to seven-syllable phrases and sentences (e.g., "fourth Monday of the month," "shut off the alarm," "best wishes for your birthday"). Mr. W will use finger occlusion of the stoma and repeat the stimulus.

Performance Summary: 80% appropriate valving while using mirror feedback

Goal 2: Using TE speech, Mr. W will use appropriate articulation during five- to seven-syllable phrases and sentences 80% of the time.

Rationale: Clear, well-articulated sounds increase the intelligibility of speech.

Baseline: 70% appropriate articulation

Procedure: The clinician will model 10 five- to seven-syllable phrases and sentences (e.g., "Please call me back tonight," "three for a dollar," "Thank you for your patience"). Mr. W will repeat each phrase.

Performance Summary: 80% appropriate articulation

---

accuracy at Level I. The client's predicted performance is 80% accuracy because the clinician will provide a model and feedback for each production. Mr. B's actual performance in the therapy task will be compared to his baseline to support or challenge the effectiveness of the therapeutic intervention.

Stimuli

Stimuli for each therapy activity are selected based on the targeted method of alaryngeal speech, the length of utterance, and the phonetic context. For ease of scoring, 10 stimuli compose a "set" for the therapy activity. LaPointe's (1985) Base-10 Response Form or an activity score sheet similar to the one shown in Chapter 16 of this text may be used. Facilitating cues and the method of monitoring are noted on the form.

Instruction and Feedback

At each level of the therapy hierarchy, the clinician's primary purpose is to provide instruction and feedback as the client learns to produce the target behaviors and to self-monitor and self-correct effectively. According to Brookshire (1997), instruction involves explaining the purpose of the activity and telling (or showing) the client what he or she is to do in the task. As with all therapeutic interventions, an explanation of the purpose of the therapy activity by the clinician may enhance client motivation. The informed client is more likely to cooperate and feel part of the rehabilitation program when he or she understands the reason for the activity (Doyle, 1994; Gilmore, 1994; see also Chapter 22 in this text). Feedback informs the individual about the accuracy of his or her behavior, either during or following the performance of the task.

Knowledge of performance is crucial to motor learning (Rosenbaum, 1991; Singer, 1980), and much of alaryngeal speech training involves motor performance. This includes oral movements for articulatory precision, placement of the artificial larynx, tongue movements required for air intake during esophageal speech, and finger positioning over the stoma to achieve TE speech. Instrumental feedback is particularly efficient for targeting certain behaviors (e.g., the mirror provides immediate information about eye contact, oral openness, or facial grimacing); a hand on the abdomen or in front of the stoma monitors for forceful exhalations, whereas a volume unit (VU) meter or the Visi-Pitch (from Kay Elemetrics, Lincoln Park, NJ) registers loudness levels. Rather than informing the client about his or her *completed* performance, instrumental feedback facilitates adjustments during the time of the performance. Feedback has the potential to be both motivational and psychologically reinforcing. Feedback during therapy is most effective when provided immediately and is based on the selected therapy goal (Yorkston, Beukelman, & Bell, 1988). The more specific the content of the analysis is, the more influence the feedback may have on subsequent responses made by the individual. Sources of feedback may also include family, friends, strangers, and other alaryngeal speakers. For some individuals, the empathetic comments of a fellow alaryngeal speaker may have a greater impact on the individual than clinician-provided feedback.

Discovery learning, in which the client determines how best to achieve the subgoals, is also an important component of therapy. According to Singer (1980), Wertz, LaPointe, and Rosenbek (1984), and Duffy (1995), self-learning may lead to better retention and generalization than learning that is highly prompted. Obviously, a balance must exist between the clinician-generated instruction and the client-generated discovery mode; however, initial instruction is required to define the subgoal and demonstrate the procedure to accomplish the task. At least for the introduction of a new subgoal, immediate, accurate, and frequent clinician-generated feedback is necessary to guide the client's performance toward the target behavior. As soon as the individual understands the task, clinician-generated instruction is faded and the client is encouraged to make decisions about his or her performance. Ultimately, the client is expected to self-monitor and self-correct appropriately within the therapy session, as well as to generalize these skills to various environmental situations.

Consistent and Variable Practice

According to Duffy (1995), both consistent and variable practice have value in the learning process. Consistent practice, or repetition of a single task, is beneficial for the stabilization of a newly learned behavior. The beginning esophageal speaker, for example, is limited in his or her capacity to inject or inhale air for speech production. Consistency of voicing may be achieved only through direct, highly structured practice involving repeated trials of moving the air back and retrieving it for the production of single-syllable words beginning with vowels (Berlin, 1963; Doyle, 1994; Graham, 1997; Snidecor, 1978b; Weinberg, 1983).

Variable practice expands the task to a broader range of related stimuli. For example, the intermediate esophageal speaker may practice consistency of voicing for a variety of words ranging in length from one- to three-syllable words and beginning with vowels or consonants. Schmidt and Bjork (1992) asserted that increasing task variability in the early stages of therapy tends to decrease performance; however, at the more advanced levels of therapy, variable practice results in better retention and generalization to other contexts. With repeated practice, the client's speech tends to increase in efficiency and naturalness, particularly if the stimuli to address the target goal are varied.

Speed Versus Accuracy

Regardless of the alaryngeal speech method being addressed, emphasis on increasing the rate of speech tends to reduce accuracy, and emphasis on accuracy tends to reduce the rate of speech (Cooper, 1977; Hoops & Noll, 1969; D. E. Martin, 1994; Shipp, 1967; Singer, 1980; Wertz et al., 1984). This suggests that, at least during the acquisition of the foundation behaviors essential to proficient alaryngeal speech, accuracy takes precedence over speed. When the rate of speech exceeds the speaker's current level of proficiency or ignores the prosodic elements of phrasing, error behavior results. Increasing the rate of speech without attention to motor control for articulatory precision almost always has a negative effect on intelligibility (Casper & Colton, 1998; Graham, 1997).

Elements of the Therapy Session

Frequency of Sessions

While still hospitalized, the clinician may see the individual as often as twice per day to establish and support one or more of the alaryngeal speech methods (Salmon, 1999). Economic factors aside, therapy sessions should be frequent, especially in the initial stages of rehabilitation. Several short practice sessions per day tend to be more effective than one or two extended practice periods (Casper & Colton, 1998; Duguay, 1999; Keith & Thomas, 1996; Salmon, 1999). In situations where such frequency cannot or does not occur, instruction for home practice supported by family members, friends, or other alaryngeal speakers is an important option (Diedrich & Youngstrom, 1966; Gilmore, 1994).

Task Hierarchy

There is wide support within clinical circles for a hierarchical organization of the session; that is, the clinician begins each session with easy and familiar tasks, advances to more challenging tasks, and closes with tasks that ensure success (Brookshire, 1972, 1976, 1997; B. Gardner & Brookshire, 1972; Graham, 1997; Rosenbek & LaPointe, 1985). Brookshire (1997) has specifically labeled these tasks the accommodation, work, cool-down, and good-bye segments. For the *accommodation* segment, the level of stimuli is simple enough that the client's performance is virtually error free. In alaryngeal speech rehabilitation, relaxation, oral-motor exercises, or repetitive drills using consonant–vowel arrangements serve as warm-ups for the more difficult tasks to follow. The *work* segment is composed of tasks that are more challenging to the client. This is the opportunity for the client to learn new behaviors. The clinician explains the task; describes and, if possible, demonstrates the target behavior; and invites the client to perform the task. The clinician provides feedback and records the performance. In the *cool-down* segment, the client engages in behaviors that are designed to elicit highly successful performance. Most often, these tasks are then assigned for carryover practice in the outside environment. In the closing, or *good-bye* segment, the clinician and client discuss the plans for the next session.

Anticipated Accuracy of Performance

Activities that result in performance levels that fall below 50% accuracy subject the individual to fatigue, discouragement, poor motivation, and a low rate of learning. There is good support in the literature for providing a hierarchical structure to therapy tasks so that the individual's performance level is maintained between 60% and 80% accuracy (Brookshire, 1972, 1997). At a rate of 6 to 8 correct behaviors for every 10 stimuli presented, the client experiences success while still being challenged sufficiently by the task for learning to occur.

A success rate of 90% or higher on the same or similar tasks over several sessions is a signal that the client is ready to move to the next level of difficulty (Berlin, 1963; Brookshire, 1972, 1997; W. N. Gardner, 1971; Graham, 1997; LaPointe, 1977; Lerman, 1991; Weinberg, 1983). Some clinicians (e.g., Doyle, 1994; Porch, 1981; Singer, 1980; Wertz et al., 1984) advocate training beyond 90% accuracy, with the explanation that overlearning may (a) lead to better retention of the target behavior and (b) potentially increase generalization of the target behavior to settings and activities beyond the clinical environment.

Individual Versus Group Therapy

In the beginning stages of teaching the various methods of alaryngeal speech, individual instruction is beneficial for the purposes of "focusing on specific aspects of performance, the opportunity to obtain a maximum number of responses, and the opportunity to alter treatment activities quickly as a function of response adequacy" (Duffy, 1995, p. 385). Furthermore, the one-on-one therapy situation may offer the opportunity for counseling about topics specific to the individual's situation (e.g., physical, psychological, social, and economic concerns).

Group therapy, on the other hand, provides individuals the opportunity to observe others and practice skills and strategies associated with various methods of alaryngeal speech. Stone and Hamilton (1986) referred to the group setting as "a 'social learning laboratory' in which clients can develop attending behavior, listening skills, turn-taking rather than interrupting a speaker, augmentation of body language, and alternative ways of expressing unpopular or threatening ideas" (p. 53).

From a hierarchical perspective, group therapy represents the transitional stage between individual therapy and the outside communication environment (Darvill, 1983; Rollin, 1987). Interactions within the group allow the alaryngeal speaker to practice communicative responsibility, role-play in preparation for carryover into the environment, and provide and receive feedback that is beneficial to speech improvement. The group situation may provide interactive support among the individuals and their families as they share information, experiences, successes, and failures related to having survived head and neck cancer. In the group environment, a variety of functions is served—education, speech improvement, social interaction, and support–counseling (Doyle, 1994; Graham, 1997; Lerman, 1999; Murphy, 1963). All of these functions may serve to increase the chance of successful rehabilitation.

Group therapy must also be lauded for its proven cost-effectiveness (Lerman, 1999; Toseland & Siporin, 1986). The fact that a number of individuals are able to receive the same information and instruction within the same time frame supports efficiency of treatment. With the professional health care system's demand for efficient, low-cost patient management, group therapy may be a viable option for alaryngeal speech rehabilitation.

THERAPY LOGS

Integral to accountability in alaryngeal speech rehabilitation is the maintenance of written records of significant interactions with the client, family members, and members of the professional rehabilitation team. These documents are subject to scrutiny by physicians, nursing personnel, insurance and Medicare examiners, health care–accrediting reviewers, and other members of the rehabilitation team. During litigation, if the client's medical records are subpoenaed, the documents serve as legal representations of the rehabilitative services performed. Because these written records serve a number of crucial roles in the rehabilitation of the client, the need for accuracy and efficiency in documentation is underscored.

Maintaining an organized and accurate written account of the client's performance during therapy is an important clinical responsibility (Brookshire, 1997; Graham, 1997; D. E. Martin, 1994). Following every therapy session, the client's performance is summarized and a written entry is made in ink, dated, and signed by the attending speech–language pathologist. Most clinicians prefer to use the SOAP format to write their notes: S = subjective information about the client (e.g., appearance, feelings, attitude); O = objective information related to goals and anticipated performance; A = activities or descriptions of stimuli and procedures used in the session, with client performance expressed in percentages or ratios; P = plans for the next session. In addition to the documentation of therapy sessions, the date and substance of telephone calls or conferences with the client, family members, or rehabilitation team members are noted. Consistent attention to the recording of dates, interactions with family and professionals, therapy procedures and results, and recommendations eliminates the frustration of trying to recall the information at a later date.

REPORT WRITING

Another avenue for recording the events of the alaryngeal speech rehabilitation process is report writing. Formal reports are used to summarize the intake evaluation, periodic reevaluations, therapy interactions and performance, and therapy logs into a cohesive representation of the particular client's communicative–rehabilitative experience.

Most often, the professional setting dictates a specific report writing protocol. At some facilities, an initial and final report are generated for each client; in other sites, periodic reevaluations are accompanied by formal reports as well. A sample therapy report outline is shown in Figure 27.7. Because not every alaryngeal speaker uses all three methods of communication, only the applicable sections are included in the individual's report.

TERMINATION OF THERAPY

The clinician will find little support in the literature regarding the criteria for terminating alaryngeal speech training. Although data are available concerning the characteristics of good or superior alaryngeal speakers (Berlin, 1963, 1965; Diedrich & Youngstrom, 1966; Filter & Hyman, 1975; Haroldson, 1999; Hoops & Guzek, 1974; Hoops & Noll, 1969; D. E. Martin, 1994; Robbins et al., 1984; Rothman, 1978; Salmon, 1994a, 1994b; Shipp, 1967; Snidecor & Curry, 1959), there are no established guidelines regarding the minimum skills needed for functional communication using alaryngeal speech methods (Carpenter, 1999).

Carpenter (1999) listed three components for establishing outcome measures:

> (1) the ultimate skill level, (2) application of the skill, and (3) satisfaction with the skill. The clinician is responsible for assessing the first component; the client evaluates the third. Both clinician and client contribute to measurement of the intermediate factor, use of the skill. (p. 71)

Using a hierarchical arrangement of goals and stimuli for the various alaryngeal speech modes, the clinician can determine, through periodic evaluation of the

THERAPY REPORT OUTLINE

Name _____   Physician _____

Address _____   Address _____

Telephone _____   Telephone _____

Date of Birth _____   Date of Surgery _____

Date of Clinic Entrance _____   Clinician _____

Date of Report _____

I. Background Information
II. Results of Evaluation
   A. Artificial Larynx
      1. Type of artificial larynx used; percent of time used; situations used
      2. Placement
      3. Coordination of the "on" control with speaking
      4. Articulation
      5. Rate and phrasing
      6. Nonverbal behaviors
   B. Esophageal Speech
      1. Method(s) of air intake used
      2. Voicing
         a. Consistency of voicing
         b. Esophageal quality
         c. Latency
      3. Intelligibility
         a. Articulation
         b. Nonverbal behaviors
         c. Rate and phrasing
         d. Intonation
         e. Loudness
   C. Tracheoesophageal Speech
      1. Valving
      2. Articulation
      3. Phrasing
      4. Rate
      5. Nonverbal behaviors
III. Goals
   A. Artificial larynx
   B. Esophageal speech
   C. Tracheoesophageal speech
IV. Progress
   A. Artificial larynx
   B. Esophageal speech
   C. Tracheoesophageal speech
V. Recommendations

FIGURE 27.7. Therapy report outline. From *The Clinician's Guide to Alaryngeal Speech Therapy* (p. 178), by M. S. Graham, 1997, Boston: Butterworth-Heinemann. Copyright 1997 by Butterworth-Heinemann. Reprinted with permission.

client's performance, the level of proficiency that has been met. The questions the clinician must ask are (a) Is this level of alaryngeal speech sufficient to meet the communication demands in this individual's daily environment? (b) Is this individual capable of achieving higher levels of alaryngeal speech? (c) Or are there medical, surgical, motivational, situational, cognitive, or psychological factors that may interfere with further progress? and (d) Is the investment of time, cost, and effort involved in helping this client to reach the next level of communication competence justified? These questions address issues that are basic to the success of the rehabilitation program.

Carpenter's (1999) second component is the client's facility in application of the alaryngeal speech skills. Questions to consider in assessing this area include these: (a) How successful is the client in communicating needs, opinions, and information in various settings and with different individuals or groups? (b) Is the client able to compensate in certain situations by using alternate or combined methods of communication? and (c) Is the client independently and consistently practicing good self-monitoring and self-correction skills?

The third area posed by Carpenter (1999) pertains to the individual's personal satisfaction with the skill. The clinician needs to ask these questions: (a) Does the alaryngeal speaker feel that he or she can engage in conversation regardless of the situation or listener? (b) How does the individual rate his or her level of communication effectiveness? (c) What are the client's expectations of the alaryngeal speech mode? and (d) Is the individual satisfied with his or her current level of alaryngeal speech?

When the results of reevaluation reveal that the client has reached a plateau or is making minimal progress, the determination of whether to continue therapy is based on the summation of all factors considered. Are there identifiable factors that can be changed, altered, improved, added, or eliminated so as to refocus the rehabilitation efforts? If not, then the outcome of the discussion may be that the therapeutic relationship is no longer viable. Carpenter (1999) suggested that the client may be the one who discontinues treatment for reasons of satisfaction or discontent with the progress achieved to date. "If this seems to be an informed, realistic decision on the client's part, the clinician is unlikely to object; ideally, this is the stopping point the clinician would choose as well" (Carpenter, 1999, p. 75). One must be mindful, however, of monitoring broader health issues for each individual (Agrawal, deSilva, Buckley, & Schuller, 2004; Doyle & White, 2004).

If the client is making progress and is interested in continuing treatment but the financial resources have been depleted, alternative services are pursued. A local New Voice Club or Lost Chord Club, the International Association of Laryngectomees, or a hospital- or university-based alaryngeal speech clinic are considerations (Graham, 1997; Haroldson, 1999; Lerman, 1999; Minear & Lucente, 1979). In lieu of providing individual therapy, the speech–language pathologist could initiate a group situation wherein the members share the cost of the therapy hour. As previously discussed in this chapter, group therapy offers the client a unique setting in which to (a) observe, listen, learn, and practice alaryngeal speech methods, and (b) offer support and be supported (Graham, 1997; Stone & Hamilton, 1986).

SUMMARY

This chapter has addressed alaryngeal speech rehabilitation with respect for the significant changes in health care that are having a profound effect on the members of adult rehabilitation teams. Speech–language pathologists are being held accountable for what they do professionally. Clinicians are being asked to document and defend their diagnostic and therapeutic techniques and to demonstrate that what they do makes a difference, not only in the individual's functional communication skills, but in his or her vocational, social, and cultural readjustments. Quality-of-life studies have underscored the idea that as communication skills increase, opportunities for the individual to make adjustments for the disability, improve social participation, and integrate into the community are enhanced (Blood, Luther, & Stemple, 1992; Brooks & Heath, 1993; Doyle, 1994; Flanagan, 1982; Kerr, 1977; O'Keefe, 1996). The future success of the profession relies on the ability of speech–language pathologists to collect and publish data supporting the idea that their evaluation and treatment methods make a significant difference in the lives of the individuals served.

REFERENCES

Agrawal, A., deSilva, B. W., Buckley B. M., & Schuller, D. E. (2004). Role of the physician versus the patient in the detection of recurrent disease following treatment for head and neck cancer. *Laryngoscope, 114,* 232–235.

American Speech-Language-Hearing Association, (1995). *Summaries of treatment efficacy technical papers.* Rockville, MD: Author.

Amster, W. W., & Amster, J. B. (1994). Developing effective communication after laryngectomy. In R. L. Keith & F. L. Darley (Eds.), *Laryngectomee rehabilitation* (3rd ed., pp. 263–281). Austin, TX: PRO-ED.

Barton, J., & Hejna, R. (1963). Factors associated with success or nonsuccess in acquisition of esophageal speech. *Journal of the Speech and Hearing Association (Virginia), 4,* 19–20.

Baum, H. (1998). Overview, definitions, and goals for ASHA's treatment outcomes and clinical trials activities (What difference do outcome data make to you?). *Language, Speech, and Hearing Services in Schools, 29,* 246–249.

Bennett, S., & Weinberg, B. (1973). Acceptability ratings of normal, esophageal, and artificial larynx speech. *Journal of Speech and Hearing Research, 16,* 608–615.

Berlin, C. I. (1963). Clinical measurement of esophageal speech: 1. Methodology and curves of skill acquisition. *Journal of Speech and Hearing Disorders, 28,* 42–51.

Berlin, C. I. (1965). Clinical measurement of esophageal speech: 3. Performance of nonbiased groups. *Journal of Speech and Hearing Disorders, 30,* 174–183.

Berry, W. R. (1978). Attitudes of speech pathologists and otolaryngologists about artificial larynges. In S. J. Salmon & L. P. Goldstein (Eds.), *The artificial larynx handbook* (pp. 35–41). New York: Grune & Stratton.

Blood, G. W., Luther, A. R., & Stemple, J. C. (1992). Coping and adjustment in alaryngeal speakers. *American Journal of Speech–Language Pathology, 1,* 63–69.

Bosone, Z. T. (1994). Tracheoesophageal fistulization/puncture for voice restoration: Presurgical considerations and troubleshooting procedures. In R. L. Keith & F. L. Darley (Eds.), *Laryngectomee rehabilitation* (3rd ed., pp. 359–381). Austin, TX: PRO-ED.

Bosone, Z. T. (1999). Tracheoesophageal speech: Treatment considerations before and after surgery. In S. J. Salmon (Ed.), *Alaryngeal speech rehabilitation* (2nd ed., pp. 105–150). Austin, TX: PRO-ED.

Brooks, W. D., & Heath, R. W. (1993). *Speech communication* (7th ed.). Madison, WI: Brown & Benchmark.

Brookshire, R. H. (1972). Effects of task difficulty on the naming performance of aphasic subjects. *Journal of Speech and Hearing Research, 15,* 551.

Brookshire, R. H. (1976). Effects of task difficulty on sentence comprehension performance of aphasic subjects. *Journal of Communication Disorders, 9,* 167.

Brookshire, R. H. (1997). *Introduction to neurogenic communication disorders* (5th ed.). Mosby-Year Book.

Carpenter, M. A. (1999). Treatment decisions in alaryngeal speech. In S. J. Salmon (Ed.), *Alaryngeal speech rehabilitation: For clinicians by clinicians* (2nd ed., pp. 55–77). Austin, TX: PRO-ED.

Casper, J. K., & Colton, R. H. (1998). *Clinical manual for laryngectomy and head/neck cancer rehabilitation* (2nd ed.). San Diego: Singular.

Connor, N. P., Hamlet, S. L., & Joyce, J. C. (1985). Acoustic and physiologic correlates of the voicing distinction in esophageal speech. *Journal of Speech and Hearing Disorders, 50,* 378–384.

Cooper, M. (1977). *Modern techniques of vocal rehabilitation.* Springfield, IL: Thomas.

Darvill, G. (1983). Rehabilitation—Not just voice. In Y. Edels (Ed.), *Laryngectomy: Diagnosis to rehabilitation* (pp. 192–217). Rockville, MD: Aspen.

Diedrich, W. M., & Youngstrom, K. A. (1966). *Alaryngeal speech.* Springfield, IL: Thomas.

Doyle, P. C. (1994). *Foundations of voice and speech rehabilitation following laryngeal cancer.* San Diego: Singular.

Doyle, P. C., Danhauer, J. L., & Reed, C. G. (1988). Listeners' perceptions of consonants produced by esophageal and tracheoesophageal talkers. *Journal of Speech and Hearing Disorders, 53,* 400–407.

Doyle, P. C., & Haaf, R. G. (1989). Perception of pre-vocalic and post-vocalic consonants produced by tracheoesophageal speakers. *Journal of Otolaryngology, 18,* 350–353.

Doyle, P. C., & White, H. D. (2004, May). *Use of the Rotterdam Symptom Checklist in laryngectomized men and women.* Paper presented at the annual conference of the Canadian Association of Speech–Language Pathologists and Audiologists, Ottawa, Ontario.

Dudley, B. L., Robbins, J. A., Singer, M. I., Blom, E. D., & Fisher, H. B. (1981, November). *An intelligibility study of tracheoesophageal speech.* Paper presented at the annual convention of the American Speech-Language-Hearing Association, Los Angeles.

Duffy, J. R. (1995). *Motor speech disorders: Substrates, differential diagnosis, and management.* St. Louis, MO: Mosby.

Duguay, M. J. (1978). Why not both? In S. J. Salmon & L. P. Goldstein (Eds.), *The artificial larynx handbook* (pp. 3–15). New York: Grune & Stratton.

Duguay, M. J. (1983). Teaching use of an artificial larynx. In W. H. Perkins (Ed.), *Voice disorders* (pp. 127–135). New York: Thieme-Stratton.

Duguay, M. J. (1999). Esophageal speech training: The initial phase. In S. J. Salmon (Ed.), *Alaryngeal speech rehabilitation: For clinicians by clinicians* (2nd ed., pp. 165–201). Austin, TX: PRO-ED.

Fagan, J. J., Lentin, R., Oyarzabal, M. F., Isaacs, S., & Sellars, S. L. (2002). Tracheoesophageal speech in a developing world community. *Archives of Otolaryngology—Head and Neck Surgery, 128,* 50–53.

Filter, M. D., & Hyman, M. (1975). Relationship of acoustic parameters and perceptual ratings of esophageal speech. *Perceptual and Motor Skills, 40,* 63–68.

Flanagan, J. C. (1982). Measurement of quality of life: Current state of the art. *Archives of Physical Medicine and Rehabilitation, 63,* 56–59.

Gallagher, T. (1998). National initiatives in outcomes measurement. In C. Frattalli (Ed.), *Outcomes measurement in speech–language pathology* (pp. 527–557). New York: Thieme Medical.

Gandour, J., & Weinberg, B. (1983). Perception of intonational contrasts in alaryngeal speech. *Journal of Speech and Hearing Research, 26,* 142–148.

Gardner, B., & Brookshire, R. H. (1972). Effects of unisensory and multisensory presentation of stimuli upon naming by aphasic patients. *Language and Speech, 15,* 342.

Gardner, W. N. (1971). *Laryngectomee speech and rehabilitation.* Springfield, IL: Thomas.

Gardner, W. N., & Harris, H. E. (1961). Aids and devices for laryngectomees. *Archives of Otolaryngology, 73,* 145–152.

Gates, G. A., Ryan, W., Cooper, J. C., Lawlis, G. F., Cantu, E., Hayashi, T., Lauder, E., Welch, R. W., & Hearne, E. (1982). Current status of laryngectomee rehabilitation: 1. Results of therapy. *American Journal of Otolaryngology, 3,* 1–7.

Gilmore, S. I. (1994). The physical, social, occupational, and psychological concomitants of laryngectomy. In R. L. Keith & F. L. Darley (Eds.), *Laryngectomee rehabilitation* (3rd ed., pp. 395–486). Austin, TX: PRO-ED.

Gilmore, S. I. (1999). Failure in acquiring esophageal speech. In S. J. Salmon (Ed.), *Alaryngeal speech rehabilitation: For clinicians by clinicians* (2nd ed., pp. 221–268). Austin, TX: PRO-ED.

Graham, M. S. (1997). *The clinician's guide to alaryngeal speech therapy.* Boston: Butterworth-Heinemann.

Haroldson, S. K. (1999). Toward advancing esophageal communication. In S. J. Salmon (Ed.), *Alaryngeal speech rehabilitation: For clinicians by clinicians* (2nd ed., pp. 203–219). Austin, TX: PRO-ED.

Hoops, H. R., & Guzek, T. J. (1974). The relationship of rate and phrasing to esophageal speech proficiency. *Archives of Otolaryngology, 100,* 190–193.

Hoops, H. R., & Noll, J. D. (1969). Relationship of selected acoustic variables to judgments of esophageal speech. *Journal of Communication Disorders, 2,* 1–13.

Hyman, M. (1955). An experimental study of artificial-larynx and esophageal speech. *Journal of Speech and Hearing Disorders, 20,* 291–299.

Hyman, M. (1994). The intermediate stage of teaching alaryngeal speech. In R. L. Keith & F. L. Darley (Eds.), *Laryngectomee rehabilitation* (3rd ed., pp. 309–321). Austin, TX: PRO-ED.

Johnston, M., & Granger, C. (1994). Outcomes research in medical rehabilitation. *American Journal of Physical Medicine & Rehabilitation, 73*(4), 296–302.

Keith, R. L., & Thomas, J. E. (1996). *A handbook for the laryngectomee* (4th ed.). Austin, TX: PRO-ED.

Kerr, N. (1977). Understanding the process of adjustment to disability. In J. Stubbins (Ed.), *Social and psychological aspects of disability: A handbook for practitioners* (pp. 305–316). Baltimore: University Park Press.

King, P. S., Fowlks, E. W., & Pierson, G. A. (1968). Rehabilitation and adaptation of laryngectomy patients. *American Journal of Physical Medicine, 47,* 192–203.

LaPointe, L. L. (1977). Base-10 programmed stimulation: Task specification, scoring, and plotting performance in aphasia therapy. *Journal of Speech and Hearing Disorders, 42,* 90–105.

LaPointe, L. L. (1985). Aphasia therapy: Some principles and strategies for treatment. In D. F. Johns (Ed.), *Clinical management of neurogenic communicative disorders* (2nd ed., pp. 179–241). Boston: Little, Brown.

Lerman, J. W. (1991). The artificial larynx. In S. J. Salmon & K. H. Mount (Eds.), *Alaryngeal speech rehabilitation* (pp. 27–45). Austin, TX: PRO-ED.

Lerman, J. W. (1999). Group therapy for laryngectomees. In S. J. Salmon (Ed.), *Alaryngeal speech rehabilitation: For clinicians by clinicians* (2nd ed., pp. 269–284). Austin, TX: PRO-ED.

Lewin, J. S. (1999). Tracheoesophageal communication: Beyond traditional speech treatment. In S. J. Salmon (Ed.), *Alaryngeal speech rehabilitation: For clinicians by clinicians* (2nd ed., pp. 151–163). Austin, TX: PRO-ED.

Martin, D. E. (1994). Evaluating esophageal speech development and proficiency. In R. L. Keith & F. L. Darley (Eds.), *Laryngectomee rehabilitation* (3rd ed., pp. 331–349). Austin, TX: PRO-ED.

Martin, H. (1963). Rehabilitation of the laryngectomee. *Cancer, 16,* 823–841.

Minear, D., & Lucente, F. D. (1979). Current attitudes of laryngectomy patients. *Laryngoscope, 89,* 1061–1065.

Murphy, G. (1963). Group psychotherapy in our society. In M. Rosenbaum & M. Berger (Eds.), *Group psychotherapy and group function: Selected readings* (pp. 33–41). New York: Basic Books.

O'Keefe, B. M. (1996). Communication disorders: Just minor inconveniences? In R. Renwick, I. Brown, & M. Nagler (Eds.), *Quality of life in health promotion and rehabilitation: Conceptual approaches, issues and applications.* Thousand Oaks, CA: Sage.

Palmer, A. D., & Graham, M. S. (2004). The relationship between communication and quality of life in alaryngeal speakers. *Journal of Speech–Language Pathology and Audiology, 28,* 3–24.

Pietranton, A., & Baum, H. (1995). Collecting outcome data: Existing tools, preliminary data, future directions. *Asha,* 36–38.

Porch, B. E. (1981). Therapy subsequent to the PICA. In R. Chapey, (Ed.), *Language intervention strategies in adult aphasia,* (2nd ed., pp. 283–296). Baltimore: Williams & Wilkins.

Putney, E. J. (1958). Rehabilitation of the post-laryngectomized patient. *Annals of Otology, Rhinology and Laryngology, 67,* 544–549.

Robbins, J. (1984). Acoustic differentiation of laryngeal, esophageal, and tracheoesophageal speech. *Journal of Speech and Hearing Research, 27,* 577–585.

Robbins, J. A., Christensen, J. C., & Kempster, G. (1986). Characteristics of speech production after tracheoesophageal puncture: Voice onset time and vowel duration. *Journal of Speech and Hearing Research, 29,* 499–504.

Robbins, J., Fisher, H. B., Blom, E. D., & Singer, M. L. (1984). A comparative acoustic study of normal, esophageal, and tracheoesophageal speech production. *Journal of Speech and Hearing Disorders, 49,* 202–210.

Robe, E. Y., Moore, P., Andrews, A. H., & Holinger, P. H. (1956). A study of the role of certain factors in the development of speech after laryngectomy: 1. Type of operation. *Laryngoscope, 66,* 173–186.

Rollin, W. J. (1987). *The psychology of communication disorders in individuals and their families.* Englewood Cliffs, NJ: Prentice Hall.

Rosenbaum, D. A. (1991). *Human motor control.* San Diego: Academic Press.

Rosenbek, J. C., & LaPointe, L. L. (1985). The dysarthrias: Description, diagnosis, and treatment. In D. F. Johns (Ed.), *Clinical management of neurogenic communicative disorders* (2nd ed., pp. 97–152). Boston: Little, Brown.

Rothman, H. B. (1978). Analyzing artificial electronic larynx speech. In S. J. Salmon & L. P. Goldstein (Eds.), *The artificial larynx handbook* (pp. 87–111). New York: Grune & Stratton.

Salmon, S. J. (1983). Artificial larynx speech: A viable means of alaryngeal communication. In Y. Edels (Ed.), *Laryngectomy: Diagnosis to rehabilitation* (pp. 142–162). Rockville, MD: Aspen.

Salmon, S. J. (1994a). Artificial larynxes: Teaching their use. In R. L. Keith & F. L. Darley (Eds.), *Laryngectomee rehabilitation* (3rd ed., pp. 179–189). Austin, TX: PRO-ED.

Salmon, S. J. (1994b). Methods of air intake and associated problems. In R. L. Keith & F. L. Darley (Eds.), *Laryngectomee rehabilitation* (3rd ed., pp. 219–234). Austin, TX: PRO-ED.

Salmon, S. J. (1994c). Pre- and postoperative conferences with laryngectomees and their spouses. In R. L. Keith & F. L. Darley (Eds.), *Laryngectomee rehabilitation* (3rd ed., pp. 133–148). Austin, TX: PRO-ED.

Salmon, S. J. (1999). Artificial larynx devices and their use. In S. J. Salmon (Ed.), *Alaryngeal speech rehabilitation: For clinicians by clinicians* (2nd ed., pp. 79–104). Austin, TX: PRO-ED.

Schaefer, S., & Johns, D. F. (1982). Attaining functional esophageal speech. *Archives of Otolaryngology, 108,* 647–649.

Schmidt, R. A., & Bjork, R. A. (1992). New conceptualizations of practice: Common principles in three paradigms suggest new concepts for training. *Psychological Science, 3*(4), 207–217.

Schultz, J. R., & Harrison, J. (1992). Defining and predicting tracheoesophageal puncture success. *Archives of Otolaryngology—Head and Neck Surgery, 118,* 811–816.

Sedory, S. E., Hamlet, S. L., & O'Connor, N. P. (1989). Comparisons of perceptual and acoustic characteristics of tracheoesophageal and excellent esophageal speech. *Journal of Speech and Hearing Disorders, 54,* 209–214.

Shanks, J. C. (1994). Developing esophageal communication. In R. L. Keith & F. L. Darley (Eds.), *Laryngectomee rehabilitation* (3rd ed., pp. 205–217). Austin, TX: PRO-ED.

Shipp, T. (1967). Frequency, duration, and perceptual measures in relation to judgments of alaryngeal speech acceptability. *Journal of Speech and Hearing Research, 10,* 417–427.

Singer, R. N. (1980). *Motor learning and human performance: An application to motor skills and movement disorders.* New York: Macmillan.

Snidecor, J. C. (1978a). The artificial larynx. In J. C. Snidecor (Ed.), *Speech rehabilitation of the laryngectomized* (2nd ed., pp. 199–208). Springfield, IL: Thomas.

Snidecor, J. C. (1978b). Speech therapy for those with total laryngectomy. In J. C. Snidecor (Ed.), *Speech rehabilitation of the laryngectomized* (2nd ed., pp. 180–193). Springfield, IL: Thomas

Snidecor, J. C., & Curry, E. T. (1959). Temporal and pitch aspects of superior esophageal speech. *Annals of Otology, Rhinology and Laryngology, 68,* 1–14.

Stone, R. E., & Hamilton, R. (1986). Laryngectomee rehabilitation in a group setting. *Seminars in Speech and Language, 7,* 53–65.

Tardy-Mitzell, S., Andrews, M. L., & Bowman, S. A. (1985). Acceptability and intelligibility of tracheoesophageal speech. *Archives of Otolaryngology, 111,* 213–215.

Tikofsky, R. S. (1965). A comparison of the intelligibility of esophageal and normal speakers. *Folia Phoniatrica, 17,* 19–32.

Toseland, R. W., & Siporin, M. I. (1986). When to recommend group treatment: A review of the clinical and research literature. *International Journal of Group Psychotherapy, 32,* 171–201.

Trudeau, M. (1994). The acoustical variability of tracheoesophageal speech. In R. L. Keith & F. L. Darley (Eds.), *Laryngectomee rehabilitation* (3rd ed., pp. 383–394). Austin, TX: PRO-ED.

Weinberg, B. (1983). Voice and speech restoration following total laryngectomy. In W. H. Perkins (Ed.), *Voice disorders* (pp. 109–125). New York: Thieme-Stratton.

Weiss, M. S., & Basili, A. G. (1985). Electrolaryngeal speech produced by laryngectomized subjects: Perceptual characteristics. *Journal of Speech and Hearing Research, 28,* 294–300.

Wepman, J. M., MacGahan, J. A., Rickard, J. C., & Shelton, N. W. (1953). The objective measurement of progressive esophageal speech development. *Journal of Speech and Hearing Disorders, 18,* 247–251.

Wertz, R. T., LaPointe, L. L., & Rosenbek, J. C. (1984). *Apraxia of speech in adults: The disorders and its management.* New York: Grune & Stratton.

Williams, S. E., Scanio, T. S., & Ritterman, S. R. (1989). Temporal and perceptual characteristics of tracheoesophageal voice. *Laryngoscope, 99,* 846–850.

Yorkston, K. M., Beukelman, D., & Bell, K. (1988). *Clinical management of dysarthric speakers.* San Diego: College-Hill.

Chapter 28

Quality of Life and Head and Neck Cancer

Candace Myers

The diagnosis and treatment of head and neck cancer has profound implications for the individual living with the disease. As Gotay and Moore (1992) aptly stated, "Head and neck cancer strikes at the most basic of human functions—the abilities to communicate, eat, and interact socially" (p. 5). For this reason, quality of life (QOL) has traditionally been of inherent fundamental importance in the field of speech–language pathology. Clinicians seek to improve their patients' QOL through intervention efforts. Although speech–language pathologists often use their own loose definitions of QOL, based on their own interpretation of how the individual is doing, there has been an increasing focus in recent years on QOL as measured from the patient's perspective. This movement has significant implications for both the speech–language pathologist and those individuals with head and neck cancers.

The purpose of this chapter is to (a) provide an overview of the concept of QOL as it is currently used in the medical literature, (b) review the impact of head and neck cancer and its treatment, (c) propose a rationale for incorporating QOL considerations in rehabilitation, and (d) provide a framework for the application of QOL assessment in the comprehensive, multidisciplinary care of head and neck cancer patients. Future research needs are also addressed.

DEFINITION AND METHODOLOGY

In the last 15 years, QOL has become an objective, measurable, definable construct that is increasingly used as a treatment outcome in health care. One of the most widely accepted definitions of QOL is that of the World Health Organization (WHO; 1947): "a state of complete physical, mental, and social well-being, and not merely the absence of disease or infirmity" (p. 100). Cella and Cherin (1988) further defined QOL as individuals' "appraisal of and satisfaction with their current level of functioning as compared to what they perceive to be possible or ideal" (p. 70). Inherent in these definitions is the notion that QOL is

- a patient-centered, subjective judgment made by the individual
- a multidimensional construct, influenced by various domains, including physical and occupational functioning, psychological state, social interaction, and somatic sensation (disease- and treatment-related symptoms)
- a dynamic concept, which changes across time and situations

The assessment of QOL is frequently accomplished by patient self-assessment tools, such as visual linear analogue scales and diary cards, and third-party assessments or interviews. Among the recommended guidelines for development and use of QOL assessments are that they should be disease specific to be sensitive to clinically important changes over time; contain items of patient importance; be designed for patient self-administration; be short, easily answered, and designed for repeated use; be amenable to statistical analysis; and have adequately demonstrated validity and reliability (Schipper, 1990a, 1990b; Schipper & Clinch, 1988; Till, 1991).

Global QOL measures assess and compare QOL across disease classes, whereas disease-specific modules are sensitive to disease- and treatment-related changes in patient functioning in several domains. Modules designed for head and neck disease assess QOL in general terms, as well as factors specific to this population—self-image, appearance and disfigurement, speech and communication, eating, and swallowing (e.g., *The Functional Assessment of Cancer Therapy Scale* [FACT-G] with head-and-neck subscale [HNS; Cella, 1994], *University of Washington QOL Questionnaire* [UW-QOL; Hassan & Weymuller, 1993], *European Organization for Research and Treatment of Cancer Core Quality of Life Questionnaire—Head and Neck Cancer Module* [EORTC QLQ–H&N37; Bjordal, Ahlner-Elmqvist et al., 1994; Bjordal, Kaasa, & Mastekaasa, 1994], and the *Head & Neck Survey* [H&NS; Gliklich, Goldsmith, & Funk, 1997]). Mount and Cohen (1995) noted that

> in many clinical situations, it is important to know more about a subset of QOL determinants related to the disease or treatment. Instruments which measure these disease- and treatment-specific variables may provide information about the patient's status, but they are informing about *possible contributors to* QOL, rather than QOL itself. Generic measures of QOL and disease- or treatment-specific measures should thus be used together when disease- or treatment-specific information is required in addition to assessment of QOL. (p. 122)

Therefore, both global and disease-specific indices contribute unique information that can be used in decisions affecting persons living with head and neck cancer.[1]

Several factors have prompted clinicians to consider the inclusion of QOL instruments in health assessment of the head and neck cancer patient (Ferrell & Hassey Dow, 1997; Gritz et al., 1999; Logemann, 1998; Morris, 1994; Schipper, 1990a, 1990b; Till, 1994). The following are the specific factors reported.

⬛ **Trade-off between quantity and quality of life.**
Treatment advances in oncology have led to increased survival and improved rates of disease control. Given the extension or quantity of life provided (Schipper, 1990a), a greater focus is needed on the quality of the patient's life. The trade-off between quantity and quality is a consideration in short-term survival, as well as in the relatively new field of cancer survivorship. Among survivors of cancer, cancer is viewed as both a life-threatening disease and a chronic illness (Ferrell & Hassey Dow, 1997).

⬛ **Individual differences.**
There is a growing body of knowledge regarding the short- and long-term effects of cancer and its treatments. With this knowledge comes a greater focus on functional limitations and the psy-

---

[1]The reader is encouraged to read King et al. (1997) for a comprehensive review of individual and global applications of the QOL paradigm in cancer care.

chosocial impact of the disease, including how individual differences *such as coping style, lifestyle factors (e.g., substance abuse), and social supports (e.g., marital status) may account for differing outcomes (Morris, 1994). The World Health Organization has proposed a framework for disability that recognizes individual variation in adjustment to physical impairment, because the degree of functional disability and social handicap can vary with similar changes in impairment (WHO, 1993). For example, two individuals who have undergone a composite resection for an oropharyngeal tumor may have a similar impairment but different degrees of disability (i.e., in terms of swallowing and speech function). Similarly, two patients who have undergone a similar surgery and have similar disability (e.g., require long-term gastrostomy tube feeding) may experience quite different levels of handicap (i.e., psychosocial adjustment to their changed function and lifestyle). In other words, individuals with the same disease and treatment can have differing effects on their degree of impairment and handicap. Recognition of the wide variation in the impact of and adjustment to a range of physical impairments can assist clinicians in identifying rehabilitation needs and guiding appropriate interventions for the individual with the disease.*

◢ Focus on treatment outcomes and efficacy.
QOL is increasingly being considered an outcome measure, *along with tumor response to treatment and survival. QOL studies are frequently endpoints in large clinical trials and can have a significant impact on the direction of treatment and rehabilitation protocols (Schipper, 1990b). In other words, if two treatments provide similar outcomes in terms of survival but result in significant differences in QOL outcomes, then subsequent treatment selection would be influenced in favor of the treatment with the more beneficial (less negative) impact on QOL. For example, the Veterans Administration chemoradiation protocol for treatment of laryngeal tumors is increasingly used because it leads to survival outcomes similar to that of surgery but allows laryngeal preservation (Woodson et al., 1996). Treatment efficacy is an increasingly important focus of both primary treatment and rehabilitation interventions. Efficacy broadly encompasses the notions of effectiveness of treatment (i.e., Does the treatment work?), efficiency (i.e., Does one treatment work better than another, and along what domains?), and effects of treatment (i.e., In what ways does treatment affect behavior?) (Olswang, 1990).*

◢ Multidisciplinary team intervention.
The movement toward continuous quality improvement *in health care has led to* multidisciplinary coordination of services, *with the*

goal of improved delivery of cancer care and rehabilitation. From the preoperative stages, treatment is planned with the individual's functional and psychosocial needs in mind (Logemann, 1998).

◢ Autonomy and increased patient participation.
Patients increasingly participate in treatment decisions as health care moves from a paternalistic model. QOL information can assist in determining patient preferences and needs. As Roy (1992) stated, "quality of life studies and measurements serve to prevent a devastating separation of a patient's body from a patient's biography during the delivery of care" (p. 4). Thus, attention to QOL measures can guide clinicians in tailoring the course of treatment and rehabilitation according to the unique and changing wishes, needs, and preferences of the individual patient (Gritz et al., 1999).

In short, QOL measures provide a structured and consistent way to more fully respect and consider the perspective of the individual patient, while capturing the benefits that clinicians strive to achieve with their patients in treatment. Furthermore, QOL measures provide indicators of efficacy that are increasingly required in health care settings. Till (1994) stated that "formal QOL assessments provide systematic, quantitative answers to the kinds of questions clinicians usually ask informally, such as 'how have you been lately?' " (p. 243). Till proposed a continuum of application of QOL measurements and their resulting benefits. At the "micro" level, QOL consideration influences treatment decisions for individual patients. Application of QOL measurements at the "meso" level is used to formulate practice guidelines for groups of patients, whereas at the "macro" level, QOL measurements can be used to assess population benefits and develop policy regarding priorities in cancer care. Therefore, the concept of QOL has a wide range of applicability in health care systems.

The use of QOL assessment in the area of head and neck cancer is a uniquely formidable undertaking. Gotay and Moore (1992) suggested that

> while research in quality of life is a challenging area, in many ways, head and neck cancer is ideally suited to such an endeavour. This disease has been characterized by a team approach to care including a variety of (health care) specialists each of which contributes to the patient's quality of life. In fact, quality of life research represents a unifying theme cutting across these somewhat disparate disciplines. While each professional can identify the effect of his/her intervention in a specific area, it is the patient who can evaluate the total impact of the treatment as a whole. The development and application of rigorous scientific research in this field holds enormous promise for the quality of life of head and neck cancer patients. (p. 15)

QOL assessment, however, is not without its challenges in the head and neck cancer population. The prevalence of aging; increased tobacco and alcohol use in this population; high rates of distress and depression; reduced compliance due to substance abuse, fatigue, or pain; and low literacy levels contribute to the difficulty in gathering sufficient QOL evidence (Gritz et al., 1999; McDonough et al., 1996; Tennstedt, 2000). Furthermore, although frequently referred to as a single entity, head and neck cancer represents a mixture of specific diagnoses and stages, each with different implications for QOL (Gotay & Moore, 1992).[2]

THE EFFECTS OF HEAD AND NECK TUMORS AND THEIR TREATMENTS

Head and neck cancers are comprised of a multitude of tumor types, stages, and anatomic sites. In addition, there is a broad range of treatment modalities, both conventional and experimental, conservative and radical (Ackerstaff et al., 2002; Carrara-de-Angelis, Feher, Barros, Nishimoto, & Kowalski, 2003). An overview of the various effects of the disease and treatments is provided to present a framework for the clinician to incorporate the current QOL concept and knowledge into clinical practice. The following is a summary gathered from the current literature on head and neck tumors.

Communication
Speech, voice, and communication disorders (Blood, 1993; Burns, Chase, & Goodwin, 1987; Doyle, 1994; Theurer & Martin, 2003)

Auditory and Vestibular Deficits
(Blakley et al., 1991; Cameron, Green, & Gulliver, 2000)

Swallowing and Nutrition
Eating, chewing, and swallowing problems (Burns et al., 1987; DeNittis et al., 2001; Eisbruch et al., 2002; Epstein et al., 1999; Graner et al., 2003; Logemann, 1997; Logemann & Bytell, 1979; McConnel, Cerenko, & Mendelsohn, 1988; McConnel, Mendelsohn, & Logemann, 1986; Robb & Lewin, 2003; Samlan & Webster, 2002; Skoner et al., 2003)

Limited Diet, Malnourishment, Loss of Appetite, Digestive Problems
(Body & Borkowski, 1987; Minasian & Dwyer, 1998; Pauloski et al., 2002; Zemel, Maves, Mickelson, & Kaplan, 1991)

---

[2]The reader is encouraged to consult Schipper and Clinch (1988) and Till (1991, 1994) for comprehensive discussions of quality of life assessment and methodology, as well as King et al. (1997) and Gotay and Moore (1992) for specific application to the head and neck cancer population and its inherent difficulties, methods, definitions, approaches to measurement, and types of findings.

Gastroesophageal Reflux
(Copper et al., 2000; Smit, Tan, Mathus-Vliegen, & Devriese, 1998)

Physical Problems
Xerostomia, dry mouth and pharynx, sticky saliva (Bjordal, Kaasa, & Mastekaasa, 1994; List, Ritter-Sterr, & Lansky, 1990; see also Chapter 10 in this text)

Mucositis and oral pain (Epstein et al., 1999; Smit et al., 1998; see also Chapter 10 in this text)

Impairment of taste and smell, loss of appetite (Moore, Getchell, Mistretta, Mozell, & Kern, 1991; Pruyn et al., 1986)

Dental Problems
Xerostomia, dental caries, osteoradionecrosis (Allison, Locker, & Feine, 1999; Clarke, 1998; Maxymiw, Rothney, & Sutcliffe, 1994; see also Chapter 13 in this text)

Trismus
(Sist, 1998; see also Chapter 7 in this text)

Excessive Mucus, Sputum
(Ackerstaff, Hilgers, Aaronson, & Balm, 1994; Hilgers, Ackerstaff, Aaronson, Schouwenburg, & van Zandwuk, 1990)

Respiratory Difficulties, Breathlessness, Coughing
(Ackerstaff et al., 1994; Fine, Krell, Ranella, Sessions, & Williams, 1991; Pruyn et al., 1986; see also Chapter 20 in this text)

Issues Related to Stoma
Cleaning, protection, hygiene, safety (Ackerstaff et al., 1994; DeSanto, Olsen, Perry, Rohe, & Keith, 1995; Pruyn et al., 1986; see also Chapter 20 in this text)

Skin Irritation
(Browman et al., 1993)

Pain or Soreness
(Campbell, Marbella, & Layde, 2000; de Graeff et al., 1999; Ingall, Saper, Kish, Kuch, & Evans, 1991)

Neck/Shoulder Pain, Reduced Range-of-Motion (ROM) or Functional Incapacity of Arm Movement
(Kuntz & Weymuller, 1999; Nowak, Parzuchowski, & Jacobs, 1989; Rathmell, Ash, Howes, & Nicholls, 1991; Schutt, 1986; Terrell et al., 2000)

Insomnia, Fatigue

(Ackerstaff et al., 1994; deBoer et al., 1995; Jones, Lund, Howard, Greenberg, & McCarthy, 1992; Rathmell et al., 1991)

Loss of Physical Capacity

(Pruyn et al., 1986)

Late Complications of Radiotherapy

Dysphagia, trismus, fatigue, skin changes, pain, osteoradionecrosis (Bjordal, Kaasa, & Mastekaasa, 1994; deBoer et al., 1995; Weissler, 1997; see also Chapter 13 in this text)

Psychosocial Problems

Psychosocial difficulties (depression, anxiety, anger, distress, loss of self-esteem) (Baile, Gibertini, Scott, & Endicott, 1992; Breitbart & Holland, 1988; Gibson & McCombe, 1999; McQuellon & Hurt, 1997; Morton, Davies, Baker, Baker, & Stell, 1984; Olson & Shedd, 1978; Pruyn et al., 1986; Rapoport, Kreitler, Chaitchik, Algor, & Weissler, 1993; Stam, Koopmans, & Mathieson, 1991; Strauss, 1989; Watt-Watson & Graydon, 1995)

Disfigurement, stigma, body image (deBoer et al., 1995; Doyle, 1994; Dropkin, 1989; Gamba et al., 1992; Strauss, 1989)

Work or Vocational Issues

Economic/financial problems (Pruyn et al., 1986)

Vocational problems (deBoer et al., 1995; Harwood & Rawlinson, 1983; Pruyn et al., 1986; Richardson, 1983; Strauss, 1989)

Loss of social and recreation interests (e.g., singing, water sports) (McQuellon & Hurt, 1997)

Social Isolation, Stigmatization, Relationship Difficulties

Reduction in social contacts, social isolation, fear of socializing with others (Breitbart & Holland, 1988; deBoer et al., 1995; Harwood & Rawlinson, 1983; Mathieson, Stam, & Scott, 1991; McDonough et al., 1996; Stam et al., 1991)

Eating in public (Campbell et al., 2000; deBoer et al., 1995; List et al., 1990; Long et al., 1996)

Impact on spouse and family (deBoer et al., 1995; Doyle & White, 2004; Gritz et al., 1999; Kreitler, Chaitchik, Rapoport, & Algor, 1993; Manne & Glassman, 2000; Mathieson et al., 1991; Silveira & Winstead-Fry, 1997)

Sexuality issues (deBoer et al., 1995; Doyle & White, 2004; Natvig, 1984; Pruyn et al., 1986; Siston, List, Schleser, & Vokes, 1997)

Other

Continued use/abuse of alcohol or tobacco (Breitbart & Holland, 1988; deBoer et al., 1995; Gritz et al., 1999; Morris, 1994)

Concerns specific to women who are laryngectomized (Brown & Doyle, 1999; Doyle & White, 2004; Stam et al., 1991)

Spiritual/existential issues among the seriously ill (hope, spirituality, suffering) (Mount & Cohen, 1995)

Long-term impact and consequences of "cancer survivorship" (deBoer et al., 1995; Ferrell & Hassey Dow, 1997)

Cancer concern/fears of recurrence (Campbell et al., 2000; Magne et al., 2001)

The multiple impacts of head and neck cancer and its treatments are indeed numerous and significant. Furthermore, the severity of impact may be even greater than previously assumed (Armstrong & Gilbert, 2004). Gritz et al. (1999) prospectively assessed QOL over a 1-year period after diagnosis and treatment of head and neck cancer in a relatively large patient group ($n = 105$) and determined predictors of QOL at 12 months posttreatment. These researchers suggested "that head and neck cancer patients have a more impaired quality of life than other populations who are not disease-free, including normative samples of male cancer patients, male nonprostate cancer patients, and female breast cancer patients" (Gritz et al., 1999, p. 357). Furthermore, they noted that "given that the subset of 105 participants on whom the data were analyzed are a group of patients *with earlier-stage disease at diagnosis than those who did not provide complete data, quality of life may be even more compromised in head and neck cancer patients than our data indicate* [italics added]" (Gritz et al., 1999, p. 357). These results indicate that QOL impairment for the person living with head and neck cancer may be even more significant than previously thought. Thus, if the goal is to improve quality of life, it is incumbent upon the clinician to give serious consideration to QOL factors affecting patients with head and neck cancer.

WHY THE SPEECH-LANGUAGE PATHOLOGIST SHOULD BE CONCERNED

QOL research has documented the likely consequences, both direct and indirect, of head and neck cancers and their associated treatments. It is well known that head and neck cancer patients experience communication problems, dental problems, difficulty with eating and swallowing, excessive mucus and sputum, dietary and nutritional changes, neck and shoulder pain, reduced range of motion, fatigue, and a multitude of psychosocial problems, any of which significantly impacts the individual's QOL. The following also have been established:

- QOL is patient-centered; that is, it must be assessed from the patient's own perspective.

- QOL is functional; that is, it deals with day-to-day activities of the individual in the areas of physical and occupational functioning, emotional or psychological functioning, and social functioning.
- QOL changes continuously in response to the symptoms of disease and treatment events affecting the patient (Schipper & Clinch, 1988; Schipper, Clinch, McMurray, & Levitt, 1984; Schipper & Levitt, 1985).

In clinical practice, however, the health care team may fail to monitor QOL issues and ultimately fail to direct patients to appropriate resources. There continues to be a tendency to evaluate QOL from the perspective of the health care professional, who is relatively young, competent, literate, well educated, independent, proactive, and healthy, rather than from the patient's perspective. The following is a rationale for the speech-language pathologist and other health care team members to monitor and address quality of life in the head and neck cancer patient. As Weiss (1993) stated, "quality of life counts for a great deal in the patients' minds. It should matter just as much to us" (p. 312).

AN ETHICAL PERSPECTIVE

From an ethical perspective, there is an emerging and heightened awareness of the ethical principles that should guide health care (Eadie & Charland, in press). As health care progresses from a paternalistic model to a more patient-centered approach, there is a greater focus on the principles of beneficence and autonomy. *Beneficence* refers to the principles of doing no harm, maximizing the possible benefits, and minimizing possible harms. The QOL movement has led to increased consideration of harms and benefits *as perceived by the individual patient.* The principle of *autonomy* considers that the individual is capable of deliberation about personal goals and consequent action: "to respect autonomy is to give weight to autonomous persons' considered opinions and choices while refraining from obstructing their actions unless they are clearly detrimental to others" (National Commission for the Protection of Human Subjects of Biomedical and Behavioral Research, 1978, p. 4). Health care professionals demonstrate respect for persons through informed consent, which refers to a provision of information to the patient related to risks, benefits, and alternatives (Eadie & Charland, in press). Furthermore, "this disclosure of information must be in a language that the patient can understand, and it should convey meanings that are relevant to the patient's concerns" (Levine, 1990, p. 157). Therefore, clinicians are ethically obliged to consider the needs and wishes of the patient, while fully informing him or her of treatments and their effects.

According to the National Commission for the Protection of Human Subjects of Biomedical and Behavioral Research (1978), "autonomous persons live according to life plans which reflect their personal conceptions of what it means to live a good life. The usually unanticipated contingency of disease often forces persons to reconsider and reevaluate their life plans" (pp. 4–5). Faced with a disease that has life-altering and life-changing effects, a patient's needs and priorities change. The growing body of QOL research has demonstrated that no one is in a better position to determine one's own priorities than the person with the disease; however, the patient must be provided with sufficient information with which to evaluate his or her own priorities. Levine (1990) stressed "the need to develop information that will enable patients to make satisfactory choices regarding the use of therapies" (p. 157).

In addition to the principles of beneficence and autonomy, Levine (1990) discussed a third ethical principle identified by the National Commission. The principle of *justice* deals with the allocation of resources, which "requires that the burdens and benefits of society be distributed fairly or equitably" (Levine, 1990, p. 160). By determining a patient's own health care priorities through consideration of QOL, health care professionals may prevent the wasted use of resources that might benefit the patient more appropriately, efficiently, and effectively at a different stage in his or her rehabilitation. Thus, consideration of individual QOL can lead to more ethical treatment of persons living with cancer, through the principles of beneficence, autonomy, and justice. For further discussion, the reader is referred to Till (1994), who raises some thoughtful issues related to ethical considerations and QOL.

REASONS WHY THE PATIENT MAY NOT RAISE QOL ISSUES AND CONCERNS

Given the importance of QOL from the patient's perspective, the health care professional must consider why some patients may not take the initiative to ask or express concern about factors affecting their own QOL. For the patient with head and neck cancer, several possible reasons emerge, as discussed in the following subsections.

Lack of Knowledge About the Effects of the Disease and Treatments

The patient's lack of knowledge is not surprising, given changing treatment protocols and the ever-evolving knowledge of the impact of new treatments on the disease. The patient may not know that the problems he or she is experiencing are related to the disease or treatment, or whether something can be done about the problems. The trend toward shorter hospital stays reduces the opportunity for thorough and coordinated education and teaching (see Chapter 24 in this text). The reasons for such a lack of knowledge may include the following

1. *Remoteness in time or from anatomical site.* Because some effects may not occur for several months after treatment has ceased, the patient may not realize that the effect is related to treatment (e.g., dental problems several months postradiotherapy, or progressive dysphagia related to development of a stricture). Patients also may not recognize related problems that are distant from the anatomical site, such as abdominal and digestive prob-

lems (e.g., gastroesophageal reflux and abdominal discomfort may be related to speech mode or a faulty swallowing status); bowel and digestive problems (gas, bloating, constipation) related to treatment or compensation (e.g., prosthesis type, swallowing pattern, changes in diet, loss of the sphincteric vocal fold function in elimination); and energy level problems related to the involvement of the thyroid gland during surgery or changes in diet due to taste aversion or dysphagia. Similarly, the patient may not know that he or she is malnourished; many factors can lead to malnourishment, and those who are malnourished have a slower and poorer recovery from treatment (Minasian & Dwyer, 1998).

2. *Assumptions about efficacy.* The patient may not be aware that something can be done to relieve his or her symptoms (e.g., excessive mucous production or coughing, limited range of motion in the shoulder following radical neck dissection, restricted manual dexterity after a forearm free flap graft, quality of eating experiences). Some patients do not address their symptom concerns, even when they persist several months after primary treatment.

3. *Education and literacy levels, and comprehension and retention of information.* Written information that has been provided as a means of patient education may not be reviewed by nonreaders or those with low or nonexistent literacy levels. In a study by Blood et al. (1994), patients following laryngectomy were grouped according to adjustment scales into "good copers" and "poorer copers." The authors noted that good copers had a mean educational level of 12.3 years, whereas poor copers had a mean educational level of 7.1 years. Given that many patient education materials are at an eighth-grade level or above (Cooley et al., 1995) and that literacy levels may not match stated educational level, it is likely that the written information routinely provided to patients as a backup resource is not as useful an educational tool as assumed. Thus, patients with low literacy levels may not have access to information that may lead to investigation and treatment of health concerns affecting their QOL.

Cooley et al. (1995) highlighted the questionable efficacy and appropriateness of materials routinely provided for patient education. The authors conducted a descriptive cross-sectional study with outpatients at an urban Veterans Administration hospital to determine whether the reading level of educational materials for patients with cancer corresponded to actual reading abilities of a sample of 63 patients. Subjects were mostly male (92%) and were free from dementias or other coexisting disorders that might affect reading ability. They found that only 27% of the sample could be expected to understand all written materials provided, and that the patients' actual reading levels were significantly less than reported grade reading levels, which, therefore, did not accurately reflect reading comprehension ability.

When asked what mode of instruction would be the most helpful, patients in Cooley et al.'s (1995) study expressed a preference for teaching methods that combined written books and pamphlets with (a) individual or group instruction or (b) movies or audiocassettes. The authors noted that with

> the increasing complexity of cancer care, shorter hospital stays, and a shift towards busy ambulatory care centers, healthcare professionals need to develop creative, innovative, and comprehensive patient educational programs that are understandable to patients and that use multiple types of instruction. (p. 1350)

The results also support the need for ongoing monitoring of patient knowledge of symptoms and concerns.

Furthermore, retention of patient information may be low due to multiple factors. Even if information is clearly and comprehensively provided in a manner in which the individual patient can understand, the patient may not retain knowledge of potential effects of the disease or treatment if presented all at one time. Health care professionals need to continually educate and repeat previously provided information, and to regularly monitor potential concerns affecting QOL. Sist (1998) stressed "the value of explaining what to expect and when to expect it" (p. 1169).

4. *Multitude of problems and variation due to disease site, tumor size and type, treatment mode, and individual differences.* The head and neck cancer patient population is far from a homogeneous group. As Cassel (1982) described in his dissertation on the nature of suffering and the goals of medicine, different patients can have the same disease but a different illness and a different experience of pain and suffering. Furthermore, generalization of QOL findings among this population is difficult due to relatively small samples, variable treatment and surgical options, and the wide range and type of possible disease and treatment effects. The patient may experience unusual symptoms that had not been discussed as part of routine pre- and postoperative education. For these reasons, the health care professional can only know what is affecting the individual patient by asking the question and finding out what the patient is most concerned about at the time. It is imperative that health care professionals regularly and consistently ask the questions that will elicit the information that will guide treatment according to each patient's values and wishes.

Concurrent Psychosocial Difficulties

Patients with head and neck cancers are at high risk for psychosocial problems, which can directly or indirectly affect QOL. Coping and adjustment difficulties were noted by Olson and Shedd (1978) in a study that assessed the extent of disability following treatment for head and neck cancer. Of the 51 patients in their study, 28 were at least 6 months or more postlaryngectomy. Of the 28 patients, 43% reported that episodes of depression occurred often or sometimes, 39% reported an adequate coping ability, and 7% reported poor coping ability. Baile et al. (1992) found that depression was equally distributed regardless of tumor stage in head and neck cancer patients. This was evident even among their patients who were "of unusually good performance and nutritional status" with few physical complaints (p. 22). Baile et al. (1992) further suggested that it is not unreasonable to assume that "patients with a more pessimistic outlook about their disease would tend to be less aggressive in seeking treatment or complying with therapy" (p. 22). McQuellon and Hurt (1997) noted that "the patient most at risk for psychological disturbance has some psychiatric comorbidity such as a history of depression and substance abuse, coexistent medical problems, poor social and family support network, few financial resources, and poorly differentiated coping skills" (p. 236). Many head and neck cancer patients have some or all of these risk factors (Breitbart & Holland, 1988; McQuellon & Hurt, 1997; Richardson, 1983).

Pain, fatigue, depression, radiation treatment schedules or side effects, distance from treatment center, economic issues, and decreased hospital stays can all potentially disrupt planned and scheduled treatments, and patients may never reinitiate. Logemann (1994) noted that 3 to 4 weeks into treatment the patient receiving postoperative radiotherapy may suffer increasing functional impairment and become depressed as he or she observes speech and swallowing function deteriorate. A prospective study of 186 oral and oropharyngeal patients treated surgically, many with postoperative radiotherapy, found that only 50% of patients received speech and swallowing therapy and less than 10% received maxillofacial prosthetic intervention (see Chapter 13 in this text). At 3 months posttreatment, 50% of the patients were lost to follow-up. One may hypothesize that these patients became disillusioned with their functional abilities and the lack of active rehabilitation and stopped trying (Logemann, 1994, p. 364). Thus, psychosocial difficulties may interfere with the patients' ability to advocate for and improve their own QOL. Lack of professional monitoring may prevent early and more effective remediation of potentially serious concerns and problems.

There is good reason to be concerned about the impact of psychosocial problems in head and neck cancer patients. Physical and psychosocial problems appear to be interrelated to a certain extent. Newell, Sanson-Fisher, Girgis, and Ackland (1999) performed a cross-sectional study of a large group of 200 patients attending an outpatient medical oncology department to assess the prevalence and predictors of physical symptoms, anxiety, depression, and perceived needs. Patients were found to experience a wide range of physical and psychosocial difficulties. Participants experiencing high levels of physical symptoms were much more likely to have elevated levels of anxiety and depression, and to report a moderate to high level of perceived needs. A reciprocal effect was also found: Patients with elevated levels of depression were more likely to have elevated anxiety levels and report four or more physical symptoms. Perceived needs included coping with fears, uncertainty, anxiety, disturbed sleep, and performance of day-to-day activities. The authors suggested that "managing one of these problems could result in improvements in the others" (Newell et al., 1999, p. 80). Similar findings were reported by de Graeff and colleagues (1999), who prospectively assessed 153 patients undergoing treatment with curative intent for cancers in the oral cavity, oropharynx, hypopharynx, and larynx. They found that patients with depressive symptoms or a low pretreatment performance status are at risk for both physical and psychological problems following treatment. The authors stressed that these patients must be followed closely during rehabilitation programs.

McQuellon and Hurt (1997) further emphasized that "the psychosocial impact of laryngeal cancer can be minimized with coordinated rehabilitation efforts [that are] initiated early by a multidisciplinary team" (p. 237). The speech–language pathologist is frequently the health care team member with the most regular and long-term contact with the patient, and may assist in the reintegration to structured multidisciplinary care. Therefore, the speech–language pathologist has the potential to offer early identification of the changing and unique needs of the individual. Logemann (1994) noted that "early and active rehabilitation is critical to the successful functioning of head and neck cancer patients" and that "the responsibility for establishing the rehabilitation plan and educating the patient and family regarding its importance falls to the members of the rehabilitation team," including the speech–language pathologist (p. 364).

Concurrent Physical Problems

A multitude of physical symptoms potentially may be experienced by the person with head and neck cancer. Fatigue, diminished energy level, and pain may contribute in varying degrees to the patient's desire or ability to participate in the overall management and improvement of his or her health status. Hwang, Chang, Corpion, Ohanian, and Kasimis (1997) noted that a strong association exists between fatigue and overall symptom burden, and that lack of energy may result from specific symptoms or a combination of symptoms. These authors further suggested that early identification and careful management of symptoms and anemia could reduce fatigue. In addition, there is frequently an interplay between such effects: Pain can affect the patient's desire or ability to obtain adequate nutrition, thus leading to dysphagia and malnourishment. This in turn can further exacerbate fatigue, influencing variables such as anxiety or depression (Sist, 1998).

Finally, various therapeutic regimes, particularly in the area of rehabilitation, may be interrupted due to medical setbacks (e.g., fatigue, infection, wound-healing problems, radiation effects, recurrences, other illnesses). In addition, logistic concerns—financial difficulties and distance from treatment—may pose further challenges for the patient. Because of the far-reaching and interactive effects of these myriad factors, such problems may interfere with or override the patient's directness in raising important QOL concerns. Through heightened awareness and judicious monitoring of the scope of QOL effects in head and neck cancer, the speech–language pathologist may play a key role in assisting the patient to identify issues of concern.

Impact of Cancer and Illness on Decision Making and Communication

The experience of cancer can negatively impact the degree to which patients will advocate on their own behalf for interventions that might improve their QOL. Ende, Kazis, Ash, and Moskowitz (1989) studied patients' desire for autonomy as measured by their desire to be informed and make medical decisions. In general, the authors found that patients preferred that decisions about their care be made principally by their physicians, rather than by themselves; however, patients—particularly older patients—had a strong desire to be informed. Furthermore, for the majority of patients, the desire to make decisions declined as they faced more serious illness.

Degner and Sloan (1992) studied the nature of decision making during serious illness among 436 newly diagnosed cancer patients and 483 members of the general public. Surveys were administered to determine what roles individuals actually want to assume in selecting their cancer treatments. The majority of patients (59%) wanted physicians to make treatment decisions on their behalf, whereas 64% of the public thought they would want to select their own treatment if they developed cancer. Age was the most significant predictor about keeping, sharing, or giving control to the physician, with older subjects preferring less control. Among cancer patients, there was also a trend for men to prefer less control over decisions about their care than women. Degner and Sloan suggested that patients may become more passive in the early stages after rather than prior to diagnosis. Furthermore, the desire to take control of decisions varies with changes in health status, that is, from the status of a healthy individual to one diagnosed with cancer. Close to the time of diagnosis, patients may play a relatively more passive role until they learn more about the disease and its treatment. This observation seems to be supported clinically, as patients seem to be more direct about their needs and desires in treatment at some period of time after diagnosis. Patients may lower their psychological distress early on by relinquishing decision making to health care professionals.

Degner and Sloan's (1992) findings reflect that of the head and neck cancer population in terms of demographics (age, gender, and education level) (Doyle, 1994; McQuellon & Hurt, 1997): Older patients preferred less control, as did males and less educated patients. Furthermore, older individuals are of a generation that often has a more paternalistic view of medicine (i.e., they are relatively non–consumer oriented and less involved with their own treatment decisions). The experience of cancer appears to change what healthy individuals may wish in terms of the level of involvement in their own health care decisions. Therefore, the health care provider may need to assume a more active role in the ongoing education of patients to assist them in making decisions affecting their care.

Individual Differences

Bjordal, Kaasa, and Mastekaasa (1994) noted the heterogeneity and high rate of variability of effects among head and neck cancer patients. This finding relates to different types of diseases in head and neck cancer, the size and location of tumors, anatomical sites involved, treatment modalities, surgical reconstruction options, and the symptom burden of disease and treatment (Curran, Irish, & Gullane, 1997). Other authors (Blood, Luther, & Stemple, 1992; Long et al., 1996; Morris, 1994) noted that variable coping styles and lifestyle factors (marital status, history of alcoholism), as well as premorbid health status, interact with disease and treatment variables to have widely differing effects on self-perceived QOL (Pauloski et al., 2002) . These factors make QOL less predictable and the assumption of specific patient needs less certain. Fayers, Hand, Bjordal, and Groenvold (1997) stated that the severity of any one symptom may be adequate to impair QOL. Similarly, Mount and Cohen (1995) stated that "the relative importance of each determinant of QOL varies tremendously from individual to individual, and over time in the same subject" (p. 123). It is clear that the experience of head and neck cancer is a truly unique and variable phenomenon. Awareness of this critical fact highlights the importance of making no assumptions about how the disease and treatments are presently affecting the patient, or the specific nature of his or her primary and current concerns (Wen & Gustafson, 2004). The speech–language pathologist must regularly and consistently "ask the questions" that will elicit this critical information and subsequently improve patient care.

Differing Perceptions

Patients receiving interventions for head and neck cancer may not raise issues of importance to their QOL if they believe the health care professional is in a better position to determine their needs and guide the direction of treatment. Substantial evidence, however, illustrates that the perception of those factors that influence an individual's QOL may differ widely between patients and healthy subjects, patients and family members, and patients and health care professionals.

Patients Versus Healthy Volunteers

McNeil, Weichselbaum, and Pauker (1981) investigated attitudes toward quality and quantity of life in 37 healthy volunteers (12 firefighters and 25 middle- and upper-management executives) to determine their preferences for longevity and voice preservation. Analysis indicated that approximately 20% of volunteers would choose radiation instead of surgery if faced with voice loss; they were willing to trade off at least 15% to 30% of their full life expectancy to preserve speech. These results suggest that treatment choices should be made on the basis of patients' attitudes toward both the quality and the quantity of survival. "Patients' attitudes toward morbidity are important, and survival is not their only consideration" (McNeil et al., 1981, p. 987). Furthermore, "normal volunteers were able to make trade-off decisions in a stress-free situation—quite different from that of a patient recently found to have laryngeal cancer" (McNeil et al., 1981, p. 986). These results highlight the difference between the perceptions of the healthy individual versus one with cancer.

Patients Versus Family Members

Rieker, Clark, and Fogelberg (1992) conducted a retrospective, descriptive study to identify patient and family perceptions about QOL and quality of care after experimental treatment such as cancer therapy. Family members differed significantly from patients in their perception of quality of care, as well as their perception of financial burden associated with care. Therefore, even those who presumably know the patient best cannot predict the issues that are most important to the patient's perceived QOL. This further reinforces the view that, whenever possible, information about pertinent QOL concerns must be elicited from the patient directly.

Patients Versus Health Care Professionals

It is not enough to be clinically familiar with the scope of problems experienced by head and neck cancer patients. Tripepi–Bova (1993) studied the perceptions of 20 postlaryngectomy patients and 20 health care professionals on issues important to laryngectomy patients. Significant differences were found between items of importance to laryngectomized individuals versus health care professionals, particularly in the areas of physical consequences, communication improvement, lifestyle changes, self-image and self-esteem, and worry or fear of cancer control. The health care professional may likely have different perceptions of what the patient's concerns are and how the patient is doing (see Gattellari, Butow, Tattersall, Dunn, & MacLeod, 1999).

In a similar study, Mohide, Archibald, Tew, Young, and Haines (1992) sought to identify postlaryngectomy QOL dimensions among patients and health care professionals. Mohide et al. surveyed 20 patients (at least 12 months after laryngectomy) and 20 health care professionals, who were asked to identify important QOL items after recovery from laryngectomy and rank and rate each item on a visual analogue scale. Health care professionals placed greater importance on communication impairment, fear of recurrence, and self-image and self-esteem issues, whereas patients emphasized lifestyle changes and the physical consequences of laryngectomy (e.g., tracheal mucous production, interference with social activities). Mohide and colleagues emphasized that laryngectomy is a highly personal and subjective experience and stressed the importance of considering QOL variables from the patient's perspective. The findings in this study are of particular importance to speech–language pathologists, because only 6 of 20 patients had successful tracheoesophageal puncture (TEP) voice rehabilitation and 12 were electrolarynx users. Use of an electrolarynx is often considered a substandard postlaryngectomy communication option, yet considerably fewer patients than health care professionals identified communication impairment as one of the five most important dimensions 12 months postlaryngectomy. One might expect patients' concerns regarding communication to be even less frequently reported if more patients had been successful TEP speakers. Mohide et al. (1992) noted, however, that their results might not be generalizeable to patients fewer than 12 months postoperatively.

The studies by McNeil et al. (1981), Mohide et al. (1992), Rieker et al. (1992), and Tripepi-Bova (1993) underscore that the experience of cancer changes what healthy individuals may wish, and stress the importance of leaving evaluation of specific determinants of QOL to the patient. Degner and Sloan (1992) noted that the experience of cancer may change what individuals think they would wish in terms of decision-making participation and control. Healthy individuals, whether health care providers or family members, even those closest to the person with cancer, should make no assumptions about what factors affect the patient's QOL, or to what degree. As concluded by Degner and Sloan (1992), "the strong effect of the presence or absence of cancer suggested that decision making preferences might be influenced by diagnosis of a life-threatening illness" (p. 949).

Uneven Relationship Between Health Care Providers and Patients

As Strauss (1989) stated, "it is the unusual patient who can question the wisdom of active treatment because this involves a challenge to professional norms" (p. 347). In other words, patients sometimes believe that the health care professional is in a better position to know their needs in terms of QOL, and may be reluctant to advocate for themselves relative to a differing direction of treatment (e.g., choosing radiotherapy vs. combination surgery and radiotherapy, requesting closure of a TEP tract, choosing to discontinue adjuvant radiotherapy). Furthermore, health care professionals are frequently perceived as busy, authoritative figures who may be difficult to challenge. Thus, patients may not raise issues of personal importance, question the direction of care, or suggest preferred alternatives.

This reluctance to voice concerns was revealed in a study by Gibson and McCombe (1999). They investigated through semistructured interview the nature and severity of problems faced by 10 laryngectomized individuals following discharge from the hospital. Study participants were interviewed in the first month following discharge and then 6 months following surgery. The authors found that 8 of the 10 patients suffered significant psychological morbidity (as indicated by low self-esteem, anhedonia, suicidal ideation, poor sleep, poor concentration, and emotional lability) in the first month following discharge. These features of psychological morbidity persisted in 7 of the 10 patients when assessed 6 months later. Gibson and McCombe suggested that subjects in their study "did not intimate their psychosocial problems to surgeons because the surgeon is perceived as the person who cured their cancer and as such is often the last to know about these problems" (p. 351). Thus, the uneven relationship between patients and health care providers, based in part on professional status, may pose barriers to patients raising issues of concern.

The uneven patient–health care provider relationship in cancer care was further revealed in a study by Lerman and colleagues (1993). These authors evaluated the perceptions of patients with breast cancer in regard to their medical interactions with health care providers. They found that a substantial proportion of patients (84%) reported difficulties communicating with the medical team. Communication problems were more common among patients who were less optimistic about their disease and had less assertive coping styles. Patients may assume a more passive role in health care interactions if they have little hope that their communicative participation will have any influence on their recovery or survival. Therefore, they may be less likely to contribute information that could potentially have a positive effect on their current QOL.

Communication

By nature, no patient group has greater difficulty communicating its needs and wishes than the patient group with tumors in the head and neck area. These patients are likely to have physical impairments as a consequence of their disease or treatment that directly relate to a communication disability or handicap. Communication, at various stages before, during, or after treatment, may be slow and inefficient, unintelligible, effortful and burdensome, fatiguing, uncomfortable, or even painful. The patient may perceive that the health care professional's time is at a premium and may be reluctant to waste the professional's time by raising concerns that may not be directly related to the disease or treatment. As Doyle (1994) stated

> for most individuals under these circumstances, the illness they suffer from and experience first-hand does not restrict their ability to verbally express their emotions to others. For individuals diagnosed with a laryngeal malignancy, treatment will frequently limit and potentially eliminate this communicative capacity. When the ability to communicate is lost, the process of recovery and rehabilitation may often be influenced appreciably. (p. 261)

The importance of communication with health care providers was illustrated in a study by Rieker et al. (1992). The authors undertook a descriptive, retrospective study that surveyed patients and families about factors that contributed to patients' ratings of their QOL and quality of care following experimental cancer therapy. They found that four components were significantly related to respondents' assessment of QOL, including adequate symptom control, availability of support services, communication with medical team members, and receipt of information about response to treatment. Therefore, communication issues in general and ease of communication specifically directly affect patients' perception of QOL (Wen & Gustafson, 2004). The issue of communication between patients and health care professionals is further complicated by the fact that head and neck cancer care often requires a multidisciplinary team with professionals from many different disciplines (Logemann, 1998). The patient may need to interact with a multitude of different health care professionals, whose roles over the longer term may be unclear to the patient, and who have different styles of interaction. Even within a professional service, the patient may need to deal with different individuals (e.g., nurses, radiation therapists). This is an immensely challenging road to navigate for the person who already has difficulty speaking and communicating needs. Many authors have noted the high degree of complexity and variability among patients and, therefore, the need for integrated multidisciplinary care and ongoing monitoring of symptoms during and after treatment (Deleyiannis, Weymuller, & Coltrera, 1997; Deleyiannis, Weymuller, Coltrera, & Futran, 1999; Logemann, 1998; McDonough et al., 1996; Minasian & Dwyer, 1998).

Health care professionals do not intend to take the responsibility away from the patient; on the contrary, health care professionals are obligated to provide ongoing information, education, and support to assist the patient in raising concerns that have an impact on his or her QOL. As Logemann (1994) stated, "an important concept for the patient to learn preoperatively is that they are in control and responsible for their own rehabilitation" (p. 363). The health care professional, however, must continue to facilitate the patient's participation in treatment in order to promote the patient's return to pretreatment activities and self-determined components of QOL.

WHAT SPEECH–LANGUAGE PATHOLOGISTS CAN DO TO IMPROVE PATIENTS' QUALITY OF LIFE

Quality of life has significant implications for the speech–language pathologist and, more important, the person living with head and neck cancer served by the clinician. The following subsections provide an overview of the range of applications of both the concept of QOL and knowledge gained from current research in this area. Suggestions apply both to direct clinical practice with individual patients and to professional involvement with this population. Application of the QOL concept can be viewed along a continuum, from informally but regularly "asking the questions" in direct individual clinical practice, to contributing to the growing body of formal research in the field of QOL research (de Graeff et al., 2000; Myers, 1995; Myers & Baird, 1992).

Familiarity with the QOL Concept and Relevant Literature

QOL is patient centered, multidimensional, functional, and changes continuously according to events affecting the patient. Awareness of this cautions the clinician against making assumptions about the patient. For example, one cannot assume that intervention is complete because the patient is intelligible; she may in fact be having considerable difficulty communicating with a mildly hearing-impaired spouse or friends in a noisy coffee shop. One must not assume that the patient who is missing several teeth and wears a dental plate may not care about or want to preserve his few remaining teeth. One cannot assume that a patient who appears well nourished would not value improvement in her mealtime experiences. Thus, an understanding of the growing body of literature related to QOL and head and neck cancers can be used to monitor patient concerns and guide the course of intervention. Clinicians who have "a firm understanding of the multiple dimensions of QOL will be in a better position to identify those concerns that may adversely affect patient outcomes" (King et al., 1997, p. 36). Identifying such concerns is a critical component of comprehensive clinical care for the individual with head and neck cancer.

Eliciting Information Through Questioning

The clinician should "ask the questions," regularly and consistently, that will elicit information on QOL issues of concern to the patient (Myers, 1995). The clinician can take small but consistent steps to change the course of practice. Asking "How can I help you?" and "What are you most concerned about today?" at each clinical visit can be an initial step. Till (1994) noted that "QOL assessments have been done informally for many years by asking the simple question, 'how have you been lately?'" (p. 244). However, a more regular and systematic approach to questioning may help to identify what is affecting the patient's present QOL. Questions should be phrased specifically, and in such a way that the patient can respond from his or her own perspective. In other words, it may not be enough to ask, "Do you have any concerns?" The patient may not know how to answer. It may not be enough to ask, "Are you getting enough to eat?" or to merely observe that the patient is maintaining his or her weight and appears well nourished. The patient may be subsisting on a diet of supplements or may have found that eating, once one of the great pleasures of life, has become joyless and burdensome.

More direct questions related to the likely consequences of the disease or treatments (e.g., "Are you having any concerns about your teeth?" "Do you have pain anywhere today?" or "Are you able to move your arm and shoulder to your satisfaction?") may elicit information about how these effects currently impact patients' lives, and enable the health care team to find the appropriate and more immediate solutions. Regularly asking such questions and eliciting responses from the patient can guide the course of clinical follow-up and maximize care of patients with head and neck cancer.

Careful clinicians will ask the appropriate questions to elicit the information that will guide the direction of treatment, rather than assuming the answers. The patient's perception of QOL should guide decision making during postoperative rehabilitation, as well as in the preoperative decision-making process. A patient undergoing such life-altering treatment must be fully informed of the consequences of treatment as they may relate to his or her individual lifestyle and preferences.

This task of eliciting information does not necessarily mean that the speech–language pathologist is doing less of the traditional speech, voice, and dysphagia therapy. It may mean, however, that through judicious questioning, the clinician identifies more pressing problems (e.g., pain management, dental, nutritional concerns) and redirects efforts to more urgently needed services so that professional clinical time is not wasted. It may also mean that opportunities to enhance the effectiveness of treatment are not wasted. For example, if a patient has identified fatigue as a primary concern, and the fatigue is found to be related to thyroid dysfunction or malnourishment, the patient may do better in therapy after these problems have been properly addressed. Gritz et al. (1999) stated that "identifying predictors of quality of life in head and neck cancer patients can assist in determining the need for early intervention immediately post treatment with the ultimate goal of reducing or preventing long-term problems" (p. 353). Early identification of patient concerns, by regularly and consistently asking questions, will lead to improved outcomes and enhanced quality of care.

Screening: Evaluation of Symptoms Within the Framework of QOL

There are pitfalls to using an informal approach in questioning the patient regarding QOL issues. For example, some important dimensions of QOL, such as emotional, social, or sexual functioning, may not be assessed systematically. A patient may be reluctant to reveal concerns of this kind. Furthermore, a health care professional "may neglect to ask about such concerns because of oversight, time limitations or embarrassment surrounding the issue" (Till, 1994, p. 244). In addition, too broad a question may miss specific concerns, and sporadic questioning may fail to address the changing variables that affect the patient from visit to visit. Till noted that informally asking patients questions is nonsystematic and does not provide quantitative information but that "formal QOL assessments assess well-defined aspects [dimensions] of QOL systematically and in quantitative terms" (p. 244). A more formal method of screening for QOL issues may be appropriate; however, it must be short and simple, and provide information from the patient's point of view, thus capturing the patient's perspective. There is a trade-off between too many questions and too little specificity (Till, 1994).

The question of which QOL variables to screen is important, given the need to capture critical information without significantly lengthening available consultation time. At a minimum, screening for psychosocial distress is warranted, given that this is one of the most commonly reported sequelae in the head and neck cancer population. McQuellon and Hurt (1997) recommended the screening of psychosocial variables specifically, and stated that the use of "a formal assessment of psychosocial difficulties with one of the quality-of-life scales may be quite useful to patients and professionals in designing individualized rehabilitation programs" (p. 238). The National Comprehensive Cancer Network (NCCN) (1999) reported that it is not uncommon for cancer patients to experience significant levels of distress, although few are referred for psychosocial counseling. Because psychosocial resources carry a stigma (as do any mental health services), patients are reluctant to express needs to their physician. Furthermore, medical professionals are perceived as too busy and too rushed to inquire about patients' psychosocial health and needs; patients are subsequently reluctant to "burden" their health care providers with their concerns (Detmar & Aaronson, 1998). It has been suggested, however, that addressing psychosocial needs can lead to a reduction in reported physical concerns and needs (Hwang et al., 1997; Newell et al., 1999).

Health care professionals may raise concerns about the time required to "open the door" to lengthy and involved patient discussions regarding psychosocial issues. Useful strategies, however, are available to assist health care providers in quickly identifying patient concerns and providing caring support (e.g., informing the patient up front about how much consultation time is available, acknowledging the patient's concerns, refocusing the patient's attention to specific issues) (Bouchard Ryan, 1996). NCCN (1999) proposed an evaluation and treatment model in which patients are rapidly assessed in the clinic on a routine basis for the presence of distress and its nature, and then referred to the appropriate resource for intervention as indicated. The recommended standards of care for management of psychosocial distress in cancer patients include the following (NCCN, 1999, p. 115):

- Distress should be recognized, monitored, documented, and treated promptly at all stages of disease.
- All patients should be screened for distress at their initial visit, at appropriate intervals, and as clinically indicated.
- Educational and training programs should be developed to ensure that health-care professionals and clergy have knowledge and skills in the management of distress.

The NCCN (1999) also generated a problem list to identify reasons for distress, which includes items in the areas of practical issues, physical symptoms, family and emotional problems, and spiritual or religious concerns. The problem list is completed by the patient and then reviewed with a team member.

The NCCN (1999) further suggested that oncology teams will vary as to who is responsible for screening for psychosocial distress. Often a nurse or social worker performs the screening. In some cases, however, the speech–language pathologist may be the member of the health care team who sees the patient most frequently over the long term (Doyle, 1994); consequently, screening for psychosocial distress may fall into the realm of the speech–language pathologist in a multidisciplinary team setting.

Another area that should be considered for regular screening is acute or chronic pain, given the high prevalence among head and neck cancer patients (Campbell et al., 2000; de Graeff et al., 1999; Ingall et al., 1991). A study by de Rond and colleagues (1999) found that daily pain assessment by nurses on medical and surgical wards is not only feasible but also appreciated by both patients and nurses. Nurses stated that daily screening allowed more insight into patients' pain, more attention paid to patients' pain, and ultimately better pain management. The authors found that screening could easily be incorporated into daily care routines. It seems possible that other health care providers, including speech–language pathologists, could also incorporate pain screening into clinical visits.

Several authors have suggested consideration of more comprehensive symptom or QOL screening (Gritz et al., 1999; Osoba, 1993; Till, 1994). Screening checklists can be used periodically to monitor QOL issues and gaps in services or a need for referral (Doyle & White, 2004). Osoba (1993) noted that in routine follow-up, "only those symptoms that seem 'relevant' are incorporated in the notes, and it is uncertain if these comprise all the symptoms a patient had at the time" and further suggested using a symptom screening checklist as a way of "documenting evidence of a systematic review of symptoms" (p. 48). The checklist can provide "a ready entry to areas of concern and also act as an 'aide memoire' ensuring that the major symptoms are reviewed in a systematic fashion at each clinic visit" (pp. 48–49). This idea is supported by a study by Detmar and Aaronson (1998), who used the EORTC QLQ-C30 (Bjordal & Kaasa, 1992; Sprangers, Cull, Bjordal, Groenvold, & Aaronson, 1993) in daily clinical oncology practice to investigate the impact on patient–physician communication. Five of 18 patients who participated in this study had head and neck cancers. A small increase was noted in the number of QOL issues per discussion; however, the most significant finding was the increased responsibility taken by physicians over three successive visits with each patient in raising specific QOL issues for discussion. Furthermore, patients believed that the use of the QOL survey had a positive influence on their communication with their doctors. Of note, the authors found that the availability to the QOL summary did not change the average length of time spent per patient.

Detmar and Aaronson (1998) and Osoba (1993) also suggested that QOL screening in daily clinical practice is feasible, does not lengthen average consultation time, is appreciated by both patients and health care providers, appears to stimulate health care providers to inquire about specific aspects of health affecting QOL, and provides a method of systematic review of symptoms and their level of change over time. The regular use of QOL screening instruments appears to sensitize health care providers to their patients' unique problems and needs in daily living. Ultimately, this should lead to earlier identification of concerns and improved care for head and neck cancer patients.

Clearly, head and neck disease–specific assessment tools such as QOL modules would be more likely to capture the specific needs of the patient with head and neck cancer. Till (1994) stated that "in addition to their potential usefulness in defining groups of patients with different needs for care, QOL scores may be helpful as indicators of the needs for care of individual patients" (p. 246). Patient self-assessment tools can provide an opportunity for individual patients to identify their own issues and concerns in an unhurried yet systematic manner, identify their own priorities, and describe concerns in their own language, which may present a more revealing picture of their circumstances (Hirshfield-Bartek, Hassey Dow, & Creaton, 1990). Although Bjordal et al. (1994) supported use of QOL instruments as screening tools, they cautioned that "these instruments should never substitute for the clinical interview" (p. 855). Furthermore, symptom screening or QOL screening does not need to detract from planned speech–language pathology interventions. Incorporated into the ongoing clinical care of patients, QOL screening tools may change the course of treatment or lead to services that are more urgently needed by patients; they can also provide a means for monitoring change over time. The role of QOL screening tools may well be suited to the speech–language pathologist in a multidisciplinary team setting who may have regular and ongoing contact with the patient. The combined use of QOL screening tools, traditional functional assessments, and the clinical interview may result in the most individualized assessment and treatment programs, giving rise to what is truly patient-centered care.

Adaptation of Rehabilitation According to Patients' Self-Determined QOL Ratings

By establishing patient-identified QOL determinants, the clinician can tailor more specific interventions. King and colleagues (1997) stressed the importance of identification of vulnerable periods during rehabilitation when interventions may need to take a different course. For example, during the period of postoperative radiotherapy, traditional speech or swallowing practice exercises may need to be put on hold due to the patient's level of fatigue, pain, or mucositis (see Chapters 13 and 14 in this text). The speech–language pathologist may provide supportive care during this period of time, with less intensive speech practice and more work on maintenance of oromotor movement and functional communication. Follow-up by other health care team members (e.g., to provide psychosocial support, nutrition services) may correspondingly increase during these periods of time.

At the same time, it is important to acknowledge self-reported, positive levels of QOL determinants while monitoring for QOL issues. For example, the clinician can draw the patient's attention to observations—such as rising levels of reported energy or lessening levels of cough and mucous production over time, or successful communication experiences, or a return to eating among other people such as a first outing to a restaurant—as markers in the journey toward recovery, improved functioning, and improved QOL. Mount and Cohen (1995) stressed the value of asking about positive contributors to QOL, thereby encouraging patient participation in activities that promote continued positive perceptions of QOL for that individual. Over time, the patient's need for various professional services will change. It is important for all members of the health care team to be sensitive to the need for assistance from other services for positive reasons, such as return-to-work or vocational issues. This client-centered focus requires a multidisciplinary team–oriented approach, with a more fluid shift between services.

Facilitation of Patient's Participation in Own Health Care

Perhaps one of the most valuable roles speech–language pathologists can assume is to assist those with communication difficulties to take a stronger role in advocating for their own self-assessed health care concerns and needs. This role requires both a knowledge of the specific posttreatment communication impairments and consequences, and an understanding of the nature of patient–professional interaction. Participating in interactions with health care professionals can be challenging, even for the cancer patient who does not have communication difficulties. An intervention strategy designed to provide decisional support for patients with cancer who want to participate in medical treatment decisions has been presented by Neufeld, Degner, and Dick (1993). Designed for and used with a patient population of women diagnosed with breast or gynecological cancer, the strategy is based on the concepts of commitment and control, and on determining the degree of involvement that each individual patient desires. The emphasis of the intervention strategy is on establishing the patient's agenda, including the extent to which she wants to participate, helping her identify questions, and supporting her in obtaining the information desired. Neufeld and colleagues (1993) successfully incorporated the strategy into a busy oncology clinic and planned to assess the impact of providing decisional support on overall QOL. These authors noted that "asking questions is not easy for many patients" (Neufeld et al., 1993, p. 634). Extension of the concerns underlying the strategy proposed by Neufeld et al. (1993) has remained an area of interest by multiple disciplines, with a variety of related complementary considerations offered by several groups of investigators (e.g., Manne & Glassman, 2000; Mellink et al., 2003; Molenaar et al., 2001; Wen & Gustafson, 2004). It is often even more difficult for the patient with head and neck cancer whose communication is impaired. The speech–language pathologist has traditionally focused on assisting the patient improve communication in a more narrow sense—that is, improving intelligibility of speech. The QOL paradigm, however, suggests a broader, and perhaps more pragmatic functional approach to communication, including facilitating interactions with health care professionals. With an increasing focus on patient autonomy and the recognition that issues affecting QOL are best identified from the patient's perspective, this role could potentially be important for the speech–language pathologist who works with this population.

Taking a Broader, More Holistic Role

Research has promoted increased knowledge of the many aspects of QOL and the changing nature of QOL throughout treatment. Furthermore, the multidisciplinary team approach has led to greater awareness of the role of other professionals and a broader view of rehabilitation. Traditionally, speech–language pathologists have focused on interventions more directly related to communication in the narrow sense, such as speech intelligibility, rate and acceptability of speech, and voice quality (see Chapter 5 in this text). Blood et al. (1992) suggested that "voice therapy serves as a necessary anchor for the patients at a time when they need some way to gain control over their lives. If this is the case, then any means of communication would be beneficial" (p. 68). Many factors, however, influence a patient's willingness or ability to communicate, including fatigue, depression, dental problems, dry mouth, pain, and so on. Speech therapy and refinement of voice may not be a priority at certain stages of treatment; therefore, "as patients with laryngectomies' reactions to their cancer differ according to what is being faced, individual therapy plans should be tailored in consultation with other members of the rehabilitation team" (Blood et al., 1992, p. 68). Furthermore, Clarke (1998) noted that "for the head and neck cancer patient with multiple rehabilitation needs, this can best be accomplished through a comprehensive, coordinated approach, utilizing interdisciplinary clinical and community resources aimed at facilitating the rehabilitation process and ultimately achieving individualized rehabilitation goals" (p. 81). Finally, Blood and colleagues (1994) also suggested that voice restoration therapy could incorporate adjustment, coping, and counseling issues in a more systematic fashion, and that "the speech language pathologist may serve as the 'door' for referral for professional counseling needs for some" (p. 43).

The speech–language pathologist may be the team member with which the patient and family have most regular and consistent contact over the long term. Therefore, the speech–language pathologist may serve as a vital identifier of more urgent needs according to the patient's perception. Whereas medical follow-up visits may address primarily evidence of recurrence of cancer, less threatening QOL issues may be overlooked. In addition, Bjordal, Ahlner-Elmqvist, et al. (1994) noted that head and neck cancer patients may experience a high level of treatment-related symptoms and psychological distress, with a corresponding impact on QOL many years after treatment.

Although the speech–language pathologist may assume a more active role in ascertaining patient QOL concerns, this is not to suggest shifting responsibility from patients or returning to a paternalistic model of intervention. Rather, it is hoped that patients will be better informed through the availability of comprehensive and improved patient education materials and methods, support groups and visitor programs, and patient newsletters, such as that published by the International Association of Laryngectomees. Patients and their families can continue to broaden their knowledge about head and neck cancer disease and its treatments, and take a more active and informed role in their health care. With support, patients with head and neck cancer and their families can express their needs and concerns, and by doing so their QOL will be enhanced.

FUTURE DIRECTIONS[3]

Continued research is needed in a variety of areas to improve the QOL of patients with head and neck cancer. The following subsections describe some suggested avenues of research.

◪ Determining Patients' QOL-Related Needs.
Further research is necessary for the continued delineation of the unique needs of patients with head and neck cancer, and the variables that affect QOL. This research is needed given the heterogeneity in this population, as well as the continued evolution

---

[3]This section is adapted from Myers (1995) and Myers and Baird (1992).

of treatment protocols. Bjordal, Ahlner-Elmqvist, et al. (1994)
stated that

> in studies where survival and tumor response are the most im-
> portant outcomes, data on QOL may give an opportunity to
> choose treatment modalities with similar survival, to reduce
> treatment-related side-effects, to improve support and reha-
> bilitation during and after treatment, and to improve the in-
> formation and communication with patients. (p. 884)

However, there are many problems with existing QOL studies: Small samples and
wide variation in disease sites and treatment options and protocols make generalization difficult. Larger sample sizes (Gritz et al., 1999) are clearly needed. Researchers need to find out more about QOL in hard-to-reach populations such
as the elderly, minorities, or those with low socioeconomic status (Curbow,
1997); in those who are unwilling to participate, illiterate, or lost to follow-up
(Gritz et al., 1999); in women who are laryngectomized (Brown & Doyle, 1999);
and in those with end-stage disease (Gritz et al., 1999). Another area of importance is how coping and lifestyle factors interact with treatment in response to
QOL (Morris, 1994). Furthermore, little has been done to formally assess the impact of rehabilitation interventions on QOL (Gritz et al., 1999; Logemann, 1994;
Long et al., 1996); the impact of specific treatment regimes (Gritz et al., 1999);
the ways in which QOL domains relate to each other (e.g., Can fatigue be offset
by spirituality? How does fatigue affect appetite?) (Curbow, 1997; Sist, 1998);
and the differences between QOL concerns among survivor subgroups, exploring culture and ethnic issues and determinants of QOL (Cook Gotay, 1997;
King et al., 1997). Despite the accumulating body of knowledge about QOL
in the head and neck cancer patient population, many unanswered questions
remain.

There is an increasing number of cancer "survivors," a unique group of patients whose needs over the long term have not been fully addressed. Bjordal,
Ahlner-Elmqvist, et al. (1994) studied a group of 204 head and neck cancer patients 7 to 11 years after radiotherapy. They found that many patients continue to
experience a reduced QOL with a high level of treatment-related symptoms and
psychological distress long after treatment has ended. Loescher, Clark, Atwood,
Leigh, and Lamb (1990) studied a group of 17 adults more than 2 years post–
cancer therapy and identified long-term physiologic, psychosocial, and economic
impacts many years after treatment. Patients had a perceived vulnerability and a
need for wellness maintenance and reassurance from health care professionals.
The authors identified ongoing needs for (a) information related to updates to
reduce anxiety and fear of recurrence, cancer cause, and prevention of recurrence; (b) support and reassurance from health care professionals; and (c) access to
medical care including rehabilitation services. Ferrrell, Hassey Dow, Leigh, Ly, and
Gulasekaram (1995) found that cancer survivors were concerned about adjustment to fatigue and aches and pains and the ongoing need for information and
support. Relatively little research has been done in the area of QOL and the
long-term needs of the patient with head and neck cancer.

Along with the need to explore QOL issues in untapped areas in patient subgroups, existing QOL research can be further improved in replications. Deleyiannis, Weymuller, and Coltrera (1997) recommended the following to further improve QOL studies: incorporating patient ratings of importance and severity of each problem within a domain; incorporating the use of two global ratings—one for overall QOL and the other for health-related QOL—to differentiate medical from nonmedical factors; and allowing patients to add supplemental items. Given small and heterogeneous patient samples and the wide range in tumor types, anatomic sites, and treatments, the replication of studies, with the addition of the above suggestions, would be of value.

Further research is needed in identifying the relatively unexplored area of positive contributors to QOL in head and neck cancer patients (Mount & Cohen, 1995). Deleyiannis et al. (1999) concluded that "although the loss of voice is disabling, the functional limitations caused by laryngectomy do not necessarily translate into a worse overall QOL" (p. 319). They stated that

> ninety percent of patients (9/10) reported that compared with one year prior to the diagnosis of cancer their general health was the same or better at two years postlaryngectomy. Seventy percent of patients (7/10) reported having good to excellent overall QOL (p. 321)

Interestingly, 7 of the 10 patients were using an electrolarynx as their method of communication, 2 were tablet writers, and 1 used TEP as his primary means of communication. Clearly, rehabilitation has improved along many dimensions and among many interrelated disciplines; however, specification of the nature of and contributors to these positive changes is not known.

Development of QOL Screening Tools.

There is a need to develop screening tools for the clinician to capture potential concerns of individual patients in the area of QOL issues. Use of such tools may change and improve the direction of treatment. Studies are needed to assess the reliability and validity of using existing QOL modules in the clinic setting to assist in decision making for individual patients in routine clinical care.

Determining Best Practice in QOL Screening.

There is a need for research in best practice in QOL screening (i.e., to determine how screening for head and neck cancer patients can best be accomplished and by whom). It would be worthwhile to compare the utility and efficacy of QOL screening by various members of the multidisciplinary team (e.g., speech–language pathologist, nurse, dietitian) to determine whether screening by different professionals changes the selection and timing of interventions, or whether multiple QOL issues are identified.

◢ Adaptation of Instruments for Certain Populations.

Existing QOL assessment and screening instruments must be adapted to capture information from those who are difficult to test (i.e., those with cognitive or language difficulties or for whom literacy or language is a barrier, or for patients for whom typical self-assessment is difficult or even impossible). QOL information should be collected from people who are physically, linguistically, or cognitively unable to complete a standard pencil-and-paper assessment tool.

◢ Assessment of Strategy Use with Patients with Communicative Impairments.

It may be of benefit to assess whether existing strategies used to facilitate communication between patients and health care providers will work with individuals with communicative impairments subsequent to head and neck cancer. Studies could explore the use by speech–language pathologists of established assessment models (e.g., Neufeld et al., 1993) and determine what modifications, if any, may be necessary. Examples of questions to research include these: Do patients with head and neck cancers need different strategies to ensure that the health care provider has clearly understood their spoken message? How effective are health care professionals who work with patients with head and neck cancer at accurately understanding patients' questions and statements? Do these patients and professionals use more or different strategies than other patients and professionals at ensuring accuracy of messages and avoiding communicative failure?

◢ Assessing Impact of Interventions on QOL.

There is a great need to assess the impact of rehabilitation interventions on QOL for head and neck cancer patients in general, as well as for subgroups of treatment modalities. Researchers need to evaluate and standardize specific rehabilitation protocols within the realm of QOL and establish outcome measures. Deleyiannis et al. (1999) noted the extreme variability of patient-specific disabilities and their effects on QOL among patients. Also, research is needed to learn more about rehabilitation needs and timing of treatment in the immediate postoperative period (Logemann, Pauloski, Rademaker, & Colangelo, 1997; Long et al., 1996). Logemann et al. (1997) stressed the importance of QOL studies to

> identify the particular types of problems of greatest concern
> to each type of patient so that interventions can be targeted

to those problems. It seems quite likely that patient complaints and concerns about their functional abilities may vary at different times following treatment. (p. 656)

Clearly, rehabilitation efforts have had a positive impact on the quality of life of the head and neck cancer patient. As stated by Mount and Cohen (1995), however,

It is clear that it is an exceedingly difficult task to accurately measure QOL. We will only be able to do so if we let the people whose QOL we are attempting to measure teach us what QOL means to them. (p. 124)

As the speech–language pathologist and other multidisciplinary team members incorporate the QOL concept into clinical practice, professional intervention efforts will improve, and health care providers can indeed claim that they can improve the QOL of individuals living with head and neck cancer.

SUMMARY

This chapter has addressed multiple issues underlying QOL and head and neck cancer. Topics included the broad concept of QOL, the parameters that contribute to one's overall QOL, and the methods by which QOL is assessed in health care generally and among persons living with head and neck cancer specifically; the multitude of impacts of head and neck cancer and its treatment in the context of QOL; a rationale for the clinician to consider both the broad QOL framework and specific QOL issues in head and neck cancer rehabilitation; the biomedical ethical concepts that support the rationale; a range of applications of the concept of QOL and the growing body of knowledge generated from QOL research, with the goal of improving patients' QOL; and ongoing research needs and future directions. It is hoped that this chapter provokes thought and provides new direction for clinicians working with this unique and challenging patient population.

ACKNOWLEDGMENTS

I am grateful to St. Boniface General Hospital and the Manitoba Cancer Treatment and Research Foundation (Cancer Care Manitoba) for their generous support and assistance, and to Agathe Bisson, Allison Baird, and Drs. Philip Doyle and Harvey Schipper who influenced my thinking in this important area of clinical practice. In addition, I am grateful to the many individuals living with head and neck cancer whom I have had the privilege to serve and who have helped shape my thoughts and beliefs about rehabilitation for the person with head and neck cancer.

REFERENCES

Ackerstaff, A. H., Hilgers, F. J., Aaronson, N. K., & Balm, A. J. M. (1994). Communication, functional disorders and lifestyle changes after total laryngectomy. *Clinical Otolaryngology, 19,* 295–300.

Ackerstaff, A. H., Tan, I. B., Rasch, C. R. N., Balm, A. J. M., Keus, R. B., Schornagel, J. H., & Hilgers, F. J. M. (2002). Quality-of-life assessment after supradose selective intra-arterial Cisplatin and concomitant radiation (RADPLAT) for inoperable stage IV head and neck squamous cell carcinoma. *Archives of Otolaryngology—Head and Neck Surgery, 128,* 1185–1190.

Allison, P. J., Locker, D., & Feine, J. S. (1999). The relationship of dental status and health-related quality of life in upper aerodigestive tract cancer patients. *Oral Oncology, 35,* 138–143.

Armstrong, T., & Gilbert, M. R. (2004). Central nervous system toxicity from cancer treatment. *Current Oncology Reports, 6,* 11–19.

Baile, W. F., Gibertini, M., Scott, L., & Endicott, J. (1992). Depression and tumor stage in cancer of the head and neck. *Psycho-oncology, 1,* 15–24.

Bjordal, K., Ahlner-Elmqvist, M., Tollesson, E., Jensen, A. B., Razavi, D., Maher, E. J., & Kaasa, S. (1994). Development of a European Organization for Research and Treatment of Cancer (EORTC) questionnaire module to be used in quality of life assessments in head and neck cancer patients. *Acta Oncologica, 33,* 879–885.

Bjordal, K., & Kaasa, S. (1992). Psychometric validation of the EORTC Core Quality of Life Questionnaire, 30-item version and a diagnosis-specific module for head and neck cancer patients. *Acta Oncologica, 31,* 311–321.

Bjordal, K., Kaasa, S., & Mastekaasa, A. (1994). Quality of life in patients treated for head and neck cancer: A follow-up study 7 to 11 years after radiotherapy. *International Journal of Radiation Oncology, Biology, Physics, 28*(4), 847–856.

Blakley, B. W., Black, F. O., Myers, S. F., Rintelmann, W. F., Schweitzer, V., & Schwan, S. A. (1991, January/February). Ototoxicity. *Head & Neck, 13,* 2.

Blood, G. W. (1993). Development and assessment of a scale addressing communication needs of patients with laryngectomies. *American Journal of Speech–Language Pathology, 27,* 82–90.

Blood, G. W., Luther, A. R., & Stemple, J. C. (1992, January). Coping and adjustment in alaryngeal speakers. *American Journal of Speech–Language Pathology, 27,* 63–69.

Blood, G. W., Simpson, K. C., Raimondi, S. C., Dineen, M., Kauffman, S. M., & Stagaard, K. A. (1994). Social support in laryngeal cancer survivors: Voice and adjustment issues. *American Journal of Speech-Language Pathology, 3,* 37–44.

Body, J. J., & Borkowski, A. (1987). Nutrition and quality of life in cancer patients. *European Journal of Cancer and Clinical Oncology, 23*(2), 127–129.

Bouchard Ryan, E. (1996). Psychosocial perspectives on discourse and hearing differences among older adults. *Journal of Speech–Language Pathology and Audiology, 20*(2), 95–100.

Breitbart, W., & Holland, J. (1988). Psychosocial aspects of head and neck cancer. *Seminars in Oncology, 15*(1), 61–69.

Browman, G. P., Levine, M. N., Hodson, D. I., Sathya, J., Russell, R., Skingley, P., Cripps, C., Eapen, L., & Girard, A. (1993). The Head and Neck Radiotherapy Questionnaire: A morbidity/quality-of-life instrument for clinical trials of radiotherapy in locally advanced head and neck cancer. *Journal of Clinical Oncology, 11*(5), 863–872.

Brown, S. I., & Doyle, P. C. (1999). The woman who is laryngectomized: Parallels, perspectives, and reevaluation of practice. *Journal of Speech–Language Pathology and Audiology, 23*(2), 54–60.

Burns, L., Chase, D., & Goodwin, W. J. (1987). Treatment of patients with stage IV cancer: Do the ends justify the means? *Otolaryngology—Head and Neck Surgery, 97*(1), 8–14.

Cameron, P., Green, W. B., & Gulliver, M. (2000). Middle ear dysfunction following laryngectomy. *Journal of Speech–Language Pathology and Audiology, 24,* 19–25.

Campbell, B. H., Marbella, A., & Layde, P. M. (2000). Quality of life and recurrence concern in survivors of head and neck cancer. *Laryngoscope, 110,* 895–906.

Carrara-de-Angelis, E., Feher, O., Barros, A. P., Nishimoto, I. N., & Kowalski, L, P. (2003). Voice and swallowing in patients enrolled in a larynx preservation trial. *Archives of Otolaryngology—Head and Neck Surgery, 129,* 733–738.

Cassel, E. J. (1982). The nature of suffering and the goals of medicine. *New England Journal of Medicine, 306,* 639–645.

Cella, D. F. (1994). *Manual for the Functional Assessment of Cancer Therapy (FACT) Scale and the Functional Assessment of HIV (FAHI) Scale (Version 3).* Chicago: Rush-Presbyterian-St. Lukes Medical Center.

Cella, D. F., & Cherin, E. A. (1988). Quality of life during and after cancer treatment. *Comprehensive Therapy, 14*(5), 69–75.

Clarke, L. K. (1998). Rehabilitation for the head and neck cancer patient. *Oncology, 12,* 81–89.

Cook Gotay, C. (1997). The Ferrell/Hassey Dow article reviewed. *Oncology, 11,* 576.

Cooley, M. E., Moriarty, H., Berger, M. S., Selm-Orr, D., Coyle, B., & Short, T. (1995). Patient literacy and the readability of written cancer educational materials. *Oncology Nursing Forum, 22,* 1345–1351.

Copper, M. P., Smit, C. F., Stanojcic, L. D., Devriese, P. P., Schouwenburg, P. F., & Mathus-Vliegen, L. M. H. (2000). High incidence of laryngopharyngeal reflux in patients with head and neck cancer. *Laryngoscope, 110,* 1007–1011.

Curbow, B. (1997). The Ferrell/Hassey Dow article reviewed. *Oncology, 11,* 572–575.

Curran, A. J., Irish, J. C., & Gullane, P. J. (1997). Recent developments in the surgical management of head and neck cancer. *Current Oncology, 4*(4), 209–214.

deBoer, M. F., Pruyn, J. F., van den Borne, B., Knegt, P. P., Ryckman, R. M., & Verwoerd, C. D. (1995). Rehabilitation outcomes of long-term survivors treated for head and neck cancer. *Head & Neck, 17,* 503–515.

Degner, L. F., & Sloan, J. A. (1992). Decision making during serious illness: What role do patients really want to play? *Journal of Clinical Epidemiology, 45,* 941–950.

de Graeff, A., de Leeuw, R. J., Ros, W. J., Hordijk, G.-J., Battermann, J. J., Blijham, G. H., & Winnubst, J. A. (1999). A prospective study on quality of life of laryngeal cancer patients treated with radiotherapy. *Head & Neck, 21,* 291–296.

de Graeff, A., de Leeuw, R. J., Ros, W. J. G., Hordijk, G.-J., Blijham, G. H., & Winnubst, J. A. M. (2000). Pretreatment factors predicting quality of life after treatment for head and neck cancer. *Head & Neck, 22,* 398–407.

Deleyiannis, F. W.-B., Weymuller, E. A., & Coltrera, M. D. (1997). Quality of life of disease-free survivors of advanced (stage III or IV) oropharyngeal cancer. *Head & Neck, 19,* 466–473.

Deleyiannis, F. W.-B., Weymuller, E. A., Coltrera, M. D., & Futran, N. (1999). Quality of life after laryngectomy. *Head & Neck, 21,* 319–324.

DeNittis, A. S., Machtay, M., Rosenthal, D. I., Sanfilippo, N. J., Lee, J. H., Goldfeder, S., Chalian, A. A., Weinstein, G. S., & Weber, R. S. (2001). Advanced oropharyngeal carcinoma treated with surgery and radiotherapy: Oncologic outcome and functional assessment. *American Journal of Otolaryngology, 22,* 329–335.

de Rond, M. E. J., de Wit, R., van Dam, F., van Campen, B., den Hartog, Y., Klievink, R., Nieweg, R., Noort, J., Wagenaar, M., & van Campen, B. (1999). Daily pain assessment: Value for nurses and patients. *Journal of Advanced Nursing, 29*(2), 436–444.

DeSanto, L. W., Olsen, K. D., Perry, W. C., Rohe, D. E., & Keith, R. L. (1995). Quality of life after surgical treatment of cancer of the larynx. *Annals of Otology, Rhinology and Laryngology, 104*(10, Pt. 1), 763–769.

Detmar, S. B., & Aaronson, N. K. (1998). Quality of life assessment in daily clinical oncology practice: A feasibility study. *European Journal of Cancer, 34,* 1181–1186.

Doyle, P. C. (1994). *Foundations of voice and speech rehabilitation following laryngeal cancer.* San Diego: Singular.

Doyle, P. C., & White, H. D. (2004, May). *Use of the Rotterdam Symptom Checklist in laryngectomized men and women.* Paper presented at the annual conference of the Canadian Association of Speech–Language Pathologists and Audiologists, Ottawa, Ontario.

Dropkin, M. J. (1989). Coping with disfigurement and dysfunction after head and neck surgery: A conceptual framework. *Seminars in Oncology Nursing, 5*(3), 213–219.

Eadie, T. L., & Charland, L. (in press). Ethics in speech–language pathology: Beyond the codes and canons. *Journal of Speech–Language Pathology and Audiology.*

Eisbruch, A., Lyden, T., Bradford, C. R., Dawson, L. A., Haxer, M. J., Miller, A. E., Teknos, T. N., Chepeha, D. B., Hogikyan, N. D., Terrell, J. E., & Wolf, G. T. (2002). Objective assessment of swallowing dysfunction and aspiration after radiation concurrent with chemotherapy for head–neck cancer. *International Journal of Radiation Oncology and Biological Physics, 53,* 23–28.

Ende, J., Kazis, L., Ash, A., & Moskowitz, M. A. (1989). Measuring patients' desire for autonomy. *Journal of General and Internal Medicine, 4,* 23–30.

Epstein, J. B., Emerton, S., Kolbinson, D. A., Le, N. D., Phillips, N., Stevenson-Moore, P., & Osoba, D. (1999). Quality of life and oral function following radiotherapy for head and neck cancer. *Head & Neck, 21,* 1–11.

Fayers, P. M., Hand, D. J., Bjordal, K., & Groenvold, M. (1997). Causal indicators in quality of life research. *Quality of Life Research, 6*(5), 393–406.

Ferrell, B., & Hassey Dow, K. (1997). Quality of life among long-term cancer survivors. *Oncology, 11,* 565–571.

Ferrell, B. R., Hassey Dow, K., Leigh, S., Ly, J., & Gulasekaram, P. (1995). Quality of life in long-term cancer survivors. *Oncology Nursing Forum, 22*(6), 915–922.

Fine, R., Krell, W., Ranella, K., Sessions, D., & Williams, M. (1991). Respiratory problems and rehabilitation in the head and neck cancer patient. *Head & Neck, 13,* 12–13.

Gamba, A., Romano, M., Grosso, I. M., Tamburini, M., Cantu, G., Molinari, R., & Ventafridda, V. (1992). Psychosocial adjustment of patients surgically treated for head and neck cancer. *Head & Neck, 14,* 218–223.

Gattellari, M., Butow, P. N., Tattersall, M. H., Dunn, S. M., & MacLeod, C. A. (1999). Misunderstanding in cancer patients: Why shoot the messenger? *Annals of Oncology, 10,* 39–46.

Gibson, A. R., & McCombe, M. D. (1999). Psychological morbidity following laryngectomy: A pilot study. *The Journal of Laryngology and Otology, 113,* 349–352.

Gliklich, R. E., Goldsmith, T. A., & Funk, G. F. (1997). Are head and neck specific quality of life measures necessary? *Head & Neck, 19,* 474–480.

Gotay, C. C., & Moore, T. D. (1992). Review: Assessing quality of life in head and neck cancer. *Quality of Life Research, 1,* 5–17.

Graner, D. E., Foote, R. L., Kasperbauer, J. L., Stoeckel, M. A., Okuno, S. H., Olsen, K. D., Sabri, A. N., Maragos, N. E., Cha, S. S., Sargent, D. J., & Strome, S. E. (2003). Swallow function in patients before and after intra-arterial chemoradiation. *Laryngoscope, 113,* 573–579.

Gritz, E. R., Carmack, C. L., de Moor, C., Coscarelli, A., Schacherer, C. W., Meyers, E. G., & Abemayor, E. (1999). First year after head and neck cancer: Quality of life. *Journal of Clinical Oncology, 17,* 352–360.

Harwood, A. R., & Rawlinson, E. (1983). The quality of life of patients following treatment for laryngeal cancer. *International Journal of Radiation Oncology, Biology, and Physics, 9,* 335–338.

Hassan, S. J., & Weymuller, E. A. (1993). Assessment of quality of life in head and neck cancer patients. *Head & Neck, 15,* 485–496.

Hilgers, F. J., Ackerstaff, A. H., Aaronson, N. K., Schouwenburg, P. F., & van Zandwijk, N. (1990). Physical and psychosocial consequences of total laryngectomy. *Clinical Otolaryngology, 15,* 421–425.

Hirshfield-Bartek, J., Hassey Dow, K., & Creaton, E. (1990). Decreasing documentation time using a patient self-assessment tool. *Oncology Nursing Forum, 17*(2), 251–255.

Hwang, S. S., Chang, V. T., Corpion, C., Ohanian, M., & Kasimis, N. J. (1997). A preliminary study of clinical predictors for lack of energy in patients with advanced cancer. *Proceedings of the Annual Meeting of the American Society of Clinical Oncologists, 16*(A241).

Ingall, J. R., Saper, J. R., Kish, J., Kuch, K., & Evans, R. (1991). Pain. *Head & Neck, 13,* 9–10.

Jones, E., Lund, V. J., Howard, D. J., Greenberg, M. P., & McCarthy, M. (1992). Quality of life of patients treated surgically for head and neck cancer. *Journal of Laryngology and Otology, 106,* 238–242.

King, C. R., Haberman, M., Berry, D. L., Bush, N., Butler, L., Hassey Dow, K., Ferrell, B., Grant, M., Gue, D., Hinds, P., Kreuer, J., Padilla, J., & Underwood, S. (1997). Quality of life and the cancer experience: The-state-of-the-knowledge. *Oncology Nursing Forum, 24*(1), 27–41.

Kreitler, S., Chaitchik, S., Rapoport, Y., & Algor, R. (1993). Psychosocial effects of level of information and severity of disease on head-and-neck cancer patients. *Journal of Cancer Education, 10*(3), 144–154.

Kuntz, A. L., & Weymuller, E. A., Jr. (1999). Impact of neck dissection on quality of life. *Laryngoscope, 109,* 1334–1338.

Lerman, C., Daly, M., Walsh, W. P., Resch, N., Seay, J., Barsevick, A., Birenbaum, L., Heggan, T., & Martin, G. (1993). Communication between patients with breast cancer and health care providers: Determinants and implications. *ACS Cancer, 72*(9), 1008–1016.

Levine, R. J. (1990). An ethical perspective. In B. Spilker (Ed.), *Quality of life assessments in clinical trials.* (pp. 156–162). New York: Raven Press.

List, M., Haraf, D., Siston, A., Stenson, K., Brockstein, B., Kies, M., & Vokes, E. (1997). A prospective study of quality of life (QL)/performance in head and neck cancer patients on an intensive chemoradiotherapy protocol (Abstract). *Proceedings of the Annual Meeting of the American Society of Clinical Oncology, 16,* A1390.

List, M. A., Ritter-Sterr, C., & Lansky, S. B. (1990). A performance status scale for head and neck cancer patients. *Cancer, 66,* 564–569.

Loescher, L. J., Clark, L., Atwood, J. R., Leigh, S., & Lamb, G. (1990). The impact of the cancer experience on long-term survivors. *Oncology Nursing Forum, 17*(2), 223–229.

Logemann, J. A. (1994). Rehabilitation of the head and neck cancer patient. *Seminars in Oncology, 21,* 359–365.

Logemann, J. A. (1997). Speech and swallowing rehabilitation for head and neck cancer patients. *Oncology, 11,* 651–658.

Logemann, J. A. (1998). The Clarke article reviewed: Response to Clarke, L. K. (1998) Rehabilitation for the head and neck cancer patient. *Oncology, 12,* 81–89, 93–94.

Logemann, J. A., & Bytell, D. E. (1979). Swallowing disorders in three types of head and neck surgical patients. *Cancer, 44*(3), 1095–1105.

Logemann, J. A., Pauloski, B. R., Rademaker, A. W., & Colangelo, L. A. (1997). Speech and swallowing rehabilitation for head and neck cancer patients. *Oncology, 11,* 651–659.

Long, S. A., D'Antonio, L. L., Robinson, E. B., Zimmerman, G., Patti, G., & Chonkich, G. (1996). Factors related to quality of life and functional status in 50 patients with head and neck cancer. *Laryngoscope, 106,* 1084–1088.

Magne, N., Marcy, P. Y., Chamorey, E., Guardiola, E., Pivot, X., Schnelder, M., Demard, F., Bensadoun, R.-J. (2001). Concomitant twice-a-day radiotherapy and chemotherapy in unresectable head and neck cancer patients: A long-term quality of life analysis. *Head & Neck, 23,* 678–682.

Manne, S., & Glassman, M. (2000). Perceived control, coping efficacy, and avoidance coping as mediators between spouses' unsupportive behaviors and cancer patients' psychological distress. *Health Psychology, 19,* 155–164.

Mathieson, C. M., Stam, H. J., & Scott, J. P. (1991). The impact of laryngectomy on the spouse: Who is better off? *Psychology and Health, 5,* 153–163.

Maxymiw, W. G., Rothney, L. M., & Sutcliffe, S. B. (1994). Reduction in the incidence of postradiation dental complications in cancer patients by continuous quality improvement techniques. *The Canadian Journal of Oncology, 4*(1), 233–237.

McConnel, F. M. S., Cerenko, D., & Mendelsohn, M. S. (1988). Dysphagia after total laryngectomy. *Otolaryngology Clinics of North America, 21*(4), 721–726.

McConnel, F. M. S., Mendelsohn, M. S., & Logemann, J. A. (1986). Examination of swallowing after total laryngectomy using manofluorography. *Head and Neck Surgery, 9,* 3–12.

McDonough, E. M., Varvares, M. A., Dunphy, F. R., Dunleavy, T., Dunphy, C. H., & Boyd, J. H. (1996). Changes in quality-of-life scores in a population of patients treated for squamous cell carcinoma of the head and neck. *Head & Neck, 18,* 487–493.

McNeil, B. J., Weichselbaum, M. D., & Pauker, S. G. (1981). Tradeoffs between quality and quantity of life in laryngeal cancer. *The New England Journal of Medicine, 305*(17), 982–987.

McQuellon, R. P., & Hurt, G. J. (1997). The psychosocial impact of the diagnosis and treatment of laryngeal cancer. *Otolaryngology Clinics of North America, 30*(2), 213–241.

Mellink, W. A. M., Dulmen, A. M. V., Wiggers, T., Spreeuwenberg, P. M. M., Eggermont, A. M. M., & Bensing, J. M. (2003). Cancer patients seeking a second surgical opinion: Results of a study on motives, needs, and expectations. *Journal of Clinical Oncology, 21,* 1492–1497.

Minasian, A., & Dwyer, J. T. (1998). Nutritional implications of dental and swallowing issues in head and neck cancer. *Oncology, 12,* 1155–1162.

Mohide, E. A., Archibald, S. D., Tew, M., Young, J. E., & Haines, T. (1992). Postlaryngectomy quality-of-life dimensions identified by patients and health care professionals. *American Journal of Surgery, 164,* 619–622.

Molenaar, S., Sprangers, M. A. G., Rutgers, E. J. T., Luiten, E. J., Mulder, J., Bossuyt, P. M. M., van Everdingen, J. J. E., Oosterveld, P., & de Haes, H. C. J. M. (2001). Decision support for patients with early-stage breast cancer. Effects of an interactive breast cancer CDROM on treatment decision, satisfaction, and quality of life. *Journal of Clinical Oncology, 19,* 1676–1687.

Moore, G. K., Getchell, T., Mistretta, C., Mozell, M., & Kern, R. (1991). Taste/smell. *Head & Neck, 13,* 7–8.

Morris, J. (1994). Widening perspectives: Quality of life as a measure of outcome in the treatment of patients with cancers of the head and neck. *Oral Oncology, European Journal of Cancer, 30*(1), 29–31.

Morton, R. P., Davies, A. D. M., Baker, J., Baker, G. A., & Stell, P. M. (1984). Quality of life in treated head and neck cancer patients: A preliminary report. *Clinics in Otolaryngology, 9,* 181–185.

Mount, B. M., & Cohen, S. R. (1995). Quality of life in the face of life-threatening illness: What should we be measuring? *Current Oncology, 2*(3), 121–125.

Myers, C. (1995, March). *Quality of life: An ethical issue in cancer treatment.* Paper presented at the First Mid-South Conference on Head and Neck Cancer, Memphis, TN.

Myers, C. L., & Baird, A. J. (1992, May). *Quality of life: Issues in communication disorders.* Paper presented at the annual conference of the Canadian Association of Speech–Language Pathologists and Audiologists, Saskatoon, Saskatchewan.

National Commission for the Protection of Human Subjects of Biomedical and Behavioral Research. (1978). *Institutional review boards: Report and recommendations* (Department of Health, Education and Welfare Publication No. OS 79–008). Washington, DC: U.S. Department of Health, Education and Welfare.

National Comprehensive Cancer Network. (1999). NCCN practice guidelines for the management of psychosocial distress. *Oncology, 13*(5A), 113–147.

Natvig, K. (1984). Laryngectomees in Norway: Study No. 1: Social, personal, and behavioral factors related to present mastery of the laryngectomy event. *Journal of Otolaryngology, 12*(3), 155–162.

Neufeld, K. R., Degner, L. F., & Dick, J. A. (1993). A nursing intervention strategy to foster patient involvement in treatment decisions. *Oncology Nursing Forum, 20*(4), 631–635.

Newell, S., Sanson-Fisher, R. W., Girgis, A., & Ackland, S. (1999). The physical and psycho-social experiences of patients attending an outpatient medical oncology department: A cross-sectional study. *European Journal of Cancer Care, 8,* 73–82.

Nowak, P., Parzuchowski, J., & Jacobs, J. R. (1989). Effects of combined modality therapy of head and neck carcinoma on shoulder and head mobility. *Journal of Surgical Oncology, 41,* 143–147.

Olson, M. L., & Shedd, D. P. (1978). Disability and rehabilitation in head and neck cancer patients after treatment. *Head & Neck Surgery, 1,* 52–58.

Olswang, L. B. (1990). Treatment efficacy: The breadth of research. In L. B. Olswang, C. K. Thompson, S. F. Warren, & N. J. Minghetti (Eds.), *Treatment efficacy research in communication disorders,* (pp. 99–104). Rockville, MD: American Speech-Language-Hearing Foundation.

Osoba, D. (1993). Self-rating symptom checklists: A simple method for recording and evaluating symptom control in oncology. *Cancer Treatment Review, 19*(Suppl A), 43–51.

Pauloski, B. R., Rademaker, A. W., Logemann, J. A., Lazarus, C. L., Newman, L., Hamner, A., MacCracken, E., Gaziano J., & Stachowiak, L. (2002). Swallow function and perception of dysphagia in patients with head and neck cancer. *Head & Neck, 24,* 555–565.

Pruyn, J. F., de Jong, P. C., Bosman, L. J., van Poppel, J. W., van den Borne, H. W., Ryckman, R. M., & de Meij, K. (1986). Psychosocial aspects of head and neck cancer: A review of the literature. *Clinical Otolaryngology, 11,* 469–474.

Rapoport, Y., Kreitler, S., Chaitchik, S., Algor, R., & Weissler, K. (1993). Psychosocial problems in head-and-neck cancer patients and their change with time since diagnosis. *Annals of Oncology, 4,* 69–73.

Rathmell, A. J., Ash, D. V., Howes, M., & Nicholls, J. (1991). Assessing quality of life in patients treated for advanced head and neck cancer. *Clinical Oncology—Royal College of Radiology, 3,* 10–16.

Richardson, J. L. (1983). Vocational adjustment after total laryngectomy. *Archives of Physical Medicine and Rehabilitation, 64,* 172–175.

Rieker, P. P., Clark, E. J., & Fogelberg, P. R. (1992). Perceptions of quality of life and quality of care for patients with cancer receiving biological therapy. *Oncology Nursing Forum, 19*(3), 433–440.

Robb, G. L., & Lewin, J. S. (2003). Speech and swallow outcomes in reconstructions of the pharynx and cervical esophagus. *Head & Neck, 25,* 232–244.

Roy, D. J. (1992). Measurement in the service of compassion. *Journal of Palliative Care, 8,* 3–4.

Samlan, R. A. & Webster, K. T. (2002). Swallowing and speech therapy after definitive treatment of laryngeal cancer. *Otolaryngology Clinics of North America, 35,* 1115–1133.

Schipper, H. (1990a). Guidelines and caveats for quality of life measurement in clinical practice and research. *Oncology, 4*(5), 51–57.

Schipper, H. (1990b). Quality of life: Principles of the clinical paradigm. *Journal of Psychosocial Oncology, 8*(2/3), 171–185.

Schipper, H., & Clinch, J. (1988). Assessment of treatment in cancer. In G. T. Smith (Ed.), *Measuring health: A practical approach* (pp. 109–155). New York: Wiley.

Schipper, H., Clinch, J., McMurray, A., & Levitt, M. (1984). Measuring the quality of life of cancer patients: The Functional Living Index—Cancer: Development and validation. *Journal of Clinical Oncology, 2*(5), 472–483.

Schipper, H., & Levitt, M. (1985). Measuring quality of life: Risks and benefits. *Cancer Treatment Reports, 69,* 1115–1123.

Schutt, A. H. (1986). Physical and occupational therapy for the patient with laryngectomy: Why and what for? In R. L. Keith & F. L. Darley (Eds.), *Laryngectomy rehabilitation* (pp. 295–308). San Diego: College-Hill Press.

Silveira, J. M., & Winstead-Fry, P. (1997). The needs of patients with cancer and their caregivers in rural areas. *Oncology Nursing Forum, 24*(1), 71–76.

Sist, T. C. (1998). The Minasian/Dwyer article reviewed. *Oncology, 12*(8), 1165–1169.

Siston, A. K., List, M. A., Schleser, R., & Vokes, E. (1997). Sexual functioning and head and neck cancer. *Journal of Psychosocial Oncology, 15*(3/4), 107–121.

Skoner, J. M., Andersen, P. E., Cohen, J. I., Holland, J. J., Nansen, E., & Wax, M. K. (2003). Swallowing function and tracheotomy dependence after combined modality treatment including free tissue transfer for advanced-stage oropharyngeal cancer. *Laryngoscope, 113*, 1294–1298.

Smit, C. F., Tan, J., Mathus-Vliegen, L. M. H., & Devriese, P. P. (1998). High incidence of gastropharyngeal and gastroesophageal reflux after total laryngectomy. *Head & Neck, 20*, 619–622.

Sprangers, M. A., Cull, A., Bjordal, K., Groenvold, M., & Aaronson, N. K. (1993). The European Organization for Research and Treatment of Cancer approach to quality of life assessment: Guidelines for developing questionnaire modules. *Quality of Life Research, 2*, 287–295.

Stam, H. J., Koopmans, J. P., & Mathieson, C. M. (1991). The psychosocial impact of a laryngectomy: A comprehensive assessment. *Journal of Psychosocial Oncology, 9*(3), 37–58.

Strauss, R. P. (1989). Psychosocial responses to oral and maxillofacial surgery for head and neck cancer. *Journal of Oral Maxillofacial Surgery, 47*, 343–348.

Tennstedt, S. L. (2000). Empowering older patients to communicate more effectively in the medical encounter. *Clinics in Geriatric Medicine, 16*, 61–70.

Terrell, J. E., Welsh, D. E., Bradford, C. R., Chepeha, D. B., Esclamado, R. M., Hogikyan, N. D., & Wolf, G. T. (2000). Pain, quality of life, and spinal accessory nerve status after neck dissection. *Laryngoscope, 110*, 620–626.

Theurer, J. A. & Martin, R. E. (2003). Effects of oral cancer treatment: Speech, swallowing, and quality of life outcomes. *Journal of Speech–Language Pathology and Audiology, 27*, 190–201.

Till, J. E. (1991). Uses (and some possible abuses) of quality-of-life measures. In D. Osoba (Ed.), *Effect of cancer on quality of life* (pp. 137–153). Boston: CRC Press.

Till, J. E. (1994). Measuring quality of life: Apparent benefits, potential concerns. *Canadian Journal of Oncology, 4*(1), 243–248.

Tripepi-Bova, K. A. (1993). Commentary on postlaryngectomy quality of life dimensions identified by patients and health care professionals. *AACN Nursing Scan in Critical Care, 3*(4), 3.

Watt-Watson, J., & Graydon, J. (1995). Impact of surgery on head and neck cancer patients and their caregivers. *Nursing Clinics of North America, 30*, 659–671.

Weiss, M. H. (1993). Head and neck cancer and the quality of life (Editorial). *Otolaryngology—Head and Neck Surgery, 108*, 311–312.

Weissler, M. C. (1997). Management of complications resulting from laryngeal cancer treatment. *Otolaryngology Clinics of North America, 30*(2), 269–278.

Wen, K. Y., & Gustafson, D. H. (2004). Needs assessment for cancer patients and their families. *Health and Quality of Life Outcomes, 2*, 11–15.

Woodson, G. E., Rosen, C. A., Murry, T., Madasu, R., Wong, F., Hengested, A., & Robbins, K. T. (1996). Assessing vocal function after chemoradiation for advanced laryngeal carcinoma. *Archives of Otolaryngology—Head and Neck Surgery, 122*, 858–864.

World Health Organization. (1947). Constitution of the World Health Organization. *WHO Chronicles, 1*, 29–43.

World Health Organization. (1993). *International classification of impairments, disabilities, and handicaps: A manual for classification relating to the consequences of disease.* Geneva, Switzerland: Author.

Zemel, M., Maves, M., Mickelson, S., & Kaplan, J. (1991). Nutrition in head and neck cancer patients. *Head and Neck, 13*, 10–12.

Chapter 29

Rehabilitation in Head and Neck Cancer
Epilogue

Philip C. Doyle

Any effort to improve the quality and completeness of health care finds its most meaningful germination in the relationships and interactions between the individual who experiences illness or disease and those professionals who will be charged with providing service to that person and members of his or her family. Clear and open communication between these individuals will create the foundation upon which any successful program of rehabilitation is built. Because health care is not a static process, particularly when serious disease is present, numerous variables and factors may influence, either positively or negatively, the eventual treatment and rehabilitative outcomes that will be realized. Within the preceding chapters of this text, a variety of topics, issues, and concerns have been identified and discussed; the information presented is deemed critical to the comprehensive care of those who are treated for head and neck cancer and must be considered if optimal health care is to be achieved. Ultimately, the quality of service provided and the success of clinical care outcomes may be influenced when a variety of dimensions, variables, and factors are carefully considered.

The dimensions, variables, and factors identified and addressed in many chapters herein have crossed numerous internal states (e.g., physical, psychological), external issues (e.g., social, recreational), and interrelated and multidimensional relationships that cross multiple domains. Because these areas of concern are diverse and multifactorial, the need for input from multiple disciplines and professions is necessary to achieve comprehensive levels of care. The first and most essential step in working toward better care and service to those with head and neck cancer requires the acknowledgment and recognition of such potential concerns. Although the preceding chapters have provided extensive coverage of many issues critical to head and neck cancer, those areas identified cannot be viewed as exhaustive. Each individual will bring a unique set of concerns and expectations to the clinical process. The purpose of this closing chapter is to provide a brief, yet broad review of thematic concerns that have been identified by the contributing authors of this text. Within this epilogue, however, a concomitant goal is to identify emerging or poorly understood themes that will serve both clinicians and health care researchers in efforts to continually improve the nature and complexion of the care provided to those individuals with cancer of the head and neck.

THE CURRENT STATUS OF HEAD AND NECK CANCER CARE

The issues addressed in preceding chapters have covered a breadth of concerns, from those involved at the point of initial diagnosis and primary treatment (Chapters 7–9, 12, and 13) to those relating to broad dimensions and considerations that hold potential to influence the person's quality of life and to affect those individuals who will eventually succumb to malignant disease (Chapters 1, 15, and 28). Cancer care requires careful examination of numerous potential concerns that span this continuum of illness. Additionally, a variety of topics that fall within the larger continuum of cancer care just noted have been presented and discussed in the specific context of head and neck cancer. These include issues that emerge from the systematic review and evaluation of documented outcomes relative to specific, yet more conservative treatment options for head and neck cancer (Chapters 10 and 11); more focused issues pertaining to disorders of voice and speech as a consequence of treatment and subsequent rehabilitation of communication (Chapters 3–5) and concerns related to swallowing disorders and relevant outcomes (Chapter 14); approaches to communication therapy (Chapters 1, 16–18, and 22) and counseling (Chapter 15); new approaches and contemporary considerations unique to the evaluation, description, and treatment of communication and related disorders secondary to treatment for cancer of the head and neck (Chapters 6, 20, and 23); efforts seeking to optimize postlaryngectomy communication through careful and systematic clinical problem solving (Chapters 19, 22, and 24); and group therapy (Chapters 25 and 26). Information on the need for a critical reevaluation of specific areas of interest that potentially influence alaryngeal outcomes (Chapter 21) also has been raised in hopes that reevaluation will occur and that past and present data will be viewed within such a context. Furthermore, topics pertaining to information provision and counseling, the utility of group support, and the personal impact of cancer also have been discussed (Chapters 22, 25, and 26), in addition to coverage regarding the important area of clinical accountability (Chapter 27). All of the previously cited chapters provide information that can assist clinicians in offering the best possible care relative to voice, speech, swallowing, and ultimately the quality of life and well-being of those diagnosed with head and neck cancer.

Together, the topics covered in this text provide a more comprehensive, albeit not exhaustive, view of the plight that individuals who experience cancer of the head and neck and their family members will experience over the course of the disease, its treatment, and ideally the patients' recovery and reintegration into society. A collective assessment of the information presented is intended to provide an enriched and expanded framework from which improvements in future health care subsequent to head and neck cancer can be achieved, ultimately improving short- and long-term posttreatment outcomes and increasing the success of rehabilitation efforts for those with cancer of the head and neck.

EXPANDING CLINICAL PROGRAMS OF HEAD AND NECK CANCER CARE

The issues identified in the previous section, in addition to others that are covered within individual chapters of this text, are indeed diverse and must be examined critically by health professionals (e.g., speech–language pathologists, physicians) desiring to provide a comprehensive, yet individualized program of health care specific to rehabilitation in the areas of voice, speech, and swallowing. Doing so may be rewarded with patients' improved perceptions of their quality of life and well-being following treatment (Ferrell & Dow, 1996). The issues and topics discussed, however, always must be considered in the context of the human condition; that is, a person's response to treatment, particularly in the case of a significant health condition such as cancer, is dynamic. The intricate relationship between body and mind, the proverbial "soma–psyche" relationship, must be fully and adequately addressed at the clinical level if comprehensive efforts at post-treatment rehabilitation are to be pursued (Dow, Ferrell, Haberman, & Eaton 1999; Folkman & Greer, 2000; see also Chapters 1, 15, and 28 in this text). The impact of disease and its effect on outcomes cannot be underestimated. Varied components and approaches to health care may optimize an individual's potential for successful rehabilitation outcomes in the broadest sense. In one respect, some professionals may identify many of the "personal" areas of concern (e.g., those that are often evaluated as components inherent to quality of life) as peripheral to cancer treatment as it traditionally has been defined. A considerable body of literature, however, suggests that to disregard such issues will significantly restrict the process of recovery and resultant long-term outcomes following treatment for cancer of the head and neck (e.g., Bjordal & Kaasa, 1995; Breitbart & Holland, 1988; De Boer, McCormick, Pruyn, Ryckman, & van den Borne, 1999; Hassan & Weymuller, 1990). Systematic attention to these personal types of issues is believed to optimize outcomes. Clinical endeavors that fail to address personal dimensions in a respectful, sensitive, and direct manner will likely observe commensurate failures in posttreatment outcomes. Therefore it is also essential that clinicians have exposure to educational resources and training opportunities in the area of head and neck cancer (Beaudin, Godes, Gowan, & Minuk, 2003).

THE PROGRAM OF CARE IN HEAD AND NECK CANCER

The nature of medical care proper as an entity of health care is by necessity quite specialized, and when changes occur, they are most frequently characterized by a transition that may be somewhat slow but quite systematic. In contrast, health care as an institution in North America today is in general a very fluid endeavor; the changes that take place at the systemic, operational level of health care are contingent on a variety of factors, including economic, social, budgetary, structural, and administration and management protocols, in addition to those of personnel requirements and constraints, and the demands of governmental and third-party agencies. This ever-changing service provision environment, coupled with professional specialization, may be seen to create an additional level of concern relative to how cancer care programs are carried out. Specifically, when rapid alterations in the structure of a given health care environment are coupled with professional and disciplinary boundaries, the outgrowth may at times create implicit barriers to specific models of practice and the ways in which programmatic, multidisciplinary services are carried out. Unfortunately, such barriers frequently do not facilitate cooperative inter- or multidisciplinary programs of care that may directly limit the character of services provided.

Certain strengths and weaknesses are inherent to specialization both within and across health care professions and disciplines, but when multiple resources coalesce, the result may be much improved outcomes for the individual. The idealized program of care has multiple professions working cooperatively to provide high-quality, individualized care that is as seamless as possible in any given setting. As noted, however, this is an idealized model, and numerous impediments to the provision of such service will at times emerge. Nevertheless, the ideal should be the target for the design and structure of all such programs. Thus, at a minimum, the provision of health care to those with head and neck cancer (and other conditions) will be influenced by the diversity of specialized professional services available, large-scale institutional considerations, and the progressive needs of the individual from the point of diagnosis through varied stages of recovery and rehabilitation, including the potential need for palliative care (Mellink et al., 2003). Although each of these areas may be considered independently (i.e., the goals of specific professions, institutional demands, and the patient's needs), they are not at all mutually exclusive—they must be considered as interdependent entities. Furthermore, professionals must always be cognizant of the multidimensional impact of any given disease and the consequences of medical treatment relative to components of any given health care program.

The impact of disease and the consequences of medical treatment cannot be discounted relative to the influence on an individual's recovery in the immediate posttreatment period, as well as relative to both short- and long-term outcomes. It also cannot be assumed that all components of a health care program or institutional protocol will be undertaken in an identical manner. Some aspects of a given rehabilitation or management program may not be pursued for a variety of reasons. For example, early participation in a support group may be deferred in some situations because the individual does not yet wish to participate. Although group support activities are viewed by many to be beneficial, such decisions rest with the individual. It is, however, not unreasonable to assume that one's ability to be actively involved in the decision-making process relative to his or her own health care has many positive attributes relative to rehabilitation. Likewise, addressing specific topics in the framework of counseling may not always follow a uniform order given the specific needs of the individual patient. In essence, programs of care should be flexible to accommodate the emergent needs of the individual.

The need to modify a program of care may occur both early and late in a patient's rehabilitation, particularly when atypical impediments to rehabilitation are observed (e.g., the patient's inability to return to work due to safety reasons, significant communication limitations). Meeting the individual's needs within the context of the health care system requires careful assessment in the hope of identifying specific needs and establishing priorities for how and when to provide services, and who will provide services to that individual and his or her family members (Blanchard, Albrecht, Rucksdeschel, Grant, & Hammick, 1995; Wen & Gustafson, 2004). The ability to meet each patient's needs is enhanced considerably with input from a variety of professional sources in direct consultation with the individual and his or her family members. This collaboration also permits consideration of various perspectives regarding a particular problem or concern in an effort to explore options so as to reduce or eliminate difficulties experienced. Multidimensional programs of care allow the traditional medical model to be expanded, with greater opportunities for comprehensive care.

MOVING BEYOND THE MEDICAL MODEL: ADDRESSING MULTIDIMENSIONAL CONSTRUCTS

A narrow viewpoint of disease is clearly inconsistent with the concept of reha-bilitation, regardless of the specific illness or disease in question. In the circum-stance of a cancer diagnosis, there is no disagreement that immediate medical in-tervention is essential. This intervention, however, must be viewed as only the initial step in the process of treatment and rehabilitation efforts (Eadie, 2003). Similarly, and perhaps more important, the absence of disease following treatment does not carry with it a return to a precancer state of being. This concept is at the heart of numerous attempts to adequately specify and define the very complex, multidimensional, and highly personalized construct of "quality of life."

Although many definitions of quality of life exist, the most comprehensive definitions specify that this construct is indeed multidimensional and that it must encompass physical, functional,[1] psychological, social, and spiritual domains (Cella & Tulsky, 1990; see also Chapter 28 in this text). The World Health Orga-nization (WHO) defined *health,* a related concept, as a "state of complete physi-cal, mental, and social well-being and not merely the absence of disease or infir-mity" (WHO, 1999, p. 100). Thus, addressing concepts of health and quality of life in the presence of illness or disease would seem to provide a more enriched foundation from which care programs then evolve. Additionally, attempts to ad-dress these concepts will likely bear fruit from the perspective of how outcomes can be effectively measured. Because the traditional biomedical model fails to provide an adequate context from which treatment success has historically been based, WHO (2000) has provided an alternative conceptual model from which a patient's functional capacity relative to changes in his or her health status can be more fully and appropriately described. This emerging model, termed the "biopsychosocial model" is guided not only by considerations of biological fac-tors, but also by the relationships that exist between biological factors and the psychological and social domains. In essence, the biopsychosocial model accounts for the influence of disease or illness on physical status, considers the effects of those changes at the psychological level of function, and views the interactive ef-fects of those factors on the individual's social participation.

There is no question that the potential for changes at physical and physio-logical levels is substantial subsequent to cancer treatment. If, however, the profes-sional were to assume that such biological changes could be addressed successfully from the standpoint of rehabilitation, other areas of concern will most certainly

---

[1]The term *functional* may cover a range of either well-defined or more broadly defined notions. These concerns may cross a wide spectrum of actions, capabilities, or activities that may fall into domains that also have been considered as physiological or activity centered. Because of this, any given definition of quality of life, and therefore any emergent data, must be evaluated with care due to potential constraints in the definition and ap-plication of such terms. This suggestion also would have a direct bearing on the interpretation and potential ap-plication of such data.

remain, with a resulting impact on the individual in other domains (i.e., those that do not fall in the biological domain). For example, it is not unreasonable to assume that if the professional disregards areas such as the patient's ability to pursue personal, vocational, avocational, or recreational interests in the posttreatment period, or to meet and engage in work-related and social demands, impediments to rehabilitation will almost certainly be encountered (see Wellisch, 1984). Similarly, individuals who become depressed due to the inability to pursue interests, work, or social activities cannot overcome the problem without acknowledging the origin of such depression (Gritz et al., 1999; Rohe, 1994; Shanks, 1995). Diverse, multidisciplinary approaches to patient care will decrease the likelihood that a cascade of insurmountable difficulties will be experienced without efforts toward amelioration through intervention.

A significant number of factors and variables may arise throughout the period of treatment and rehabilitation. Those areas that historically have been considered primary levels of concern (e.g., physical alterations) now require interpretation within the larger context of what might be termed secondary or collateral concerns (e.g., concerns related to sexuality and intimacy) that influence one's quality of life (Doyle, 1999).[2] Therefore, the information presented in chapters of this text may facilitate the clinician's understanding of both primary and secondary levels of concern (Doyle, 1999) as a consequence of head and neck cancer treatment. The information presented provides a framework from which multiple domains and perspectives can be considered in the context of each individual who presents in the clinic for services. The recognition of the multidimensional character of cancer, its treatment, and myriad concerns in the posttreatment period is essential.

By recognizing the larger framework from which individualized programs of treatment may be structured, the professional can appreciate the importance of contributions from multiple professional sources (e.g., Doyle, 1994, 1999; Eadie, 2001, 2003; Salmon, 1986; Shanks, 1995; see also Chapter 1 in this text). Professionals from multiple professions and disciplines should evaluate a broader expanse of issues specific to head and neck cancer and seek to understand the role and scope of practice of other professionals. Doing so serves to reduce territorial chaos and creates the opportunity for improved programs of care relative to each person and members of his or her family or significant others. Furthermore, understanding the value of multidisciplinary input into an individual's care provides an ideal opportunity for the development and design of strategies that will foster an environment conducive to optimizing rehabilitation efforts. Using a simple analogy, although the big picture or forest of issues must be carefully considered, it is critical to consider the trees that make up the forest—the inability to do so will result in generic (i.e., nonindividualized) levels of care that are unlikely to

---

[2]Use of the term *collateral* does not imply that concerns falling in such a grouping of behaviors are less important than those deemed as primary. In fact, contemporary thinking suggests that many concerns that traditionally have been considered secondary or collateral may have an even more dramatic impact on the individual's perceived well-being and overall quality of life (see WHO, 2000).

meet realistic expectations or may restrict the clinician's ability to access additional professional services that may be readily available in a given setting. As programs of health care in general, and those related to head and neck cancer care in specific, are devised and pursued in the context of each person, the likelihood of being able to address unique dimensions is increased commensurately (Reuille, 2004). This increase may be inferred to result in better levels of care, the increased potential for social reentry, and consequently a more successful rehabilitative outcome and improved well-being and related quality of life.

A NEW PARADIGM OF CARE

As noted in earlier sections of this chapter, information provided in the historical literature on head and neck cancer has been strongly guided by the medical model. Although the historic application of this model is understandable, it is becoming clear that the medical model is at best an incomplete one (Eadie, 2001, 2003), and possibly one that restricts the potential for realizing maximum rehabilitation gains. As Reed (1983) stated, the ultimate goal of any rehabilitation effort subsequent to treatment for head and neck cancer is to return the individual to as normal a life as possible. Thus, the more contemporary paradigm, which finds its conceptual foundation in that of the biopsychosocial model, may be seen to evolve from the recognition and acceptance of a greater and more encompassing set of dimensions that actively considers and addresses varied components of disease, illness, and health (see Chapter 1 in this text).

As acknowledged in many chapters of this text, the domains of importance are many and multifold when one considers the potentially expansive consequences (physical, psychological, etc.) of head and neck cancer. Although historical reference domains for head and neck cancer existing in the speech pathology literature have included physical and communicative domains, and intermittently and to a lesser extent the psychological domain, other domains such as those in the social, psychosocial, and psychiatric areas have been less frequently addressed (Blood, Luther, & Stemple, 1992; Doyle, 1994; Langius, Bjorvell, & Lind, 1994; Plumb & Holland, 1977; Rohe, 1994; Salmon, 1986; Shanks, 1995; Shapiro & Kornfeld, 1987).[3] Data in the literature do suggest that psychological status must be carefully evaluated with respect to functional status and the perceived impact of "sickness" (e.g., Brooks, Jordan, Divine, Smith, & Neelon, 1993), as well as in

---

[3]The historical literature in the discipline of communication disorders has focused largely on direct physical changes secondary to head and neck cancer and subsequent disruption in voice, speech, and swallowing. Few published sources have fully addressed issues that concern the alteration in social participation or other contextually bound factors. Thus, the domains specific to physical and communication changes have served as frequent points of reference secondary to the treatment of head and neck cancer. In this specific case, a disease or health condition is seen to lead to changes in body function or structures, which lead to potential disruptions in individual activity (see WHO, 2000), without consideration of the disease's or condition's impact on social and participatory activities.

relation to social performance and perceived satisfaction with one's life (LoBello et al., 2003). In this vein, optimized programs of care and rehabilitation for those treated for head and neck cancer must, at a minimum, consider multiple primary and collateral domains that hold potential to negatively affect treatment and subsequent rehabilitation outcomes.

Whereas the traditional medical model has fallen short of addressing the multidimensional impact of head and neck cancer, the emergence of the biopsychosocial model (WHO, 2000) holds substantial promise for those professionals involved in all levels of health care. With this in mind, professionals must now seek to critically evaluate the current state of the art relative to how rehabilitation efforts are designed, structured, and carried out.[4] Doing so will permit professionals to examine what is done well, as well as to identify where changes can be made to improve the care of those with head and neck cancer. When such changes occur, the benefits of these efforts may be evident in the improved success as perceived by the individual who experiences disease, as well as through various clinical outcome measures and instruments that may be used.

THE PSYCHOSOCIAL IMPACT OF HEAD AND NECK CANCER

Those working in oncology often observe that a diagnosis of cancer frequently results in some level of isolation, a change that has been suggested to relate directly to the disease (Ablon, 1981). Stigmatization is a common observation related to many illnesses and disease types, not only cancer (Doyle, 1994; Folkman & Greer, 2000; see also Chapter 1 in this text). For example, there is a long history of information related to the stigmatizing effects of mental illness (e.g., Cumming & Cumming, 1965; Link, Cullen, Frank, & Woyneale, 1987). Similarly, in the past two decades, an ever-present and multifactorial process of stigmatization has been identified and reported relative to acquired immune deficiency syndrome/human immunodeficiency virus (AIDS/HIV) and related disorders as an illness and disease class. Findings specific to individuals with AIDS/ HIV indicate that stigma may be substantial; however, perhaps more important, the stigma may be relative to factors external to the disease itself. Specifically, stigma associated with AIDS/HIV arises in part from factors that reflect on lifestyle issues or sexual preference. The point of interest here is that not only may the disease and any changes that emerge subsequent to its treatment create stigmatization, but also, in some instances, other factors may directly influence how society perceives the individual who experiences the disease. Clearly, stigma may be attached to the lifestyle factors—that is, smoking and drinking—that have been reported in association with many head and neck cancers. Regardless of the origin of stigma,

---

[4]The reader is strongly encouraged to consult the excellent review by Eadie (2003) concerning the application of the International Classification of Functioning (ICF) to those with laryngeal cancer.

multiple levels of social penalty may create challenges to the person's self-image and identity, with substantially negative consequences.

The idea of a "virtual identity," one that is defined by society, has been elegantly presented by Goffman (1963); the value of this concept to those with cancer of the head and neck is clearly of interest to the present discussion. Questions regarding the potential existence of multiple levels of stigma following the diagnosis and treatment of laryngeal cancer have been raised previously in the literature (Doyle, 1994). The premise underlying Doyle's suggestion was specific to the belief that any consideration of stigma must account for aspects of the disease itself, in addition to those factors that emerge subsequent to and as a direct consequence of the method(s) of disease treatment (e.g., altered verbal communication, physical disfigurement). Although Doyle's (1994) premise was indeed specific to cancer of the larynx and the sequelae of its management, its application to other head and neck cancers is not unreasonable as the potential long-term negative consequences of stigma can be devastating. As stated by Fife and Wright (2000, p. 51), stigma secondary to disease or illness "increases the stress," which in turn increases "secondary psychological and social morbidity," which then affects the person's quality of life and social well-being. The concerns are further expanded when one evaluates the possible extension of stigma to family members and friends, with the resulting potential for further isolation. Thus, and in the context of the present collection of works, it should be clear that a diverse, well-designed, and systematic program of care considers factors that extend beyond that of the medical condition proper (see Eadie, 2001, 2003; WHO, 2000).

FACILITATING REHABILITATION

A comprehensive program of rehabilitation for those individuals with head and neck cancer is multifaceted. Although medical management remains primary, the myriad issues that emerge in the period following treatment (whether surgical, radiotherapy, or combined approaches are pursued) require careful consideration. Rigid models of care are not seen to optimize health care and rehabilitation; flexible and individualized components of a treatment and rehabilitation program are essential to foster improved outcomes. Substantial and long-standing information in the literature suggests and supports the value of multidisciplinary approaches to rehabilitation efforts (e.g., Johnson, Casper, & Lesswing, 1979). Including multiple professionals is of value because the varied issues that emerge following treatment for head and neck cancer then may be addressed in an expedited fashion by those with adequate levels of education and training. Through collaboration, the true nature of comprehensive care may be realized.

I do not mean to imply, however, that high-quality, comprehensive levels of care cannot be provided outside of the "ideal" clinical environment. In fact, very good, comprehensive, and highly individualized care may be provided in what might at first observation be judged as a less than perfect setting (e.g., centers outside of major health care or hospital environments, centers that are not found in larger metropolitan settings). One example of such a setting would be a small center that is distant from the site where primary care was provided. In this situation, the individual must receive follow-up care in the small facility where multiple resources may not be readily available. Therefore, one or more professionals at the small center need to facilitate the acquisition of appropriate information through secondary and often distant resources. Additional and often excellent resources also may be accessed through the Internet by the professional, individual patients, and family members. These resources are of particular benefit to those individuals who may experience significant communication problems secondary to treatment or those who seek information on any variety of topics that might not commonly be addressed.

Other components of care programs that must be considered, but are also poorly understood, are the influence of different treatment options on the health-related quality-of-life outcomes of those treated for head and neck cancer (Finizia & Bergman, 2001) and concerns regarding how to measure the level of "sickness" experienced by these individuals (Bergner, Bobbitt, Carter, & Gilson, 1981; Eadie, Myers, & Doyle, 2003). Different methods of treatment certainly have their own advantages and disadvantages when viewed within the context of the individual (see Chapters 4 and 23 in this text). Although specific to those with laryngeal cancer who undergo conservative surgical treatments for laryngeal malignancies, voice quality as an isolated postoperative feature may carry differential weightings of burden to individuals (Doyle, 1994, 1997).[5] Furthermore, Doyle raised the issue of differential societal penalty when one considers gender (i.e., men may be less penalized than women for abnormal vocal quality), and this suspicion has been confirmed experimentally (Eadie & Doyle, 2004). Such effects may also be persistent, with a long-term negative influence on treatment (Morgan, Robinson, Marsh, & Bradley, 1988). Finally, anticipated or expected post-treatment outcomes relative to voice and voice quality may not always be observed clinically, which ultimately threatens the ability to adequately prepare a patient for what is forthcoming (Fung et al., 2001; see also Chapters 10 and 11 in this text). The primary issue of importance in this discussion is that the disease, its treatment, and the eventual outcome from such treatment must be assessed within the larger social context, because outcomes are not always predictable (see Chapters 4–6 in this text). These concerns must also be evaluated in view of different modes of communication and their relative impact on perceived quality of life (Finizia & Bergman, 2001; Krizek, Roberts, Ragan, Ferrara, & Lord, 1999). In fact, the commonalities that are observed and identified across methods of alaryngeal voice and speech provide a framework for reexamination while pursuing programs of treatment and long-term follow-up (see Chapter 3 in this text).

---

[5]The issue of changes in voice quality may become more prevalent for both men and women in the future given the potential for increased application of conservation methods of treatment.

For many individuals diagnosed and treated for head and neck cancer, an effort toward curative treatment is the primary and most urgent concern. Closely coinciding with this concern when treatment results in a communication disorder is the critical matter of initiating timely and complete therapeutic programs to restore some form of functional verbal communication (see Chapters 3, 17–19, 22, and 24). The ability to speak is a critical aspect of recovery and rehabilitation. In essence, and with few exceptions (e.g., brain cancer), communication disorder is what distinguishes those with head and neck cancer from other individuals who have cancer; despite the presence of a malignant disease, communication is not disrupted from the anatomical and physiological perspective for many other forms of cancer. Those with head and neck cancer may be unable to adequately express their fears, anger, frustration, and other human emotions at a time of extreme emotional burden (see Chapters 15 and 28 in this text), resulting in what has been referred to as a form of trauma. Additionally, a reduction in or the loss of verbal communication will isolate and restrict efforts by the individual to actively seek information, assistance, and support. How a patient adapts to his or her situation may be of particular importance as a predictor variable in outcomes (Krouse, Krouse, & Fabian, 1989).

The trauma experienced by those with head and neck cancer has been the topic of widespread discussion in the literature (e.g., Langius et al., 1994), and the effects of this trauma at multiple levels of the personality may be reflected in one's demeanor toward the care he or she receives. In most instances, the person who has been treated for head and neck cancer will actively work toward understanding what will happen or what has already taken place and, with adequate information, will become more compliant relative to components of his or her own care. Active participation in the health care process is essential if a successful outcome is desired and can potentially influence and facilitate social reintegration and the resumption of many normal activities and an improved quality of life.

McDonough, Boyd, Varvares, and Maves (1996) stated that compliance to health care in those with cancer of the head and neck is a multidimensional construct. These authors identified areas that have been incidentally noted in the past, but are areas of concern that have potential to exert a substantial influence on the person's level of compliance. McDonough et al. identified diet, exercise, medication use, and one's ability to alter lifestyle behaviors, specifically those relating to the cessation of smoking and reduction in alcohol use, to be important variables influencing health care.[6] These factors, among others, might not always be seen to be obvious concerns that may impact a patient's compliance to health care. Nevertheless, outcome measures must be employed during head and neck cancer rehabilitation to carefully assess a divergent although likely interrelated set of factors and variables and to more accurately and validly assess the patient's response to rehabilitation efforts. These factors have not been explored adequately

---

[6]These issues also may exhibit differential levels of social penalty as a function of gender.

up to this point and, therefore, require additional evaluation and exploration at the clinical level.

EMERGENT THEMES IN THE REHABILITATION OF INDIVIDUALS WITH HEAD AND NECK CANCER

Based on the reviews of literature that cross many disciplines and professions, it appears that rehabilitation programs may benefit from closer attention to a number of emergent themes and domains that do not fall in the traditional model of care. In particular, clinicians may now need to address varied issues ranging from aspects of general cancer surveillance, to assessments of psychological status, to the monitoring of alcohol use or abuse in relation to issues of patient compliance. Further information concerning the best methods of assessing quality of life will prove to be invaluable as clinicians work to improve the structure of care programs. When this range of divergent concerns is assessed in the context of the clinical setting, the demands and expectations associated with efforts to provide the highest level of care may be challenged at the levels of both practice and personnel. McDonough and colleagues (1996) suggested that not only must the optimal course of treatment be identified, but also levels of patient compliance must be actively monitored in regard to efficient care protocols. Of particular importance here is that McDonough et al. proposed that health care professionals may misdirect their efforts in working with patients with cancers of the head and neck; they stated: "It is our belief that more emphasis is generally placed on the physical rather than the psychological ramifications of treatment" (p. 273). Doyle (1994) posited that success or failure of treatment is influenced considerably by what occurs in the postoperative period as the patient begins to deal with the effects of treatment; the provision of timely, honest, and easily understood (avoidance of jargon) information is critical throughout all stages of rehabilitation if successful clinical interactions are to be achieved. In many instances, information may be a critical factor related to patients' "psychological health."

Psychological concerns must always be addressed as part of a comprehensive program. Often, depression is first observed during the early postoperative period (Sanchez-Salazar & Stark, 1972); therefore, consideration of a patient's psychological status is essential relative to long-term effects on quality of life (e.g., D'Antonio et al., 1998; Mathieson, Stam, & Scott, 1990; Mellette, 1989; O'Young & McPeek, 1987; Quigley, 1989; Weismann & Worden, 1975; Welsh-McCaffrey, Hoffman, Leigh, Loescher, & Meyskens, 1989). Nevertheless, questions pertaining to the validity and value of differences that exist in judgments of depression by patients and physicians have been raised by several groups of researchers (e.g., D'Antonio et al., 1998; Slevin, Plant, Lynch, Drinkwater, & Gregory, 1988), and this issue requires additional research in the future. At the level of face validity, however, the determination of one's well-being and quality of life appear to be best defined in the eyes of the beholder.

SUMMARY

This epilogue has attempted to provide a brief summary of the myriad issues and concerns that are believed to influence the short- and long-term outcomes of individuals treated for head and neck cancer. Although many areas of general concern that may directly and indirectly influence clinical care have been raised in this chapter, many others have not been specifically addressed. It is clear, however, that multidisciplinary efforts are required to achieve the most successful rehabilitation outcomes possible—those that also serve to optimize the individual's perceived quality of life. Furthermore, the need for the adoption of the more contemporary biopsychosocial model of health care (WHO, 2000), as compared to the traditional medical model, has been identified and discussed specific to the model's relative merits. Some novel and many long-standing facets of care have been identified as areas of emerging or continuing issues of importance. The diversity of expertise necessary to adequately meet the concerns of those with head and neck cancer, however, cannot be understated. Although not all areas can be addressed in all settings, the acknowledgment of the potential influence of many factors and variables is a critical dimension if the quality of care is to be enhanced. A desire to provide broad-based care programs that meet the diverse needs of the patient and his or her family also must be considered in the context of numerous external factors, such as rapidly changing health care environments. Thus, idealized programs of care must consider multidimensional and multifactorial aspects of disease, its treatment, and the short- and long-term consequences specific to the individual and his or her social milieu. At a minimum, this suggestion spans physical, physiological, psychological, communicative, social, psychosocial, emotional, and spiritual domains. Attempts to better address the relationship between disease, the person affected by that disease, and the response of society to the individual and the disease may offer significant advantages to improving the rehabilitation process. Therefore, the ability to successfully offer expanded and, perhaps better stated, individualized care to those treated for cancers of the head and neck can be achieved only through recognition of such factors and themes and, ultimately, through the open and cooperative interactions between professionals and those they serve.

REFERENCES

Ablon, J. (1981). Stigmatized health conditions. *Social Science and Medicine, 15B,* 5–9.

Beaudin, P. G., Godes, J. R., Gowan, A. C., & Minuk, J. L. (2003). An education and training survey of speech–language pathologists working with individuals with cancer of the larynx. *Journal of Speech–Language Pathology and Audiology, 27,* 144–157.

Bergner, M., Bobbitt, R. A., Carter, W. B., & Gilson, B. S. (1981). The Sickness Impact Profile: Development and final revision of a health status measure. *Medical Care, 19,* 787–805.

Bjordal, K., & Kaasa, S. (1995). Psychological distress in head and neck cancer patients 7–11 years after curative treatment. *British Journal of Cancer, 71,* 592–597.

Blanchard, C. G., Albrecht, T., Rucksdeschel, J., Grant, D., & Hammick, R. (1995). The role of social support in adaptation to cancer and to survival. *Journal of Psychosocial Oncology, 13,* 75–95.

Blood, G. W., Luther, A. R., & Stemple, J. C. (1992). Coping and adjustment in alaryngeal speakers. *American Journal of Speech–Language Pathology, 1,* 63–69.

Breitbart, W., & Holland, J. (1988). Psychosocial aspects of head and neck cancer. *Seminars in Oncology, 15,* 61–69.

Brooks, W. B., Jordan, J. S., Devine, G. W., Smith, W. E., & Neelon, F. A. (1993). The impact of psychological factors on measurement of functional status: Assessment of the Sickness Impact Profile. *Medical Care, 28,* 793–804.

Cella, D. F., & Tulsky, D. S. (1990). Measuring quality of life today: Methodological aspects. *Oncology, 4,* 29–38.

Cumming, J., & Cumming, E. (1965). On the stigma of mental illness. *Community Mental Health Journal, 1,* 135–143.

D'Antonio, L. L., Long, S. A., Zimmerman, G. J., Peterman, A. H., Petti, G. H., & Chonkich, G. D. (1998). Relationship between quality of life and depression in patients with head and neck cancer. *Laryngoscope, 108,* 806–811.

deBoer, M. F., McCormick, L. K., Pruyn, J. F. A., Ryckman, R. N., & van den Borne, B. W. (1999). Physical and psychosocial correlates of head and neck cancer: A review of the literature. *Otolaryngology—Head and Neck Surgery, 120,* 427–436.

Dow, K. H., Ferrell, B. R., Haberman, M. R., & Eaton, L. (1999). The meaning of quality of life in cancer survivorship. *Oncology Nursing Forum, 26,* 519–528.

Doyle, P. C. (1994). *Foundations of voice and speech rehabilitation following laryngeal cancer.* San Diego, CA: Singular.

Doyle, P. C. (1997). Voice refinement following conservation surgery for carcinoma of the larynx: A conceptual model for therapeutic intervention. *American Journal of Speech-Language Pathology, 6,* 27–35.

Doyle, P. C. (1999). Postlaryngectomy speech rehabilitation: Contemporary considerations in clinical care. *Journal of Speech–Language Pathology and Audiology, 23,* 109–116.

Eadie, T. L. (2001). The ICIDH–2: Theoretical and clinical implications for speech-language pathology. *Journal of Speech–Language Pathology and Audiology, 25,* 193–211.

Eadie, T. L. (2003). The ICF: A proposed framework for comprehensive rehabilitation of individuals who use alaryngeal speech. *American Journal of Speech–Language Pathology, 12,* 189–197.

Eadie, T. L., & Doyle, P. C. (2004). Auditory–perceptual scaling and quality of life in tracheoesophageal speakers. *Laryngoscope, 114,* 753–759.

Eadie, T. L., Myers, C., & Doyle, P. C. (2003, May). *New perspectives on the clinical care of persons with head and neck cancer.* Seminar presented at the annual meeting of the Canadian Association of Speech–Language Pathologists and Audiologists, St. John's, Newfoundland.

Ferrell, B., & Dow, K. (1996). Portraits of cancer survivorship: A glimpse through the lens of survivors' eyes. *Cancer Practice, 4,* 76–80.

Fife, B. L., & Wright, E. R. (2000). The dimensionality of stigma: A comparison of its impact on the self of persons with HIV/AIDS and cancer. *Journal of Health and Social Behavior, 41,* 50–67.

Finizia, C., & Bergman, B. (2001). Health-related quality of life in patients with laryngeal cancer: A post-treatment comparison of different modes of communication. *Laryngoscope, 111,* 918–923.

Folkman, S., & Greer, S. (2000). Promoting psychological well-being in the face of serious illness: When theory, research and practice inform each other. *Psycho-Oncology, 9,* 11–19.

Fung, K., Yoo, J., Leeper, H. A., Hawkins, S., Heeneman, H., Doyle, P. C., & Venkatesan, V. M. (2001). Vocal function following radiation for non-laryngeal versus laryngeal tumors of the head and neck. *Laryngoscope, 111,* 1920–1924.

Goffman, E. (1963). *Stigma: Notes on the management of a spoiled identity.* Englewood Cliffs, NJ: Prentice Hall.

Gritz, E. R., Carmack, C. L., de Moor, C., Coscarelli, A., Schacherer, C. W., Meyers, E. G., & Abemayor, E. (1999). First year after head and neck cancer: Quality of life. *Journal of Clinical Oncology, 17,* 352–360.

Hassan, S. J., & Weymuller, E. A. (1990). Assessment of quality of life in head and neck cancer patients. *Head & Neck, 15,* 485–496.

Johnson, J. T., Casper, J., & Lesswing, N. J. (1979). Toward the total rehabilitation of the alaryngeal patient. *Laryngoscope, 89,* 1813–1819.

Krizek, C., Roberts, C., Ragan, R., Ferrara, J. J., & Lord, B. (1999). Gender and cancer support group participation. *Cancer Practice, 7,* 86–92.

Krouse, J. H., Krouse, H. J., & Fabian, R. L. (1989). Adaptation to surgery for head and neck cancer. *Laryngoscope, 99,* 789–794.

Langius, A., Bjorvell, H., & Lind, M. G. (1994). Functional status and coping in patients with oral and pharyngeal cancer before and after surgery. *Head & Neck, 16,* 559–568.

Link, B. G., Cullen, F. T., Frank, J., & Woyneale, J. F. (1987). The social rejection of former mental patients: Understanding why labels matter. *American Journal of Sociology, 92,* 1461–1500.

LoBello, S. G., Underhil, A. T., Valentine, P. V., Stroud, T. P., Bartolucci, A. A., & Fine, P. R. (2003). Social integration and life and family satisfaction in survivors of injury at 5 years postinjury. *Journal of Rehabilitation Research and Development, 40,* 293–300.

Mathieson, C. M., Stam, H. J., & Scott, J. P. (1990). Psychosocial adjustment after laryngectomy: A review of the literature. *Journal of Otolaryngology, 19,* 331–336.

McDonough, E. M., Boyd, J. H., Varvares, M. A., & Maves, M. D. (1996). Relationship between psychological status and compliance in a sample of patients treated for cancer of the head and neck. *Head & Neck, 18,* 269–276.

Mellette, S. J., (1989). Rehabilitation issues for cancer survivors: Psychosocial challenges. *Journal of Psychological Oncology, 7,* 93–110.

Mellink, W. A. M., Dulmen, A. M. V., Wiggers, T., Spreeuwenberg, P. M. M., Eggermont, A. M. M., & Bensing, J. M. (2003). Cancer patients seeking a second surgical opinion: Results of a study on motives, needs, and expectations. *Journal of Clinical Oncology, 21,* 1492–1497.

Morgan, D. A., Robinson, H. F., Marsh, L., & Bradley, P. J. (1988). Vocal quality 10 years after radiotherapy for early glottic cancer. *Clinical Radiology, 39,* 295–296.

O'Young, J., & McPeek, B. (1987). Quality of life variable in surgical trials. *Journal of Chronic Diseases, 40,* 513–522.

Plumb, M. J., & Holland, J. (1977). Comparative studies of psychological function in patients with advanced cancer: I. Self-reported depressive symptoms. *Psychosomatic Medicine, 39,* 264–276.

Quigley, K. M. (1989). The adult cancer survivor: Psychosocial consequences of cure. *Seminars in Oncology Nursing, 5,* 63–69.

Reed, C. G. (1983). Surgical-prosthetic techniques for alaryngeal speech. *Communicative Disorders, 8,* 109–124.

Reuille, R. (2004). An evaluation of the Moffitt Cancer Center's laryngectomee visitor program. *Journal of Oncology Management, 13,* 12–18.

Rohe, D. E. (1994). Loss, grief, and depression after laryngectomy. In R. L. Keith & F. L. Darley (Eds.), *Laryngectomy rehabilitation* (3rd ed., pp. 487–514). Austin, TX: PRO-ED.

Salmon, S. J. (1986). Adjusting to laryngectomy. *Seminars in Speech and Language, 7,* 67–94.

Sanchez-Salazar, V., & Stark, A. (1972). The use of crisis intervention in the rehabilitation of laryngectomees. *Journal of Speech and Hearing Disorders, 37,* 323–328.

Shanks, J. C. (1995). Coping with laryngeal cancer. *Seminars in Speech and Language, 16,* 180–190.

Shapiro, P. A., & Kornfeld, D. S. (1987). Psychiatric aspects of head and neck cancer surgery. *Psychiatric Clinics of North America, 10,* 87–100.

Slevin, M. L., Plant, H., Lynch, D., Drinkwater, J., & Gregory, W. M. (1988). Who should measure quality of life, the doctor or the patient? *British Journal of Cancer, 57,* 109–112.

Weismann, A., & Worden, J. (1975). Psychosocial analysis of cancer deaths. *OMEGA, 6,* 62–75.

Wellisch, D. K. (1984). Work, social, recreational, family, and physical states. *Cancer, 53,* 2290–2302.

Welsh-McCaffrey, D., Hoffman, B., Leigh, S. A., Loescher, L. J., & Meyskens, F. L. (1989). Surviving adult cancers: Part 2. Psychosocial implications. *Annals of Internal Medicine, 111,* 517–523.

Wen, K. Y., & Gustafson, D. H. (2004). Needs assessment for cancer patients and their families. *Health and Quality of Life Outcomes, 2,* 11–15.

World Health Organization. (1999). *Constitution of the World Health Organization.* Geneva, Switzerland: Author.

World Health Organization. (2000). *ICIDH–2: International classification of functioning, disability, and health* (Prefinal draft, short version). Geneva, Switzerland: Author.

Author Index

Subject Index

About the Authors

Annemieke H. Ackerstaff, PhD, is a research psychologist in the Department of Otolaryngology—Head & Neck Surgery at the Netherlands Cancer Institute/ Antoni van Leeuwenhoek Hospital in Amsterdam. Ackerstaff received her doctorate from the University of Amsterdam. Her research focuses primarily on the quality of life of individuals treated for head and neck cancer. Specific interests include vocal and pulmonary rehabilitation of laryngectomized individuals and quality of life aspects of those treated with concomitant chemoradiation protocols.

J. E. A. Armstrong, DDS, MSc, is currently an oral and maxillofacial surgeon at the London Health Sciences Centre in London, Ontario, Canada. He also serves as a clinical consultant at the London Regional Cancer Centre. Armstrong received his DDS from the University of Toronto and his MSc from Dalhousie University, Halifax, Nova Scotia, Canada. His research interests include problems related to oral cancer. He also is actively investigating various systems for the fixation of fractures of bones of the facial skeleton and less morbid means of fracture repair.

Daniel G. Deschler, MD, FACS, is an assistant professor of otology and laryngology at the Harvard Medical School, is director of the Division of Head and Neck Surgery in the Department of Otology and Laryngology at the Massachusetts Eye and Ear Infirmary, and director of the Division of Head and Neck Oncology at the Massachusetts General Hospital in Boston, Massachusetts. He specializes in head and neck oncology surgery and microvascular reconstruction. Deschler received his MD with honors from Harvard Medical School, Boston, Massachusetts, and trained at the University of California, San Francisco, and completed a fellowship in head and neck oncology and reconstructive surgery. His research interests focus on voice rehabilitation following laryngopharyngectomy and reconstruction, as well as microvascular thrombosis prophylaxis.

Philip C. Doyle, PhD, is a professor in the Department of Communication Sciences and Disorders and is director of the Voice Production and Perception Laboratory at the University of Western Ontario, London, Ontario, Canada. He also holds academic appointments in the Department of Otolaryngology, Schulich School of Medicine, and serves as the chair of the Doctoral Program in Rehabilitation Sciences. Doyle received his doctorate in speech and hearing sciences from the University of California, San Francisco School of Medicine and the University of California, Santa Barbara. His research work and numerous publications address acoustic, physiologic, and psychophysical (auditory–perceptual) aspects of voice and speech communication following treatment for head and neck cancer and issues influencing posttreatment quality of life. Doyle is an elected Fellow of the American Speech-Language-Hearing Association.

Tanya L. Eadie, PhD, is an assistant professor in the Department of Speech and Hearing Sciences at the University of Washington. She teaches courses in voice disorders and anatomy and physiology. Eadie received her doctorate from the University of Western Ontario, London, Ontario, Canada. Her research interests include auditory–perceptual evaluation of voice and communication disorders related to head and neck cancer, including those issues related to quality of life.

Leslie E. Glaze, PhD, CCC-S, is director of clinical programs in the Department of Communication Disorders at the University of Minnesota. She teaches courses in voice and alaryngeal speech disorders, cleft palate and craniofacial anomalies, counseling, and professional issues. Glaze received her doctorate at the University of Wisconsin–Madison and has clinical and research interests in normal and disordered vocal fold physiology, alaryngeal speech rehabilitation, and treatment efficacy in voice disorders. She is a former coordinator of the American Speech-Language-Hearing Association's Special Interest Division 3: Voice and Voice Disorders.

Minnie S. Graham, PhD, is an associate professor in and director of the Communicative Disorders Program at San Francisco State University. She teaches courses in voice disorders, counseling in communicative disorders, and neurology for the speech–language pathologist. She supervises the Alaryngeal Speech Clinic, a therapy program for teaching esophageal, tracheoesophageal, and artificial larynx methods to individuals postlaryngectomy. She received her doctorate in Speech and Hearing Sciences from the University of California, San Francisco–Santa Barbara. Graham actively presents at state and national conferences related to speech–language pathology and alaryngeal speech rehabilitation. She is the author of *The Clinician's Guide to Alaryngeal Speech Therapy* and a number of articles in professional journals.

David G. Gratton, DDS, MS, is an assistant professor in the Department of Prosthodontics, College of Dentistry, at the University of Iowa, Iowa City. He teaches fixed, removable, implant, and maxillofacial prosthodontics at both the undergraduate and graduate levels, both didactically and clinically. Gratton received his DDS from the University of Michigan and his MS and Certificate in Prosthodontics from the University of Iowa. He was previously affiliated with the Department of Prosthodontics in the School of Medicine and Dentistry at the University of Western Ontario, London, Ontario, Canada, where he also provided maxillofacial prosthodontic care at the Oral and Maxillofacial Rehabilitation Unit, Department of Dentistry, London Health Sciences Centre. His research interests include micromotion and dynamic fatigue pertaining to dental implants and dental ceramics.

Carla DeLassus Gress, ScD, CCC-SLP, is a speech pathologist in private practice in Lynchburg, Virginia. Gress received a doctorate in speech pathology from Boston University following a decade of clinical practice. She has held appointments as a research associate at the Voice and Speech Laboratory of the Massachusetts Eye and Ear Infirmary, Instructor in Otolaryngology/Head and Neck Surgery at Harvard Medical School, and assistant professor in Otolaryngology/Head and Neck Surgery and director of the Voice Center at the University of California, San Francisco. Gress has clinical and research interests in the areas of head and neck cancer, voice disorders, and the use of acoustic, aerodynamic and videoendoscopic procedures.

James T. Heaton, PhD, received his doctorate in psychology from the University of Maryland, College Park in 1997. He joined the faculty of Harvard Medical School later that year in the Department of Otology and Laryngology, where he is currently an assistant professor. He also holds an adjunct faculty position in the Department of Communication Sciences and Disorders at the Massachusetts General Hospital Institute of Health Professions, where he teaches anatomy and physiology to graduate students in speech–language pathology, and is affiliated with the Center for Voice Surgery and Rehabilitation at the Massachusetts General Hospital. Heaton is a member of the Society for Neuroscience, and his research interests include the neural mechanisms of vocal learning and vocal production in birds and mammals. His recent research projects have focused on human larynx innervation (neurolaryngology) and exploring new methods for quantitative assessment of laryngeal function, as well as the feasibility of using neck surface electromyographic signals to control the onset, offset, and pitch of an electrolarynx for hands-free prosthetic speech.

Frans J. M. Hilgers, MD, PhD, is chair of the Department of Otolaryngology—Head and Neck Surgery of the Netherlands Cancer Institute/Antoni van Leeuwenhoek Hospital in Amsterdam, and a staff member of the Department of Otolaryngology—Head and Neck Surgery of the Academic Hospital of the University of Amsterdam. Hilgers received his doctorate from the University of Amsterdam. His research is focused on postlaryngectomy rehabilitation issues, including vocal, pulmonary, and olfactory rehabilitation of laryngectomized individuals. Hilgers's research on prosthetic voice and speech quality is conducted in close collaboration with the Institute of Phonetic Sciences of the University of Amsterdam.

Robert E. Hillman, PhD, currently holds positions as co-director/research director at the Center of Laryngeal Surgery and Voice Rehabilitation at the Massachusetts General Hospital, professor in communication sciences and disorders at the Massachusetts General Hospital Institute of Health Professions, associate professor in surgery at Harvard Medical School, and member of the affiliated faculty of the Harvard–MIT Division of Health Sciences and Technology. He received his doctorate in speech science from Purdue University. His research and numerous publications have focused on mechanisms for normal and disordered voice production, evaluation and development of methods for alaryngeal (laryngectomy) speech rehabilitation, development of objective physiologic and acoustic measures of voice and speech production, and evaluation of methods used to treat voice disorders. Hillman is a fellow of the American Speech-Language-Hearing Association and an associate fellow of the American Laryngological Association.

Kenneth M. Houston, SB, MEng, is a principal member of technical staff at the Charles Stark Draper Laboratory in Boston, Massachusetts. He has been with CSDL since 1992, where he has worked on a wide range of projects related to acoustics and signal processing. Houston is currently group leader of the Analog Systems Group within Draper's Electronics Division. He received his undergraduate degree from Harvard University in Boston, Massachusetts; Master of Engineering degree in Computer and Systems Engineering from Rensselaer Polytechnic Institute in Troy, New York; and Master of Engineering Management degree from the Gordon Institute of Tufts University, Medford, Massachusetts.

Robert L. Keith, MS, CCC, is an associate professor and supervisor of speech pathology emeritus at the Mayo Medical School, Rochester, Minnesota. Keith continues to work as an on-call speech pathologist at the Mayo Clinic and also serves as a chaplaincy volunteer at St. Mary's Hospital in Rochester. He is well regarded for his contributions to the care of individuals with head and neck cancer and has published several texts in the area of therapy for individuals with communicative disorders.

Gail B. Kempster, PhD, CCC-SLP, is an associate professor in the Department of Communication Disorders and Sciences at Rush University, Chicago, Illinois. She teaches courses in voice disorders, research methods, and anatomy and physiology of the speech mechanism, and serves as a part-time clinical staff member, working with individuals with voice disorders at Rush University Medical Center. Kempster received her PhD from Northwestern University, and is a former associate editor for speech for the *Journal of Speech, Language and Hearing Research*. Her research interests center around the perceptual analysis of vocal quality. Her experience in the area of head and neck cancer was obtained primarily during 4 intensive years of clinical service as a speech–language pathologist at Cook County Hospital in Chicago.

James Kobler, PhD, is an assistant professor in the Department of Otology and Laryngology at Harvard Medical School and director of the H. P. Mosher Laryngological Research Laboratory at the Massachusetts Eye and Ear Infirmary in Boston, Massachusetts. Kobler received his PhD in neuroscience from the University of North Carolina, Chapel Hill. He is also a member of the affiliated faculty of the Harvard–MIT Division of Health Sciences and Technology, where he teaches head and neck anatomy. He works as an assistant physiologist in the Laryngeal Surgery and Voice Rehabilitation Laboratory at the Massachusetts General Hospital in Boston. His research interests include laryngeal anatomy and physiology and clinical applications of technology for enhancing diagnosis and treatment of voice disorders.

Howard B. Lampe, MD, is a professor in and former chair of the Department of Otolaryngology at the University of Western Ontario, London, Ontario, Canada. He received his medical training at the University of Western Ontario and undertook fellowship training at the University of Michigan. Lampe is a head and neck surgeon with research interests in head and neck oncology, use of fine needle aspiration, and development of clinical pathways.

Henry J. Lapointe, DDS, PhD, FRCD(C) is an associate professor in and chair of the Division of Oral and Maxillofacial Surgery, School of Dentistry, the University of Western Ontario and Chief of Dentistry, St. Joseph's Health Centre, London, Ontario, Canada. He teaches undergraduate courses in oral and maxillofacial surgery and supervises interns, residents, and graduate students. Lapointe received his DDS and PhD from the University of Western Ontario and undertook oral surgery training at the University of Toronto. His clinical interests include the dental care of those with head and neck cancer, as well as the management of congenital and acquired dentofacial deformities.

Cathy L. Lazarus, PhD, is an associate professor in the Department of Otolaryngology at New York University School of Medicine and is director of the Hearing and Speech Department at Bellevue Hospital Center in New York City. Lazarus received her doctorate from Northwestern University, Evanston, Illinois. Her research interests include swallowing disorders in individuals with head and neck cancer and the treatment for swallowing disorders.

Herbert A. Leeper, PhD, was a professor in the School of Communication Sciences and Disorders, University of Western Ontario, London, Ontario, Canada, where he taught courses in craniofacial disorders and resonance disorders. He received his doctorate from Purdue University in West Lafayette, Indiana. Prior to his untimely death in May 2001, he conducted research in the area of voice and resonance disorders and communication disorders related to maxillofacial cancer. Leeper was an elected Fellow of the American Speech-Language-Hearing Association.

Jan S. Lewin, PhD, is an associate professor in and director of the Speech Pathology and Audiology Section in the Department of Head and Neck Surgery and director of the Voice Laboratory at the University of Texas M.D. Anderson Cancer Center in Houston, Texas. Lewin received her undergraduate and graduate degrees from the University of Michigan in Ann Arbor and her doctorate from Michigan State University in East Lansing. She is a recognized expert in rehabilitation following total laryngectomy, with specific interest in tracheoesophageal voice restoration, and has lectured extensively on this subject. Her research has encompassed the area of functional restoration of speech and swallowing in persons with head and neck cancer.

T. Wayne Matthews, MD, FRCS(C), is an otolaryngologist—head and neck surgeon in the Department of Otolaryngology at the University of Western Ontario in London, Ontario, Canada. He received his medical degree from the University of Toronto, undertook residency training at the University of Ottawa, and completed fellowships in head and neck oncology and microvascular surgery at the University of Toronto. Matthews has clinical and academic interests in head and neck oncology and reconstructive surgery.

Geoffrey Meltzner, PhD, is a senior engineer in the Advanced Technologies unit of BAE Systems in Burlington, Massachusetts, where is he currently conducting research on space–time adaptive processing for radar applications, speech coding, and subvocal speech. Meltzner received his doctorate in speech and hearing biosciences and technology from the Massachusetts Institute of Technology in 2003. His research interests include electrolarynx speech enhancement, speech processing, and general digital signal processing.

Gail Monahan, MS, is head speech pathologist at the Jerry L. Pettis Veterans Administration Medical Center, Loma Linda, California, and an associate clinical professor in the Department of Communicative Disorders at Loma Linda University. She has been a practicing clinician for 30 years. Monahan began working with tracheoesophageal puncture voice restoration in 1980 and has been a faculty member at the Annual Laryngectomy Rehabilitation Training Conference at the University of California, San Francisco Voice Center since 1995.

Candace Myers, MSc, SLP(C), is senior speech–language pathologist in patient and family support services at CancerCare Manitoba in Winnipeg, Manitoba, Canada. She has worked with people with head and neck cancers for over 15 years, and provides clinical services in an interdisciplinary head and neck disease site group. Myers has presented numerous papers and workshops locally and nationally. Her clinical and research interest areas include dysphagia assessment and management, palliative care, and health ethics.

Robert F. Orlikoff, PhD, served as a voice pathologist and director of the Laryngology Laboratory at Memorial Sloan-Kettering Cancer Center until 1999, when he assumed his current position as an associate professor in the Communication Sciences Program at Hunter College of the City University of New York. Orlikoff received his doctorate from Columbia University in New York City, with a specialization in speech and voice physiology. He teaches courses in voice disorders, physiologic and acoustic phonetics, research methods, and developmental speech disorders. Orlikoff has authored more than 30 professional publications on normal and abnormal speech and voice and is the coauthor of the second edition of the text *Clinical Measurement of Speech and Voice.*

Yingyong Qi, PhD, is a principal engineer at QUALCOMM, Inc., in San Diego, California. Prior to joining QUALCOMM, he was an associate professor at the University of Arizona in Tucson. He received his first doctoral degree in speech and hearing sciences from Ohio State University and his second in electrical engineering from the University of Arizona. His current research interests focus on wireless multimedia applications and embedded systems.

William J. Ryan, PhD, is an associate professor in and chair of the Department of Communication Sciences and Disorders at Texas Christian University (TCU) in Fort Worth, Texas, and is director of the Miller Speech and Hearing Clinic on the TCU campus. He received his doctorate from Purdue University in West Lafayette, Indiana. Ryan teaches courses in voice disorders, orofacial pathologies, and augmentative and alternative communication. His research interests include communication disorders related to head and neck cancer and age-related changes in speech and voice.

Shirley J. Salmon, PhD, served as a speech pathologist at the Veterans Administration Medical Center in Kansas City, Kansas, and is a professor emeritus at the University of Kansas. Salmon received her doctorate in speech pathology from the University of Iowa, Iowa City. She is widely recognized as a master clinician in the area of postlaryngectomy speech rehabilitation and has had a longstanding affiliation with the International Association of Laryngectomees. Salmon has lectured extensively, provided numerous workshops, and published numerous papers and books related to speech rehabilitation following treatment for cancer of the larynx. Salmon is an elected fellow of the American Speech-Language-Hearing Association.

James C. Shanks, PhD, is formerly chief of speech pathology and professor emeritus of otolaryngology–head and neck surgery in the Indiana University School of Medicine and of orthodontics in the Indiana University School of Dentistry in Indianapolis. Shanks's professional career has encompassed many decades of continuous clinical service to individuals with laryngeal cancer. He is regarded as one of the foremost master clinicians in speech rehabilitation following laryngeal cancer and total laryngectomy. Shanks has presented and authored numerous articles and chapters addressing multiple issues related to postlaryngectomy communication rehabilitation. Shanks is an elected fellow of the American Speech-Language-Hearing Association.

Mark I. Singer, MD, FACS, is the Robert K. Werbe Distinguished Professor of Head and Neck Cancer at the University of California, San Francisco (UCSF), and an associate member at the UCSF Comprehensive Cancer Center. Singer received his medical degree from the Columbia University College of Physicians and Surgeons in New York City and undertook additional training at Northwestern University Medical School in Evanston, Illinois. He is internationally recognized for his contributions to the development of the tracheoesophageal voice restoration technique. His research interests are in the broad area of head and neck cancer. Singer has published widely in multiple clinical areas pertaining to otolaryngology and head and neck surgery and has won awards from the American Laryngologic Association and has received the James Newcome Award of the American Laryngologic Association.

Corina J. van As, PhD, is a speech–language pathologist and phonetic scientist in the Department of Otolaryngology—Head and Neck Surgery of the Netherlands Cancer Institute/Antoni van Leeuwenhoek Hospital in Amsterdam. She received her doctorate from the University of Amsterdam. She specializes in head and neck cancer rehabilitation, with interests in postlaryngectomy speech and dysphagia issues. Her postdoctoral research focuses on voice and speech quality and olfaction rehabilitation in laryngectomized individuals. She conducts her research in close collaboration with the Institute of Phonetic Sciences of the University of Amsterdam.

Michael J. Walsh, MEd, is chief of the Audiology/Speech Pathology Service at the Veterans Administration Boston Healthcare System and a clinical instructor of speech pathology at the Boston University School of Medicine. Walsh received his graduate education at Northeastern University in Boston, Massachusetts. He has taught courses in voice and swallowing disorders. His research interests include evaluation of voice disorders and functional outcomes following treatment of voice and communication disorders related to head and neck cancer.

Steven M. Zeitels, MD, is an associate professor in the Department of Otology and Laryngology at Harvard Medical School in Cambridge, Massachusetts; co-director of the Center for Laryngeal Surgery and Voice Rehabilitation at the Massachusetts General Hospital; and president-elect of the American Broncho-Esophagological Association. His research efforts in phonosurgery have led to many new procedures to treat a spectrum of benign and malignant lesions, as well as paralytic/paretic dysphonia. Zeitels directs the postresidency Laryngology Fellowship at Harvard and has received more than 40 awards and honored lectureships for his achievements, including the Casselberry Award from the American Laryngological Association.